MW00624011

2nd Edition

Nursing2004

HERBAL MEDICINE HANDBOOK

2nd Edition

Nursing2004

HERBAL MEDICINE HANDBOOK

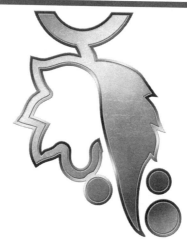

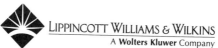

LIPPINCOTT WILLIAMS & WILKINS
A **Wolters Kluwer** Company

Philadelphia • Baltimore • New York • London
Buenos Aires • Hong Kong • Sydney • Tokyo

Staff

Publisher
Judith A. Schilling McCann, RN, MSN

Editorial Director
William J. Kelly

Senior Art Director
Arlene Putterman

Art Director
Elaine Kasmer

Clinical Manager
Eileen Cassin Gallen, RN, BSN

Drug Information Editor
Melissa M. Devlin, PharmD

Project Editor
Karen C. Comerford

Clinical Project Editor
Minh N. Luu, RN, BSN, JD

Editors
Stacey Follin, Carol Turkington

Clinical Editors
Ann M. Barrow, RN, MSN;
Christine M. Damico, RN, MSN;
Kimberly A. Zalewski, RN, MSN

Copy Editors
Beth Pitcher, Trish Turkington,
Doris Weinstock

Manufacturing
Patricia K. Dorshaw (manager),
Beth Janae Orr

Digital Composition Services
Diane Paluba (manager),
Donald G. Knauss (project manager),
Joy Rossi Biletz (senior desktop assistant)

Editorial Assistants
Danielle J. Barsky, Carol A. Caputo,
Arlene P. Claffee

Indexer
Karen C. Comerford

Visit our Web site at NDHnow.com

ISSN 1543-7841
ISBN 1-58255-231-2
NDHHMH-D N O S A J J
05 04 03   10 9 8 7 6 5 4 3 2 1

Contents

Clinical contributors and consultants

At the time of publication, the contributors and consultants held the following positions.

Michael Briggs, RPh, PharmD
Co-owner
Lionville Natural Pharmacy &
    Health Food Store
Exton, Pa.

Dina Cheiman, PharmD
Clinical Communication Scientist
Pfizer Global Research and
    Development
Ann Arbor, Mich.

Linda M. Eugenio Clark,
PharmD, CDE
Pharmacist
St. Luke's Hospital
New Bedford, Mass.

Jason Cooper, PharmD
Clinical Pharmacist
Bon Secours-St. Francis Hospital
Charleston, S.C.

Ami Dansby, RPh
Pharmacist, Natural Medicine
    Consultant
Natural Health Consulting
Charlottesville, Va.

Lana Dvorkin, RPh, PharmD
Assistant Professor of Clinical
    Pharmacy
Massachusetts College of
    Pharmacy and Health Sciences
Boston

Marie Fasano-Ramos, RN, MN,
MA
Holistic Nursing Consultant
InterAge
Ventura, Calif.

AnhThu Hoang, PharmD
Medical Director
    IntraMed Educational Group
New York

Susan Holcomb, RN-CS, MN,
FNP
Nursing Practitioner &
    Nutritional Counseling
Sastun Center of Integrative
    Health Care
Mission, Kansas

Mary Kate Kelly, PharmD
Publications Director
Institute for Safe Medication
    Practices
Huntingdon Valley, Pa.

Yun Lu, RPh, PharmD, MS, BCPS
Clinical Specialist
Hennepin County Medical Center
Minneapolis

Kristy Lucas, PharmD
Assistant Professor of Clinical
    Pharmacy and Internal
    Medicine
West Virginia University,
    Charleston (W.V.) Division

Bonnie Mackey, ARNP, MSN,
MTC, HNC
Holistic Nurse Practitioner
Mackey Health Institute, Inc.
West Palm Beach, Fla.
Medical University of South
    Carolina
Charleston, S.C.

Jolynne Myers, RNCS, MSN, MSEd, ANP
Adult Nurse Practitioner
Gastroenterology Clinic of St. Joseph
St. Joseph, Mo.

Steven G. Ottariano, RPh
Clinical Herbal Specialist
V.A. Medical Center
Manchester, N.H.

Robert Lee Page II, PharmD, BCPS
Assistant Professor
University of Colorado Health Sciences Center, School of Pharmacy
Denver

June Riedlinger, RPh, PharmD
Assistant Professor
Director, Center for Integrative Therapies in Pharmaceutical Care
Massachusetts College of Pharmacy and Health Sciences
Boston

Marsha Silkroski, RD
Executive Director, Owner
Nutrition Advantage
Chester Springs, Pa.

Laurie Willhite, PharmD
Clinical Associate Professor
University of Minnesota
Minneapolis

Pamela S. Yee, MD
Santa Barbara Cottage Hospital
Santa Barbara, Calif.

Preface

Disillusioned with traditional medicines, their costs, and their adverse effects, many people take treatment into their own hands and turn to herbal medicine. About 80% of the world's population use herbs and nutraceuticals for a variety of ailments. And nearly three-quarters of these people never inform their health care providers that they use herbs or nutraceuticals.

Such unmonitored use can cause several problems. Whenever a patient adds a prescription medicine to the alternative medicine mixture he's already taking, the potential exists for the herbal base to raise or lower the levels of the prescribed drug significantly. Herbs and nutraceuticals contain many pharmacologically active chemicals, which can conflict with the therapeutic goals of conventional drug regimens. Enhanced adverse effects can result if the alternative medicine and conventional drug contain similar compounds. These facts raise many questions. For example, should a patient with diabetes or heart disease avoid a certain herb? Could there be an interaction between an herb and the conventional drug regimen the patient is following?

As a nurse, your first challenge is to elicit a detailed history from your patient, including his use of alternative medicines. Your second challenge is to find a reliable nursing reference that will give you information about the herb or nutraceutical the patient is using and practical patient-teaching advice that you can give your patient.

Now, *Nursing2004 Herbal Medicine Handbook,* which covers over 300 herbs and 16 nutraceuticals, helps you meet these needs. The logical format of these two sections lists herbs and nutraceuticals by their popular names, and the consistent layout of each monograph helps you locate the specific information you need right away.

You'll find the information you need to teach your patient about the actions, common uses and dosages, adverse reactions, possible effects on lab test results, and interactions of the herb or nutraceutical he's using. Facts about actual and potential drug, herb, food, and lifestyle interactions are at your fingertips. You'll find out which herbs and which foods or medicines your patient should avoid or which lifestyles he should modify if he's taking a certain herb or nutraceutical because of the unpredictable, and potentially harmful, ways these substances can interact. In some cases, an entire herb is toxic, and only very small doses of it or certain parts of it can be tolerated.

This handbook is intended to give you information about herbs and nutraceuticals your patients may be using. But because these substances haven't been approved by the Food and Drug Administration and have no standard indications or dosages, this book neither recommends nor endorses their use.

If you keep this book handy during patient assessment, and remember to ask about your patient's herb or nutraceutical intake early on, you'll be able to quickly spot potential dangers hidden in the use of these natural remedies.

How to use this book

The *Nursing2004 Herbal Medicine Handbook* provides comprehensive information on almost every herb and nutraceutical used today, arranged alphabetically in two separate sections by popular name for easy access. This information was written and reviewed by pharmacists and nurses to provide a much-needed practical nursing handbook on herbs and nutraceuticals. The important facts for each herb and nutraceutical are listed, to give nurses a solid background on everything from basic pharmacology to management of toxicity and overdose.

In each self-inclusive entry, the popular name of each herb and nutraceutical is followed by a list of alternative popular names, which precedes an alphabetical list of common trade names. Abbreviations used in the entries are spelled out on pages xiii and xiv.

Next, *Available forms* describes the forms in which each herb and nutraceutical is available and provides information on the parts of the herb and nutraceutical that are used to manufacture the product. The preparations available for each herb and nutraceutical are listed (for example, tablets, capsules, elixirs, teas, and extracts) with known dosage forms and strengths.

Actions & components details how each herb and nutraceutical works, including its actions on body systems. An herb's anesthetic or stimulating effects, if any, can be found in this section. An asterisk following a liquid herbal formulation (such as tincture) indicates that the liquid may contain alcohol, an important fact when your patient is a child, a recovering alcoholic, or someone with other alcohol-related problems.

Uses lists the therapeutic claims for each herb and nutraceutical. This section may help you determine why your patient is using the herb.

Dosage & administration includes information on the various forms of the herbs and nutraceuticals and the amounts reported to achieve the desired effects. Keep in mind that dosages may vary widely, depending on the indication, herbal form used, and literature cited.

Adverse reactions lists the undesirable effects that may result from use of the herb or nutraceutical. These effects are arranged by body system (CNS, CV, EENT, GI, GU, Hematologic, Hepatic, Metabolic, Musculoskeletal, Respiratory, Skin, and Other). Adverse reactions not specific to a single body system (for example, the effects of hypersensitivity) are listed under Other. Life-threatening reactions are presented in ***bold italic*** type.

The *Interactions* section provides cautions against potentially significant additive, synergistic, and antagonistic effects that may result from combined use of the herb or nutraceutical with other elements. Interactions are broken down into four categories: drug, herb, food, and lifestyle. The interacting agent is italicized.

Effects on lab test results offers a bulleted listing of changes in laboratory test results that may occur if the patient is taking the herb or nutraceutical.

Cautions lists situations in which the patient shouldn't use the herb or nutraceutical. These include hypersensitivity, pregnancy, breast-feeding, and certain diseases as well as the presence of other drugs, herbs, or nutraceuticals.

Nursing considerations offers practical information regarding use of the herb or nutraceutical. An "Alert" logo signals cautionary tips and warnings on the danger of confusing herb or plant names, the toxic effects of certain herbs, life-threatening results of taking an herb in high doses, and herbs that have poisonous components.

Patient teaching contains points for the patient who is taking a particular herb or nutraceutical, such as the signs of toxicity and the importance of alerting his pharmacist to any alternative medicine he's taking before having a new prescription filled.

The appendices include supplemental vitamins and minerals, herb-drug interactions, common uses of herbs and nutraceuticals, monitoring of patients using herbs, the Food and Drug Administration's list of toxic herbs, selected references, and an herbal resource list. A helpful glossary is also included.

The index lists popular names for each herb and nutraceutical plus synonyms, brand names, and indications.

To earn continuing education contact hours based on the information in this book, visit NDHnow.com, the Web site of the Nursing Drug Handbook series.

Guide to abbreviations

AIDS	acquired immuno-deficiency syndrome	DNA	deoxyribonucleic acid
		ECG	electrocardiogram
ALT	alanine aminotrans-ferase	EEG	electroencephalogram
AST	aspartate aminotrans-ferase	FDA	Food and Drug Admin-istration
ATP	adenosine triphosphate	g	gram
AV	atrioventricular	G	gauge
AZT	zidovudine	GFR	glomerular filtration rate
b.i.d.	twice a day	GGT	gamma glutamyl-transferase
BPH	benign prostatic hyper-plasia	G6PD	glucose-6-phosphate dehydrogenase
BUN	blood urea nitrogen	GI	gastrointestinal
cAMP	cyclic 3',5' adenosine monophosphate	gtt	drops
CBC	complete blood count	GU	genitourinary
CK	creatine kinase	HIV	human immuno-deficiency virus
CNS	central nervous system		
COPD	chronic obstructive pulmonary disease	h.s.	at bedtime
CPR	cardiopulmonary resuscitation	I.D.	intradermal
		I.M.	intramuscular
CSF	cerebrospinal fluid	INR	international normal-ized ratio
CV	cardiovascular	IU	international unit
CVA	cerebrovascular accident	I.V.	intravenous
CVP	central venous pressure	kg	kilogram
DIC	disseminated intravas-cular coagulation	L	liter
		LDH	lactate dehydrogenase

m^2	square meter	SIADH	syndrome of inappropriate antidiuretic hormone
MAO	monoamine oxidase		
mcg	microgram	S.L.	sublingually
mEq	milliequivalent	SSRI	selective serotonin reuptake inhibitor
mg	milligram		
MI	myocardial infarction	T_3	triiodothyronine
ml	milliliter	T_4	thyroxine
mm^3	cubic millimeter	TCA	tricyclic antidepressant
ng	nanogram (millimicrogram)	t.i.d.	three times a day
		UTI	urinary tract infection
NG	nasogastric	WBC	white blood cell
NSAID	nonsteroidal anti-inflammatory drug		
OTC	over-the-counter		
P.O.	by mouth		
P.R.	per rectum		
p.r.n.	as needed		
PT	prothrombin time		
PTT	partial thromboplastin time		
PVC	premature ventricular contraction		
q	every		
q.d.	every day		
q.i.d.	four times a day		
RBC	red blood cell		
RNA	ribonucleic acid		
SA	sinoatrial		
S.C.	subcutaneous		

Overview of Herbal Medicine

For thousands of years, cultures around the world have used herbs and plants to treat illness and maintain health. What's more, archaeological evidence shows that prehistoric humans selected remedies from a variety of basic healing flora.

Many drugs prescribed today are derived from plants that earlier cultures used for medicinal purposes. (The word "drug" comes from the Old Dutch word *drogge,* meaning "to dry," because pharmacists, doctors, and ancient healers commonly dried plants for use as medicines.) In fact, about one-fourth of all conventional drugs—including about 120 of the most commonly prescribed modern drugs—contain at least one active ingredient derived from plants. The rest are chemically synthesized. (See *Common plant-based drugs,* page 2.)

Herbs and plants are valuable not only for their active ingredients but also for their minerals, vitamins, volatile oils, glycosides, alkaloids, acids, alcohols, and esters. These components come from all parts of the plant, including the leaves, flowers, stems, berries, seeds, fruit, bark, and roots.

The World Health Organization estimates that 80% of the world's population uses some herbal remedy. Still, health care providers in the United States are generally unaware of which herbal remedies are effective, and many patients are reluctant to reveal their use of such remedies.

Today, however, renewed interest in all forms of alternative medicine is encouraging patients, health care providers, and drug researchers to reexamine the value of herbal remedies. One of the most newsworthy plants being studied is St. John's wort. This perennial herb is commonly used in Europe as a tonic for anxiety and mild depression; its effectiveness as an antidepressant is currently being studied by the U.S. government.

Because of the staggering number of stories touting herbal remedies in the media, you're likely to encounter patients who have read claims about certain herbs and who want your opinion about them. This chapter provides a general overview of the subject.

History of herbal medicine

Also known as *phytotherapy* or *phytomedicine* (especially in Europe), herbal medicine has been practiced since the beginning of recorded history, with specific remedies being handed down from generation to generation. In ancient times, medicinal plants were first prescribed because of their color or the shape of their leaves. For example, heart-shaped leaves were used for heart problems, and plants with red flowers were used to treat bleeding disorders. This approach is known as the *Doctrine of Signatures.* The best use for each plant was determined by trial and error.

The formal study of herbs, known as *herbology,* can be traced back to the ancient cultures of the

Common plant-based drugs

Drug	Therapeutic class	Botanical origin
aspirin	analgesic	white willow bark and acid meadow-sweet plant
atropine	antiarrhythmic	belladonna leaves
codeine, morphine	potent narcotics	opium poppy
colchicine	antigout drug	autumn crocus
digoxin	antiarrhythmic	foxglove, a poisonous plant
ephedrine	bronchodilator	ephedra
paclitaxel	antineoplastic	yew tree
quinine	antimalarial	cinchona bark
vinblastine, vincristine	anticarcinogens	periwinkle
warfarin	anticoagulant	sweet clover, contains dicumarol (a hemorrhagic agent)

Middle East, Greece, China, and India. These cultures revered the power of nature and developed herbal remedies based on plants that grew locally. Written evidence of the medicinal use of herbs has been found on Mesopotamian clay tablets and ancient Egyptian papyrus.

The first known compilation of herbal remedies was ordered by the king of Sumeria around 2000 B.C. and included 250 medicinal substances, including garlic. Ancient Greek and Roman healers produced their own collections, including the *De Materia Medica,* written in the 1st century A.D. Of the 950 medicinal products described in this work, 600 are derived from plants and the rest are from animal or mineral sources.

Arab herbalists added their own discoveries to the Greco-Roman texts, resulting in a collection of more than 2,000 substances that was eventually reintroduced to Europe by Christian doctors traveling with the Crusaders.

Herbal therapy is also a major component of India's Ayurvedic medicine, traditional Chinese medicine, Native American medicine, homeopathy, and naturopathy.

In the United States, herbal remedies handed down by European settlers and learned from Native Americans were a mainstay of medical care until the early 1900s. The rise of technology and the biomedical approach to health care eventually led to the decline of herbal medicine. However, interest in herbal preparations has been revitalized in the United States for various reasons, including a general disillusionment with modern medicine, the high cost and adverse effects of prescription drugs, the widespread availability of herbal drugs, and an increased interest in self care.

Regulation

In 19th century America, many bogus remedies were sold to gullible, desperate people. The federal government finally took action against disreputable purveyors of phony remedies with the Food and Drug Act of 1906. This law addressed problems of mislabeling and adulteration of plant remedies but didn't address safety and effectiveness.

Today, the U.S. Food and Drug Administration (FDA) regulates herbal remedies as dietary supplements, not drugs. This means the FDA can challenge any herbal product that is proven to be harmful, as opposed to drugs, which must be proven to be safe and effective before they reach the consumer. The Dietary Supplement Health and Education Act of 1994 (DSHEA) requires that the contents of herbal remedies be indicated on the label. It also permits manufacturers and marketers of dietary supplements to make limited claims regarding their health benefits. For herbs and other supplements that don't provide nutritional support conventionally, the law allows the manufacturer to make claims about how the product affects the body's structure or function. However, labels can't claim that the herbal remedy can treat, mitigate, prevent, or cure a disease or condition, nor can they mention a specific pathologic condition. Although the DSHEA provides a regulatory framework for the labeling and safety of herbal products, at present herbal products don't need approval from the FDA before they are marketed. There are no FDA regulations that establish a minimum standard of practice for manufacturing them.

This means that when it comes to buying herbal remedies in the United States, the message is: "Buyer beware." Consumers should be well educated about the herbal products they plan to use and should seek advice from a trained practitioner before trying a product, especially for a serious condition. (See *Herbal remedies: Patient precautions,* pages 4 and 5.)

In Europe, millions of people use herbal and homeopathic remedies. Government bodies and the scientific community are much more open to natural remedies, especially those that have a long history of use. In Great Britain and France, traditional medicines that have been used for years with no serious adverse effects are approved for use under the "doctrine of reasonable certainty" when scientific evidence is lacking.

In addition, the European Economic Community has established guidelines that standardize the quality, dosage, and production of herbal remedies. These guidelines are based on the World Health Organization's (WHO) 1996 publication *Guidelines for the Assessment of Herbal Medicines,* which ad-

(Text continues on page 6.)

Herbal remedies: Patient precautions

Many patients take for granted the safety of the foods and drugs they purchase. However, if your patient is taking or is considering taking any herbal remedies, let him know that no U.S. government agency reviews these products for quality, dosage, safety, or efficacy. Also, advise him of the general precautions and specific warnings listed below.

General precautions

• Advise your patient to consult a health care provider before using any herbal product, especially if he's also taking a prescription drug. Also, tell him to inform his herbalist of any prescription drugs he's taking. Many herbal remedies contain chemical substances that can interact with other drugs.

• Caution your patient that the FDA regulates herbal products only as food supplements, not as drugs. The patient and his health care provider are responsible for keeping informed and monitoring the risks, adverse effects, and possible harmful interactions with other substances.

• Tell your patient that herbal products may contain ingredients other than those indicated on the label.

• Remind your patient that each person metabolizes and absorbs botanical and synthetic drugs differently, so there's no way to know if the herb is in a form that his body can absorb or if the recommended dosage on the label is right for him.

• Tell your patient that commercially grown herbs may be contaminated from pesticides, polluted water, or car exhaust fumes.

• Inform your patient that the quantity of the active ingredient varies from brand to brand—and possibly from bottle to bottle—within a particular brand. Advise him to read the label carefully for this information.

• Caution your patient that products promising to cure specific health problems should be suspect. Labeling laws prohibit claims of treating, mitigating, preventing, or curing any disease or condition.

• Advise your patient not to take herbal products for serious or potentially serious medical conditions without first seeking medical evaluation.

• Advise your patient to seek guidance from a knowledgeable health care provider before using herbal preparations before, during, or after pregnancy or breast-feeding. There is a lack of scientific studies to support any indications in the first trimester of pregnancy.

• Caution your patient that many herbal remedies containing two or more herbs (also known as compounded herbal remedies) haven't been adequately researched.

• Advise your patient to be informed of reputable herbal companies and cautious about products sold through magazines, brochures, the broadcast media, or the Internet.

• Tell your patient to talk to a health care provider who is well-trained in herbology when in doubt about using herbal remedies—and to remember that the clerk at the health food store is a salesperson, not a trained practitioner.

Herbal remedies: Patient precautions *(continued)*

Specific warnings

• *Bloodroot* is promoted as an expectorant, antimicrobial, anti-inflammatory, antiplaque agent, mouthwash for gingivitis, and for the treatment of diarrhea and rheumatism. It has an emetic effect in doses above 0.03 g; however, doses greater than 0.03 g can cause dangerous and fatal symptoms of vomiting, diarrhea, colic, and collapse.

• *Chaparral tea,* promoted as an antioxidant and a pain reliever, may cause liver failure.

• *Indian herbal tonics* may cause lead poisoning.

• *Jin bu huan,* an ancient Chinese sedative and analgesic, contains morphinelike substances and may cause liver inflammation. It has been associated with life-threatening bradycardia and toxicity in children.

• *Kombucha tea,* made from mushroom cultures and used as a cure-all, can cause death from acidosis.

• *Lobelia,* used to treat respiratory congestion, may contribute to respiratory paralysis and death.

• *Kava* has been linked to serious liver injury, including hepatitis, cirrhosis, and liver failure. The FDA advises patients with liver problems or who are taking drugs that can harm the liver to check with a health care provider before taking kava. Those taking kava should contact their health care provider at the first signs of liver damage, such as jaundice, dark urine, or yellowing of the eyes.

• *Ma huang,* or *ephedra,* an ingredient in many diet pills, is a potentially dangerous drug because it can raise blood pressure and produce an ir-regular heartbeat. Also sold under such names as Herbal Ecstasy, Cloud 9, and Ultimate Xphoria as a way of inducing a high, it can cause heart attacks, seizures, psychotic behavior, and even death.

• *Mistletoe* has been falsely touted as a cure for cancer.

• *Pau d'arco tea* has been falsely touted as a cure for cancer and AIDS.

• *Pennyroyal,* which is used to treat coughs and upset stomach, may have toxic effects on the liver, inhibiting blood clotting. Use of its essential oil has been fatal.

• *Sassafras,* which is a tonic used for fever reduction, skin disorders, and rheumatism, has been banned in the United States for causing liver damage and has been implicated in narcotic poisoning and accidental abortion.

• *St. John's wort,* used for treating mild depression, anxiety, and unrest, may prolong the sedative effects of anesthesia. Patients undergoing elective surgery should stop taking herb 2 weeks before procedure. Using St. John's wort rather than a prescription drug to treat depression may be dangerous because the dosage and purity of the herb may be unknown.

• *Yohimbe bark,* which is used as an aphrodisiac, can severely lower blood pressure and may contribute to psychotic behavior.

dresses concerns about the safety and efficacy of herbal medicines and establishes guidelines for pharmacopoeia monographs. (See *World Health Organization guidelines.*) The usefulness of these guidelines has been recognized and most of the material published separately by WHO's expert committee in Chapter 2 of *Quality Assurance of Pharmaceuticals: A Compendium of Guidelines and Related Materials, Volume 1* (1997).

Therapeutic uses

Herbal remedies are used primarily to treat minor health problems, such as nausea, colds and flu, coughs, headaches, aches and pains, constipation and diarrhea, menstrual cramps, insomnia, skin disorders, and dandruff. These therapeutic uses also serve as a way to categorize herbal remedies. (See *Herbal classifications,* page 8.)

Some herbalists have also reported success in treating certain chronic conditions such as peptic ulcers, colitis, rheumatoid arthritis, hypertension, and respiratory problems, such as bronchitis and asthma. Others even use herbs with some illnesses usually treated only with prescription drugs, such as heart failure, hepatitis, and cirrhosis. However, advise any patient with a serious disorder who expresses an interest in herbal remedies not to discontinue ongoing medical treatment and to consult a health care provider about possible interactions between prescribed drugs and herbal remedies.

Numerous studies have been done on herbal remedies in Europe and Asia, where phytomedicine has a long history. European studies have shown that such herbs as ginkgo, bilberry, and milk thistle are beneficial in treating various chronic disorders. Chinese researchers have done extensive studies on many herbs, such as ginseng, ginger, foxglove, licorice, and wild chrysanthemum. Indian researchers using modern scientific methods recently studied various Ayurvedic herbs, including Indian gooseberry and turmeric. In addition, European researchers have published a comprehensive herbal guidebook, *The Complete German Commission E Monographs: Therapeutic Guide to Herbal Medicines,* which has been adopted by many health care providers, pharmaceutical companies, schools, and universities in the United States.

The United States lags behind other countries in herbal medicine research for a number of reasons:

- Until the establishment of the National Institutes of Health's Office of Alternative Medicine (OAM) in 1992, there was no federal support for research on natural remedies.
- Pharmaceutical companies have little financial incentive to develop herb-based drugs because botanical products can't be patented; therefore, the companies could never recoup their research investment.
- Western pharmaceutical standards call for the isolation of single active ingredients, but herbs may contain several active ingredients that work together to produce a specific effect.

World Health Organization guidelines

In 1996, the World Health Organization (WHO) published revised *Guidelines for the Assessment of Herbal Medicines*, which establishes standards for determining the safety, quality, and efficacy of herbal preparations and the development of pharmacopoeia monographs. A summary of these guidelines appears below.

Safety
• If the product traditionally has been used without demonstrated harm, no specific restrictive action should be taken unless new evidence demands a revised risk-benefit assessment.
• Prolonged and apparently uneventful use of a substance is considered testimony to its safety.

Efficacy
• For treatment of minor disorders and for nonspecific indications, some relaxation is justified in the requirements for proof of efficacy, taking into account the extent of traditional use.
• The same considerations can apply to prophylactic use.

Pharmacopoeia monographs
• If a pharmacopoeia monograph exists, it should be sufficient to make reference to this monograph.
• If a monograph doesn't exist, one must be supplied and should be prepared in the same way as in an official pharmacopoeia.

World Health Organization monographs
The WHO also published the WHO Monographs on Selected Medicinal Plants, which is used to validate the increasing use of herbs, phytomedicines, and medicinal plant preparations as official medicines. An international team of scientific experts assembled by the WHO extensively reviewed the monographs. These monographs contain most of the elements needed to determine baseline standards for identity and quality and to assess the relative safety and efficacy of each medicinal plant. Monographs also have a therapeutics section that includes levels of medicinal uses—that is, those supported by clinical data, those described in pharmacopoeias and traditional systems of medicines, and those described in folk medicine but not supported by experimental or clinical data.

In 1997, WHO published *Quality Assurance of Pharmaceuticals: A Compendium of Guidelines and Related Materials, Volume 1*. Chapter 2 reproduces separately published guidelines relating to national drug regulation, product assessment, registration and distribution, *The International Pharmacopeia*, basic tests for drugs, and other information relevant to pharmacy faculties and the pharmaceutical industry.

Herbal classifications

Herbs are commonly classified by their effects on patients, as follows:

- *Adaptogenic herbs* work on the adrenal gland to increase the body's resistance to illness.
- *Anthelmintic herbs* eliminate intestinal worms from the body.
- *Anti-inflammatory herbs* reduce the tissues' inflammatory response.
- *Antimicrobial herbs* boost the immune system by destroying disease-causing organisms or helping the body resist them.
- *Antispasmodic herbs* ease skeletal and smooth muscle cramps and tension.
- *Astringent herbs*, applied externally, reduce inflammation, irritation, and the risk of infection on the mucous membranes, skin, and other tissues.
- *Bitter herbs* affect the CNS to increase the secretion of digestive juices, stimulate the appetite, and promote liver detoxification.
- *Carminative herbs* (aromatic oils) stimulate proper function of the digestive system, soothe the lining of the GI tract, and reduce gas, inflammation, and pain.
- *Demulcent herbs* are rich in mucilage, soothing and protecting irritated or inflamed tissue and mucous membranes.
- *Diuretic herbs* increase the production and elimination of urine.
- *Emmenagogic herbs* stimulate menstrual flow.
- *Expectorant herbs* help eliminate mucus from the lungs.
- *Hepatic herbs* increase the strength and tone of the liver, increase the flow of bile, and increase the production of hepatocytes.
- *Hypotensive herbs* decrease abnormally high blood pressure.
- *Laxative herbs* relieve constipation and promote digestion.
- *Nervine herbs* are divided into three groups based on their role in helping the nervous system: those that strengthen and restore, those that ease anxiety and tension, and those that stimulate nerve activity.
- *Stimulating herbs* stimulate the body's physiologic and metabolic activities.
- *Tonic herbs*, the foundation of traditional Chinese and Ayurvedic (Indian) medicine, enliven and invigorate by promoting the "vital force," the key to health and longevity.

Despite these reasons, many herbal medicine clinical trials are underway in the United States. The OAM supports more than 110 research centers throughout the United States that use credible scientific research methods related to complementary medicine and health care. Collaborative research efforts continue among the OAM, National Institutes of Health, Office of Dietary Supplements, and many other organizations.

Forms of herbal preparations

Herbs are available in various forms, depending on their medicinal purpose and the body system involved. They may be bought individually or in mixtures formulated for specific conditions. Herbs may be prepared as tinctures, extracts, capsules, tablets, lozenges, teas, juices, vapor treatments, and bath products. Some herbs are applied topically with a poultice or compress; others are rubbed into the skin as an oil, ointment, or salve.

Tinctures and extracts

An herb placed in alcohol or liquid glycerin and reduced over time is known as a *tincture* or an *extract*. (Tinctures contain more alcohol than extracts.) The alcohol draws out the active chemical properties of the herb, concentrates it, and helps preserve it. The body easily absorbs alcohol. The full flavor of the herb isn't masked by the alcohol, so it can taste strong or unpleasant. Alcohol-based tinctures and extracts have a shelf life of 3 to 5 years.

Liquid glycerin extracts called *glycerites* are an alternative to alcohol extracts and are better suited to some patients. Glycerites usually taste sweet and feel warm on the tongue. Glycerin is processed in the body as a fat, not a sugar, which is important for the patient with diabetes, who must limit sugar intake. The patient should be aware that taking more than 1 ounce (30 ml) of glycerin can have a laxative effect. In general, glycerin isn't an efficient solvent for most herbs, especially those that contain resins and gums. These herbs require alcohol for extraction.

Glycerin-based extracts should contain at least 60% glycerin with 40% water to ensure preservation.

The shelf life of these extracts is shorter than that of alcohol-based extracts. An extract that contains citric acid can last for more than 2 years if stored properly.

Tinctures or extracts may be taken as drops in a tea, diluted in spring water, used in a compress, or applied during body massage. If the alcohol content of a tincture is a concern—for example, when giving the remedy to a child—a few drops may be placed in ¼ cup of very hot water and left to stand for 5 minutes. During this time, most of the alcohol evaporates and the mixture becomes cool enough to drink.

To make an herbal tincture, the consumer fills a glass bottle or jar with carefully calculated and weighed plant parts (cut fresh herbs or crumbled dry herbs); adds the appropriate amount of natural ethanol, such as vodka; seals the container; and places it in a warm area (70° to 80° F [21° to 27° C]) for 3 to 4 weeks. The mixture should be shaken daily. After 3 to 4 weeks, the mixture is strained, separating the herbs from the residue that contains the chemical constituents of the herb.

Consumers may also purchase prepared extracts, made with alcohol, water, or both, to bring out the herb's essence. The product label should indicate which base was used. Extracts have about the same advantages and disadvantages as tinctures, except they're more concentrated and usually require less of a dose to be effective. Because of their strong herbal taste, they're usually diluted in juice or water.

Capsules and tablets

Capsules and tablets contain the ground or powdered form of the raw herb and are much less potent than tinctures; however, they're easier to transport and generally tasteless. The best products use fresh herbs (those made within 24 hours of milling the herb because herbs degrade very quickly). The use of fresh herbs should be indicated on the label. Capsules can be a hard or soft gel made of animal or vegetable gelatin. Most patients find capsules easier to swallow than tablets.

The patient should be aware that both capsules and tablets may contain a large amount of filler, such as soy or millet powder. Filler makes the herb difficult to identify in the powdered form, and a poorer quality herb may be substituted without the patient's knowledge. Tablets may also contain a binder, such as magnesium stearate or dicalcium phosphate, which may contain lead. Binders are used to help the herb absorb water and break down more readily for easy absorption by the body.

Capsules or tablets can be swallowed whole, or they may be mixed with a spoonful of cream-style cereal or applesauce. They may also be dissolved in sweet fruit juice.

Lozenges

Herbal lozenges are nutrient-rich, naturally sweetened preparations that dissolve in the mouth. They're available in various formulations, such as cough suppressants, decongestants, or cold fighters. Most lozenges have added vitamin C.

One type that has become popular is the horehound lozenge, used to relieve coughs and minor throat irritation.

Lozenges should be taken as directed by a knowledgeable practitioner or as indicated on the package.

Teas

Teas can be made from most herbs, and are used for various specific purposes. These teas are generally prepared by infusion or decoction. For an *infusion,* a dried herb is steeped in hot water for 3 to 5 minutes. For a *decoction,* the herb is placed into gently boiling water for 15 to 20 minutes; this method is preferable for denser plant materials, such as roots or bark. Teas may be steeped in a muslin or conventional tea bag or tea ball or used in loose form for their fragrant, aromatic flavor.

Some teas, such as barberry, taste bitter because they contain alkaloids or, like oak bark, highly astringent tannins. In some cases, the bitterness promotes the digestive reflex, thereby stimulating the production of gastrin and cholecystokinin. The digestive reflex is commonly altered in people with liver, colon, or other digestive problems. Tasting the bitterness of the tea, then, becomes an important part of the treatment. For other patients, teas may be sweetened with the herbal sweetener Stevia or with honey. However, honey should not be given to children younger than age 1 because of the risk of infant botulism.

For infants, tea may be mixed with breast milk or formula, then put into a bottle, an eyedropper, or an empty syringe without a needle and gently squirted into the infant's mouth. If a breast-feeding mother takes an adult dose of an herbal remedy, the effect may be transmitted to her child through her breast milk.

Chinese herbalists teach that the heat of the water and the taste of the herb enhance its effectiveness. Steeping an herb in hot water draws out its therapeutic essence. Generally, 1 to 2 heaping tablespoons of dried herb are used for each cup of tea, unless the product label says otherwise. The herbs should be placed in 8 ounces of freshly boiled water per cup in a covered china or glass teapot or cup (plastic and metal containers are considered unsuitable for steeping).

Leaf or flower herbs are generally steeped for 5 to 10 minutes. Roots or bark are simmered or boiled for 10 minutes, then steeped for 5 more minutes. After steeping, the tea is strained and allowed to cool to a comfortable temperature before serving. If a tincture or extract is being placed in the tea, the cup of hot water should sit for 5 minutes to allow the alcohol to evaporate. Teas may be served hot, cold, or iced, depending on the purpose and according to instructions.

Five parts of a fresh herb generally equal one part of a dry herb. Bark, root, seeds, and resins must be powdered to break down the cell walls before they're added to water. Seeds should be slightly bruised to release the volatile oils from the cells. An aromatic herb

may be infused in a pot with a tight lid to decrease the loss of volatile oil through evaporation. Because roots, wood, bark, nuts, and certain seeds are tough and their cell walls strong, they should be gently boiled in water to release their properties.

Juices

Juices are produced by washing fresh herbs under cold running water, cutting them with scissors into smaller pieces, and then running them through a juice extractor until they turn into a liquid. Juices are usually administered by placing a few drops in tea or spring water. They also may be applied externally by dabbing on the affected part of the body. Ideally, fresh juices should be taken immediately after extraction; however, they may be stored in a small glass bottle, corked tightly, and refrigerated for several days without appreciable oxidation and loss of vital properties.

Vapor and inhalation treatments

Used primarily for respiratory and sinus conditions, vapor and inhalation treatments open congested sinuses and lung passages, help discharge mucus, and ease breathing. One inhalation method requires a sink and an herbal oil. In this method, the sink is filled with very hot water and 2 to 5 gtt of the herbal oil are added. Hot water should be allowed to trickle into the sink to keep the water steaming. As the mixture becomes diluted, a few more drops of the herbal oil may be needed. The patient should deeply inhale the steam for 5 minutes and repeat three or four times a day.

Another method involves heating a large, wide pot of water, adding a handful of dried or fresh herbs, and bringing the pot to a low boil. After the herbs have simmered for 5 minutes, the pot is removed from the heat and placed on a trivet to cool slightly. If an aromatic oil is being used, the water is first heated to just short of boiling and then removed from the heat. With the pot on a trivet, the patient adds 4 or 5 gtt of the oil, then drapes a towel over the head to form a tent and leans over the pot, inhaling the steam for 5 minutes. If the vapor is too hot, it can burn the nasal passages.

Herbal baths

If the herb is in a soluble medium, such as baking soda or aloe gel, it may be dissolved in hot bath water. If the herb is an oatmeal-type preparation, it may be finely milled or whirled into a powder in a blender. Fresh or dried herbs also can be bagged in a square of cheesecloth or placed in a washcloth and tied securely. The goal is maximum release of the herbal essence without having parts of the herb floating in the bath water. Full baths require about 6 ounces of dried or fresh herbs.

As the tub fills with water, the bagged herbs are placed under a forceful stream of comfortably hot water, then dragged through the bath water to better distribute the herbal essence. Squeezing the bag releases a rich stream of essence that may be directed to the affected body part. The bag may also be gently rubbed over itching skin. Herbs with pointed or rough edges may be too irritating to use in this manner.

An herbal infusion can also be added to bath water. To make the infusion, 6 tablespoons of dried or fresh herbs should be soaked overnight in 3 cups of boiled water. The cup is usually covered with a saucer. The next morning, the strained infusion can be poured directly into the bath water.

Poultices and compresses

A *poultice* is a moist paste made from crushed herbs that is either applied directly to the affected area or wrapped in cloth to keep it in place and then applied. Poultices are especially useful in treating bruises, wounds, and abscesses.

Only fresh herbs should be used for poultices. One preparation method involves wrapping the herbs in a clean white cloth, such as gauze, linen, cotton, or muslin; folding the cloth several times; and then crushing the herbs to a pulp with a rolling pin. Pulping the herb directly onto the poultice cloth helps to retain its juices and improves the effectiveness of the poultice. The pulp is then exposed and applied to the affected area. Wrapping the entire area with a woolen cloth or towel will trap the herbal juices and hold them in place. This type of poultice can remain in place overnight.

A poultice also may be prepared by placing the herbs in a steamer, colander, strainer, or sieve over a pot of rapidly boiling water and allowing the steam to penetrate and wilt the herbs. After 5 minutes, the softened, warmed herbs are spread on a clean white cloth (such as loosely woven cheesecloth) and applied to the affected area. Wrapping the poultice with a woolen cloth or towel helps retain the heat. This type of poultice can be left on for 20 minutes or overnight if the patient finds the wrap comforting and soothing.

A *compress* is made by soaking a soft cloth in an herbal infusion and then wringing it out and applying it to the affected area. Compresses are very effective for bleeding, bruises, muscle cramps, and headaches. A bandage or plastic wrap may be used to hold the compress, which may be hot or cold, in place.

Oils, ointments, salves, and rubs

Herbal oils are usually expressed from the peels of lemons, oranges, or other citrus fruits. Because they may irritate the skin, they're commonly diluted in fatty oils or water before being applied topically. Essential oils are used in massage and aromatherapy; diluted oils can be used to prevent skin irritation.

To make an oil, the fresh herbs are washed, left to dry overnight, and then sliced. If using dry herbs, they are crumbled, placed in a glass bottle or jar, and covered by about 1″ of light virgin olive, almond, or sesame oil. The container is covered tightly and allowed to stand in a very warm area, such as on a stove or in the sunshine, for 2 weeks. The oil should be strained before use.

Herbal ointments, salves, and rubs are applied topically for various conditions. For example, calendula ointment may be used for broken skin and wounds; goldenseal is helpful in treating infections, rashes, and skin irritations; aloe vera gel may be used to treat minor burns; and heat-producing herbs are a good choice for muscle aches and strains.

Ointments can be made in a ceramic or glass double-boiler by heating 2 ounces of vegetable lanolin or beeswax until it liquefies. When the lanolin or wax has melted, 80 to 120 gtt of tincture are added and the compound is mixed together. The formula should then be poured into a glass container and refrigerated until it hardens.

Visiting an herbalist

A visit to an herbalist begins with an evaluation that includes the patient's history. The herbalist may perform a physical assessment, including a check of the patient's pulse and tongue, to help reach a diagnosis. Some herbalists also assess the iris, a technique known as iridology, to aid in diagnosis; this procedure involves correlating minute markings on the iris with specific parts of the body.

Most herbalists also ask which drugs and herbs the patient is already taking, to help guard against interactions. For example, the herb St. John's wort, which is used as an antidepressant, shouldn't be taken before surgery and shouldn't be combined with prescription antidepressants.

The herbalist will ask whether the patient is pregnant or breast-feeding because certain herbs can induce miscarriage or be transmitted to the infant in breast milk, causing adverse reactions.

After the evaluation, the herbalist will suggest individual plants or herbal combinations to treat a particular condition. Medicinal plants may be combined to increase their therapeutic effect, alter the individual actions of each herb, or minimize or negate toxic effects of stronger herbs. As with traditional drug combinations, herbal compounds may have a synergy that allows the remedy to function more effectively. The art of herbal compounding has been practiced for more than 5,000 years and is the basis of today's herbal practice.

Determining dosages

Dosages for herbal remedies have been established over the years, but these guidelines for quantity and frequency must be adjusted for each individual, based on factors such as age, weight, and use of other herbs or drugs. (See *Understanding herbal dosages*.)

Herbal remedies take time to work. The length of time a particular herb is used depends on whether it's being used as a therapy to relieve symptoms, a tonic to build strength, or both. An herb that is being used therapeutically may only be taken for a brief period—typically, 1 to 4 weeks. As with other drugs, herbs should be taken at specific times of the day. Some herbs are more effective when taken in the morning; others work better in the evening.

An herbal remedy that is being used as a tonic generally requires a longer period of use—usually 4 to 6 months or longer. For example, hawthorn, a cardiovascular tonic, is most effective when used for 6 to 12 consecutive months.

Some herbs work best if used with a resting cycle. For example, the patient might use an herb for 6 days, followed by 1 day off, 6 weeks on and 1 week off, 6 months on and 1 month off, or some similar pattern. The theory behind a resting cycle is that each period of rest from the herb treatment allows its effect to become integrated into the patient's physiology. If the desired effect doesn't appear in the specified time, or if adverse effects develop, the dosage or herb may be changed.

Nursing perspective

Although the overall risk of herbal remedies to public health appears to be low, some traditional remedies have been associated with potentially serious adverse effects. For example, ma huang, an ingredient in numerous diet pills, contains the same active ingredient that is in the bronchodilator ephedrine and can cause irregular heartbeats, seizures, and even death.

The patient taking, or considering taking, an herbal remedy should know the potential risks involved in self-treatment. These risks include misdiagnosis, taking the wrong herb, worsening a condition by delaying conventional treatment, having the herbal drug counteract or interact with prescribed medical treatment, and aggravating other disorders.

Make sure your patient is aware of the actions and adverse effects

Understanding herbal dosages

Age and weight dosing
The *age-dosing guidelines,* useful for treating infants and young children, are based on organ maturity—the organ's ability to metabolize, use, and eliminate herbs. The *weight-to-dose guidelines* are based on the principle that the herb is distributed to different parts of the body. This method is used for patients who fall outside the normal weight range, requiring either an increased or a decreased dose; however, it may not be reliable for very young children. It's similar to Clark's rule, which is used to verify pediatric dosages.

Homeopathic prescribing
Homeopathic prescribing is based on the homeopathic principle of "like cures like." For example, cantharis or apis causes burning urination and kidney damage in high doses but is given in low doses to treat UTIs and kidney disease.

Pharmacologic prescribing
Most herbal dosages are set by a method called *pharmacologic prescribing,* in which the amount of a botanical preparation is enough to induce definite, visible, strong, sustained changes in the patient. The oldest dosage method that's best represented by the British herbal tradition, pharmacologic prescribing can mask symptoms if the dose is improper or used for too long.

Physiologic prescribing
In *physiologic prescribing,* the herbalist recommends the minimum dosage of an herb required to induce a physiologic change. For example, he'd give a laxative only until a change in bowel action occurs.

Prescribing herbal extracts
The standard dose of herbal extracts for the average adult is 6 g per day. However, this dose is only a guideline and may be modified for patients who aren't average sized.

Wise woman prescribing
Based on ancient wisdom, *wise woman prescribing* is also known as folk herbalism. Herbs are taken in large doses like foods. The herbalist avoids strong, toxic, and rare plants, choosing those that grow freely and are close at hand.

---

of the herb he'll be taking *before* he begins taking it. Possible signs and symptoms of sensitivity or an adverse reaction include headache, upset stomach, and rash. Also, some patients are predisposed to react to particular herbs. For example, a patient with depressive symptoms shouldn't take certain herbs that treat insomnia—hops, for example—because they can heighten symptoms of depression. This warning may appear on the herbal remedy package, but there is no guarantee that all remedies will carry adequate warnings.

Advise your patient to stop using an herb and to notify a health care provider if an adverse reaction, such as headache, upset stomach, or rash occurs.

Tell your patient that if his response to an herb is favorable but too intense, he should decrease the dose or stop taking the herb altogether. For example, if a laxative causes diarrhea, the laxative should be discontinued.

If the patient experiences adverse effects, make sure the correct herb is being taken in the proper amounts at the correct intervals. Sometimes symptoms are related to incorrect dosage. For example, chamomile taken orally daily over an extended period may cause an allergy to ragweed. Also, taking black licorice in moderate to large quantities daily can lead to high blood pressure or increased intraocular pressure.

Many patients, disillusioned with conventional medicine, have turned to self-treatment using alternative remedies. As a nurse, you're in a position to learn about drug interactions and adverse reactions caused by herbal therapy and to educate and caution your patient about potential dangers.

Herbal medicines

acacia gum

Acacia senegal

Common trade names
Acacia Vera, Cape Gum, Egyptian Thorn, Gum Acacia, Gum Arabic, Gum Senegal, Gummae Mimosae, Gummi Africanum, Kher, Somali Gum, Sudan Gum Arabic, Yellow Thorn

AVAILABLE FORMS
Available as flakes, granules, powder, and spray-dried formulations.

As a component in a drug preparation, amount varies with the preparation. For periodontal use, concentrations range from 0.5% to 1%.

ACTIONS & COMPONENTS
Derived from the sap of the acacia tree, *A. senegal*. Naturally appears as odorless, white or yellow-white to pale amber brittle tears. The main component of the gum is arabin, which is the calcium salt of arabic acid. It's almost completely soluble in water, but it doesn't dissolve in alcohol and is hydrolyzed to form arabinose, galactose, and arabinosic.

USES
The dry powder form is commonly used as a stabilizer in drug emulsions and as an additive in various oral combinations.

Acacia gum is dissolved in water to make a mucilage. Although acacia gum is commonly used to reduce cholesterol levels, it may actually increase these levels in serum and tissue.

Acacia is used to soothe throat and stomach irritation, to treat diarrhea, and to interfere with absorption of certain substances. It's also used in cough drops.

Chewing acacia-based gum may limit development of periodontal disease and may also prevent plaque deposit. Whole gum mixtures of 0.5% to 1% may prevent growth of periodontal bacteria, and mixtures of 0.5% may inhibit bacterial protease enzyme.

Acacia also masks acrid substances such as capsicum, and is used as a treatment for catarrh, as a mild stimulant, as a food stabilizer, and as a film-forming agent in peel-off skin masks. It's also used in some wound-healing preparations.

DOSAGE & ADMINISTRATION
Mucilage: Usual dose is 1 to 4 teaspoons P.O.

ADVERSE REACTIONS
Respiratory: *severe bronchospasm.*
Skin: skin lesions.

INTERACTIONS
Herb-drug. *Alkaloids:* When mixed, acacia gum may partially degrade certain alkaloids. Monitor patient closely.
Ethyl alcohol: Acacia is insoluble in substances containing ethyl alcohol concentrations of more than 50%. Advise patient not to mix the two together.

---

*Liquid contains alcohol.

Iron: Ferric iron salt solutions may gelatinize acacia. Monitor patient closely.

Oral drugs: The fiber component of acacia may impair absorption of oral drugs. Monitor patient for loss of therapeutic effect.

EFFECTS ON LAB TEST RESULTS
None reported.

CAUTIONS
Patients who are allergic or sensitive to acacia dust should avoid using herb. Pregnant and breast-feeding patients should avoid using acacia because the effects of the herb are unknown.

NURSING CONSIDERATIONS
• Explore patient's knowledge of this herb.
• Acacia gum, which is essentially nontoxic, has no significant systemic effects when taken orally.
• Monitor patient for allergic reactions to acacia dust, including severe bronchospasm and skin lesions.
• **ALERT:** Don't confuse acacia gum with sweet acacia (*A. farnesiana*) or products from trees of the genus *Albizia*. These products may not be substituted for one another.
• Dry powder, flake, and granule formulations should be stored in tightly closed containers.

PATIENT TEACHING
• Advise patient to consult a health care provider before using an herbal preparation because another treatment may be available.
• Tell patient that when filling a new prescription he should inform pharmacist of any herbal or dietary supplement he's taking.
• Inform patient that if he delays seeking diagnosis and treatment from a health care provider, conditions such as high fat levels in the blood, periodontal infection, and GI or throat irritation could worsen.
• Advise patient allergic to acacia dust not to use acacia gum because severe reactions may occur.
• Inform patient that acacia gum may affect the absorption of other oral drugs and that he should notify a health care provider before using the herb.
• Advise patient to store dry powder, granule, or flake formulations in tightly closed containers.

aconite

Aconitum napellus, aconite, friar's cap, helmet flower, monkshood, soldier's cap, wolfsbane

Common trade names
Aconiti, Aconiti Tuber, Blue Rocket, Mousebane

AVAILABLE FORMS
Available as the dried tuberous root of *A. napellus*.

ACTIONS & COMPONENTS
Root contains many alkaloids; aconite is the most pharmacologically active. Other alkaloids include hypaconitin and mesaconitin.

Aconitin increases membrane permeability of sodium ions and slows repolarization. Initially, aconitin is stimulating, but then it paralyzes the CNS and other nerve

---

Bold italic type indicates that reaction may be life-threatening.

endings. In small doses, aconitin causes bradycardia and hypotension; in higher doses, it has an initial positive inotropic effect, then causes tachycardia, cardiac arrhythmias, and cardiac arrest.

The other alkaloids have comparable effects, with hypaconitin being the strongest.

USES
Liniments made from aconite are used for neuralgia, sciatica, and rheumatism.

Aconite is used as a cardiac depressant and as a component in some cough mixtures.

In traditional Chinese medicine, aconite is used to treat everything from sciatica to nephritis. In homeopathic preparations, aconite is used as an analgesic, antipyretic, and hypotensive.

DOSAGE & ADMINISTRATION
External use: Average dose of Aconiti tinctura is 0.1 to 0.2 g, applied topically with a brush. Maximum daily dose is 0.6 g.

ADVERSE REACTIONS
CV: *heart failure, arrhythmias, paralysis of cardiac muscle.* **Respiratory:** *paralysis of respiratory center.*

INTERACTIONS
None reported.

EFFECTS ON LAB TEST RESULTS
None reported.

CAUTIONS
Oral use of aconite isn't recommended.

Liniments absorbed through the skin may produce serious poisoning. Liniments containing aconite should never be applied to wounds or abrasions because of the potential for enhanced absorption, which could cause systemic toxicity.

NURSING CONSIDERATIONS
• Explore patient's knowledge of this herb.

▨**ALERT:** Because of aconite's toxic effects, it's rarely used in the United States. These effects may be partially decreased by some manufacturing processes; however, inability to predict toxic effects among available products should discourage use.

• Several fatal poisonings and numerous nonfatal toxic effects have been reported, perhaps because aconite's therapeutic index is narrow and its potency varies. Even as little as 1 teaspoon of the root may cause paralysis of the respiratory center and cardiac muscle, leading to death.

▨**ALERT:** Immediate symptoms of toxic reaction include burning sensation of lips, tongue, mouth, and throat. Numbness of the throat and inability to speak may follow. Numbness of fingers and toes and eventually the entire body may progress to a furry sensation. Body temperature may significantly decline. Excessive salivation, nausea, vomiting, urination, hypotension, and blurred vision with yellow-green visual disturbance may also follow initial symptoms.

• The onset of aconite poisoning is almost immediate, with the delay of symptom onset being as long as 1 hour. Death from aconite poison-

---

*Liquid contains alcohol.

ing may occur from minutes to days after ingestion, depending on the dose.

• Treatment of aconite poisoning is symptomatic. Atropine has been used to treat aconite-induced heart problems in severe cases. Arrhythmias may not respond to procainamide and may worsen with verapamil. Gastric lavage or induced vomiting may need to be performed.

PATIENT TEACHING
☑ALERT: Warn patient that use of this herb isn't recommended because it may have toxic effects and cause death.

agrimony

Agrimonia eupatoria, A. procera, burr marigold, church steeples, cocklebur, common agrimony, liverwort, philanthropos, sticklewort, stickwort

Common trade names
Fragrant Agrimony, Herba eupatoriae
Combination products: *Gall & Liver Tablets, Potter's Piletabs, Rhoival*

AVAILABLE FORMS
Available as pulverized or powdered herb and as other preparations used to make compresses, gargles, poultices, teas, and various bath preparations.

ACTIONS & COMPONENTS
The dried above-ground parts of the plant are harvested during flowering season.

Contains flavonoids and 4% to 10% condensed tannins, which give the herb astringent properties. The ethanolic extracts of agrimony are thought to have antiviral properties.

USES
Probably safe and effective as a mild topical antiseptic or astringent, and may be effective for mild, nonspecific acute diarrhea and gastroenteritis.

Specifically used for sore throat, inflammation of mouth and pharynx, inflammation of the skin, and diabetes. Also used as an antitumorigenic, cardiotonic, antihistamine, antasthmatic, diuretic, sedative, dye or flavoring agent, and coagulant for skin rashes or cuts.

Historically, agrimony was used for gallbladder disorders (in "liver and bile" teas), tuberculosis, corns and warts, and catarrh (mucous membrane inflammation with discharge).

DOSAGE & ADMINISTRATION
External use: Topical poultices using 10% water extract can be made by boiling agrimony at low heat for 10 to 20 minutes. Poultice may be applied several times daily.
Oral use: Average daily dose is 3 g P.O.

ADVERSE REACTIONS
CV: hypotension.
GI: GI upset, constipation.
Metabolic: *hypoglycemia.*
Skin: photodermatitis.

Bold italic type indicates that reaction may be life-threatening.

INTERACTIONS
Herb-drug. *Anticoagulants:* High doses of agrimony may influence anticoagulant effects. Monitor patient closely.
Antihypertensives: High doses of agrimony may cause added hypotensive effects. Monitor blood pressure.
Insulin, oral antidiabetics: Increases risk of hypoglycemia. Monitor glucose level.
Herb-lifestyle. *Sun exposure:* Increases risk of photosensitivity reactions. Advise patient to wear protective clothing and sunscreen and to limit his exposure to direct sunlight.

EFFECTS ON LAB TEST RESULTS
• May decrease glucose level.
• May increase PT and INR.

CAUTIONS
Oral use of agrimony may be unsafe in women who are pregnant. Because of the tannin content of agrimony, this herb may be unsafe when taken in high topical or oral doses.

NURSING CONSIDERATIONS
• Explore patient's knowledge of this herb.
• Short-term use of agrimony in appropriate doses is considered safe.
• Monitor patient taking high doses for nausea and vomiting.
• Monitor diabetic patients for hypoglycemia.
• Monitor blood pressure in patients taking high doses.

PATIENT TEACHING
• Advise patient to consult a health care provider before using an herbal preparation because another treatment may be available.
• Tell patient that when filling a new prescription he should inform pharmacist of any herbal or dietary supplement he's taking.
• Caution patient that if he delays seeking medical diagnosis and treatment, his condition could worsen.
• Inform diabetic patient that agrimony may decrease blood glucose level, so if he's taking a conventional antidiabetic drug the dosage of that drug may need to be adjusted.
• Inform patient that agrimony may affect the menstrual cycle.
• Advise patient that high doses of this herb may cause nausea and vomiting.
• Caution patient not to exceed recommended doses because high doses may cause low blood pressure.
• Advise patient that long-term use isn't recommended because of the risk of adverse reactions.
• Warn patient of potential adverse effects, particularly if he's also taking a drug for blood pressure, an antidiabetic drug, or a blood thinner.

alfalfa

Medicago sativa

Common trade names
*Alfalfa Concentrate, Alfalfa
Fortified, Alfalfa Natural, Alfalfa
Organics, Alfalfa Whole Juice
Concentrate, Alfamin, Feuille De
Luzerne, Lucerne, Medicago,
Phytoestrogen, Purple Medick*

AVAILABLE FORMS
Available as capsules, tablets, and
alfalfa seeds, leaves, and tea bags.
The applicable parts of alfalfa are
the parts that grow above the
ground.
Capsules: 380 mg, 405 mg,
490 mg
Tablets: 10 grains, 430 mg,
500 mg

ACTIONS & COMPONENTS
Alfalfa leaf contains saponins that
act on the CV, nervous, and digestive systems. These saponins appear to decrease plasma cholesterol without creating a change in
HDL cholesterol level. Constituents of alfalfa seem to decrease
cholesterol absorption, and increase excretion of neutral steroids
and bile acids. Alfalfa also contains manganese, which also might
be responsible for the hypoglycemic effects, and medicagol,
which appears to have antifungal
properties. Alfalfa also contains
coumetrol, genistein, biochanin A,
and daidzein, all of which seem to
have estrogenic properties.

USES
In general, alfalfa has been used
for kidney, bladder, and prostate
conditions, asthma, diabetes, indigestion, thrombocytopenic purpura, and as a diuretic. Alfalfa has
also been suggested to lower cholesterol level.
  In folk medicine, alfalfa is used
to treat diabetes and thyroid dysfunction.

DOSAGE & ADMINISTRATION
Oral: 5 to 10 g of dried herb, or as
steeped strained tea, t.i.d.
Liquid extract (1:1 in 25% alco-
hol):* 5 to 10 ml t.i.d.

ADVERSE REACTIONS
GI: diarrhea, digestive upset.
Hematologic: *pancytopenia.*
Skin: photosensitivity.

INTERACTIONS
Herb-drug. *Anticoagulants:* Excessive use of alfalfa may interfere
with anticoagulant therapy. Discourage use together.
Chlorpromazine: Excessive doses
of alfalfa may potentiate drug-
induced photosensitivity. Discourage use together.
*Hormonal contraceptives or hor-
mone therapy:* Excessive doses of
alfalfa may interfere with hormone
therapy. Discourage use together.
Herb-herb. *Herbs with clotting
potential (such as alfalfa, parsley,
nettle, and plantain):* Excessive
use of herbs that contain vitamin K
can increase the risk of clotting in
people using anticoagulants. Discourage use together.
Vitamin E: Alfalfa contains
saponins, which interfere with the
absorption or activity of vitamin E.
Discourage use together.

Bold italic type indicates that reaction may be life-threatening.

EFFECTS ON LAB TEST RESULTS
• May lower cholesterol and glucose levels.

CAUTIONS
Large consumption of alfalfa seeds can cause pancytopenia.

Pregnant women should avoid excessive amounts of alfalfa because constituents may act like estrogens in the body. Estrogenic constituents of alfalfa may interfere in therapy of patients with hormone-dependent conditions.

Patients with a history of systemic lupus erythematosus (SLE) should avoid use because consuming alfalfa seeds may reactivate latent SLE. Alfalfa leaves and stems are reportedly free of substances in the seeds that trigger SLE.

NURSING CONSIDERATIONS
• Explore patient's knowledge of this herb.
• Monitor glucose regularly if patient has diabetes.
• Monitor patients with SLE for signs and symptoms of reactivation of disease.

PATIENT TEACHING
• Advise patient to consult a health care provider before using an herbal preparation because another treatment may be available.
• Tell patient that when filling a new prescription he should inform pharmacist of any herbal or dietary supplement he's taking.

allspice

clove pepper, Jamaica pepper, pimenta, pimento

Common trade names
Allspice

AVAILABLE FORMS
Available as aqueous extract, oil, and powder, which consists of ground dried fruit.

ACTIONS & COMPONENTS
Allspice berries and leaves contain a volatile oil that's 60% to 80% eugenol. The leaves contain more eugenol than the berries (up to 96%). The oil also contains caryophyllene, cineole, levophellandrene, and palmitic acid.

Eugenol is responsible for the herb's effects on the GI system and its analgesic properties. It works by depressing the CNS and inhibiting prostaglandin activity in the lining of the colon. It also increases the activity of some digestive enzymes, such as trypsin.

Eugenol has antioxidant properties and in vitro activity against yeast and fungi. Eugenol inhibits platelet activity.

USES
Allspice is commonly used to enhance the taste of food and toothpaste and the smell of cosmetics. In herbal medicine, it's used for GI problems such as indigestion, stomachache, and flatulence; it's also used as a purgative. Topically, it's used as an analgesic for muscle pain or toothache and as an antiseptic for teeth and gums.

---

*Liquid contains alcohol.

DOSAGE & ADMINISTRATION
Antiflatulent: 0.05 to 0.2 ml all-spice oil P.O.

ADVERSE REACTIONS
CNS: CNS depression, *seizures* (with high doses).
EENT: mucous membrane irritation (with topical use).
GI: nausea, vomiting.

INTERACTIONS
Herb-drug. *Anticoagulants, anti-platelet drugs:* Enhances effect of drug. Monitor patient for bleeding.

EFFECTS ON LAB TEST RESULTS
None reported.

CAUTIONS
Patients with intestinal disorders should avoid use because allspice and its extracts stimulate the GI tract and may irritate mucous membranes.

NURSING CONSIDERATIONS
• Explore patient's knowledge of this herb.
• Allspice is safe when used topically or when consumed in amounts typically found in foods.
⚠ **ALERT:** Ingestion of large quantities may cause toxic reaction. Ingestion of more than 5 ml of allspice oil can cause nausea, vomiting, CNS depression, and seizures.

PATIENT TEACHING
• Advise patient to consult a health care provider before using an herbal preparation because another treatment may be available.
• Tell patient that when filling a new prescription he should inform pharmacist of any herbal or dietary supplement he's taking.
• Advise patient not to ingest large amounts of allspice.
• Advise patient not to delay treatment for an illness that persists after taking allspice.

aloe

Aloe barbadensis, A. capensis, A. vera, Barbados aloes, burn plant, Curacao aloe, elephant's gall, first-aid plant, Hsiang-dan, lily of the desert, lu-hui, socotrine, Zanzibar

Common trade names
Aloe Gel, Aloe Latex, Aloe Vera, Cape Aloe

AVAILABLE FORMS
Available as dried latex for internal use, extract capsules, juice (99.7% of whole leaf aloe vera juice), tincture* (1:10, 50% alcohol), and topical gel.
Extract capsules: 75 mg, 100 mg, 200 mg
Topical gel: 98%, 99.5%, 99.6%, and 100% purity strengths

ACTIONS & COMPONENTS
A solid residue is obtained by evaporating aloe latex. It contains aloinosides, which irritate the large intestine, increasing peristalsis, thereby producing a laxative effect. Water and electrolyte reabsorption is inhibited. Aloe can cause potassium loss.
   Aloe gel is a clear, thin, viscous material obtained by crushing the mucilaginous cells found in the leaf. The gel contains a polysaccharide similar to guar gum.

The gel's wound-healing ability comes from its moisturizing effect, which prevents air from drying the wound. Mucopolysaccharides and sulfur and nitrogen compounds also stimulate healing.

Aloe gel may work as an antibacterial against *Staphylococcus aureus, Escherichia coli,* and *Mycobacterium tuberculosis,* but information is conflicting.

Aloe also contains bradykinase, which is a protease inhibitor that relieves pain and decreases swelling and redness. The anti-itching effect of aloe may be related to the antihistamine properties of magnesium lactate.

USES
Used orally, aloe latex is a potent cathartic. It's used to treat constipation; to provide evacuation relief for patients with anal fissures, hemorrhoids, or recent anorectal surgery; and to prepare a patient for diagnostic testing of the GI tract.

Aloe gel is used to treat minor burns and skin irritation and to aid in wound healing. It may also be effective as an antibacterial.

DOSAGE & ADMINISTRATION
Laxative: 100 to 200 mg of aloe capsules, 50 mg of aloe extract, or 1 to 8 ounces of juice h.s. Or, 30 ml of aloe gel or 15 to 60 gtt of aloe tincture *(1:10, 50% alcohol), p.r.n.
Topical use: Apply gel liberally three to five times daily, p.r.n.

ADVERSE REACTIONS
CV: arrhythmias, edema.
GI: cramps, diarrhea.
GU: albuminuria, hematuria, nephropathy.
Metabolic: electrolyte abnormalities, weight loss.
Musculoskeletal: muscle weakness, accelerated bone deterioration.
Skin: nummular eczematous, papular dermatitis.

INTERACTIONS
Herb-drug. *Antiarrhythmics, cardiac glycosides such as digoxin:* May lead to toxic reaction. Monitor patient closely.
Beta blockers, corticosteroids, diuretics: May enhance potassium loss. Monitor potassium level.
Disulfiram: Any herbal preparation that contains alcohol can precipitate a disulfiram-like reaction. Discourage use together.
Herb-herb. *Licorice:* Increases risk of potassium deficiency. Discourage use together.

EFFECTS ON LAB TEST RESULTS
● May decrease potassium level.

CAUTIONS
Patients with intestinal obstruction, Crohn's disease, ulcerative colitis, appendicitis, or abdominal pain of unknown origin; pregnant women; and children younger than age 12 should avoid taking aloe orally.

Products derived from the latex of aloe's outer skin should be used cautiously.

NURSING CONSIDERATIONS
● Explore patient's knowledge of this herb.
● Aloe's laxative effects are apparent within 10 hours of taking aloe.

*Liquid contains alcohol.

• Monitor patient for signs of dehydration. Elderly patients are particularly at risk.
• Monitor electrolyte levels, especially potassium, after long-term use.
• If patient is using aloe topically, monitor wound for healing.

PATIENT TEACHING
• Advise patient to consult a health care provider before using an herbal preparation because another treatment may be available.
• Tell patient that when filling a new prescription he should inform pharmacist of any herbal or dietary supplement he's taking.
• Caution patient that his condition could worsen if he delays seeking medical diagnosis and treatment.
• If patient is taking digoxin or another drug to control his heart rate, a diuretic, or a corticosteroid, he shouldn't take aloe without consulting a health care provider.
• Advise patient to reduce dose if cramping occurs after a single dose, and not to take aloe for longer than 1 or 2 weeks at a time without consulting a health care provider.
• Advise patient to notify a health care provider immediately if he experiences symptoms of dehydration, including weakness, thirst, decreased urination, dry mouth, or confusion.

American cranesbill

Geranium maculatum, alum bloom, alumroot, American kino, chocolate flower, crowfoot, dove's-foot, old maid's nightcap, shameface, spotted cranesbill, stinking cranesbill, storksbill, wild cranesbill, wild geranium

Common trade names
None known

AVAILABLE FORMS
Available as dried herb, essential oil, liquid extract*, mouthwash, and tincture.

ACTIONS & COMPONENTS
High in tannins, which likely accounts for its antidiarrheal activity. May have some antiviral and antibacterial properties. A preparation with extract and 80% ethanol may inhibit the growth of some gram-negative bacteria.

USES
Used for diarrhea, dysentery, Crohn's disease, inflammation of the mouth, liver and gallbladder disease, calculosis, and inflammation of the mouth, kidney, and bladder.
 Used as a gargle or mouthwash. Fresh leaves are commonly chewed.

DOSAGE & ADMINISTRATION
Liquid extract: 1 to 2 ml P.O. t.i.d.
Tea: 1 to 2 g P.O. Prepared by adding 1 teaspoon of herb to ½ quart of cold water, bringing that to a boil, and leaving it to draw.

Bold italic type indicates that reaction may be life-threatening.

Daily dose is 2 or 3 cups between meals.
Tincture: 3 ml P.O. t.i.d.

ADVERSE REACTIONS
GI: upset stomach.

INTERACTIONS
Herb-drug. *Disulfiram:* Any herbal preparation that contains alcohol can trigger a disulfiram-like reaction. Discourage use together.

EFFECTS ON LAB TEST RESULTS
None reported.

CAUTIONS
Those with digestive disorders should avoid use because of the herb's high tannin content.

NURSING CONSIDERATIONS
• Explore patient's knowledge of this herb.
• Relatively little information is available on this herb.

PATIENT TEACHING
• Advise patient to consult a health care provider before using an herbal preparation because another treatment may be available.
• Tell patient that when filling a new prescription he should inform pharmacist of any herbal or dietary supplement he's taking.
• Caution patient not to delay seeking medical evaluation for symptoms that may indicate a serious medical condition.
• Inform patient with a sensitive stomach that herb could cause nausea or vomiting.
• Tell patient not to take a higher dose than is recommended.

• Advise patient not to take cranesbill for longer than 1 or 2 weeks at a time without consulting a health care provider.

angelica

Angelica archangelica, angelica root, angelique, dong quai, engelwurzel, European angelica, garden angelica, heiligenwurzel, root of the Holy Ghost, tang-kuei, wild angelica

Common trade names
Nature's Answer Angelica Root Liquid

AVAILABLE FORMS
Available as liquid extract, tincture, and essential oil.

ACTIONS & COMPONENTS
The root and fruit seeds of angelica are used to extract the medicinally active part of the plant. Angelica contains alpha-angelica lactone, which augments calcium binding and calcium turnover. Its action may involve increasing the contraction-dependent calcium pool to be released upon systolic depolarization. The coumarins and furanocoumarins may induce photosensitivity and may be photocarcinogenic and mutagenic.

USES
Angelica seed is used as a diuretic and diaphoretic. It's also used to treat conditions of the kidneys and the urinary, GI, and respiratory tracts as well as rheumatic and neuralgic symptoms.
　Angelica root is used orally for loss of appetite, GI spasm, and

*Liquid contains alcohol.

flatulence. It has been used topically to treat neuralgia. Other uses include treatment for coughs and bronchitis, anorexia, dyspepsia with intestinal cramping, and menstrual, liver, and gallbladder complaints.

Angelica seed has also been used as a flavoring in gin, some regional wines, candied leaves, and cake and pastry decorations.

DOSAGE & ADMINISTRATION
Crude root: 4.5 g P.O. daily.
Essential oil: 10 to 20 gtt P.O. daily.
Liquid extract (1:1): 0.5 to 3 g P.O. daily.
Tincture (1:5): 1.5 g P.O. daily.

ADVERSE REACTIONS
Skin: photosensitivity reactions.

INTERACTIONS
Herb-drug. *Antacids, H₂ blockers, proton pump inhibitors, sucralfate:* Angelica may increase acid production in the stomach and so may interfere with absorption of these drugs. Advise patient to separate administration times.
Anticoagulants: Potentiated effects of anticoagulants with excessive doses of angelica. Monitor patient for bleeding.
Herb-lifestyle. *Sun exposure:* Increases risk of photosensitivity reactions. Advise patient to wear protective clothing and sunscreen and to limit direct exposure to sunlight.

EFFECTS ON LAB TEST RESULTS
None reported.

CAUTIONS
Pregnant and breast-feeding patients should avoid using angelica because it appears to stimulate menstruation and the uterus.

NURSING CONSIDERATIONS
- Explore patient's knowledge of this herb.
- Monitor patient for persistent diarrhea, which may be a sign of something more serious.
- Monitor patient for dermatologic reactions.
- Photodermatosis is possible after contact with the plant juice or plant extract.

PATIENT TEACHING
- Advise patient to consult a health care provider before using an herbal preparation because another treatment may be available.
- Tell patient that when filling a new prescription he should inform pharmacist of any herbal or dietary supplement he's taking.
- Caution patient not to delay seeking medical treatment for symptoms that may be related to a serious medical condition.
- Advise patient not to take angelica if pregnant or if taking a gastric acid blocker or anticoagulant.
- Advise patient to notify his health care provider if he develops a skin rash.

Bold italic type indicates that reaction may be life-threatening.

anise

Pimpinella anisum, aniseed, anise oil, semen anisi, sweet cumin

Common trade names
None known

AVAILABLE FORMS
Available as dried fruit, essential oil, and tea.

ACTIONS & COMPONENTS
Anise oil is obtained from fruits of the herb. The highest quality oil comes from anise seeds. The major component of the oil is trans-anethole, which is responsible for the taste, smell, and medicinal properties of anise.

Structurally, anise is comparable to catecholamines (such as dopamine, epinephrine, and norepinephrine) and the hallucinogenic compound myristicin.

Bergapten, another component of anise, may cause photosensitivity reactions and may be carcinogenic.

USES
Anise is used to treat coughs and colds and to decrease bloating and gas. In higher doses, anise is used as an antispasmodic and antiseptic for cough, asthma, and bronchitis.

Anise also has weak antibacterial effects against gram-positive and gram-negative organisms. The oil has been used for lice, scabies, and psoriasis.

Anise has also been used as flavoring in alcohols, various foods, perfumes, and soaps.

DOSAGE & ADMINISTRATION
Antiflatulent: For adults, 1 tablespoon of tea several times daily; for breast-feeding babies, 1 teaspoon of tea P.O. p.r.n.
Dried fruit: 0.5 to 1 g P.O. Maximum daily dose is 3 g.
Essential oil: 50 to 200 ml P.O. daily.
Expectorant: 1 cup of tea P.O. in the morning or the evening.
Tea: Prepared by steeping 1 to 2 teaspoons of crushed seed in water for 10 to 15 minutes and then straining. Tea may be taken t.i.d.

ADVERSE REACTIONS
CNS: *seizures.*
GI: nausea, vomiting, stomatitis.
Respiratory: pulmonary edema.
Skin: erythema, scaling, vesiculation, photosensitivity reactions.

INTERACTIONS
Herb-drug. *Anticoagulants, MAO inhibitors, oral contraceptives:* High doses of anise can interfere with these drugs. Monitor patient closely.
Herb-lifestyle. *Sun exposure:* Increases risk of photosensitivity reactions. Advise patient to wear protective clothing and sunscreen and to limit exposure to direct sunlight.

EFFECTS ON LAB TEST RESULTS
None reported.

CAUTIONS
Those allergic to anise or anethole should avoid use. Pregnant patients should avoid using anise because it may cause abortion. Patients with dermatitis or inflammatory or al-

---

*Liquid contains alcohol.

lergic skin reactions should avoid using anise because it may cause photosensitivity.

Patients with coagulation problems should use anise cautiously.

NURSING CONSIDERATIONS
• Explore patient's knowledge of this herb.
• Preparations containing 5% to 10% essential oil can be used externally.
✒ **ALERT:** Don't confuse anise with Chinese star anise.
• If overdose occurs, monitor patient for neurologic changes and provide supportive measures for nausea and vomiting.

PATIENT TEACHING
• Advise patient to consult a health care provider before using an herbal preparation because another treatment may be available.
• Tell patient that when filling a new prescription he should inform pharmacist of any herbal or dietary supplement he's taking.
• If patient is pregnant, instruct her not to use anise.
• If patient is taking an anticoagulant or an antiplatelet drug, advise him not to take anise.
• Instruct patient not to exceed the daily recommended dose.
• Advise patient to report any skin changes to his health care provider.

arnica

Arnica montana, arnica flowers, arnica root, common arnica, Leopard's bane, mountain snuff, mountain tobacco, sneezewort, wolfsbane

Common trade names
Arnica Flowers Extract, Arnica Gel, Arnicalm, Arnica Ointment, Arnica-Si, Weleda Massage Balm

AVAILABLE FORMS
Available, for external use only, as ointment, semisolid cream, and tincture for poultice preparation. Also available in tablets for homeopathic preparations.

ACTIONS & COMPONENTS
Typically, the dried yellow to orange-yellow flower heads of the plant are used to extract the active compounds. Parts of the rhizome at the base of the plant also may be used.

The plant contains many chemical compounds, including oils and fatty acids. Its sesquiterpene lactones have mild analgesic and anti-inflammatory effects. Helenalin and dihydrohelenalin, additional sesquiterpenes, may also have antibacterial and additional anti-inflammatory effects. Some components may reduce bleeding times and inhibit platelet function. Arnica may also have antifungal effects.

Arnica, which has some immunostimulatory activity, contains a group of polysaccharides that can modify the immune response.

Bold italic type indicates that reaction may be life-threatening.

USES
Poultices and ointments have been used topically to treat skin inflammation, acne, bruises, sprains, blunt injuries, and rheumatic muscle and joint problems.

Oral rinses have been used to treat inflammation of the mouth and pharynx; however, ingestion of arnica can cause a severe toxic reaction, including death, so its use as an oral rinse should be avoided or carefully monitored.

Arnica has also been used to treat heart problems, improve circulation, stimulate the CNS, ease pain, and treat surgical or accidental trauma, postoperative thrombophlebitis, and pulmonary emboli.

DOSAGE & ADMINISTRATION
Oral rinse: Tincture diluted 10 times with water.
Poultice preparation: Tincture diluted 3 to 10 times with water.

ADVERSE REACTIONS
CNS: *coma,* drowsiness.
CV: *cardiac arrest*.
GI: stomach pain, diarrhea, vomiting, gastroenteritis.
Respiratory: dyspnea.
Skin: contact dermatitis, irritation of mucous membranes, and eczema (with prolonged use of topical preparation).

INTERACTIONS
Herb-drug. *Aspirin, heparin, warfarin:* Increases risk of bleeding. Monitor patient closely.
Herb-herb. *Angelica, anise, asafoetida, bogbean, boldo, capsicum, celery, chamomile, clove, danshen, fenugreek, feverfew, garlic, ginger, ginkgo, ginseng, horse chestnut, horseradish, licorice, meadowsweet, onion, papain, passion flower, poplar bark, prickly ash, quassia wood, red clover, turmeric, wild carrot, wild lettuce, willow:* May increase bleeding times or alter platelet function. Discourage use together.

EFFECTS ON LAB TEST RESULTS
None reported.

CAUTIONS
Pregnant and breast-feeding patients and those allergic to arnica, tansy, sunflowers, or chrysanthemums should avoid use.

Any patient taking a drug that affects coagulation or platelet function should use arnica cautiously.

NURSING CONSIDERATIONS
• Explore patient's knowledge of this herb.
• The typical extract strength of the tincture is ⅛ ounce of flower heads in 3½ ounces of water.
• Arnica oil is usually made with 1 part herb extract to 5 parts vegetable-fixed oil.
• Frequent topical use of arnica increases the likelihood of contact dermatitis. Eczema may also be caused by prolonged contact with arnica-containing external dressings.
✓ ALERT: Arnica should be used only externally because internal use may cause severe toxic reaction or death.
• Signs and symptoms of overdose include vomiting, diarrhea, drowsiness, dyspnea, and cardiac arrest.

- If overdose occurs, perform gastric lavage or induce vomiting, and follow with supportive treatment.
- In tablet form, the active ingredient is extremely diluted.

PATIENT TEACHING
- Advise patient to consult a health care provider before using an herbal preparation because another treatment may be available.
- Tell patient that when filling a new prescription he should inform pharmacist of any herbal or dietary supplement he's taking.
- Warn patient that arnica should only be used externally.
- Advise patient with a history of skin reactions to perfumes, cosmetics, hair tonics, and antidandruff preparations to use arnica cautiously because many of these products contain arnica, to which he might be allergic.
- If patient is taking an anticoagulant or using long-term aspirin therapy, instruct him to use arnica cautiously and to notify his health care provider of any unusual bleeding or bruising.
- Warn patient that only a diluted tincture should be used as a dressing.
- Advise patient that prolonged or frequent use of arnica dressings can increase the risk of skin reactions.
- Advise patient to store ointment and undiluted tincture out of children's reach and away from pets.

artichoke

Cynara scolymus, garden artichoke, globe artichoke, inulin Jerusalem artichoke powder

Common trade names
Artichoke Extract, Artichoke Hrt with Water, Artichoke Power, Cynara-SL Artichoke, Inuflora, Psta Spag Artichoke

AVAILABLE FORMS
Available as fresh pressed juice or fresh or dried leaf, stem, root, and capsules.

ACTIONS & COMPONENTS
Although the active component of artichoke hasn't been identified, cynarin or a mono-caffeoylquinic acid may have some cholesterol-lowering effects. Cynarin may also have some liver-protective qualities, and it increases bile production.

USES
Used to treat dyspepsia, abdominal and gallbladder problems, and nausea. Also used as an antidiabetic, antilipemic, diuretic, and liver protectant. However, it isn't known whether artichokes reduce cholesterol in patients with types IIa or IIb familial hypercholesterolemia.

Artichoke also has been used to prevent the return of gallstones.

DOSAGE & ADMINISTRATION
Dried leaf, stem, or root: 1 to 4 g P.O. daily.
Dry extract: 500 mg P.O. daily in a single dose.

Bold italic type indicates that reaction may be life-threatening.

ADVERSE REACTIONS
Skin: contact dermatitis.

INTERACTIONS
Herb-drug. *Insulin, oral antidiabetics:* Increases risk of hypoglycemia because both drug and herb have glucose-lowering effects. Avoid using together.

EFFECTS ON LAB TEST RESULTS
None reported.

CAUTIONS
Patients allergic to artichokes, marigolds, daisies, or chrysanthemums and those with bile duct obstruction should avoid use.

Patients with gallstones should use artichoke cautiously.

NURSING CONSIDERATIONS
• Explore patient's knowledge of this herb.
• Bile duct obstruction should be ruled out before artichoke is used medicinally.
• Artichoke preparations should be stored in a tightly closed container, away from light.
• Monitor glucose level in patients with diabetes.

PATIENT TEACHING
• Advise patient to consult a health care provider before using an herbal preparation because another treatment may be available.
• Tell patient that when filling a new prescription he should inform pharmacist of any herbal or dietary supplement he's taking.
• Advise patient to avoid medicinal use of artichoke if he's allergic to artichokes, marigolds, daisies, or chrysanthemums.
• If patient has gallstones, advise him to consult a health care provider before using artichoke medicinally.
• Advise patient to store artichoke preparations in a tightly closed container away from light.
• Advise diabetic patient that artichokes may have a hypoglycemic effect. If he's taking an antidiabetic drug, inform him that his dosage may need to be adjusted.

asparagus

Asparagus officinalis, garden asparagus, sparrowgrass

Common trade names
Hy-C (Bu Yin), Tian Men Dong, Ultimate Urinary Cleanse
Combination products:
ClearLung

AVAILABLE FORMS
Available as cut rhizome or root, fresh stalks, root powder, and tea.

ACTIONS & COMPONENTS
Rich in vitamin A; also contains folic acid. It has saponin components that act as mucous membrane irritants. The shoots have several sulfur-containing acids that can cause urine to become strong smelling.

USES
Used with large amounts of liquid as irrigation therapy. Used to treat UTIs and rheumatic joint pain and swelling, to prevent kidney or blad-

der stones, and to provide contraception.

The seeds and root extracts are used in the production of alcoholic beverages. The seeds are also used in coffee substitutes, diuretic preparations, laxatives, and remedies for neuritis and rheumatism. The seeds may relieve toothaches, stimulate hair growth, and treat cancer. Topical preparations may have drying effects on acne.

Despite these varied uses, irrigation therapy is the only treatment with clinical supporting evidence of its effectiveness.

DOSAGE & ADMINISTRATION
Daily dose: 45 to 80 g P.O. daily.
Root powder: 10 to 50 g mixed with milk and sugar P.O. b.i.d.
Tea: 40 to 60 g of cut rhizome or root P.O. daily. The tea is prepared by steeping the herb in 5 ounces of boiling water for 5 to 10 minutes and then straining the mixture.

ADVERSE REACTIONS
GI: mucous membrane irritation.
GU: malodorous urine.
Skin: contact dermatitis (with external use).

INTERACTIONS
Herb-drug. *Diuretics:* May increase drug effects. Monitor patient closely.

EFFECTS ON LAB TEST RESULTS
None reported.

CAUTIONS
Patients with inflammatory kidney diseases should avoid use. Those with edema caused by heart or kidney disorders shouldn't use asparagus as an irrigant. Pregnant women should avoid medicinal use of asparagus because the effects on the developing fetus are unknown.

NURSING CONSIDERATIONS
• Explore patient's knowledge of this herb.
• Patients using asparagus as a urinary irrigant should drink plenty of fluids.
• Asparagus may also be applied topically; however, no guidelines for concentration or dosage exist.

PATIENT TEACHING
• Advise patient to consult a health care provider before using an herbal preparation because another treatment may be available.
• Tell patient that when filling a new prescription he should inform pharmacist of any herbal or dietary supplement he's taking.
• Encourage patient to drink plenty of fluids while taking asparagus.
• Inform patient that asparagus may cause his urine to develop a strong odor, and that the smell may be stronger after eating fresh asparagus as opposed to taking the rhizome or root as a tea.
• If patient is pregnant, advise her to avoid using asparagus medicinally, but assure her that consuming fresh asparagus should be safe.

Bold italic type indicates that reaction may be life-threatening.

astragalus

Astragalus membranaceus, A. mongholicus

Common trade names
Alvita Astragalus Root, Astragali, Astragalus Extract, Astragalus Root, Astragalus Vegicaps, Beg Kei, Bei Qi, Buck Qi, Huang-Qi, Hwanggi, Membranous Milk, Milk Vetch Root, Mongolian Milk, Ogi, Superior Chinese Astragalus, Tragacanth

AVAILABLE FORMS
Available as tea, liquid, and capsules. The applicable part of astragalus is the root.
Capsules: 200 mg, 250 mg, 400 mg, 450 mg, 470 mg, 500 mg, 520 mg

ACTIONS & COMPONENTS
Astragalus contains varied constituents including more than 40 saponins (such as astragaloside), several flavonoids, polysaccharides, multiple trace minerals, amino acids, and coumarins.

A. membranaceus interferes with the replication of coxsackie B-3 virus (CB3V), which causes myocarditis in animals, and significantly improves survival rates in animals infected with CB3V. Astragalus stimulates macrophages, promotes antibody formation, and increases T lymphocyte proliferation.

Astragalus is an antioxidant, inhibiting free radical production, increasing superoxide dismutase and decreasing lipid peroxidation.

The herb has demonstrated fibrinolytic activity and various effects on the heart, GI tract, and liver. Astragaloside, an active constituent of astragalus, relieves symptoms and improves exercise tolerance in patients with heart failure.

Aqueous extracts of astragalus have also been shown to improve memory acquisition and retrieval.

USES
In general, astragalus has been used for respiratory infections, immune suppression, cancer, heart failure, viral infections, liver disease, and kidney disease. Astragalus also has been used for chronic nephritis and diabetes, and as a diuretic, antioxidant, anti-inflammatory, and hypotensive drug.

Astragalus has also reportedly been used in combination with *Ligustrum lucidum* (glossy privet) for treating breast, cervical, and lung cancers.

Topically, astragalus is used as a vasodilator and to speed healing.

In Chinese medicine, astragalus is used alone or in combination for liver fibrosis, acute viral myocarditis, heart failure, small cell lung cancer, amenorrhea, and as an antiviral drug.

DOSAGE & ADMINISTRATION
Dried root: Decoction of 1 teaspoon (5 ml) per cup (250 ml) t.i.d.
Dry extract (1:8): 250 mg t.i.d.
Fluidextract: 4 to 12 ml daily
Powder: 9 to 30 g daily; 30 to 60 g daily for serious conditions
Powdered root capsule: 500 to 1,000 mg t.i.d.
As a soup: Mix 30 g in 3.5 L of soup and simmer with other food ingredients.
Tincture* (1:8): 2 to 4 ml t.i.d.

*Liquid contains alcohol.

ADVERSE REACTIONS
Hematologic: Immunosuppression (with doses greater than 28 g).

INTERACTIONS
Herb-drug. *Acyclovir:* May cause additive antiviral effects. Balance effectiveness with incidence of adverse effects.
Anticoagulants, antithrombotics, antiplatelet agents: Fibrinolytic activity may be additive and may increase the risk of bleeding. Discourage use together.
Cyclophosphamide: When used together, astragalus isn't effective for cyclophosphamide-induced myelosuppression and may reduce immunosuppression caused by cyclophosphamide. Discourage use together.
Immunosuppressants: May interfere with immunosuppression therapy. Discourage use together.
Herb-herb. *Glossy privet:* Increases survival rates in individuals receiving radiation therapy for breast cancer and in those receiving chemotherapy for lung cancer. May be used together for therapeutic effect.

EFFECTS ON LAB TEST RESULTS
• May increase PT and INR.

CAUTIONS
Patients with autoimmune disorders should avoid using astragalus because this herb may increase immune system activity, which may not be appropriate.
  Astragalus contains trace amounts of selenium, and toxic doses may cause neurologic dysfunction leading to paralysis. Patients with a history of neurologic diseases should avoid use.
  Organ transplant recipients should avoid using astragalus because it may interfere with immunosuppressive therapy.

NURSING CONSIDERATIONS
• Explore patient's knowledge of this herb.
• Astragalus is most commonly used together with other herbs.
• Closely monitor patient for bleeding complications if he's taking anticoagulants or antiplatelet or antithrombotic drugs.

PATIENT TEACHING
• Advise patient to consult a health care provider before using an herbal preparation because another treatment may be available.
• Tell patient that when filling a new prescription he should inform pharmacist of any herbal or dietary supplement he's taking.
• Caution patient to avoid doses above 28 g because this may suppress the immune system.

autumn crocus

Colchicum autumnale, crocus, fall crocus, meadow saffron, mysteria, naked ladies, vellorita, wonder bulb

Common trade names
None known

AVAILABLE FORMS
Available as pulverized herb, freshly pressed juice, and other preparations for oral use.

Bold italic type indicates that reaction may be life-threatening.

ACTIONS & COMPONENTS

Contains colchicine and other alkaloids. These components act as antichemotactics, antiphlogistics, and antimitotics. Overall, the herb decreases inflammation and collagen synthesis and inhibits cell division.

USES

The plant and extracts have been used to treat arthritis, rheumatism, prostate enlargement, and gonorrhea. Extracts have also been used to treat cancer.

The FDA has approved the use of colchicine, the active ingredient in autumn crocus, for the treatment of gout.

Colchicine has also been used to treat multiple sclerosis, familial Mediterranean fever, hepatic cirrhosis, and primary biliary cirrhosis and as an adjunct therapy in primary amyloidosis, Behçet's disease, pseudogout, skin manifestations of scleroderma, psoriasis, palmoplantar pustulosis, and dermatitis herpetiformis.

DOSAGE & ADMINISTRATION

For acute gout attack: One dose equivalent to 1 mg of colchicine P.O., followed by 0.5 to 1.5 mg P.O. q 1 to 2 hours until the pain diminishes. Total daily dose shouldn't exceed 8 mg of colchicine equivalent.
For Mediterranean fever: 0.5 to 1.5 mg of colchicine equivalent P.O. as a single dose.

ADVERSE REACTIONS

CNS: peripheral neuritis, numbness of fingertips.

EENT: irritation of the nose and throat.
GI: GI disturbances.
Hematologic: *agranulocytosis,* aplastic anemia.

INTERACTIONS

Herb-drug. *Colchicine:* May have additive adverse and toxic effects. Discourage use together.

EFFECTS ON LAB TEST RESULTS

• May decrease hemoglobin and hematocrit. May decrease granulocyte count.

CAUTIONS

Pregnant and breast-feeding patients should avoid use because of drug's potential teratogenic effects and antimitotic properties.

NURSING CONSIDERATIONS

• Explore patient's knowledge of this herb.
✍**ALERT:** Because of plant's toxicity, internal use isn't recommended. Advise patient to consult a knowledgeable practitioner before use.
• Because many autumn crocus preparations aren't evaluated for colchicine content the way prescription colchicine products are, overdose is a concern.
• If patient insists on taking autumn crocus, advise him to alert his health care provider first and then to obtain the product from a reputable source.
• Monitor patient for agranulocytosis, aplastic anemia, and peripheral neuritis with prolonged use.
✍**ALERT:** Any patient who experiences nausea, vomiting, intense

---

*Liquid contains alcohol.

thirst, burning in the mouth, abdominal pain, or diarrhea after taking autumn crocus should immediately contact the poison control center. Diarrhea may be persistent and may lead to hypovolemic shock, renal impairment, and oliguria. Treatment for toxic reaction includes fluid replacement, induction of vomiting, and gastric lavage.

• Postmenopausal women and those using adequate contraceptive measures are the only women who should use autumn crocus. Any patient who may be pregnant should perform a pregnancy test before beginning therapy.

• Slicing the fresh corm can irritate the nose and throat and cause numbness of the fingers holding the corm.

PATIENT TEACHING
• Advise patient to consult a health care provider before using an herbal preparation because another treatment may be available.

• Tell patient when filling a new prescription he should remind pharmacist of any herbal or dietary supplements he's taking.

• Advise any patient who's pregnant, breast-feeding, or not using birth control and who could become pregnant not to use autumn crocus. Further, instruct her to immediately discontinue herb and notify her health care provider if pregnancy occurs.

• Advise any patient taking colchicine, NSAIDs, or allopurinol to avoid autumn crocus.

• Warn patient that the entire plant is toxic and that he shouldn't take it orally, unless his health care provider has instructed him to do so.

• Advise any patient using autumn crocus to obtain it from a reputable source that clearly identifies the amount of colchicine in each dose.

• Advise patient to call a poison control center immediately if he experiences nausea, vomiting, burning in the mouth, or abdominal pain after taking a dose.

avens

Geum urbanum, avens root, blessed herb, city avens, clove root, colewort, European avens, gariophilata, goldy star of the earth, herb bennet, St. Benedict's herb, way bennet, wild rye, yellow avens

Common trade names
None known

AVAILABLE FORMS
Available as aerial parts and root, dried and made into a tea for oral consumption, and liquid extract* containing alcohol for oral consumption.

ACTIONS & COMPONENTS
Contains tannins and phenolic glycosides, including eugenol, which give avens roots a clovelike odor. Both components have astringent properties that cause tissues to contract.

USES
Used to treat diarrhea, digestive complaints, ulcerative colitis, intermittent fever, sore throat, gingivitis, and halitosis.

Bold italic type indicates that reaction may be life-threatening.

DOSAGE & ADMINISTRATION
Extract* (contains 25% alcohol): 1
to 4 ml P.O. t.i.d.
Tea: 1 to 4 g, steeped in boiling
water and strained, P.O. t.i.d.

ADVERSE REACTIONS
None known.

INTERACTIONS
None reported.

EFFECTS ON LAB TEST RESULTS
None reported.

CAUTIONS
Pregnant and breast-feeding patients should avoid use because of
unknown effects.

NURSING CONSIDERATIONS
• Explore patient's knowledge of
this herb.
🗹 **ALERT:** Don't confuse avens
with water avens (*Geum rivale,*
chocolate root).
• Avens is rarely used in herbal
medicine.

PATIENT TEACHING
• Advise patient to consult a health
care provider before using an
herbal preparation because another
treatment may be available.
• Tell patient that when filling a
new prescription he should inform
pharmacist of any herbal or dietary
supplement he's taking.
• If patient is pregnant, breast-
feeding, or planning pregnancy,
advise her not to use avens and to
notify her health care provider if
she becomes pregnant during therapy.
• If patient is using avens to treat
diarrhea, advise him to contact his

health care provider if the diarrhea
persists.

*Liquid contains alcohol.

B

balsam of Peru

Myroxylon balsamum, balsam tree, Peruvian balsam, tolu balsam

Common trade names
None known

AVAILABLE FORMS
Available in shampoo, lotions, and syrups.

ACTIONS & COMPONENTS
Contains 50% to 70% ester mixtures; benzyl ester of benzoic, cinnamein, and cinnamic acid appear in the greatest amount.

USES
Used externally to help heal infected and poorly healing wounds, burns, pressure ulcers, frostbite, sore nipples, leg ulcers, bruises from prostheses, and hemorrhoids. Used to stimulate the heart, raise blood pressure, and reduce mucous secretions. Used as an antiparasitic to treat scabies, and for fevers, colds, cough, bronchitis, vulnerability to infection, and mouth and pharynx inflammation. This herb is also used to treat itching and later stages of acute eczema.

DOSAGE & ADMINISTRATION
Daily topical dosage: Preparations containing 5% to 20% Peruvian balsam may be used for up to 1 week.
Extensive application: Preparations containing not more than 10% Peruvian balsam may be used for up to 1 week.
Tolu balsam for internal use: The average dosage is 0.5 g P.O. daily.

ADVERSE REACTIONS
GI: aphthoid oral ulcers.
GU: renal damage.
Skin: allergic skin reactions, urticaria, purpura, photosensitivity reaction, phototoxicity.
Other: *angioedema.*

INTERACTIONS
Herb-drug. *Sulfur-containing products:* Causes additive effects. Advise patient to use cautiously.
Herb-lifestyle. *Sun exposure:* Increases risk of photosensitivity reactions. Advise patient to wear protective clothing and sunscreen and to limit exposure to direct sunlight.

EFFECTS ON LAB TEST RESULTS
None reported.

CAUTIONS
Patients with a propensity for allergies shouldn't use this herb.
   Patients with hypertension should use balsam of Peru cautiously because it may increase blood pressure if ingested.

NURSING CONSIDERATIONS
• Explore patient's knowledge of this herb.
• Advise patient to stop use if skin reaction occurs.

PATIENT TEACHING
• Advise patient to consult a health care provider before using an

---

Bold italic type indicates that reaction may be life-threatening.

herbal preparation because another treatment may be available.
• Tell patient that when filling a new prescription he should inform pharmacist of any herbal or dietary supplement he's taking.
• Warn patient to seek appropriate medical evaluation before using balsam of Peru to treat wound infection or pressure ulcers, to avoid a delay in healing and a worsening of the condition.
• Advise patient not to use herb with products containing sulfur.
• Advise patient to discontinue use if skin reaction occurs.
• Instruct any patient using the herb externally to treat sore nipples to remove residue from her breasts before breast-feeding.
• Advise patient to limit external application to 1 week or less.

barberry

Berberis vulgaris, berberry, jaundice berry, mountain grape, Oregon grape, pepperidge bush, pipperidge, sour-spine, sow berry, trailing mahonia, wood sour

Common trade names
Barberry-Berberis Vulgaris

AVAILABLE FORMS
Available as liquid extract, tablets, and tea.
Tablets: 400 mg

ACTIONS & COMPONENTS
Contains isoquinolone alkaloids in the root and bark, including the alkaloid berberine, which is effective in managing bacteria-induced diarrhea. In small doses, it stimu-

lates the respiratory system; in large doses, it may produce dyspnea and lethal respiratory system paralysis.

USES
Used to dilate blood vessels and stimulate the circulatory system, to treat GI ailments, and to relieve or reduce fever. May be beneficial as a bactericidal and for cholera-induced diarrhea, may stimulate uterine contractions, and may have some laxative effects.

DOSAGE & ADMINISTRATION
Dried root: 2 to 4 g P.O.
For cholera-induced diarrhea: 100 mg of berberine P.O. q.i.d. or 400 mg P.O. daily, alone or with tetracycline. Maximum daily dose, 500 mg.
Fluidextract (1:1): 2 to 4 ml P.O.
Solid (powdered dry) extract (4:1) or 8% to 12% alkaloid content: 250 to 500 mg P.O.
Tea: Prepared by pouring 5 ounces of hot water onto 1 to 2 teaspoons whole or squashed barberries and straining after 10 to 15 minutes. Dose is 2 to 4 g P.O. or 2 g in 8½ ounces.
Tincture (1:5): 6 to 12 ml P.O.
Tincture (1:10): 20 to 40 gtt P.O. daily.

ADVERSE REACTIONS
CNS: stupor, lethargy.
CV: hypotension.
EENT: epistaxis, eye irritation.
GI: diarrhea.
GU: nephritis.
Respiratory: dyspnea.
Skin: skin irritation.

*Liquid contains alcohol.

INTERACTIONS
Herb-drug. *Antihypertensives:* May increase effects. Monitor blood pressure closely.
Herb-herb. *Berberine-containing herbs (amur cork tree, bloodroot, Chinese cork tree, goldenseal, goldthread, Oregon grape):* May increase berberine toxicity. Discourage use together.

EFFECTS ON LAB TEST RESULTS
None reported.

CAUTIONS
Pregnant women should avoid using barberry because it may stimulate uterine contractions.

Patients with heart failure or respiratory diseases should use barberry cautiously.

NURSING CONSIDERATIONS
• Explore patient's knowledge of this herb.
• If patient is using barberry to treat diarrhea, monitor him to ensure the therapy is working.
• Ingestion of berberine in doses greater than 500 mg can produce lethargy, nosebleeds, dyspnea, and skin and eye irritation.
⚡ALERT: Signs of toxic reaction include stupor, diarrhea, and nephritis. If signs or symptoms of toxic reaction occur, patient should stop using barberry and notify a health care provider.
⚡ALERT: Don't confuse barberry with bayberry or bearberry.

PATIENT TEACHING
• Advise patient to consult a health care provider before using an herbal preparation because another treatment may be available.
• Tell patient that when filling a new prescription he should inform pharmacist of any herbal or dietary supplement he's taking.
• Advise patient to avoid use during pregnancy and to discontinue use if she becomes pregnant during barberry therapy.
• If patient is taking high blood pressure medication, advise him to contact a health care provider before taking barberry.
• Caution patient that herb may be useful in treating bacteria-induced diarrhea only, so he shouldn't delay seeking appropriate medical evaluation for persistent diarrhea or diarrhea of unknown cause.
• Advise patient not to take more than 500 mg of barberry daily because this may increase the risk of adverse reactions, such as lethargy, nosebleeds, difficulty breathing, and skin and eye irritation.
• Inform patient of the signs and symptoms of toxic reaction, and advise him to stop using barberry if he experiences any of these reactions.

basil

Ocimum basilicum, common basil, holy basil, St. Josephwort, sweet basil

Common trade names
None known

AVAILABLE FORMS
Available as an oil and a spice.

ACTIONS & COMPONENTS
Contains estragole (70% to 85% of essential oil) as a major component and smaller amounts of safrole.

Bold italic type indicates that reaction may be life-threatening.

Estragole may possess mutagenic effects if taken internally in massive quantities, but it's safe to use as a spice. In vitro, basil is antimicrobial.

USES
Used as an antiseptic, antimicrobial, diuretic, insect repellant, and antihypertensive. Also used to stimulate digestion and to treat halitosis.

DOSAGE & ADMINISTRATION
Insect repellant: Patient should rub oil on exposed areas before going outdoors.

ADVERSE REACTIONS
CNS: dizziness, confusion, headache, trembling.
CV: palpitations.
Hepatic: *hepatocarcinoma.*
Metabolic: *hypoglycemia.*
Skin: diaphoresis.

INTERACTIONS
Herb-drug. *Antihypertensives:* May further reduce blood pressure. Monitor blood pressure.
Insulin, oral antidiabetics: May worsen hypoglycemia. Monitor glucose level.

EFFECTS ON LAB TEST RESULTS
• May decrease glucose level.

CAUTIONS
Pregnant or breast-feeding women, infants, and young children should avoid using basil.

Patients with diabetes and those taking an antihypertensive should use basil cautiously because it may increase the therapeutic effect of conventional drugs.

NURSING CONSIDERATIONS
• Explore patient's knowledge of this herb.
• Estragole and safrole are procarcinogens with weak carcinogenic effects in the liver. Although the risk of developing cancer from using basil is slight, long-term or high-dose therapy isn't recommended.
• If a patient is taking both an antihypertensive and basil and his blood pressure stabilizes, the dosage of the conventional antihypertensive may need to be adjusted once he stops taking the herb.
• Taking medicinal doses of basil may disrupt a previously stable antidiabetic regimen.
• Monitor patient for signs and symptoms of hypoglycemia, such as dizziness, weakness, sweating, tachycardia, headache, confusion, and trembling.

PATIENT TEACHING
• Advise patient to consult with a health care provider before using an herbal preparation because a standard treatment that has been proven effective may be available.
• Tell patient that when filling a new prescription he should inform pharmacist of any herbal or dietary supplement he's taking.
• Tell patient that this herb isn't recommended for use in large quantities because it may cause cancer; however, the amounts used in cooking appear to be safe.
• Advise pregnant or breast-feeding women to avoid medicinal use of basil.
• Advise patient to avoid use in infants and children.

*Liquid contains alcohol.

• Advise diabetic patient to consult a health care provider before using basil because it can lower blood glucose levels.
• If patient is taking medication for high blood pressure, inform him that basil may also lower blood pressure; these two products together could cause a dangerously low blood pressure level.

bay

Laurus nobilis, bay laurel, bay leaf, bay tree, Daphne, Grecian laurel, Indian bay, laurel, noble laurel, Roman laurel, sweet bay, true laurel

Common trade names
None known

AVAILABLE FORMS
Available as berries, extracts, leaves, oils, ointments, and soaps.

ACTIONS & COMPONENTS
Contains 1,8-cineol, which may be bactericidal, and parthenolides, which may help prevent migraine. Lowers the glucose level by helping the body use insulin more effectively.

USES
Used as an antiseptic and a stimulant. Used to treat the common cold and to relieve muscle spasms. Also found in some toothpastes because it may help prevent tooth decay.

DOSAGE & ADMINISTRATION
Not well documented.

ADVERSE REACTIONS
Metabolic: *hypoglycemia.*
Respiratory: asthma.
Other: allergic reactions, including contact dermatitis.

INTERACTIONS
Herb-drug. *Antidiabetics, insulin:* Bay may intensify the intended therapeutic effects of conventional drugs. Monitor glucose level.

EFFECTS ON LAB TEST RESULTS
• May decrease glucose level.

CAUTIONS
Patients shouldn't take bay internally. Pregnant and breast-feeding patients should avoid this herb.
    Patients with diabetes who are taking an antidiabetic should use bay cautiously because it may worsen hypoglycemia, disrupting a previously stable antidiabetic regimen.

NURSING CONSIDERATIONS
• Explore patient's knowledge of this herb.
• Internal use may cause allergic reactions, including asthma.
• Monitor patient for signs and symptoms of hypoglycemia, such as confusion, dizziness, sweating, and trembling.

PATIENT TEACHING
• Advise patient to consult a health care provider before using an herbal preparation because another treatment may be available.
• Tell patient that when filling a new prescription he should remind pharmacist of any herbal or dietary supplement that he's taking.

Bold italic type indicates that reaction may be life-threatening.

• Tell patient that bay isn't recommended for internal use because it can cause allergic reactions, including asthma.

• If patient has diabetes, advise him to consult a health care provider before using bay because it can cause low blood glucose levels.

• Advise patient to avoid use if she's pregnant or breast-feeding and to notify her health care provider if she becomes pregnant while taking bay.

bayberry

Myrica cerifera, M. cortex, bog myrtle, candleberry, Dutch myrtle, sweet gale, tallow shrub, vegetable tallow, wachsgagle, waxberry, wax myrtle

Common trade names
Bayberry Bark, Bayberry Root Bark

AVAILABLE FORMS
Available as capsules, liquid extract*, powder, and tea.
Capsules: 450 mg, 475 mg

ACTIONS & COMPONENTS
Contains tannins, triterpenes, myricadiol, taraxerol, taraxerone, and flavonoid glycoside myricitrin.

Tannins give bayberry its astringent properties. Myricadiol may have mineralocorticoid activity. Myricitrin may stimulate the flow of bile, and the dried root may help lower a fever.

USES
Used as a tea to treat diarrhea and as a gargle to treat sore throats.

Also used internally for coughs and colds and for its antipyretic and circulatory stimulant properties. Used topically for its astringent properties.

DOSAGE & ADMINISTRATION
Liquid extract (1:1) in 45% alcohol: 0.6 to 2 ml or 10 to 90 gtt P.O. t.i.d.
Powdered bark: 600 mg to 2 g P.O. t.i.d. by infusion or decoction.

ADVERSE REACTIONS
EENT: sneezing.
GI: stomach upset, vomiting.
Respiratory: cough.

INTERACTIONS
Herb-drug. *Antihypertensives, corticosteroids:* Using these drugs with bayberry may have an additive effect. Bayberry may interfere with the intended therapeutic effects of conventional drugs. Discourage use together.
Iron: Decreases absorption of iron. Advise patient to separate times of use by 2 hours.

EFFECTS ON LAB TEST RESULTS
None reported.

CAUTIONS
Patients shouldn't take bayberry internally. Pregnant patients, breast-feeding patients, and patients allergic to bayberry should avoid the herb. Patients who are taking corticosteroids, or who have hypertension, peripheral edema, heart failure, or another condition in which mineralocorticoid use isn't recommended should also avoid using herb.

---

*Liquid contains alcohol.

NURSING CONSIDERATIONS
- Explore patient's knowledge of this herb.
- Bayberry has a high tannin content and commonly causes gastric distress and liver damage after long-term use.
- Long-term use of bark extract may cause malignant tumors.
- Heat, moisture, and light may cause bayberry to break down, so it should be stored in a dry, moisture, and cool place.
- Large doses have mineralocorticoid effects, such as sodium and water retention and hypertension.
  ⚡ALERT: Don't confuse bayberry with barberry or bearberry.

PATIENT TEACHING
- Advise patient to consult a health care provider before using an herbal preparation because another treatment may be available.
- Tell patient that when filling a new prescription he should inform pharmacist of any herbal or dietary supplement he's taking.
- If patient has high blood pressure or heart disease, advise him to consult a health care provider before using bayberry.
- Caution patient to avoid using bayberry if she's pregnant or breast-feeding, and to notify her health care provider if she becomes pregnant while taking the herb.
- Caution patient that ingesting bayberry isn't recommended because this can cause stomach upset and vomiting.
- Advise patient to avoid using bayberry for extended periods because it can cause tumors or adverse reactions.

- Advise patient to store bayberry in a dry, dark, cool place.

bearberry

Arctostaphylos uva-ursi, arberry, bear's grape, kinnikinnick, manzanita, mealberry, mountain box, mountain cranberry, redberry leaves, rockberry, sagackhomi, sandberry, upland cranberry, uva-ursi

Common trade names
Uva-Ursi, Uva-Ursi Leaf, Standardized Uva-Ursi Extract

AVAILABLE FORMS
Available as capsules, dried leaves, liquid extract, and tea bags.
Capsules: 455 mg, 460 mg (with dandelion), 500 mg, 505 mg capsules that contain 335 mg of leaf extract and 150 mg of uva-ursi leaves and millet
Liquid extract (prepared from dried leaves): Cold processed biochelated extract made from freshly manufactured uva-ursi leaves, vegetable glycerin, and grain neutral spirits (12% to 14% by volume)
Tea bags: Caffeine free

ACTIONS & COMPONENTS
Bearberry leaves contain the hydroquinone derivatives arbutin and methyl arbutin, in levels ranging from 5% to 15%. Arbutin is hydrolyzed to hydroquinone when it comes in contact with gastric fluid, which acts as a mild astringent and antimicrobial in alkaline urine.
   Large amounts of bearberry must be ingested to achieve a significant antiseptic effect. The herb is effective against *Escherichia*

Bold italic type indicates that reaction may be life-threatening.

coli, *Proteus mirabilis, P. vulgaris, Pseudomonas aeruginosa, Staphylococcus aureus,* and 70 other urinary tract bacteria.

Bearberry also contains ursolic acid and isoquercetin, which contribute to the plant's mild diuretic effect.

Bearberry may help treat hepatitis; reduce polyphagia, polydipsia, and weight gain resulting from diabetes; inhibit melanin production; and have anti-inflammatory effects.

USES
Used as a urinary antiseptic and a mild diuretic. Also used to treat contact dermatitis, allergic-type hypersensitivity reactions, and arthritis.

DOSAGE & ADMINISTRATION
Capsules: Doses vary depending on the formulation. Capsules should be taken with a meal or a glass of water.
Cold maceration: 3 g in 5 ounces of water P.O. up to q.i.d. or 400 to 840 mg of hydroquinone derivatives calculated as water-free arbutin.
Concentrated infusion: 2 to 4 ml P.O.
Dried leaves infusion: Prepared by pouring boiling water over 2.5 g of finely cut or coarse powdered herb or placing the herb in cold water and rapidly bringing the mixture to a boil. Tea is strained after 15 minutes. (1 teaspoon is equivalent to 2.5 g of drug.)
Liquid extract*: 1.5 to 4 ml (1:1 in 25% alcohol) P.O. t.i.d. Typically, 5 to 10 gtt of extract are mixed in a small amount of spring or purified water b.i.d. or t.i.d.

Tea bag infusion: 1.5 to 4 g by infusion t.i.d. Prepared by placing one tea bag into a cup, adding no more than 6 ounces of boiling water, and steeping for 3 minutes. Tea bag is pressed before it's removed to enhance the flavor. Cold water, instead of hot water, is poured over the leaves to minimize the tannin content of the infusion. The tea steeps for 12 to 24 hours before the patient drinks it.

ADVERSE REACTIONS
CNS: *seizures.*
EENT: tinnitus.
GI: nausea, vomiting.
GU: inflammation and irritation of the bladder and urinary tract mucous membranes, green-brown urine.
Hepatic: *hepatotoxicity.*
Other: cyanosis, collapse.

INTERACTIONS
Herb-drug. *Dexamethasone, prednisolone:* Arbutin increases the inhibitory action of prednisolone and dexamethasone on contact dermatitis, allergic-type hypersensitivity reactions, and arthritis. Discourage use together.
Disulfiram: Herbal products prepared with alcohol may cause a disulfiram-like reaction. Discourage use together.
Diuretics: Enhances drug effect. Monitor patient closely.
Drugs known to acidify urine such as ascorbic acid or methenamine or to increase uric acid levels such as diazoxide, diuretics, or pyrazinamide: May inhibit bearberry's effects because bearberry needs an alkali environment. Discourage use together.

*Liquid contains alcohol.

Herb-food. *Foods known to increase uric acid levels in the bladder, such as those rich in vitamin C:* May inhibit bearberry's effects because bearberry needs an alkali environment and the urinary acidifier may inhibit the conversion of herb's arbutin to the active hydroquinone component. Discourage use together.

EFFECTS ON LAB TEST RESULTS
None reported.

CAUTIONS
Pregnant patients, breast-feeding patients, and children younger than age 12 should avoid using bearberry because of its oxytocic effects. Patients with kidney disease shouldn't use bearberry because its tannin components may be excreted in the urine.

NURSING CONSIDERATIONS
• Explore patient's knowledge of this herb.
• Bearberry shouldn't be used for longer than 10 days at a time or more than five times per year.
• Bearberry contains 15% to 20% tannin, which may trigger nausea and vomiting.
• A bearberry dose of 9 g is equivalent to 400 to 700 mg of arbutin daily.
• Signs and symptoms of overdose include inflammation and irritation of the bladder and urinary tract mucous membranes. Prolonged use (over 2 weeks) isn't recommended.
• Prolonged use or overdose can cause nausea, vomiting, tinnitus, cyanosis, seizures, delirium, and even death.

• Liver toxicity may occur with prolonged use, especially in children.
⚡**ALERT:** Don't confuse bearberry with barberry or bayberry.

PATIENT TEACHING
• Advise patient to consult a health care provider before using an herbal preparation because another treatment may be available.
• Tell patient that when filling a new prescription he should inform pharmacist of any herbal or dietary supplement he's taking.
• Patients with kidney disease or who are pregnant or breast-feeding shouldn't use bearberry.
• Advise patient to take bearberry with a meal or a glass of water.
• Inform patient that urine pH must be alkaline for bearberry to be effective and that a diet high in milk, vegetables (especially tomatoes), fruit, fruit juice, and potatoes can help keep urine alkaline. A patient may take 6 to 8 g of sodium bicarbonate a day to help keep the urine alkaline.
• Inform patient that the hydroquinone in the herb may temporarily discolor urine green-brown but that this is harmless.
• Advise patient to consult a health care provider if symptoms persist for more than 7 days or if he experiences high fever, chills, nausea, vomiting, diarrhea, or severe back pain.
• Inform patient that pouring hot water over the leaves when preparing a bearberry beverage may increase the tannin content of the infusion and, thus, increase the risk of stomach discomfort. Advise him instead to pour cold water over the

---

Bold italic type indicates that reaction may be life-threatening.

leaves and to allow the mixture to steep for 12 to 24 hours before drinking it.

• Advise patient not to take bearberry for more than 10 days at a time or more than five times per year.

bee pollen

buckwheat pollen, maize pollen

Common trade names
Bee Pollen, Health Honey, Super Bee Pollen Complex

AVAILABLE FORMS
Available as capsules, chewable tablets, cream (in combination with other moisturizers), jelly, liquid (manufactured bee pollen extract, vegetable glycerin, and grain-neutral spirits), powder, raw granules, soft gel caps, and tablets.
Capsules: 265 mg, 500 mg, 580 mg, 586 mg
Granules: 154 servings per container
Jelly: 3,000 mg in 10-ounce jar of honey
Powder: 5 g per heaping teaspoon
Soft gel cap: 100 mg
Tablets: 378 mg, 500 mg, 1,000 mg
Tablets (chewable): 500 mg

ACTIONS & COMPONENTS
Contains about 30% protein, 55% carbohydrates, 1% to 2% fat, 3% minerals, and trace vitamins. Components vary depending on plant source, geographic region, harvest methods, and season of the year. May contain up to 100 vitamins, minerals, enzymes, amino acids, and other substances, but the phys-

iologic benefit of many of these components is unclear. Some bee pollen supplements also contain 3.6% to 5.9% vitamin C.

USES
Used to enhance athletic performance, minimize fatigue, and improve energy.

May relieve cerebral hemorrhage, brain damage, body weakness, anemia, enteritis, colitis, constipation, and indigestion. May be beneficial in treating chronic prostatism and relieving symptoms of radiation sickness in those being treated for cervical cancer. May also be an effective prenatal vitamin and aid in weight loss.

Although bee pollen is used to treat allergic disorders, this isn't recommended because bee pollen commonly causes allergic reactions.

DOSAGE & ADMINISTRATION
Granules: Directions vary depending on product. One manufacturer recommends ingesting 1 teaspoon or more P.O. daily or sprinkling on food or mixing in drinks. Another manufacturer recommends ingesting 1 granule at lunchtime, increasing by 1 granule with each meal until 1 teaspoon is being eaten each meal.
Liquid: 10 to 12 gtt of extract mixed in a little water, b.i.d. or t.i.d.
Oral use: 1 to 3 g daily. Dosage varies depending on product and manufacturer.
Powder: 1 to 2 teaspoons P.O. daily. May be consumed as sold or may be blended or mixed with other foods.

*Liquid contains alcohol.

Soft gel cap: 1 cap or more P.O. daily

Tablets: Dosage varies depending on the formulation and manufacturer. Tablets may be swallowed or dissolved with warm water and honey.

ADVERSE REACTIONS
Hepatic: *hepatitis.*
Other: *acute anaphylactoid reactions,* including sneezing, *angioedema,* itching, dyspnea, and lightheadedness; chronic allergic symptoms, including hypereosinophilia; and neurologic and GI complaints.

INTERACTIONS
None reported.

EFFECTS ON LAB TEST RESULTS
• May increase alkaline phosphatase, ALT, AST, LDH, and total bilirubin levels.
• May increase PT.

CAUTIONS
Patients sensitive or allergic to pollen should avoid bee pollen.

Patients allergic to apples, carrots, or celery should use this herb cautiously because of the potential for adverse reaction.

NURSING CONSIDERATIONS
• Explore patient's knowledge of this herb.
• Bee pollen in general hasn't been found to have significant nutritional or therapeutic benefit over more easily and safely administered nutritional products.
• Some bee pollen products also contain bee propolis extract and numerous other ingredients and vitamins.
• Doses as low as 1 tablespoon can cause acute anaphylactoid reactions, including sneezing, generalized angioedema, itching, dyspnea, and light-headedness. Ask patient how much herb he uses daily.
• Patients taking bee pollen for longer than 3 weeks may experience chronic allergic symptoms, such as hypereosinophilia and neurologic and GI complaints; however, such symptoms are likely to gradually disappear after the patient stops taking the bee pollen.

PATIENT TEACHING
• Advise patient to consult a health care provider before using an herbal preparation because another treatment may be available.
• Tell patient that when taking a new prescription, he should remind pharmacist of any herbal or dietary supplement he's taking.
• Inform patient that bee pollen should be taken between meals, with a full glass of water.

betel palm

Areca catechu, piper betle

Common trade names
Areca Nut, Betel Nut, Bunga, Jambe, Pinang, Pinlang, Supari

AVAILABLE FORMS
Available as quids, made from powdered or sliced areca nut, tobacco, and slaked lime (calcium hydroxide), obtained from powdered snail shells, and wrapped in the betel vine leaf.

Bold italic type indicates that reaction may be life-threatening.

ACTIONS & COMPONENTS
Contains arecoline, arecaidine, arecaine, arecolidine, guvacine, isoguvacine, and guvacoline, which cause CNS stimulation.

Chewing the nut increases salivary flow and aids digestion.

USES
Used as a mild CNS stimulant and digestive aid. It also can be used to treat coughs, stomach complaints, diphtheria, middle ear inflammation, and worm infestation.

Some patients steam the leaves and apply them as a facial dressing, but this isn't recommended because of adverse dermatologic reactions.

DOSAGE & ADMINISTRATION
Quid: 4 to 15 quids chewed daily, for 15 minutes each.

ADVERSE REACTIONS
CNS: *tetanic seizures.*
GI: gingivitis, oral lichen planuslike lesion, oral cancer including leukoplakia and squamous cell carcinoma, periodontitis.
Musculoskeletal: chronic osteomyelitis.
Respiratory: asthma exacerbation.
Skin: contact leukomelanosis characterized by immediate bleaching, hyperpigmentation, and confetti-like depigmentation.
Other: tooth discoloration, resorption of oral calcium.

INTERACTIONS
Herb-drug. *Anticholinergic drugs, procyclidine:* May cause tremor, stiffness, akathesia because of decreased effectiveness of the drugs in the presence of herb's choliner-gic alkaloid, arecoline. Discourage use together.
Prednisone, salbutamol: May worsen asthma. Discourage use together.

EFFECTS ON LAB TEST RESULTS
None reported.

CAUTIONS
Patients with a history of asthma should avoid using betel palm because it constricts the bronchial passages. Pregnant patients should avoid the herb because of possible cancerous or toxic effects on the fetus.

NURSING CONSIDERATIONS
• Explore patient's knowledge of this herb.
⚡**ALERT:** Arecaine, a compound of the herb, is poisonous. It affects respiration and heart rate and may cause seizures. Seed doses of 8 g can be fatal.
• Warn patient that chewing betel palm may cause severe oral mucosal changes, including cancerous lesions, and that he should consult a health care provider immediately if lesions appear. Chewing the betel palm–slaked lime mixture may place patient at higher risk for oral lesions than chewing betel palm alone.
• Monitor patient for asthmalike symptoms.
• Betel palm leaf facial dressings can cause severe dermatologic reactions, such as contact leukomelanosis, which occurs in three stages—immediate bleaching, hyperpigmentation, and confetti-like depigmentation.

---

*Liquid contains alcohol.

PATIENT TEACHING
• Advise patient to consult a health care provider before using an herbal preparation because another treatment may be available.
• Tell patient that when filling a new prescription he should inform pharmacist of any herbal or dietary supplement he's taking.
• Chewing betel nuts stains feces red and may interfere with stool tests.
• Advise patient who chews betel nut to contact a health care provider if he develops asthmalike symptoms.
• Advise patient not to apply betel palm leaves as a facial dressing because this may cause adverse skin reactions.

bethroot

Trillium erectum, T. pendulum, birthroot, coughroot, ground lily, Indian balm, Indian shamrock, jew's-harp plant, lamb's quarters, milk ipecac, nightshade, pariswort, purple trillium, rattlesnake root, snakebite, stinking benjamin, three-leaved, wakerobin

Common trade names
None known

AVAILABLE FORMS
Available as ground drug and liquid extract.

ACTIONS & COMPONENTS
Contains a fixed oil, a volatile oil, a saponin called trillarin, a glycoside, tannic acid, and starch. The saponin glycosides have antifungal activity.

USES
Used internally to treat long, heavy menstrual periods; to relieve pain; to control postpartum bleeding; and to manage diarrhea. Also used as an expectorant.

Used externally for varicose veins and ulcers, hematomas, and hemorrhoids. Also used externally as an astringent to minimize topical bleeding and irritation.

DOSAGE & ADMINISTRATION
Ground drug and liquid extract are used for infusions and poultices.

ADVERSE REACTIONS
GI: nausea, vomiting.
Skin: irritation at the application site.

INTERACTIONS
None reported.

EFFECTS ON LAB TEST RESULTS
None reported.

CAUTIONS
Pregnant patients should avoid this herb because it stimulates the uterus.

NURSING CONSIDERATIONS
• Explore patient's knowledge of this herb.
• Monitor application site for irritation.

PATIENT TEACHING
• Advise patient to consult a health care provider before using an herbal preparation because another treatment may be available.
• Tell patient that when filling a new prescription he should inform

Bold italic type indicates that reaction may be life-threatening.

pharmacist of any herbal or dietary supplement he's taking.
- Discourage use during pregnancy.
- Inform patient that high doses of bethroot can cause nausea.
- Advise patient to discontinue use if skin irritation develops.

betony

Betonica officinalis, Stachys officinalis, bishopswort, wood betony

Common trade names
Betony, Wood Betony

AVAILABLE FORMS
Available as a tincture*, powder, or in 450-mg capsules.

ACTIONS & COMPONENTS
The basal leaves—which contain betaine, caffeic acid derivatives, and flavonoids—are the medicinal part of the herb. They're collected and dried in the shade at a maximum temperature of 40° F (4.4° C).

Betony contains 15% tannins, which give the herb its astringent effects. Mixtures of flavonoid glycosides have hypotensive and sedative effects. Stachydrine is a systolic depressant and can decrease rheumatic pain.

USES
Used as an antidiarrheal, a sedative, and an expectorant for coughs, bronchitis, and asthma. Also used to treat catarrh, heartburn, gout, nervousness, kidney stones, and inflammation of the bladder.

Used with other herbs such as linden as a sedative, a mild hypo-tensive for treating neuralgia and anxiety, and a decongestant for treating sinus headache and congestion.

DOSAGE & ADMINISTRATION
Oral use: 1 to 2 g daily in three divided doses.
Topical use: Extract or infusion is applied to the skin as an astringent or as a treatment for wounds. Or, fresh leaves are boiled and cooled and the liquid applied to skin.

ADVERSE REACTIONS
CNS: drowsiness.
GI: GI irritation.

INTERACTIONS
Herb-drug. *Antihypertensives:* May increase therapeutic drug effect. Advise patient to use cautiously.
CNS depressants: Causes additive effects. Advise patient to use cautiously.
Disulfiram, metronidazole: Tincture contains up to 40% ethyl alcohol and may cause a disulfiram or disulfiram-like reaction. Discourage use together.
Herb-lifestyle. *Alcohol use:* Causes additive effects. Advise patient to use cautiously.

EFFECTS ON LAB TEST RESULTS
None reported.

CAUTIONS
Pregnant and breast-feeding patients should avoid use.

NURSING CONSIDERATIONS
- Explore patient's knowledge of this herb.

*Liquid contains alcohol.

• Large oral dosage may cause GI irritation because of the tannin content.

• Don't confuse *Stachys officinalis* with *S. alpina*.

PATIENT TEACHING

• Advise patient to consult a health care provider before using an herbal preparation because another treatment may be available.

• Tell patient that when filling a new prescription he should inform pharmacist of any herbal or dietary supplement he's taking.

• Warn patient not to exceed the recommended dosage.

• Caution patient that ingesting betony may cause drowsiness.

• A patient taking betony to treat diarrhea should consult a health care provider if it continues for longer than 2 days.

• If patient is taking betony to treat headache and it doesn't improve, advise him to discontinue use and consult a health care provider.

bilberry

Vaccinium myrtillus, airelle, black whortles, bleaberry, bog bilberries, burren myrtle, dwarf bilberry, dyeberry, European blueberry, huckleberry, hurtleberry, hurts, trackleberry, whortleberry, wineberry

Common trade names
Bilberry, Bilberry Fruit, Bilberry Power, Bilberry Tincture, Dried Bilberry

AVAILABLE FORMS
Available as dried fruit, 10% decoction for topical use, dry extract (25% anthocyanosides) in an 80-mg capsule, and fluidextract 1:1.

ACTIONS & COMPONENTS
The fruit of the bilberry contains 5% to 10% tannins, which act as an astringent; these tannins may help treat diarrhea.

The anthocyanidins in bilberry help prevent angina episodes, reduce capillary fragility, and stabilize tissues that have collagen-like tendons and ligaments. They also inhibit platelet aggregation and thrombus formation by interacting with vascular prostaglandins.

The anthocyanidins also help regenerate rhodopsin, a light-sensitive pigment found on the rods of the retina, so bilberry may help treat degenerative retinal conditions, macular degeneration, poor night vision, glaucoma, and cataracts.

Bilberry may have vasoprotective, antiedemic, and hepatoprotective properties because of its antioxidant effects from anthocyanidins. The anthocyanidin pigment in the herb may increase the gastric mucosal release of prostaglandin E_2, accounting for the antiulcerative and gastroprotective effects.

USES
Used to treat acute diarrhea and mild inflammation of the mucous membranes of the mouth and throat. Used to provide symptomatic relief from vascular disorders (including capillary weakness, venous insufficiency, and hemorrhoids) and to prevent macular de-

---

Bold italic type indicates that reaction may be life-threatening.

generation. Also used for its potential ability to protect the liver.

DOSAGE & ADMINISTRATION
Dried fruit: 4 to 8 g P.O. with water several times daily.
Fluidextract: 2 to 4 ml P.O. t.i.d.
For eye disorders: 80 to 160 mg dry extract (25% anthocyanosides) P.O. t.i.d.
For inflammation: 10% decoction. Prepared by boiling 5 to 10 g of crushed dried fruit in 5 ounces of cold water for 10 minutes and then straining while hot. Applied topically as an astringent.
For treatment of acute diarrhea: 20 to 60 g of dried fruit P.O. daily.

ADVERSE REACTIONS
None known.

INTERACTIONS
Herb-drug. *Warfarin:* May cause additive effects. Monitor patient for bleeding or loss of therapeutic anticoagulation.

EFFECTS ON LAB TEST RESULTS
• May decrease glucose level.

CAUTIONS
The herb is unsuitable in patients with a bleeding disorder because it may inhibit platelet aggregation.

NURSING CONSIDERATIONS
• Explore patient's knowledge of this herb.
• Because bilberry may reduce a diabetic patient's glucose level, dosage of conventional antidiabetics may need to be adjusted if patient is also using this herb.

• Consistent dosing of bilberry is needed when using the herb to treat vascular or ocular conditions.
• Bilberry should be safe for pregnant and breast-feeding patients to use.
• Bilberry may be taken without regard to food.

PATIENT TEACHING
• Advise patient to consult a health care provider before using an herbal preparation because another treatment may be available.
• Tell patient that when filling a new prescription he should inform pharmacist of any herbal or dietary supplement he's taking.
• Tell patient that bilberry may be taken without regard to food.
• Advise any patient using the dried fruit to take each dose with a full glass of water.
• If patient is using bilberry to treat diarrhea, advise him to consult a health care provider if the condition doesn't improve in 3 to 4 days.

birch

Betula lenta, betula

Common trade names
Birch, Birch Leaf, Birch Tea

AVAILABLE FORMS
Available as dried leaves for tea, freshly pressed plant juices for internal use, and ointment and birch tar for topical use.

ACTIONS & COMPONENTS
Birch leaves are collected in spring and dried at room temperature in the shade. The leaves contain tannin and gaultherine oil which,

when mixed with water, yields methyl salicylate. Other components of the leaves are triterpene alcohol, flavonoids (1.5%), proanthocyanidins, and caffeic acid derivatives. These substances have a diuretic effect.

USES
Used as a gentle stimulant and astringent. Warm water infusion is used to stimulate diaphoresis, to flush out kidney stones, and to treat diarrhea, dysentery, cholera infantum, and UTIs.

Applied topically, birch may temporarily relieve rheumatic pain because of its methyl salicylate content. Infusion is used to treat dandruff. Birch tar oil, or pix betulina, is used to treat scabies and skin infections.

DOSAGE & ADMINISTRATION
Dried herb: Average daily dose is 2 to 3 g several times a day.
Infusion: Taken between meals t.i.d. or q.i.d.
Tea: Prepared from dry leaves or fresh plant juice and used internally as is, or used to make an infusion that is taken internally.

ADVERSE REACTIONS
Skin: irritation from topical use.

INTERACTIONS
Herb-drug. *Diuretics:* Birch leaf may increase sodium retention and interfere with diuretic therapy. Monitor patient.

EFFECTS ON LAB TEST RESULTS
• May increase sodium level.

CAUTIONS
Patients who are dehydrated or allergic to birch trees should avoid use. Patients with compromised cardiac or renal function shouldn't use birch to treat edema.

NURSING CONSIDERATIONS
• Explore patient's knowledge of this herb.
• Make sure any patient taking the herb orally drinks plenty of fluids because birch has a diaphoretic effect.
• Birch ointment and oil could be lethal if used internally.
• Birch tar is a toxic substance that kills scabies. It shouldn't be overused because of the risk of systemic absorption.

PATIENT TEACHING
• Advise patient to consult a health care provider before using an herbal preparation because another treatment may be available.
• Tell patient that when filling a new prescription he should inform pharmacist of any herbal or dietary supplement he's taking.
• Advise patient not to exceed the average daily dose without consulting a health care provider.
• Advise patient to drink plenty of fluids if taking birch orally.
• Advise patient to consult with a health care provider if the condition doesn't improve in a few days.
• Instruct patient to discontinue use if the skin becomes irritated.

Bold italic type indicates that reaction may be life-threatening.

bistort

Persicaria bistorta, adderwort, dragonwort, Easter giant, Easter mangiant, oderwort, osterick, patience dock, snakeweed, sweet dock

Common trade names
None known

AVAILABLE FORMS
Available as a powder, which is used to make an extract, infusion, ointment, or tincture for external use.

ACTIONS & COMPONENTS
The powder is made from the leaves and rhizome of older plants; the parts are harvested, cleaned, freed from green parts, cut up, and dried in the sun.

Bistort contains 13% to 36% tannins, which give the herb the astringent effects that are helpful in treating diarrhea and sore or dry throat.

USES
Used to treat digestive disorders, particularly diarrhea. Used as a gargle for mouth and throat infections and as an ointment for minor wounds.

DOSAGE & ADMINISTRATION
Tincture: 10 to 40 gtt diluted in a small amount of water and used as a gargle.
To treat minor mouth and throat irritations or infections: An infusion is made with cold water and used as a gargle or a rinse.

ADVERSE REACTIONS
None reported.

INTERACTIONS
Herb-drug. *Disulfiram, metronidazole:* Tincture contains alcohol and may trigger a disulfiram or disulfiram-like reaction, including flushing, dyspnea, vomiting, syncope, and confusion. Discourage use together.

EFFECTS ON LAB TEST RESULTS
None reported.

CAUTIONS
Pregnant and breast-feeding patients should avoid the herb.

NURSING CONSIDERATIONS
• Explore patient's knowledge of this herb.
• Bistort is rarely used, and dosage information for internal use is lacking.
• Because of the tannin content, overuse may increase mucus formation and irritate the intestines.

PATIENT TEACHING
• Advise patient to consult a health care provider before using an herbal preparation because another treatment may be available.
• Tell patient that when filling a new prescription he should inform pharmacist of any herbal or dietary supplement he's taking.
• If patient is pregnant or breast-feeding, advise her not to use bistort.
• Warn patient that this herb is rarely used and that few dosage guidelines exist.
• Because of bistort's high tannin content, tell patient to separate the

*Liquid contains alcohol.

use of bistort and drug by the longest appropriate period of time.
● Instruct patient to keep herb away from children and pets.

bitter melon

Momordica charantia, art pumpkin, balsam apple, balsam pear, bitter cucumber, bitter gourd, carilla cundeamor, cerasee, karela

Common trade names
Bitter Melon, Bitter Melon Extract, Bitter Melon Juice, Bitter Melon Power

AVAILABLE FORMS
Available as juice or as an extract in gel caps.

ACTIONS & COMPONENTS
The hypoglycemic effect of bitter melon is the result of the melon's charantin, polypeptide P, and vicine components. These substances reduce the glucose level and improve glucose tolerance. The seeds of the bitter melon contain alpha-momorcharin and beta-momorcharin, which are abortifacients.

Bitter melon may have antimicrobial effects and may inhibit viruses, including polio, herpes simplex 1, and HIV. It may also have anti-inflammatory effects and improve GI ailments, such as flatus, ulcers, constipation, and hemorrhoids.

USES
Used to treat diabetes symptoms. May help treat GI disorders.

DOSAGE & ADMINISTRATION
To lower the glucose level: 2 ounces of the fresh juice daily or the equivalent of 15 g of the aqueous extract in gel cap form.

ADVERSE REACTIONS
CNS: headache, ***coma.***
GI: abdominal pain.
GU: uterine bleeding, uterine contractions, abortion.
Hepatic: *hepatotoxicity.*
Metabolic: *hypoglycemia.*
Other: fever.

INTERACTIONS
Herb-drug. *Chlorpropamide, insulin, oral antidiabetics:* May increase hypoglycemic effect and cause rapid drop in glucose level. Monitor patient for signs of hypoglycemia.
Herb-herb. *Stimulant laxative herbs, potassium-depleting herbs.* Increases risk of potassium depletion. Discourage use together.

EFFECTS ON LAB TEST RESULTS
● May decrease glucose level.

CAUTIONS
Parents shouldn't give bitter melon to children because the red arils around the seeds may cause a toxic reaction. Pregnant women should avoid using the herb because it may cause uterine bleeding or miscarriage.

NURSING CONSIDERATIONS
● Explore patient's knowledge of this herb.
● The juice of bitter melon has a bitter taste.

Bold italic type indicates that reaction may be life-threatening.

• Bitter melon should be taken only in small doses, for no longer than 4 weeks.

• The hypoglycemic effects of bitter melon are dose related, so dosage should be adjusted gradually.

⚡ALERT: Bitter melon seeds contain vicine, which may cause an acute condition characterized by headache, fever, abdominal pain, and coma.

PATIENT TEACHING

• Advise patient to consult a health care provider before using an herbal preparation because another treatment may be available.

• Tell patient that when filling a new prescription he should inform pharmacist of any herbal or dietary supplement he's taking.

• Inform pregnant or breast-feeding patients not to use bitter melon.

• Advise patient to keep doses low and not to take bitter melon for longer than 4 weeks.

• Inform diabetic patient that herb may cause low blood glucose levels.

⚡ALERT: Advise patient to store herb out of reach of children and pets because it can have toxic effects, including death.

• Instruct patient to immediately report headache, fever, and abdominal pain.

bitter orange

Citrus aurantium, bigarade orange, corteza de naranja amarga, neroli, orange, pomeranzenschale, zhi shi

Common trade names
Bitter Orange Extract, Bitter Orange Peel, Oil of Bitter Orange

AVAILABLE FORMS
Available as a crude, dry orange peel for use in tea and traditional Chinese medicine, capsules and tablets in weight-loss preparations, essential oil, and extracts for topical use.

ACTIONS & COMPONENTS
An aromatic bitter with a spicy aroma and taste that consists of the dry outer peel of both ripe and unripe fruits of *C. aurantium,* minus the white, spongy parenchyma. Contains the flavanone glycosides naringin and neohesperidin, which are responsible for the bitter flavor. The volatile oils limonene, jasmone, linalyl acetate, geranyl acetate, and citronellyl acetate contribute to the aroma.

A bitter orange aqueous extract may have vasoactive effects. Topical bitter orange has antifungal effects and may be useful as an antiseptic.

The plant that bitter orange comes from contains synephrine and other sympathomimetics that cause CNS stimulation, insomnia, hypertension, and tachycardia. Bitter orange may also have these effects.

*Liquid contains alcohol.

USES
Used to stimulate appetite, aid digestion, and relieve bloating. Used as an antifungal and as a gargle for sore throat. May also help patients lose weight.

In traditional Chinese medicine, it's used to treat prolapsed uterus, prolapsed anus or rectum, dysentery, abdominal pain, and other GI conditions.

It is also used to improve the taste and smell of herbal teas, and is often added to sedative teas containing valerian or balm leaves.

It also may be used to treat sleep disorders, high blood pressure, and regulation of lipid levels and glucose in diabetic patients.

DOSAGE & ADMINISTRATION
Extract: 1 to 2 g P.O. daily
Herb: 4 to 6 g P.O. daily
Tea: Prepared by steeping peel in 5 ounces of boiling water for 10 to 15 minutes and then straining.
Tincture: 2 to 3 g P.O. daily

ADVERSE REACTIONS
Skin: photosensitivity, erythema, blisters, pustules, dermatoses leading to scab formation, pigment spots.

INTERACTIONS
Herb-drug. *Antihypertensives, anxiolytics, sedatives:* May decrease effectiveness. Discourage use together.
Herb-lifestyle. *Sun exposure:* Increases risk of photosensitivity reactions. Advise patient to wear protective clothing and sunscreen and to limit exposure to direct sunlight.

EFFECTS ON LAB TEST RESULTS
• May decrease glucose level.

CAUTIONS
Pregnant and breast-feeding patients should avoid this herb because the effects are unknown. Patients with stomach or intestinal ulcers should avoid bitter orange because of its toxic effect on the GI tract.

Patients with CV disease, anxiety, or insomnia should use bitter orange cautiously.

Parents shouldn't give bitter orange to children because large amounts can cause intestinal colic, seizures, and death.

NURSING CONSIDERATIONS
• Explore patient's knowledge of this herb.
• Frequent contact with the peel or oil, such as with occupational exposure, can cause erythema, blisters, pustules, dermatoses leading to scab formation, and pigment spots.
• Monitor glucose level in patients with diabetes.
• Monitor blood pressure of patients taking antihypertensives.

PATIENT TEACHING
• Advise patient to consult a health care provider before using an herbal preparation because another treatment may be available.
• Tell patient that when filling a new prescription he should inform pharmacist of any herbal or dietary supplement he's taking.
• Warn patient not to postpone seeking appropriate medical evaluation for indigestion, abdominal pain, or bloating because this could

---

Bold italic type indicates that reaction may be life-threatening.

delay diagnosis of a potentially serious medical condition.

• Advise women not to use bitter orange if they are (or may be) pregnant, breast-feeding, or planning to get pregnant.

• Advise patient to wash hands after handling the dry peel and oil, and to avoid touching the eyes because frequent contact with the skin can cause blistering and irritation.

• Advise patient that bitter orange may be unsafe for children.

• Tell patient to avoid driving or other activities that require alertness until CNS effects are known.

black catechu

Acacia catechu, catechu, cutch, gambier, gambir

Common trade names
Black Catechu, Cutch, Diarcalm, Elixir Bonjean, Enterodyne, Spanish Tummy Mixture

AVAILABLE FORMS
Available as dry powder, extract, lozenge, and tincture*.

ACTIONS & COMPONENTS
Comes from *A. catechu,* a tree native to Burma and India. Dried extract is prepared from the bark and sapwood of the tree and boiled in water; this decoction is then evaporated in syrup, cooled in molds, and broken into pieces. Contains 20% to 35% of catechutannic acid, 2% to 10% of acacatechin, quercetin, and red catechu.

The therapeutic properties of black catechu come from its tannic acid content. Tannic acid is an as-tringent with antisecretory properties.

USES
Used to treat diarrhea and other GI disorders. As a gargle or lozenge, the herb is used for its astringent effects on mucous membranes and to treat sore throat.

Externally, it's incorporated into ointments for boils, ulcers, and skin lesions. At one time tannic acid was widely used to treat burns, but cases of fatal liver toxicity from systemic absorption ended this practice.

DOSAGE & ADMINISTRATION
Dried extract: 0.3 to 2 g P.O. or by infusion, as tea.
Tincture: 2.5 to 5 ml of 1:5 dilution in 45% alcohol.

ADVERSE REACTIONS
GI: nausea, vomiting, abdominal pain.
Hematologic: *hemolytic anemia* caused by catechin content.
Hepatic: *liver damage* caused by tannin content (with excessive ingestion).

INTERACTIONS
Herb-drug. *Cardiac glycosides:* May reduce effectiveness of digoxin. Monitor patient closely.
Disulfiram, metronidazole: Tincture contains alcohol. Discourage use together.
Iron: May interfere with iron absorption. Encourage patient to separate times of use.

*Liquid contains alcohol.

EFFECTS ON LAB TEST RESULTS
• May increase liver function test values. May decrease hemoglobin and hematocrit.

CAUTIONS
Pregnant and breast-feeding patients should avoid use because the effects are unknown. Patients with liver disease should avoid the herb because of its tannin content.

Patients with liver disease or a history of alcoholism should use black catechu cautiously.

NURSING CONSIDERATIONS
• Explore patient's knowledge of this herb.
• Black catechu may exacerbate the intended therapeutic effects of conventional drugs such as antihypertensives.
☑ALERT: Ingesting large amounts of tannic acid can cause nausea, vomiting, abdominal pain, and liver damage. Tannic acid barium enemas and tannic acid burn treatments may cause fatal liver toxicity from systemic absorption. It isn't known how much black catechu is needed to cause these reactions.
• Many tinctures contain between 15% and 90% alcohol and may be unsuitable for children, alcoholic patients, and patients with liver disease.

PATIENT TEACHING
• Advise patient to consult a health care provider before using an herbal preparation because another treatment may be available.
• Tell patient that when filling a new prescription he should inform

pharmacist of any herbal or dietary supplement he's taking.
• Warn patient not to postpone seeking appropriate medical evaluation for symptoms of GI disorders because doing so may delay diagnosis of a potentially serious medical condition.
• Advise patients not to use black catechu if they are pregnant, breast-feeding, or planning pregnancy.
• Advise patient that safe oral dosing information is unknown.
• Instruct patients with a history of alcoholism or liver disease to check label of black catechu products carefully because they may contain alcohol.
• Advise patient not to apply black catechu to burned, damaged, or abraded skin.

black cohosh

Cimicifuga racemosa, baneberry, black snake root, bugbane, bugwort, cimicifuga, rattle root, rattleweed, richweed, squaw root

Common trade names
Black Cohosh Liquid Extract, Black Cohosh Root Powder, One-A-Day Menopause Health Tablets, NuVeg Black Cohosh Root, Remifemin, Wild Countryside Black Cohosh

AVAILABLE FORMS
Available as capsules, liquid extract*, powder, tablets, and tincture*.

ACTIONS & COMPONENTS
Obtained from the fresh or dried rhizome with attached roots of *C. racemosa.* Triterpene glycosides—

Bold italic type indicates that reaction may be life-threatening.

including actein, cimicifugoside, and 27-deoxyactein—may produce the therapeutic effects. Black cohosh also contains salicylic acid.

May affect hormones such as estradiol, luteinizing hormone, follicle-stimulating hormone, and prolactin. However, the herb probably isn't estrogenic.

USES

The German Commission E has approved black cohosh for premenstrual discomfort, dysmenorrhea, and menopausal symptoms of the autonomic nervous system.

Black cohosh (specifically, the Remifemin product) is effective in treating symptoms of menopause, including hot flashes, sweating, sleep disturbances, and anxiety. Because it doesn't affect the vaginal epithelium, black cohosh may be ineffective in treating menopausal vaginal dryness.

May be safe for women with a history of breast cancer and other estrogen-sensitive cancers, although such studies have not been done.

DOSAGE & ADMINISTRATION

Dried root: 0.3 to 2 g t.i.d.
Liquid extract (1:1 in 90% alcohol): 0.3 to 2.0 ml P.O.
Remifemin: 20 mg P.O. b.i.d.
Tincture (1:10 in 60% alcohol): 2 to 4 ml P.O.

ADVERSE REACTIONS

CNS: headache, *seizures.*
GI: GI discomfort.
Other: weight gain.

INTERACTIONS

Herb-drug. *Antihypertensives:* May potentiate effects of antihypertensives, causing hypotension. Discourage use together.
Disulfiram, metronidazole: Tinctures contain alcohol and may cause a disulfiram or disulfiram-like reaction. Discourage use together.
Estrogen replacement therapy: May lead to estrogen excess. Discourage use together.
Ferrous fumarate, ferrous gluconate, ferrous sulfate: Decreases iron absorption. Advise patient to separate uses.
Sedatives: May have additive effects. Discourage use together.
Tamoxifen: May have an antiproliferative effect. Monitor patient.

EFFECTS ON LAB TEST RESULTS

• May decrease luteinizing hormone level.
• May decrease platelet count.

CAUTIONS

Pregnant patients should avoid use because large doses may cause miscarriage or premature birth. Breast-feeding patients should avoid using the herb because its effects aren't understood.

Patients who are sensitive to salicylates—including those with asthma, gout, peripheral vascular disease, diabetes, hemophilia, and kidney and liver disease—should use black cohosh cautiously.

NURSING CONSIDERATIONS

• Explore patient's knowledge of this herb.
• Effective doses are equivalent to 40 mg per day of crude drug.

*Liquid contains alcohol.

• The adverse reactions of and precautions for salicylates may apply to black cohosh.

⚠️**ALERT:** Don't confuse black cohosh with blue or white cohosh.

• Black cohosh has no known benefits for osteoporosis or CV disease.

• Tincture may contain up to 90% alcohol and so may be unsuitable for children, alcoholic patients, and those with liver disease.

• Black cohosh should not be used for more than 6 months.

• Signs and symptoms of overdose include nausea, vomiting, dizziness, nervous system and visual disturbances, slowed pulse rate, and increased perspiration.

PATIENT TEACHING

• Advise patient to consult with his health care provider before using an herbal preparation because a treatment with proven efficacy may be available.

• Tell patient that when filling a new prescription he should inform pharmacist of any herbal or dietary supplement he's taking.

• Advise patient not to use the herb if she is pregnant, breast-feeding, or planning a pregnancy.

• Encourage patient to have a proper medical evaluation before treating symptoms of menopause.

• Inform patient with history of alcoholism or liver disease that tincture contains alcohol.

• Inform patient that he shouldn't use black cohosh for longer than 6 months.

• Advise patient to keep black cohosh away from children and pets.

black haw

Viburnum prunifolium, American sloe, cramp bark, dog rowan tree, European cranberry, guelder rose, high cranberry, King's crown, May rose, red elder, rose elder, silver bells, snowball tree, stagbush, viburnum, water elder, Whitsun bosses, Whitsun rose, wild guelder rose

Common trade names
Black Haw Bark

AVAILABLE FORMS
Available as dried black haw bark and tincture*.

ACTIONS & COMPONENTS
Obtained from the root and stem bark of the plant, which contain scopoletin, tannins, oxalic acid, salicin, and salicylic acid. Scopoletin may be a uterine relaxant.

USES
Used to relieve menstrual cramps. Used as an antidiarrheal, diuretic, antispasmodic, and antasthmatic. Also used to prevent miscarriage.

DOSAGE & ADMINISTRATION
Tea: 2 teaspoons of dried bark boiled and simmered in 1 cup of water for 10 minutes, and then strained, t.i.d.
Tincture: 5 to 10 ml P.O. t.i.d.

ADVERSE REACTIONS
Hepatic: Possible liver damage caused by tannin content (with excessive ingestion).

Bold italic type indicates that reaction may be life-threatening.

INTERACTIONS

Herb-drug. *Anticoagulants such as heparin, low-molecular-weight heparin, and warfarin; antiplatelets such as aspirin, clopidogrel, dipyridamole, NSAIDs, and ticlopidine:* Enhances effects of these drugs. Advise patient to use cautiously.

Digoxin: May reduce effect of digoxin caused by tannin content of herb. Monitor patient.

Disulfiram, metronidazole: Tincture contains alcohol and may cause a disulfiram or disulfiram-like reaction. Discourage use together.

Iron: Decreases absorption. Separate times of use.

Herb-herb. *Feverfew, garlic, ginger, ginkgo, ginseng:* Black haw may have antiplatelet effects, which may interact with anticoagulant or antiplatelet herbs, and produce increased bleeding tendencies. Advise patient to use cautiously.

EFFECTS ON LAB TEST RESULTS

• May increase liver function test values. May decrease platelet count.

CAUTIONS

Pregnant patients shouldn't use black haw without the consent of an obstetrician. Breast-feeding patients should avoid use because the effects aren't known.

Patients with liver disease or history of alcoholism should use herb cautiously. Patients with history of kidney stones should use cautiously because black haw contains oxalic acid.

NURSING CONSIDERATIONS

• Explore patient's knowledge of this herb.

• Tincture may contain up to 90% alcohol and so may be unsuitable for children, alcoholic patients, and those with liver disease.

• Black haw may have antiplatelet effects, which can increase a patient's tendency for bleeding. Monitor patient for bleeding.

• Black haw may increase the intended therapeutic effect of conventional drugs.

PATIENT TEACHING

• Advise patient to consult a health care provider before using an herbal preparation because another treatment may be available.

• Tell patient that when filling a new prescription he should inform pharmacist of any herbal or dietary supplement he's taking.

• Warn patient not to postpone seeking appropriate medical evaluation because doing so may delay diagnosis of a potentially serious medical condition.

• Advise patient with history of kidney stones to consult his health care provider before using black haw.

• Advise pregnant or breast-feeding patient to avoid use of black haw unless directed by her health care provider.

• Inform patient with a history of liver disease or alcoholism to use tincture cautiously because it contains alcohol.

• Tell patient to report unusual bleeding or bruising.

• Instruct patient to keep herb away from children and pets.

---

*Liquid contains alcohol.

black root

Leptandra virginica, beaumont root, Bowman's root, Culveris root, hini, oxadoddy, physic root, tall speedwell, tall veronica, whorlywort

Common trade names
Black Root Tincture, Dried Black Root, Powdered Black Root Bark

AVAILABLE FORMS
Available as dried root, powdered root bark, and tincture*.

ACTIONS & COMPONENTS
Derived from the whole root or root bark, which contains tannic acid, volatile oils, gum, resin, a crystalline principle, a saccharine principle resembling mannite, and a glucoside-resembling senegin. Tannic acid has astringent and antisecretory properties.

USES
The fresh root is used as an emetic. The dried root has a gentler action and is used to treat constipation and liver and gallbladder disease, and to increase bile flow.

Historically, black root was used to treat bilious fever.

DOSAGE & ADMINISTRATION
Powdered root bark: 1 to 4 g P.O.
Tea: Prepared by steeping 1 teaspoon of black root in 1 cup boiling water for 30 minutes, and then straining. Dosage is ⅓ cup before each meal, not to exceed 1 cup of tea per day.
Tincture: 2 to 4 gtt P.O. in water.

ADVERSE REACTIONS
GI: nausea, vomiting, abdominal cramps, excessive diarrhea.
Hepatic: *hepatotoxicity* caused by tannin content (with excessive ingestion).

INTERACTIONS
Herb-drug. *Cardiac glycosides such as digoxin:* May reduce effectiveness of digoxin. Monitor patient closely.
Disulfiram, metronidazole: Herbal products that contain alcohol may cause a disulfiram-like reaction. Discourage use together.
Iron: Decreases absorption. Encourage patient to separate times of use.
Laxatives: May increase the cathartic effects of black root. Hypokalemia also increases the risk of digoxin toxicity. Monitor patient for dehydration and hypokalemia.
Herb-herb. *Herbs with laxative effects such as aloe, blue flag rhizome, butternut, cascara sagrada bark, castor oil, colocynth fruit, manna bark exudate, podophyllum root, rhubarb root, senna, wild cumber fruit, yellow dock root:* Increases cathartic effects of black root. Monitor patient for dehydration and hypokalemia.
Herbs with potassium-wasting effects such as gossypol, horsetail, and licorice: Causes additive effects. Monitor patient for hypokalemia.

EFFECTS ON LAB TEST RESULTS
- May decrease potassium levels.
- May increase liver function test values.

Bold italic type indicates that reaction may be life-threatening.

CAUTIONS

Patients with gallstones or bile duct obstruction should avoid using black root because it may worsen these diseases. Pregnant patients should avoid this herb because the fresh root may induce an abortion or harm the fetus. Breast-feeding patients should avoid this herb because the effects on the infant are unknown.

Patients with GI diseases, such as colitis or irritable bowel syndrome, Crohn's disease, and gallstones, should use this herb cautiously because the cathartic effects of black root may aggravate these conditions. Patients with a history of liver disease or alcoholism should use the herb cautiously because of its tannin content.

NURSING CONSIDERATIONS

• Explore patient's knowledge of this herb.

• A patient using black root should use only the dry root, not the fresh root.

🗹 **ALERT:** Ingesting tannic acid in large amounts can cause nausea, vomiting, abdominal pain, and liver damage. Tannic acid barium enemas and tannic acid burn treatments can cause fatal liver toxicity after systemic absorption. It isn't known how much black root is required to cause these symptoms.

• Monitor patient for excessive diarrhea.

• Many tinctures and extracts contain alcohol and may be unsuitable for children or patients with a history of alcoholism or liver disease.

PATIENT TEACHING

• Advise patient to consult a health care provider before using an herbal preparation because another treatment may be available.

• Tell patient that when filling a new prescription he should inform pharmacist of any herbal or dietary supplement he's taking.

• Warn patient not to postpone seeking appropriate medical evaluation because doing so may delay diagnosis of a potentially serious medical condition.

• Advise patient not to use this herb if she is pregnant, breast-feeding, or planning to get pregnant.

• Caution patient to use only dried, not fresh, black root.

• Advise patient not to drink more than 1 cup of black root tea per day.

• Advise patient to use caution when combining black root with other herbal, OTC, or prescription laxatives.

• Inform patients with a history of alcoholism or liver disease to be aware that some products may contain alcohol.

• Tell patient to take black root and iron at different times.

*Liquid contains alcohol.

blackthorn

Berry: *Prunus spinosa fructus,*
blackthorn fruit, sloe, sloe berry

Flower: *Prunus spinosa flos,*
sloe flower, wild plum flower

Common trade names
None known

AVAILABLE FORMS
Available as dried flowers and
fresh or dried fruit of *P. spinosa,*
juice, marmalade, syrup, tea, and
wine.

ACTIONS & COMPONENTS
The tannins in blackthorn berry
have astringent effects, which help
reduce mucous membrane inflammation. Blackthorn flower contains
cyanogenic glycosides.

USES
Blackthorn berry is added to
mouth rinses and used to treat mild
inflammation of the oral and pharyngeal mucosa.

Blackthorn syrup and wine are
used to purge the bowels and induce sweat; blackthorn marmalade
is used to relieve symptoms of dyspepsia.

Blackthorn flower is used orally
to prevent gastric spasms and to
treat common colds, respiratory
tract disorders, bloating, general
exhaustion, dyspepsia, rashes, skin
impurities, and kidney and bladder
ailments. It's used for its laxative,
diuretic, diaphoretic, and expectorant effects.

Blackthorn flower is also a component of blood-cleansing teas,
which may help purify the blood.

DOSAGE & ADMINISTRATION
Oral berry: Mouth rinse up to
b.i.d. Daily dose is 2 to 4 g.
Oral flower: 1 or 2 cups of tea during the day, or 2 cups in the
evening.
Tea: Both berry and flower teas are
prepared by steeping and stirring 1
or 2 g of blackthorn in 5 ounces of
water for 10 minutes, and then
straining.

ADVERSE REACTIONS
None reported.

INTERACTIONS
Herb-drug. *Digoxin*: May have
additive effects. Avoid using herb
and drug together.
Disulfiram, metronidazole: Herbal
products that contain alcohol may
cause a disulfiram-like reaction.
Discourage use together.
Iron-containing products: Decreases absorption. Patient should separate administration times.

EFFECTS ON LAB TEST RESULTS
• May increase liver function test
values.

CAUTIONS
Pregnant patients should avoid using this herb because its cyanogenic compounds may harm the fetus. Breast-feeding patients also
should avoid using this herb.

Patients with a history of alcoholism or liver disease should use
herb cautiously.

NURSING CONSIDERATIONS
• Explore patient's knowledge of
this herb.
• Blackthorn isn't recommended
for long-term use.

Bold italic type indicates that reaction may be life-threatening.

• Many tinctures and extracts contain alcohol and may be unsuitable for children or patients with a history of alcoholism or liver disease.

• Blackthorn flower could be toxic because it contains cyanogenic glycosides.

• Blackthorn may be stored for up to 1 year, away from light and moisture.

PATIENT TEACHING

• Advise patient to consult a health care provider before using an herbal preparation because another treatment may be available.

• Tell patient that when filling a new prescription he should inform pharmacist of any herbal or dietary supplement he's taking.

• Advise patient not to use blackthorn if she is pregnant or breast-feeding.

• Warn patient that blackthorn is for short-term use only.

• Tell patient to take iron and blackthorn at different times.

• Tell patient that although the safety and effectiveness of the herb are uncertain, use as a coloring agent for tea is regarded as safe.

• Inform patients with a history of alcoholism or liver disease to be aware that some products may contain alcohol.

• Inform patient that blackthorn may be stored for up to 1 year, away from light and moisture.

blessed thistle

Cnicus benedictus, benediktenkraut, cardin, holy thistle, spotted thistle, St. Benedict thistle

Common trade names
Blessed Thistle Combo, Blessed Thistle Herb

AVAILABLE FORMS
Available as capsules, decoction, dried herb, fluidextract*, infusion, oil, tea, and tincture. Extracts appear in "healing" skin lotions, creams, and salves.
Capsules: 325 mg, 340 mg
Dried herb: 1-ounce packets
Tincture: 1-ounce containers

ACTIONS & COMPONENTS
Contains the sesquiterpene lactones cnicin and salonitenolide. Also contains 8% tannins.

The glycoside cnicin is responsible for the herb's bitterness, which stimulates the appetite and aids in digestion by encouraging the secretion of saliva and gastric juices. It also may act directly on the stomach and part of the small intestine.

Blessed thistle stimulates menstruation. It's characterized as a bitter tonic, astringent, diaphoretic, antibacterial, expectorant, antidiarrheal, antihemorrhagic, vulnerary, antipyretic, and galactagogue. The antibacterial properties come from the volatile oil and the cnicin component.

USES
Used orally to treat digestive problems such as liver and gallbladder

*Liquid contains alcohol.

diseases, loss of appetite, indigestion and heartburn, constipation, colic, diarrhea, dyspepsia, and flatulence. May also improve memory, relieve menstrual complaints and amenorrhea, regulate the menstrual cycle, increase perspiration, lower fever, increase lactation, dissolve blood clots, control bleeding, and reduce rheumatic pain. It's also used as an expectorant and antibiotic.

Topically, blessed thistle poultice is used for boils, wounds, ulcers, and hemorrhages.

Blessed thistle is added to alcoholic beverages as a flavoring during manufacturing.

DOSAGE & ADMINISTRATION

Capsules: 2 capsules P.O. t.i.d.
Decoction: 1 cup P.O. 30 minutes before meals. Prepared using 1.5 or 2 g of finely chopped herb in a cup of water.
Extract*: 1.5 to 3 ml t.i.d. (1:1 in 25% alcohol).
Mean daily dose: 4 to 6 g of herb or equivalent preparations.
Tea: 3 cups P.O. daily—that is, 2 g of dried herb added to 1 cup of boiling water and steeped for 10 to 15 minutes.
Tincture: 1 to 2 ml P.O. t.i.d.

ADVERSE REACTIONS

GI: nausea, vomiting, diarrhea.
Hepatic: *liver damage* caused by tannin content (with excessive ingestion).
Skin: contact dermatitis.

INTERACTIONS

Herb-drug. *Antacids, H_2 antagonists, proton pump inhibitors, sucralfate:* Because the herb increases stomach acidity, it may interact with these drugs. Monitor patient closely.
Disulfiram, metronidazole: Herbal products that contain alcohol may cause a disulfiram-like reaction. Discourage use together.
Iron-containing products: Decreases absorption. Advise patient to separate times of use.
Herb-herb. *Echinacea:* May potentiate the antibiotic activity of echinacea. Monitor patient closely.
Herbs from the Compositae *family, such as mugwort and cornflower:* May cause cross-sensitivity. Discourage use together.

EFFECTS ON LAB TEST RESULTS

• May increase liver function test values.

CAUTIONS

Pregnant and breast-feeding patients should avoid using blessed thistle because it may promote menstruation. Patients with acute stomach inflammation, ulcers, or hyperacidity shouldn't use the herb because it stimulates gastric juices.

Patients with a history of contact dermatitis, especially if it's caused by other members of the Compositae family (including ragweed, chrysanthemums, marigolds, and daisies) and those with diabetes, ulcers, acute stomach inflammation, or hyperacidity of the GI tract should use blessed thistle cautiously.

Patients with a history of liver disease or alcoholism should use herb cautiously.

Bold italic type indicates that reaction may be life-threatening.

NURSING CONSIDERATIONS
- Explore patient's knowledge of this herb.
- Infusions of more than 5 g per cup may cause vomiting and diarrhea.
- Blessed thistle may cross-react with mugwort and cornflower.
- Many tinctures and extracts contain alcohol and may be unsuitable for children or patients with a history of alcoholism or liver disease.

 ⚡ALERT: Don't confuse blessed thistle with the closely named milk thistle *(Silybum marianum)*.

PATIENT TEACHING
- Advise patient to consult a health care provider before using an herbal preparation because another treatment may be available.
- Tell patient that when filling a new prescription he should inform pharmacist of any herbal or dietary supplement he's taking.
- Warn patient not to postpone seeking appropriate medical evaluation for indigestion, anorexia, or heartburn because doing so may delay diagnosis of a potentially serious medical condition.
- Advise patients who are pregnant or breast-feeding not to use blessed thistle.
- If patient is taking a drug for ulcers or heartburn, instruct him to contact a health care provider before taking blessed thistle.
- If patient is collecting blessed thistle himself, advise him to wear protective clothing and glasses because the plant can cause inflammation of the skin, eyes, and mucous membranes.
- Advise patient not to add milk or cream to blessed thistle tea; doing

so may mute the gastric acid secretion.
- Inform patients with a history of alcoholism or liver disease to be aware that some products may contain alcohol.

bloodroot

Sanguinaria canadensis, coon root, Indian plant, Indian red plant, paucon, pauson, red Indian paint, red puccoon, red root, sanguinaria, snakebite, sweet slumber, tetterwort

Common trade names
Combination products: *Lexat, Viadent*

AVAILABLE FORMS
Available for external use as decoction, extract*, ointment, powder, and tincture*. Available for internal use as decoction and tincture. Extracts appear in commercial mouthwashes and toothpastes.

ACTIONS & COMPONENTS
Isoquinolone alkaloid components (primarily sanguinarine) have antimicrobial, antiseptic, antiinflammatory, antihistamine, expectorant, antispasmodic, emetic, cathartic, pectoral, and cardiotonic effects.

Sanguinarine converted to a negatively charged iminium ion helps to block plaque from settling on tooth enamel. Antibacterial properties of bloodroot fight organisms responsible for bad breath.

Another alkaloid, cholerythrine, may have some anticarcinogenic effects.

---

*Liquid contains alcohol.

USES
Used as an emetic, cathartic, anti-spasmodic, decongestant, digestive stimulant, laxative, expectorant, dental analgesic, and general tonic. Also used to treat bronchitis, asthma, croup, laryngitis, pharyngitis, congestion, deficient capillary circulation, nasal polyps, rheumatism, warts, ear and nose cancer, fever, sore throat, skin burns, and fungal infections.

Topically, it's used as an irritant and debriding agent.

DOSAGE & ADMINISTRATION
Extract (1:1 in 60% alcohol): 0.06 to 0.3 ml (1 or 2 ml for emetic dose) P.O. t.i.d.
Rhizome: 0.06 to 0.5 g (1 or 2 g for emetic dose) P.O. t.i.d.
Tea: 1 cup P.O. several times a day. Prepared by boiling 1 or 2 tablespoons of chopped rhizome in 17 ounces of water for 15 minutes.
Tincture: 0.3 to 2 ml (2 to 8 ml for emetic dose) P.O. t.i.d. (1:5 in 60% alcohol).
Wine: Prepared by steeping chopped drug in brandy, and then filtering.

ADVERSE REACTIONS
CNS: headache, CNS depression, ataxia, reduced activity, ***coma.***
CV: hypotension.
EENT: eye and mucous membrane irritation.
GI: nausea, vomiting.
Other: ***shock, oral leukoplakia.***

INTERACTIONS
Herb-drug. *Antihypertensives, dopamine, ganglionic or peripheral adrenergic blockers such as tubocurarine and norepinephrine:*
May potentiate the action of these drugs. Advise patient to use cautiously.
CNS depressants: May cause additive effects. Discourage use together.
Corticotropin, corticosteroids: May produce hypokalemia. Monitor potassium level.
Disulfiram, metronidazole: Herbal products that contain alcohol may cause a disulfiram-like reaction. Discourage use together.
Herb-food. *Sanguinarine products containing zinc:* Increases antimicrobial activity of sanguinarine. Discourage use together.
Herb-lifestyle. *Alcohol use:* May increase CNS effects. Discourage use together.

EFFECTS ON LAB TEST RESULTS
None reported.

CAUTIONS
Pregnant and breast-feeding patients and those with infections or inflammatory GI conditions should avoid this herb.

Patients with GI irritation should use bloodroot cautiously because it can irritate the GI tract. Patients with glaucoma should avoid the herb because it can affect glaucoma treatment.
☑**ALERT:** The FDA lists *S. canadensis* in its poisonous plant database.

NURSING CONSIDERATIONS
• Explore patient's knowledge of this herb.
• In most countries, the drug isn't used orally.
☑**ALERT:** Powdered rhizome or juice can destroy live tissue. Large

---

Bold italic type indicates that reaction may be life-threatening.

doses of the internal formulations can be poisonous. The FDA has classified bloodroot as unsafe.

• Oral use can cause CNS depression and narcosis because of bloodroot's relaxant effect on smooth muscle.

• At higher doses, bloodroot produces interactions similar to diuretics and cathartics.

• If patient is taking an antihypertensive, monitor his blood pressure.

• If overdose occurs or if patient ingests a large quantity of bloodroot, perform gastric lavage or induce vomiting and treat other symptoms.

• Many tinctures and extracts contain alcohol and may be unsuitable for children or patients with a history of alcoholism or liver disease.

PATIENT TEACHING

• Advise patient to consult a health care provider before using an herbal preparation because another treatment may be available.

• Tell patient that when filling a new prescription he should inform pharmacist of any herbal or dietary supplement he's taking.

⚠ALERT: Inform patient that bloodroot isn't recommended for oral use and that large doses can be poisonous.

• Advise pregnant patients not to use bloodroot.

• Advise patient to avoid contact with the eyes and mucous membranes because of bloodroot's irritant properties, and to be careful not to inhale the herb during crude herb processing.

• Tell patient that toothpastes and mouthwashes containing bloodroot extracts are unlikely to cause harm if they aren't swallowed.

• Tell patient to avoid alcohol while using bloodroot because the herb may depress the CNS.

• Warn patient that a component of the herb may cause cataracts.

• Inform patients with a history of alcoholism or liver disease to be aware that some products may contain alcohol.

blue cohosh

Caulophyllum thalictroides, beechdrops, blueberry, blueberry root, blue ginseng, papoose root, squawroot, yellow ginseng

Common trade names
Blue Cohosh Root Liquid

AVAILABLE FORMS
Available as capsules, decoction, dried powder, liquid extract*, tablets, tea, and tincture.
Capsules: 500 mg
Liquid extract: 0.5 to 1 ml (1:1 in 70% alcohol)
Tinctures: 1-ounce and 2-ounce containers

ACTIONS & COMPONENTS
Made from the aerial parts of the plant, its roots, and its rhizomes. Pharmacologic effects are attributed to several glycosides and alkaloids, such as caulosaponin and methylcytisine.

Caulosaponin is responsible for the herb's oxytocic effects and its effects on coronary vasculature as well as its ability to stimulate intestinal contractions.

*Liquid contains alcohol.

Methylcytisine produces nicotinic effects—for example, it raises blood pressure and glucose level, stimulates respiration, and causes peristalsis.

USES

Used to treat colic, sore throat, cramps, hiccups, epilepsy, hysterics, UTIs, inflammation of the uterus, asthma, memory problems, high blood pressure, muscle spasms, worm infestation, anxiety, restlessness and pain during pregnancy, and labor pains. Used to stimulate uterine contractions and induce menstruation, and as an antispasmodic, antirheumatic, diaphoretic, expectorant, and laxative.

May also have some antimicrobial activity. Low doses of the extract may interfere with ovulation.

The roasted seeds of the herb are commonly used as a coffee substitute.

DOSAGE & ADMINISTRATION

Dried rhizome or root: 0.3 to 1 g P.O. t.i.d.
Liquid extract (1:1 in 70% alcohol): 0.5 to 1 ml P.O. t.i.d.
Tea: Prepared by steeping the herb in 5 ounces of boiling water, and then straining. Daily dose is t.i.d.

ADVERSE REACTIONS

CV: chest pain, hypertension, vasoconstriction, hypotension.
EENT: mucous membrane irritation.
GI: GI irritation, severe diarrhea, cramping.
Metabolic: hyperglycemia.

INTERACTIONS

Herb-drug. *Aminosalicylic acid, antihistamines, disulfiram, halothane, isoniazid, methylphenidate, phenothiazines, propoxyphene, sulfa drugs, troleandomycin:* May decrease metabolism of blue cohosh. Monitor patient closely.
Antacids, mineral oil: May reduce anthelmintic effect of blue cohosh. Monitor patient closely.
Antianginals, nicotine replacement therapy: Blue cohosh may interact with these drugs. Discourage use together.
Antihypertensives, peripheral adrenergic blockers: Diuretic activity of blue cohosh may potentiate the action of these drugs. Monitor patient closely.
Barbiturates, diazoxide, loxapine, and vitamin B_6: May induce metabolism of blue cohosh. Monitor patient closely.
Clindamycin: May enhance neuromuscular relaxing action of blue cohosh. Monitor patient closely.
Corticosteroids, digoxin, fluroxene, hormonal contraceptives, methadone, metyrapone, phenytoin, tetracyclines: May increase metabolism of these drugs. Monitor patient closely.
Disulfiram, metronidazole: Herbal products that contain alcohol may cause a disulfiram-like reaction. Discourage use together.
Lithium: May reduce renal clearance of lithium. Monitor patient for toxic reaction.
Sparteine: May produce synergistic oxytocic activity when used with blue cohosh. Monitor patient closely.
Vasoconstrictors such as ephedrine, methoxamine, phenylephrine:

Bold italic type indicates that reaction may be life-threatening.

May cause severe hypertension. Discourage use together.

Herb-lifestyle. *Alcohol use:* May induce metabolism of blue cohosh, thus decreasing pharmacologic effects. Discourage use together.

EFFECTS ON LAB TEST RESULTS
• May increase glucose level.

CAUTIONS
Blue cohosh shouldn't be used during labor. Several adverse effects have been reported to the U.S. Food and Drug Association Special Nutritionals Adverse Event Monitoring System, including fetal toxicity, neonatal stroke and aplastic anemia after maternal use of herb during labor, and neonatal acute MI associated with heart failure and shock.

Pregnant patients should avoid use of blue cohosh because it may stimulate menstruation. Cardiac patients and those with GI conditions also should avoid use.

Patients with hypertension or diabetes should use blue cohosh cautiously.

NURSING CONSIDERATIONS
• Explore patient's knowledge of this herb.
• Blue cohosh has held official drug status in the past, and was listed in the USP and the National Formulary; however, because of serious safety concerns, its use isn't recommended.
• The root of this herb can be toxic, and the danger associated with its use seems to outweigh the reported medicinal benefits.
• **ALERT:** Raw blue cohosh berries are poisonous to children.

• Many tinctures and extracts contain alcohol and may be unsuitable for children or patients with a history of alcoholism or liver disease.
• Blue cohosh may increase the intended therapeutic effects of conventional drugs.
• Despite the common last name, blue cohosh isn't related to black cohosh.
• Monitor blood pressure and glucose, BUN, uric acid, and protein-bound iodine levels.
• Signs and symptoms of overdose resemble those of nicotine toxicity. Monitor patient for evidence of these signs and symptoms.
• If overdose occurs, perform gastric lavage or induce vomiting, if needed.

PATIENT TEACHING
• Advise patient to consult a health care provider before using an herbal preparation—especially if patient has diabetes, high blood pressure, or is taking other drugs—because a standard treatment that has been proven effective may be available.
• Tell patient that when filling a new prescription he should inform pharmacist of any herbal or dietary supplement he's taking.
• Warn patient to avoid using blue cohosh during pregnancy, labor, and breast-feeding.
• Inform patients with a history of alcoholism or liver disease to be aware that some products may contain alcohol.

*Liquid contains alcohol.

blue flag

Iris versicolor, dagger flower, daggers, dragon flower, flaggon, flag lily, fleur-de-lis, fliggers, Florentine orris, flower-de-luce, gladyne, iris, Jacob's sword, liver lily, myrtle flower, orris root, poison flag, segg, sheggs, snake lily, water flag, white flag root, wild iris, yellow flag, yellow iris

Common trade names
Irisin

AVAILABLE FORMS
Fluidextract: 0.5 to 1 fluidram
Powdered root: 20 grains
Solid extract: 10 to 15 grains
Tincture: 1 to 3 fluidrams

ACTIONS & COMPONENTS
Blue flag preparations are obtained from the rhizome portion of the plant. Primary components are iridin (a glycoside) and oleoresin. It may also contain salicylic acid and tannins.

Blue flag may stimulate the flow of bile from the gallbladder to the duodenum. It's used as an anti-inflammatory, diuretic, laxative, and sialagogue, as well as a hepatic and dermatologic herb.

USES
Used to purify toxins from the blood. Used to treat heartburn, belching, nausea, and headaches resulting from digestive disorders as well as disorders of the respiratory tract and thyroid gland. Used for its cathartic, emetic, and diuretic effects.

Applied externally on sores and bruises to decrease inflammation.

DOSAGE & ADMINISTRATION
Decoction: 1 cup of preparation P.O. t.i.d. Prepared by placing ½ to 1 teaspoon of dried herb in 1 cup of boiling water and simmering for 10 to 15 minutes.
Solid extracts, powdered root: 10 to 20 grains P.O.
Tincture: 2 to 4 ml P.O. t.i.d.

ADVERSE REACTIONS
CNS: headache.
EENT: lacrimation, eye inflammation, throat irritation.
GI: iridin poisoning, severe nausea and vomiting after consumption of fresh root.
Other: mucous membrane irritation from the furfural component.

INTERACTIONS
Herb-drug. *Anticoagulants:* May potentiate these drugs by reducing absorption of vitamin K from the gut. Monitor patient for bleeding.
Antihypertensives, ganglionic, or peripheral adrenergics: May potentiate the action of these drugs. Monitor patient closely.
Antiplatelet drugs: May increase risk of bleeding. Monitor patient closely.
Aspirin-containing drugs: May cause additive effects or toxicity. Avoid using together.
Beta blockers such as meprobamate, phenobarbital, propranolol, and other sedative hypnotics such as chloral hydrate: May decrease blue flag's anti-inflammatory effects. Monitor patient closely.
Digoxin: May reduce effectiveness of digoxin. Monitor patient closely.

Iron: May interfere with iron absorption. Encourage patient to separate times of use.

Lithium: May reduce renal clearance. Monitor patient for toxic reaction and discourage concomitant use.

Herb-herb. *Stimulant laxative herbs such as aloe, buckthorn fruit and bark, butternut, cascara sagrada bark, castor oil, colocynth fruit pulp, gamboge bark exudate, podophyllum root, rhubarb root, senna leaves and pods, yellow dock root, potassium-wasting herbs such as horsetail plant and licorice rhizome, and wild cucumber fruit:* Blue flag may increase depletion of potassium when used with listed herbs. Monitor patient for hypokalemia.

EFFECTS ON LAB TEST RESULTS
• May increase glucose level.
• May increase liver function test values, PT, and INR.

CAUTIONS
Patients who are pregnant or breast-feeding should avoid this herb.

Patients with infectious or inflammatory conditions of the GI tract should use blue flag cautiously because it can irritate the GI tract. Patients with a history of liver disease or alcoholism should use herb cautiously.

NURSING CONSIDERATIONS
• Explore patient's knowledge of this herb.

 ALERT: The fresh root of blue flag is poisonous, so if patient chooses to use the herb, he should use only small doses of the dried root.

• If patient is also taking digoxin, monitor his blood digoxin levels.
• Monitor blood pressure and glucose, electrolyte, and uric acid levels.
• If patient is also taking an anticoagulant, monitor PT and INR.

PATIENT TEACHING
• Advise patient to consult a health care provider before using an herbal preparation because another treatment may be available.
• Tell patient that when filling a new prescription he should inform pharmacist of any herbal or dietary supplement he's taking.
• Advise patient to avoid taking blue flag internally.
• Advise patient not to use blue flag if she is pregnant or breast-feeding.
• Caution patient that blue flag can cause severe irritation if it touches the eyes, ears, nose, or mouth.

bogbean

Menyanthes trifoliata, bean trefoil, bitterworm, bog hop, bog myrtle, bog nut, brook bean, buck bean, marsh clover, marsh trefoil, moonflower, trefoil, water shamrock, water trefoil

Common trade names
Bogbean Extract, Bogbean Leaf, Bogbean Herb

AVAILABLE FORMS
Available as a fluidextract*, tincture*, tablet, powder, and whole leaf.

---

*Liquid contains alcohol.

ACTIONS & COMPONENTS
Obtained from the dried rhizome of *M. trifoliata*. Main components are a small quantity of volatile oil and the glucoside menyanthin.

Menyanthin is reported to stimulate saliva production and gastric secretion.

USES
Used to treat loss of appetite, dyspepsia, gout, rheumatoid arthritis, osteoarthritis, rheumatism, and skin diseases. Used as a bitter to promote gastric secretion. In large doses, it's also used as an emetic.

DOSAGE & ADMINISTRATION
Infusion: ½ cup P.O., unsweetened, before each meal.
Liquid extract (1:1 in 25% alcohol): 1 or 2 ml P.O. t.i.d.
Tea: Prepared by steeping 1 to 3 g of leaf in boiling water (or in cold water that is rapidly heated) for 5 to 10 minutes; then strain.
Tincture (1:5 in 45% alcohol): 1 to 3 ml P.O. t.i.d.

ADVERSE REACTIONS
CV: *hemolytic anemia.*
GI: stomach upset.

INTERACTIONS
Herb-drug. *Antacids, histamine$_2$ antagonists, proton pump inhibitors, sucralfate:* May negate the effects of these drugs because herb promotes gastric secretion. Discourage use together.
Anticoagulants, antiplatelet drugs: May increase risk of bleeding. Avoid using them together.
Disulfiram, metronidazole: Herbal products that contain alcohol may cause a disulfiram-like reaction. Discourage use together.
Stimulant laxatives: May potentiate effects. Discourage use together.

EFFECTS ON LAB TEST RESULTS
• May decrease hemoglobin and hematocrit.

CAUTIONS
Patients with diarrhea, dysentery, and colitis shouldn't use herb. Pregnant patients shouldn't use herb because it may stimulate menstruation and act as a stimulant laxative. Patients with history of bleeding or anemia should avoid bogbean because of reported hemolytic activity.

NURSING CONSIDERATIONS
• Explore patient's knowledge of this herb.
• Bogbean may alter the intended therapeutic effect of conventional drugs.
• If overdose occurs, induce vomiting.
• Many tinctures and extracts contain alcohol and may be unsuitable for children or patients with a history of alcoholism or liver disease.

PATIENT TEACHING
• Advise patient to consult a health care provider before using an herbal preparation because another treatment may be available.
• Tell patient that when filling a new prescription he should inform pharmacist of any herbal or dietary supplement he's taking.
• Warn patient not to use bogbean to treat symptoms of appetite loss, indigestion, or pain before seeking

---

Bold italic type indicates that reaction may be life-threatening.

medical evaluation because doing so may delay diagnosis of a potentially serious medical condition.
- Educate patient about possible adverse effects that result from overdose, such as vomiting.
- Advise patient with diarrhea, dysentery, or colitis not to use the herb.
- Advise patient to avoid herb during pregnancy or breast-feeding.
- Inform patients with a history of alcoholism or liver disease to be aware that some products may contain alcohol.
- Tell patient to stop taking herb if bleeding or easy bruising occurs.

boldo

Peumus boldus, boldea, boldoa, boldu, boldus

Common trade names
Boldo Extract, Boldo Leaf, Boldo Leaf Powder, Tincture of Boldo

AVAILABLE FORMS
Available as capsules, fluidextract*, tablets, and tincture* of varying potencies.
Capsules: 250 mg, 400 mg; also in combination with other vitamins and herbal preparations

ACTIONS & COMPONENTS
Comes from the dried leaves of *P. boldus.* Contains boldine, an isoquinoline alkaloid of the aporphine type and a volatile oil that contains ascaridiole.

Boldine may be effective as an antispasmodic, choleretic, and diuretic; it may also increase gastric secretions. The pharmacologic effects of the volatile oil are similar

to those of boldine. Ascaridiole is an anthelmintic.

USES
Used to treat liver and gallbladder complaints, loss of appetite, dyspepsia, and mild spastic complaints.

Boldo leaves, which are included in herbal teas for their diuretic and laxative effects, can cause significant diuresis. The oil is used to treat GU inflammation, gout, and rheumatism.

DOSAGE & ADMINISTRATION
Boldo oil: 5 gtt P.O.
Fluidextract (1:1 in 45% alcohol): 0.1 to 0.3 ml P.O. t.i.d.
Pulverized herb for infusions: Average daily dose is 3 g P.O.
Tincture (1:10 in 60% alcohol): 0.5 to 2 ml P.O. t.i.d.

ADVERSE REACTIONS
CNS: exaggerated reflexes, disturbed coordination, *seizures,* paralysis of motor and sensory nerves and muscle fibers.
Respiratory: *respiratory depression.*

INTERACTIONS
Herb-drug. *CNS depressants:* May increase risk for respiratory depression. Avoid using together.
Disulfiram, metronidazole: Herbal products that contain alcohol may cause a disulfiram-like reaction. Discourage use together.
Diuretics: Causes additive effects. Discourage use together.

EFFECTS ON LAB TEST RESULTS
None reported.

*Liquid contains alcohol.

CAUTIONS
Patients should avoid using this herb if they have seizures, respiratory conditions such as asthma and pneumonia, bile duct obstruction, severe liver diseases, or if they are pregnant.

NURSING CONSIDERATIONS
• Explore patient's knowledge of this herb.

⚡ALERT: In large doses, boldo stimulates the CNS, causing exaggerated reflexes, disturbed coordination, and seizures. In large doses, it may also paralyze motor and sensory nerves and muscle fibers, eventually causing death as a result of respiratory depression.

• Ascaridiole is a known toxin, and preparations of the volatile oil or distillates of the leaf should be avoided.

• Patients with gallstones or bile duct obstruction should not use boldo.

• Overdose may lead to respiratory depression; patient may require intubation and respiratory support.

• Many tinctures and extracts contain alcohol and may be unsuitable for children or patients with a history of alcoholism or liver disease.

PATIENT TEACHING
• Advise patient to consult a health care provider before using an herbal preparation because another treatment may be available.

• Tell patient that when filling a new prescription he should inform pharmacist of any herbal or dietary supplement he's taking.

• Discourage use in pregnant patients.

• Inform patients with gallstones to consult a health care provider before using boldo.

• Advise patient to avoid preparations with the volatile oil of boldo because of the toxic effects of ascaridiole.

• Inform patient that preparations with virtually no ascaridiole are available.

• Inform patient not to delay seeking medical intervention if symptoms persist after taking this herb.

• Caution patient that overdose may lead to neurologic and respiratory symptoms that, if severe enough, may cause death.

• Inform patients with a history of alcoholism or liver disease to be aware that some products may contain alcohol.

boneset

Eupatorium perfoliatum, agueweed, crosswort, eupatorium, feverwort, Indian sage, sweating plant, teasal, thoroughwort, vegetable antimony, wood boneset

Common trade names
Alvita Tea, Boneset Extract, Boneset Herb Organic Alcohol, Boneset Leaf, Boneset Tops

AVAILABLE FORMS
Available as capsules, dried leaf or powder, fluidextract*, tincture*, and tablets.
Capsules: 430 mg

ACTIONS & COMPONENTS
Obtained from the complete aerial part of *E. perfoliatum.* Contains the following components: a glu-

---

Bold italic type indicates that reaction may be life-threatening.

coside (eupatorin), volatile oil, resin, inulin, wax, sterols, triterpenes, and flavonoids. Also contains pyrrolizidine alkaloids, which cause hepatic impairment if consumed over a prolonged period, and tremetol, an unsaturated alcohol that lowers the glucose level.

Boneset acts as a diaphoretic, an antiphlogistic, and a bitter, which stimulates the appetite, aids digestion, and stimulates the body's immune system. Small doses of boneset may have diuretic and laxative effects, whereas large doses may result in vomiting and catharsis.

USES
Used as a tonic to help restore systemic vitality and as a nutritional tonic to rejuvenate the body while recovering from any debilitating condition. Also used to treat colds, catarrh, influenza, rheumatism, most fevers, and inflammation of the nose, throat, or tongue.

DOSAGE & ADMINISTRATION
Fluidextract (1:1 in 25% alcohol): 1 to 2 ml P.O. t.i.d.
Infusion: Prepared by steeping 2 teaspoons to 2 tablespoons of crushed dried leaves and flowering tops in 8 to 16 ounces of boiling water. Infusion should be administered t.i.d.
Tincture (1:5 in 45% alcohol): 2 to 3 ml P.O. t.i.d.

ADVERSE REACTIONS
GI: *GI hemorrhage,* diarrhea.
GU: fatty degeneration of the kidneys.
Hepatic: fatty degeneration of the liver, hepatic dysfunction.

Metabolic: *hypoglycemia.*
Skin: contact dermatitis.

INTERACTIONS
Herb-drug. *Disulfiram, metronidazole:* Herbal products that contain alcohol may cause a disulfiram-like reaction. Discourage use together.
Insulin, oral antidiabetics: Increases risk of hypoglycemia. Monitor glucose level.

EFFECTS ON LAB TEST RESULTS
• May decrease glucose level.
• May increase liver function test values.

CAUTIONS
Patients should avoid long-term use of boneset. Patients with liver disease and pregnant or breast-feeding patients should avoid use.

NURSING CONSIDERATIONS
• Explore patient's knowledge of this herb.
• The herb contains pyrrolizidine alkaloids, which are hepatotoxic and hepatocarcinogenic, and so may cause hepatic dysfunction.
• If patient is diabetic and is taking an oral antidiabetic, closely monitor his glucose level.
• Symptoms of overdose include weakness, nausea, lack of appetite, thirst, and constipation. Severe poisoning may result in muscle trembling and loss of motor control, progressing to paralysis and death. For a toxic effect to occur, the cytochrome P-450 system must activate one of the herb's toxic components.
• Many tinctures and extracts contain alcohol and may be unsuitable

---

*Liquid contains alcohol.

for children or patients with a history of alcoholism or liver disease.

PATIENT TEACHING

• Inform patient that the FDA has classified boneset as an "herb of undefined safety." Discourage use.

• Advise patient to consult a health care provider before using an herbal preparation because another treatment may be available.

• Tell patient that when filling a new prescription he should inform pharmacist of any herbal or dietary supplement he's taking.

• Warn patient to seek medical evaluation promptly so as not to delay diagnosis of a potentially serious medical condition.

• Advise pregnant patients not to use boneset.

• Advise diabetic patient who's also taking an antidiabetic to monitor his glucose level closely because the tremetrol component of the herb may lower blood glucose level.

• Inform patients with a history of alcoholism or liver disease to be aware that some products may contain alcohol.

borage

Borago officinalis, beebread, bugloss, burage, burrage, oxtongue, starflower

Common trade names
Borage Bio-EFA Capsules, Borage Extract, Borage Leaf, Borage Leaf Powder, Borage Oil, Borage Oil Softgels, Borage-Power, GLA-320 Borage Capsules, Ultra GLA Capsules

AVAILABLE FORMS
Available as dried leaf or powder, fluidextract, oil, and tablets.
Oil: 90-mg, 240-mg, 300-mg, 500-mg, and 1,000-mg capsules and softgels, in liquid form, and in combination with other vitamins in capsule and powder forms

ACTIONS & COMPONENTS
Oil comes from the fatty oil of the seeds and flower of *B. officinalis.* Borage oil may contain between 17% and 25% gamma-linolenic acid (GLA). GLA has anti-inflammatory effects because of increased production of 15-hydroxy fatty acid and prostaglandin E_1, both metabolites of GLA, and astringent and sequestering effects. GLA is an essential fatty acid.

Leaves are the dried leaves and flower clusters of *B. officinalis.* They're harvested during the flowering period and are artificially dried at 104° F (40° C). They contain pyrrolizidine alkaloids, which are hepatotoxic and hepatocarcinogenic, and so may cause hepatic dysfunction. They also contain tannins, mucilage, malic acid, and potassium nitrate. In small amounts, borage may cause constipation because of its tannin content.

Borage's mucilage component may contribute to its expectorant effect; the malic acid and potassium nitrate components may cause its mild diuretic effect.

USES
Used externally as an astringent, a poultice for inflammation, and a treatment for eczema. The oil is

used as treatment for neurodermatitis and as a GLA supplement.

Used for its sequestering and mucilaginous effects in treating coughs and throat illnesses, as an anti-inflammatory for kidney and bladder disorders, and for rheumatism. It is also used as an analgesic, cardiotonic, sedative, and diaphoretic, to enhance performance, and to treat phlebitis and menopausal complaints.

DOSAGE & ADMINISTRATION
Borage oil: Usually administered in vitamin capsules, 1 g P.O. daily or b.i.d. with meals.
Dried borage leaves: For internal use, 1 ounce of leaves is infused in 16 ounces of boiling water and is taken in doses of one wine glass (60-ml).
Fluidextract: 2 to 4 ml P.O.

ADVERSE REACTIONS
GI: constipation.
Hepatic: *hepatotoxicity.*

INTERACTIONS
Herb-drug. *Anticoagulant, antiplatelet drugs:* Use of oil may increase risk for bleeding. Monitor patient.
Anticonvulsants: May lower the seizure threshold. Discourage use together.

EFFECTS ON LAB TEST RESULTS
• May increase liver function test values, PT, and INR. May alter CBC with differential.

CAUTIONS
Patients should avoid long-term use of borage. Patients with liver disease or seizure disorders and pregnant or breast-feeding patients should avoid use.

NURSING CONSIDERATIONS
• Explore patient's knowledge of this herb.
• Some borage seed oil products *don't* contain the potentially toxic unsaturated pyrrolizidine alkaloids (UPAs). Encourage patient to use these to avoid toxicity. Products that *do* contain UPAs, dosed at 1 or 2 g/day, provide 10 times the recommended dose of UPAs.
• Liver function tests may be needed to help monitor patient for liver toxicity. The potential for liver damage increases with larger doses and longer use.
• If patient has a history of seizures and is taking an anticonvulsant, monitor him for seizure activity because borage may lower the seizure threshold.
• Borage leaves should be protected from light and moisture.

PATIENT TEACHING
• Advise patient to consult a health care provider before using an herbal preparation because another treatment may be available.
• Tell patient that when filling a new prescription he should inform pharmacist of any herbal or dietary supplement he's taking.
• Advise patients who are pregnant or breast-feeding not to use borage.
• Warn patient of the potential for liver problems and cancerous effects of borage plant preparations.
• Advise patient that UPA-free borage oil is usually safe and free

---

*Liquid contains alcohol.

from adverse effects when taken in therapeutic doses.
• Advise patient not to delay seeking medical treatment if symptoms persist after taking borage.
• Advise patient to store dried leaves away from light and moisture.

boswellia

Boswellia carteri

Common trade names
Frankincense, Olibanum

AVAILABLE FORMS
Available as essential oils and tablets.
Tablets: 250 mg

ACTIONS & COMPONENTS
The applicable part of boswellia is the resin. The resin gum is collected by tapping the bark and leaves of *B. carteri* for 3 months, during which time the resin will slightly harden.

Contains about 60% resin components, including alpha- and beta-boswellic acids. In vitro, alpha- and beta-boswellic acids showed antimicrobial activity and inhibited the complementary system. The triterpene and essential oil content (about 20% mucin) makes use in respiratory conditions and wound care plausible.

USES
Traditionally, boswellia is used for colic and flatulence. The oils have been used for centuries in aromatherapy for relaxation and to slow and deepen respiration. The oils were believed to support the respiratory and immune systems during colds, flu, bronchitis, coughs and laryngitis. Other reported uses include as an anti-inflammatory, antiseptic and astringent. Boswellia is commonly used in topical hand creams.

DOSAGE & ADMINISTRATION
There is no consensus on dosage.

ADVERSE REACTIONS
Skin: mild irritation with topical use.

INTERACTIONS
None known.

EFFECTS ON LAB TEST RESULTS
None reported.

CAUTIONS
Pregnant and breast-feeding patients should avoid this herb because of the lack of available data.

Patients with sensitive skin shouldn't use boswellia externally because it may cause mild skin irritation.

NURSING CONSIDERATIONS
• Explore patient's knowledge of this herb.
⚠ **ALERT:** Don't confuse *B. carteri* with *B. serrata*, also called Indian frankincense.

PATIENT TEACHING
• Advise patient to consult a health care provider before using an herbal preparation because another treatment may be available.
• Advise patient to discontinue external use if rash develops.
• Tell patient to dilute the essential oil before use.

Bold italic type indicates that reaction may be life-threatening.

broom

Cytisus scoparius, basam, besenginsterkraut, besom, bizzom, breeam, broom top, browme, brum, ginsterkraut, green broom, hogweed, Irish broom top, Irish tops, sarothamni herb, Scotch broom, Scotch broom top

Common trade names
Broomtops, Scotch Broom

AVAILABLE FORMS
Available as an aqueous essential oil extract, liquid extract*, and tincture*. Also available as root and herb.

ACTIONS & COMPONENTS
Derived from the dried and stripped flowers, the dried aerial parts, and the freshly picked flowers of *C. scoparius.*

The main alkaloid in broom is sparteine, a transparent, oily liquid that is colorless when fresh, turning brown on exposure to air. It has an aniline-like odor and a very bitter taste. It's slightly soluble in water, but readily dissolves in alcohol and ether. Sparteine is a powerful oxytocic once used for inducing uterine contractions. It also has antiarrhythmic and bradycardic effects.

Scoparin, the other principal component, is a glucoside that occurs in pale yellow crystals, is tasteless, and is soluble in alcohol and hot water. It's responsible for broom's diuretic effect.

Broom also contains flavonoids, biogenic amines, isoflavonoids, and other alkaloids.

USES
Aqueous essential oil extracts are used internally. Broom is used to treat hypertension and CV and circulatory disorders, as well as to stabilize circulation and to elevate blood pressure. Used as a cathartic and diuretic and, in large doses, as an emetic.

Also used to treat pathologic edema, cardiac arrhythmia, nervous cardiac complaints, menorrhagia, hemorrhage after birth, uterine contraction stimulant, low blood pressure, bleeding gums, hemophilia, gout, rheumatism, sciatica, gall and kidney stones, splenomegaly, jaundice, snake bites, and bronchial conditions.

Prepared as a cigarette and smoked like marijuana to produce euphoria and relaxation.

DOSAGE & ADMINISTRATION
Infusion: 1 cup fresh infusion P.O. t.i.d.
Liquid extract (1:1 in 25% alcohol): 1 or 2 ml P.O. daily
Tincture (1:5 in 45% alcohol): 0.5 to 2 ml P.O.

ADVERSE REACTIONS
CNS: vertigo, dizziness, headaches, drowsiness.
CV: tachycardia, *arrhythmias.*
EENT: pupil dilation.
GI: nausea, vomiting.
GU: uterine contraction and stimulation.
Respiratory: *decreased respirations, respiratory arrest.*

INTERACTIONS
Herb-drug. *Antihypertensives:* Causes additive effects. Discourage use together.

*Liquid contains alcohol.

Disulfiram, metronidazole: Herbal products prepared with alcohol may cause a disulfiram-like reaction. Discourage use together.

MAO inhibitors: May cause a hypertensive crisis. Discourage use together.

Quinidine, haloperidol: Causes additive effects. Discourage use together.

Herb-lifestyle. *Nicotine, smoking:* Causes additive effects. Discourage smoking while using herb.

EFFECTS ON LAB TEST RESULTS
- May increase creatinine levels.
- May increase liver function test values.

CAUTIONS
Patients taking an MAO inhibitor; those with high blood pressure, kidney or liver disease, or AV block; and those who are pregnant should avoid use.

NURSING CONSIDERATIONS
- Explore patient's knowledge of this herb.
- Monitor blood pressure.
- Broom has the potential for abuse.
- Doses that contain more than 300 mg sparteine, or 30 g of drug, may cause dizziness, headache, palpitations, weakness, sweating, sleepiness, pupil dilation, or ocular palsy.
- If overdose occurs and patient doesn't vomit on his own, perform gastric lavage and administer activated charcoal. Treat spasms with chlorpromazine or diazepam. If patient starts to suffocate, intubation and oxygen respiration may be needed.

- Many tinctures and extracts contain alcohol and may be unsuitable for children or patients with a history of alcoholism or liver disease.

PATIENT TEACHING
- Advise patient to consult a health care provider before using an herbal preparation because another treatment may be available.
- Tell patient that when filling a new prescription he should inform pharmacist of any herbal or dietary supplement he's taking.
- Warn patient not to put off seeking medical evaluation for swelling or heart problems because doing so may delay diagnosis of a potentially serious medical condition.
- Advise patients who are pregnant or taking an MAO inhibitor not to use broom.
- Advise patient that broom should be used only under a health care provider's supervision.
- Inform patients with a history of alcoholism or liver disease to be aware that some products may contain alcohol.

buchu

Barosma (synonym *Agathosma*) *betulina, B. crenulata, B. serratifolia,* bookoo, bucco, bucku, buku, long buchu, round buchu, short buchu

Common trade names
Buchu Leaf Bulk

AVAILABLE FORMS
Available as capsules, extract*, herbal tea, tablets, and tincture*. Also found in commercial herbal blends used for diuresis.

Bold italic type indicates that reaction may be life-threatening.

ACTIONS & COMPONENTS

Consists of the dried leaves of *B. betulina*, *B. crenulata*, and *B. serratifolia*. Contains flavonoids, resin, and mucilage, and volatile oil that is made up of more than 100 identified compounds. The principal component in the distilled oil is diosphenol, which crystallizes at room temperature (buchu camphor). Other major components of the oil include pulegone, limonene, and menthone.

Buchu is reported to have urinary antiseptic, antibacterial, diuretic, anti-inflammatory, and carminative properties. Diosphenol is thought to exert an antibacterial effect, similar to that of bearberry leaves. Like bearberry, this phenol is excreted as a glucuronic acid conjugate, which may account for similar antibacterial properties. Volatile oil and flavonoid components may be responsible for the anti-inflammatory effects.

Weak diuretic activity similar to coffee or tea may come from the flavonoids, diosphenol and terpinen-4-ol present in buchu leaf. Terpinen-4-ol increases glomerular filtration rate and may irritate the kidneys.

Pulegone is a hepatotoxin and an abortifacient that stimulates uterine contractions and may cause increased menstrual flow.

USES

Used since the 16th century in Europe and popular among advocates of herbs, particularly in South Africa. However, German Commission E lists buchu as an unapproved herb whose effectiveness isn't documented.

Used to treat mild inflammation and infection of the kidneys and urinary tract in those with cystitis, urethritis, prostatitis, and venereal disease. Used to treat bladder irritation, gout, stomachache, and constipation. Also used as a mild diuretic, antiseptic, tonic, and stimulant.

A douche prepared from an infusion of the leaves is used to treat yeast infections and leukorrhea.

DOSAGE & ADMINISTRATION

Fluidextract: 0.3 to 1.2 ml P.O. t.i.d.
For diuresis: Tea is prepared by steeping 1 g of herb in boiled water, covered, for 10 minutes, and then straining. Taken P.O. several times a day.
Oral use: Daily dosage is 1 or 2 g.
Tincture: 2 to 4 ml P.O., up to t.i.d.

ADVERSE REACTIONS

GI: stomach or bowel irritation.
GU: kidney irritation, increased menstrual flow.

INTERACTIONS

Herb-drug. *Anticoagulants:* May enhance the effects of anticoagulants. Monitor patient for bleeding.
Disulfiram: Herbal products prepared with alcohol may cause a disulfiram-like reaction. Discourage use together.

EFFECTS ON LAB TEST RESULTS

• May increase AST and ALT levels.
• May increase PT, INR, and PTT.

CAUTIONS

Pregnant patients and those planning pregnancy should avoid use

*Liquid contains alcohol.

because of buchu's abortifacient effects. Patients with kidney inflammation should avoid use.

Patients with liver disease should use buchu cautiously because it may cause liver toxicity.

NURSING CONSIDERATIONS
• Explore patient's knowledge of this herb.
• Ingesting large amounts of buchu or its oil can irritate the GI tract and kidneys.
• Buchu may alter the intended therapeutic effect of conventional drugs.
• If patient is taking an anticoagulant, consider monitoring INR, PT, PTT, liver function, and menstruation.

PATIENT TEACHING
• Advise patient to consult a health care provider before using an herbal preparation because another treatment may be available.
• Tell patient that when filling a new prescription he should inform pharmacist of any herbal or dietary supplement he's taking.
• Warn patient not to put off seeking medical evaluation because doing so may delay diagnosis of a potentially serious medical condition.
• Advise patient not to use buchu if she is pregnant or is planning pregnancy.
• If patient is taking a blood thinner such as warfarin, advise him to tell a health care provider that he is using buchu because the herb can enhance the effects of such drugs.
• Advise patient to alert her health care provider if she experiences profuse menstrual flow or kidney, stomach, or bowel irritation after using buchu.

buckthorn

Rhamnus catharticus, R. frangula, alder buckthorn, alder dogwood, arrow wood, black alder bark, black dogwood, buckthorn bark, dogwood, frangula, frangula bark, glossy buckthorn, hartshorn, highwaythorn, purging buckthorn, ramsthorn, waythorn

Common trade names
None known

AVAILABLE FORMS
Available as capsules, liquid formulations, and tablets. It's also an ingredient in various teas.

ACTIONS & COMPONENTS
Dried bark comes from the stems and branches of the *R. frangula* tree, which is imported from the Commonwealth of Independent States (formerly USSR), the Federal Republic of Yugoslavia, and Poland. Contains anthranoids and 3% to 9% anthraquinone glycosides, which include glucofrangulin A and B and frangulin A and B, which have a laxative effect.

The fresh bark contains the reduced forms of anthrones and anthrone glycosides, which have an emetic component. Use of the untreated fresh herb can irritate the stomach mucosa, causing severe vomiting, colic, and bloody diarrhea.

Buckthorn's stimulant and irritant laxative effect on the large intestine is similar to, yet milder

---

Bold italic type indicates that reaction may be life-threatening.

than, that of cascara sagrada. It has weaker antiabsorptive and hydragogic properties. The herb takes effect 6 to 8 hours after it has been administered. Unlike bulk-forming laxatives, stimulant laxatives act directly on the intestinal mucosa and commonly result in gripping and loose stools.

Anthraquinones stimulate active chloride secretion and increase the amount of water and electrolytes discharged into the large intestine and passed in stool. The motility of the colon is increased, as stationary and stimulating propulsive contractions are inhibited, which results in faster bowel movements.

USES
Used orally to treat cancer. Used as a laxative to treat constipation and to ease bowel evacuation in those who have anal fissures or hemorrhoids and in those who have had rectal-anal surgery. Also used as a tonic.

Extracts of buckthorn bark are used topically in sunscreen products.

DOSAGE & ADMINISTRATION
Daily dose: The daily dose of buckthorn bark is based on the quantity of its key component (anthranoid), not on the quantity of dry herb. The average daily dose based on its hydroxyanthracine content is 20 to 180 mg; however, some sources list the daily dose as 20 to 30 mg of hydroxyanthracine derivative, calculated as glucofrangulin A.
Tea, infusion: Prepared by pouring boiling water over 2 g of finely ground herb and straining after 10 to 15 minutes. A cold infusion can be prepared by letting the herb steep for 12 hours at room temperature. (1 teaspoon equals about 2.4 g; 1 scant teaspoon is about 2 g.)

ADVERSE REACTIONS
GI: GI cramping or gripping.
GU: dark yellow or red urine.

INTERACTIONS
Herb-drug. *Antiarrhythmics:* Overuse or abuse may interfere with the effects of antiarrhythmics because of potassium loss. With extended use of both, monitor potassium level.
Cardiac glycosides such as digoxin: Overuse or abuse may potentiate the adverse effects of cardiac glycosides because of potassium loss. With extended use of both, monitor potassium level.
Corticosteroids: Increases risk of hypokalemia, which may cause arrhythmias. With extended use of both, monitor potassium level.
Thiazide diuretics such as furosemide: Increases risk of hypokalemia, which may cause arrhythmias. With extended use of both, monitor potassium level.
Herb-herb. *Licorice:* May increase the risk of hypokalemia. With extended use of both, monitor potassium level.
Potassium-wasting herbs such as horsetail herb, stimulant laxative herbs such as aloe, black root, blue flag rhizome, butternut bark, cascara sagrada bark, castor oil, colocynth fruit pulp, gamboge bark exudate, jalap root, manna bark exudate, podophyllum root, rhubarb root, senna leaves and

---

*Liquid contains alcohol.

pods, wild cucumber fruit (Ecballium elaterium)*, and yellow dock root:* May increase the risk of hypokalemia. With extended use of both, monitor potassium level.

EFFECTS ON LAB TEST RESULTS
• May decrease potassium level.

CAUTIONS
Patients with intestinal obstruction, abdominal pain of unknown origin, or acute inflammatory intestinal disease including appendicitis, colitis, Crohn's disease, and irritable bowel syndrome should avoid use. Pregnant and breast-feeding patients and children younger than age 12 should avoid use.

Patients with fluid or electrolyte imbalances should use buckthorn cautiously because long-term use or abuse can cause hypokalemia and loss of fluid.

NURSING CONSIDERATIONS
• Explore patient's knowledge of this herb.
• If buckthorn is being used as a laxative, advise patient to use the smallest dose required to produce a soft stool.
• Buckthorn may alter the intended therapeutic effect of conventional drugs.
• Advise patient not to exceed the recommended dose or to use buckthorn for longer than 2 weeks.
• Because buckthorn takes effect 6 to 8 hours after it's used, it isn't suitable for rapid emptying of the bowels.
• Patient can decrease the adverse GI effects of buckthorn by reducing the dosage.

• If patient experiences diarrhea or watery stools, he should stop using buckthorn.
• Long-term use of buckthorn can cause loss of fluid and electrolytes, especially potassium, and eventual hyperaldosteronism. Consequences of chronic hypokalemia include aggravated constipation, accelerated bone deterioration, nephropathies, albuminuria, hematuria, damage to the renal tubules, heart function disorders, and muscular weakness, especially when patient is also taking a cardiac glycoside or a diuretic.
• Buckthorn may cause pigment changes in the intestinal mucosa that may be precancerous.
• It's unknown if the anthranoid level in buckthorn is high enough to cause diarrhea in breast-feeding infants.
⚡ **ALERT:** Don't confuse buckthorn bark with buckthorn berry (*R. cathartica*), which is also an anthranoid laxative used for constipation.
• Signs and symptoms of overdose include vomiting and severe GI spasms.

PATIENT TEACHING
• Advise patient to consult a health care provider before using an herbal preparation because another treatment may be available.
• Tell patient that when filling a new prescription he should inform pharmacist of any herbal or dietary supplement he's taking.
• Warn patient not to postpone seeking medical evaluation because doing so may delay diagnosis of a potentially serious medical condition.

Bold italic type indicates that reaction may be life-threatening.

- Advise patient not to use buckthorn if she is pregnant, breastfeeding, or planning pregnancy, or has abdominal pain or diarrhea.
- Advise patient not to use buckthorn for longer than 2 weeks without consulting a health care provider because overuse can lead to severe electrolyte imbalances and intestinal sluggishness.
- Suggest that the patient try lifestyle changes to restore normal bowel function—such as increasing dietary fiber and fluid intake and increasing exercise—or even a bulk laxative as opposed to using buckthorn.
- Tell patient to report planned or suspected pregnancy to a health care provider.
- Warn patient not to exceed the recommended dose and to discontinue use if he develops diarrhea or watery stools.
- Inform patient that many so-called dieter's teas contain buckthorn.
- Advise patient that herb may change urine color to dark yellow or red.

bugleweed

Lycopus europaeus, L. virginicus, archangel, green ashangee, gypsy weed, gypsywort, Paul's betony, sweet bugle, water bugle, water hoarhound, water horehound, wolf's foot, wolfstrappkraut

Common trade names
Bugleweed Herb Vcaps

AVAILABLE FORMS
Available as capsules, freshly pressed juice, powdered herb, tea, water-ethanol extract, and other galenic preparations for internal use.
Capsules: 350 mg

ACTIONS & COMPONENTS
Consists of the fresh or dried leaves and tops of *L. europaeus* or *L. virginicus.* Contains flavonoids and hydrocinnamic and caffeic acid derivatives, including rosmaric acid, lithospermic acid, and their oligomerics, created through oxidation.

Herb may have antithyrotropic activity—specifically, it may inhibit peripheral deiodination of T_4. Herb may also have hypoglycemic and antigonadotropic activity and may also decrease prolactin levels.

USES
Used for mild hyperthyroidism with disturbances of the autonomic nervous system, nervousness, insomnia, premenstrual syndrome, and breast pain.

Tinctures and infusions were once used to decrease bleeding of menorrhagia and nosebleeds.

DOSAGE & ADMINISTRATION
Teas: 1 to 2 g P.O. daily.
Water-ethanol extracts: Equivalent of 20 mg of herb P.O. daily.

ADVERSE REACTIONS
Other: thyroid enlargement, increased prolactin secretion.

INTERACTIONS
Herb-drug. *Insulin, oral antidiabetics:* May increase the risk of

*Liquid contains alcohol.

hypoglycemia. Monitor glucose level.

Iodine: May interfere with metabolism of iodine. Discourage use together.

Thyroid hormones: Reduces effectiveness of thyroid hormones, blocking peripheral conversion of thyroxin to T_3. Discourage use together.

Herb-herb. *Thyroid-suppressing herbs such as balm leaf and wild thyme plant:* May have additive effects. Discourage use together.

EFFECTS ON LAB TEST RESULTS
• May decrease prolactin and glucose levels.

CAUTIONS
Patients with hypothyroidism or thyroid enlargement without functional disturbance, those receiving other thyroid treatments, and pregnant or breast-feeding patients should avoid use.

NURSING CONSIDERATIONS
• Explore patient's knowledge of this herb.
• Because every patient's optimal level of thyroid hormone is different, the dosages provided are only rough estimates. Both age and weight should be considered when determining dose.
• Bugleweed may interfere with control of the glucose level and may cause hypoglycemia. Monitor glucose level if patient has hypoglycemia or diabetes.
• Bugleweed therapy shouldn't be stopped abruptly because sudden withdrawal can lead to increased prolactin secretion or exacerbation of the disorder being treated.

• Bugleweed may interfere with diagnostic procedures using radioisotopes.

PATIENT TEACHING
• Advise patient to consult a health care provider before using an herbal preparation because another treatment may be available.
• Tell patient that when filling a new prescription he should inform pharmacist of any herbal or dietary supplement he's taking.
• Advise patient with hyperthyroidism to consult a health care provider for treatment of condition.
• Advise patients using other thyroid treatments not to use bugleweed.
• If patient is pregnant, breast-feeding, or planning pregnancy, advise her not to use bugleweed unless a health care provider who is an expert in the use of this herb has directed otherwise.
• If patient is diabetic or has low blood glucose levels, advise him to alert a health care provider about taking this herb. Bugleweed may lower blood glucose level.
• Advise patient not to stop taking bugleweed abruptly. It should be discontinued gradually unless a health care provider has directed otherwise.

Bold italic type indicates that reaction may be life-threatening.

burdock

Arctium lappa, bardana, bardane root, beggar's buttons, burr seed, clot-bur, cocklebur, cockle buttons, edible burdock, fox's clote, great burr, happy major, hardock, hareburr, lappa, lappa root, love leaves, personata, philanthropium, thorny burr

Common trade names
Combination products: *Arth Plus Capsules, Burdock Liquid Extract, Catarrh Mixture (oral liquid), Potter's G.B. Tablets and Gerard House Blue Flag Root Compound Tablets, Seven Seas Rheumatic Pain Tablets, Skin Eruptions Mixture (oral liquid), Tabritis Tablets*

AVAILABLE FORMS
Available as capsules, liquid extract*, fresh root, tinctures*, and various topical formulations for cosmetic and toiletry-type products.
Capsules: 460 mg, 475 mg, 500 mg, 625 mg

ACTIONS & COMPONENTS
Consists of the fresh or dried, first-year root of great burdock, *A. lappa;* common burdock, *A. minus;* or woolly burdock, *A. tomentosum.* The leaves and fruits also may be used.

Contains volatile oil, fatty oil, sucrose, resin, tannin, and large amounts of carbohydrates, specifically inulin. Active constituents include podophyllin-type lignan derivatives and guanidinobutyric acid.

The fresh root and root extracts may have mild bacteriostatic and fungistatic activity and also may stimulate the flow of bile from the gallbladder to the duodenum.

Polyacetylenes (specifically, arctiopiricin) may be responsible for the gram-positive and gram-negative antimicrobial properties.

Burdock may have antimutagenic, antitumorigenic, hypoglycemic, and uterine stimulant activity, and it may increase carbohydrate tolerance. The hypoglycemic and antimutagenic component may be a polyanionic, lignan-like compound. It's speculated that guanidinobutyric acid, a substance found in fruit extracts derived from burdock, may be responsible for the hypoglycemic activity.

Burdock may also have antipyretic, diuretic, and diaphoretic properties. It may inhibit HIV-1 infection, antagonize platelet-activating factor, prevent tumors, and affect the digestion of dietary fiber.

USES
Used orally to treat cancers, renal or urinary calculi, GI tract disorders, constipation, catarrh, fever, infection, gout, arthritis, and fluid retention. Also used as a blood purifier, aphrodisiac, and diaphoretic.

Used topically to promote healing and to treat various skin conditions, including hair loss, dandruff, eczema, scaly skin, psoriasis, acne, dry skin, and impure skin.

In traditional Chinese medicine, the fruits are commonly combined with other herbs to treat coughs, sore throat, tonsillitis, colds, sores, and abscesses. In Asia, the root is

*Liquid contains alcohol.

considered nutritious and is part of the diet.

German Commission E doesn't recommend burdock's use because of a lack of data and lists burdock as an unapproved herb.

DOSAGE & ADMINISTRATION
Liquid extract (1:1 in 25% alcohol): 2 to 8 ml P.O. t.i.d.
Oral: 2 to 6 g of dried root P.O. t.i.d.
Tea: Prepared by placing 1 to 2.5 g of finely chopped or coarsely powdered herb into 5 ounces of boiling water for 10 to 15 minutes, and then straining. 1 teaspoon equals 2 g of herb. Tea is consumed t.i.d.
Tincture (1:10 in 45% alcohol): 8 to 12 ml P.O. t.i.d.

ADVERSE REACTIONS
CNS: headache, drowsiness, loss of coordination, slurred speech, incoherent speech, restlessness, hallucinations, hyperactivity, ***seizures,*** disorientation.
CV: flushing.
EENT: blurred vision, dry mouth and nose.
Skin: rash, lack of sweating, allergic dermatitis (topical).
Other: fever.

INTERACTIONS
Herb-drug. *Disulfiram:* Herbal products prepared with alcohol may cause a disulfiram-like reaction. Discourage use together.
Insulin, oral antidiabetics: May interfere with control of glucose level. Monitor patient for hypoglycemia. Drug dosage may need to be adjusted.
Herb-lifestyle. *Alcohol use:* Causes additive effects when used with alcohol-containing products. Discourage use together.

EFFECTS ON LAB TEST RESULTS
• May decrease glucose level.

CAUTIONS
Pregnant patients should avoid this herb because it may cause uterine contractions. Breast-feeding patients should avoid the herb because it isn't known whether burdock appears in breast milk.

Patients allergic to ragweed, chrysanthemums, marigolds, and daisies should use burdock cautiously.

NURSING CONSIDERATIONS
• Explore patient's knowledge of this herb.
• Burdock is native to Europe but is now grown in the United States.
• In the past, burdock capsules, tinctures, and extracts appeared in the official monographs in the National Formulary and USP.
• None of the herb's properties have been proven to exist in the dried commercial product.
• Liquid extract and tincture contain alcohol and may be inappropriate for alcoholic patients or those with liver disease.
• Burdock should only be used when the fresh root or greens are collected by an expert with sufficient botanical knowledge.
• Burdock root closely resembles the toxic *Atropa belladonna,* commonly known as deadly nightshade.
• Burdock may cause or exacerbate hypoglycemia. Monitor patient for hypoglycemia and changes in the glucose level. Dosage of insulin or

---

Bold italic type indicates that reaction may be life-threatening.

antidiabetic may need to be adjusted.

• Adverse reactions are related to atropine poisoning, which can occur if burdock is contaminated with the root of belladonna. Monitor patient for signs of belladonna toxicity.

PATIENT TEACHING

• Advise patient to consult a health care provider before using an herbal preparation because another treatment may be available.

• Tell patient that when filling a new prescription he should inform pharmacist of any herbal or dietary supplement he's taking.

• Warn patient not to put off seeking medical evaluation because doing so may delay treatment of a potentially serious medical condition.

• Advise patient not to use burdock if she is pregnant, breast-feeding, or planning pregnancy.

☑ALERT: Caution patient that burdock can cause poisoning if contaminated with belladonna (atropine, or deadly nightshade). Advise him to immediately report blurred vision, headache, drowsiness, slurred speech, loss of coordination, incoherent speech, restlessness, hallucinations, hyperactivity, seizures, disorientation, flushing, dry mouth or nose, rash, lack of sweating, and fever.

• Instruct patient to report any allergic symptoms to a health care provider.

• Inform patient with diabetes or low blood glucose levels that burdock may lower the glucose level.

• Inform patient that some liquid formulations contain alcohol.

butcher's broom

Ruscus aculeatus, Jew's myrtle, knee holly, kneeholm, pettigree, sweet broom

Common trade names
None known

AVAILABLE FORMS

Available as capsules, extracts, ointments, and suppositories.
Capsules: 75 mg, 100 mg, 370 mg, 470 mg, 475 mg, 675 mg

ACTIONS & COMPONENTS

Consists of the dried rhizome and root of *R. aculeatus,* an evergreen shrub native to the Mediterranean. Contains the steroid saponins ruscin, ruscoside, aglycones, neoruscogenin, and ruscogenin. Also contains benzofuranes including euparone and ruscodibenzofurane.

Ruscogenin and neoruscogenin cause vasoconstriction by directly stimulating postjunctional alpha$_1$ and alpha$_2$ receptors of the smooth-muscle cells in the vascular wall. Two other steroid saponins may have cytostatic activity on a leukemic cell line.

Butcher's broom has diuretic, antipyretic, and anti-inflammatory properties. It may also be effective in treating venous disorders.

USES

Used extensively in Europe to treat circulatory disorders and has gained popularity in the United States.

Used orally to treat conditions of venous insufficiency, such as pain, cramps, heaviness, and itching and swelling in the legs. Used

*Liquid contains alcohol.

to prevent atherosclerosis and to help mend broken bones. Also used as a laxative, a diuretic, and an anti-inflammatory.

Ointments and suppositories are used to relieve itching and burning from hemorrhoids.

In early cultures, the asparagus-like shoots of butcher's broom were eaten as food.

DOSAGE & ADMINISTRATION
Raw extract: 7 to 11 mg P.O. daily based on the total ruscogenin content, determined as the sum of neoruscogenin and ruscogenin components.
Root powder: 100 to 3,000 mg P.O. daily.

ADVERSE REACTIONS
GI: GI discomfort, nausea.

INTERACTIONS
None known.

EFFECTS ON LAB TEST RESULTS
None reported.

CAUTIONS
Pregnant and breast-feeding patients should avoid this herb.

NURSING CONSIDERATIONS
● Explore patient's knowledge of this herb.
⚠ ALERT: Don't confuse butcher's broom with the following herbs: Scotch broom, broom, *Cytisus scoparius* L., or Spanish broom, *Spartium junceum* L.

PATIENT TEACHING
● Advise patient to consult a health care provider before using an herbal preparation because another treatment may be available.
● Tell patient that when filling a new prescription he should inform pharmacist of any herbal or dietary supplement he's taking.
● Warn patient not to put off seeking medical evaluation because doing so may delay treatment of a potentially serious medical condition.
● Advise patients who are pregnant or breast-feeding to avoid use.
● Advise patient not to use with other treatments for circulatory disorders without consulting a health care provider.
● Inform patient that although products containing butcher's broom may claim to be effective for treating circulatory problems of the legs, these products aren't approved by the FDA, and may be ineffective for these conditions.

butterbur

Petasites hybridus, bladderdock, bog rhubarb, bogshorns, butterdock, butterfly dock, capdockin, flapperdock, langwort, petasites, umbrella leaves

Common trade names
Butterbur Herb, Butterbur Root, Petadolex Standardized Extract

AVAILABLE FORMS
Available as capsules, dried herb, and dried root.
Capsules: 50 mg of butterbur root extract (Petadolex)

ACTIONS & COMPONENTS
Derived from the rhizome, rootstock, and leaves of this perennial shrub. Contains sesquiterpene lac-

tones including pestacins, angeli-coyleneopetasol, fukinolide, and fukione. The antispasmodic and analgesic actions may be caused by the effects of pestacins on prostaglandin synthesis. The herb also contains volatile oils, pectin, mucilage, inulin flavonoids, and tannins.

Butterbur contains pyrrizolidine alkaloids, which are carcinogens and hepatotoxins.

USES
Used as an antispasmodic and analgesic. As an antispasmodic, it's used to treat urinary tract spasms, mild kidney stone disease, bile flow obstruction, dysmenorrhea, colic, bronchospasm, and cough.

As an analgesic, it's used for backache and migraine headache.

DOSAGE & ADMINISTRATION
Capsules containing 50 mg of butterbur root extract—Petadolex: 50 mg b.i.d. for migraine headache.
GI disorders: 5 to 7 g of dried herb daily.

ADVERSE REACTIONS
CNS: sedation.
Hepatic: *hepatotoxicity.*
Other: *cancer.*

INTERACTIONS
Herb-drug. *Antihistamines, atropine, phenothiazines, scopolamine, TCAs:* May have added anticholinergic adverse effects. Monitor patient closely.

EFFECTS ON LAB TEST RESULTS
• May increase liver function test values.

CAUTIONS
Pregnant patients, breast-feeding patients, and those with liver disease should avoid this herb because of its pyrrizolidine alkaloid content and antispasmodic effect.

NURSING CONSIDERATIONS
• Explore patient's knowledge of this herb.
• A reduction in migraine severity and frequency has occurred after 4 weeks of treatment.
⚠**ALERT:** Butterbur's pyrrizolidine alkaloids are known hepatotoxins and carcinogens.
• Because the pyrrizolidine alkaloids in butterbur are toxic, patient shouldn't use herb for longer than 4 to 6 weeks annually.
• Monitor liver function test results, as indicated.
• Butterbur may be unsafe for children.

PATIENT TEACHING
• Advise patient to consult a health care provider before using an herbal preparation because another treatment may be available.
• Tell patient that when filling a new prescription he should inform pharmacist of any herbal or dietary supplement he's taking.
• Advise patients who are pregnant, breast-feeding, or planning pregnancy not to use butterbur.
• Warn the patient not to delay treatment for an illness that doesn't get better after taking butterbur.
• Instruct patient to stop using butterbur immediately if he experiences skin discoloration, abdominal pain, nausea, or vomiting.

---

*Liquid contains alcohol.

C

cacao tree

Theobroma cacao, chocolate tree, cocoa bean, kakao, theobroma

Common trade names
Cocoa, Cocoa Butter, Cocoa Powder, Cocoa Seed, Theobroma Oil

AVAILABLE FORMS
Cacao seed is roasted and then pressed to express cocoa butter, also known as theobroma oil. The remaining cocoa cake is ground into cocoa powder. Cocoa, chocolate, and cocoa butter are derived from this plant.

ACTIONS & COMPONENTS
Contains 0.5% to 2.7% theobromine and 0.25% caffeine; also contains other methylxanthine alkaloids. Unsweetened dark chocolate contains 47 mg of caffeine and 450 mg of theobromine per ounce. Milk chocolate contains about 6 mg caffeine and 45 mg of theobromine per ounce.

Theobromine has weaker stimulant effects than caffeine but is a more potent diuretic, CV stimulant, and coronary dilator. Cocoa contains the antioxidant catechin.

USES
Cocoa powder and butter are widely used in food products; cocoa butter is also used as a base for moisturizers, cosmetics, and suppositories.

Cocoa seed and seed coat are used to treat a wide variety of illnesses, such as intestinal conditions; diarrhea; liver, bladder, and renal disease; and diabetes.

DOSAGE & ADMINISTRATION
Dosage varies with the preparation.

ADVERSE REACTIONS
CNS: CNS stimulation, tremor, insomnia.
CV: tachycardia.

INTERACTIONS
Herb-drug. *Acetaminophen, aspirin:* May increase the analgesic effects of these drugs. Monitor patient.
Alendronate: Decreases alendronate bioavailability. Advise patient to separate uses by 2 hours.
Barbiturates: Decreases caffeine effects because of increased metabolism and CNS depression. Monitor patient.
Beta agonists such as albuterol, isoproterenol, terbutaline: Increases CNS and CV stimulation. Monitor patient.
Cimetidine, disulfiram, fluoroquinolones, such as ciprofloxacin, hormonal contraceptives, mexiletine, norfloxacin: Increases caffeine effects resulting from decreased metabolism. Monitor patient closely.
Clozapine: Increases clozapine levels, increasing risk of adverse reactions. Monitor patient closely.

Bold italic type indicates that reaction may be life-threatening.

Iron, zinc: Decreases absorption of vitamins. Advise patient to separate uses by 2 hours.

Lithium: Increases lithium clearance. Monitor lithium levels closely.

MAO inhibitors, such as isocarboxazid, phenelzine, tranylcypromine: Large amounts of caffeine may result in hypertensive crisis. Discourage use of large doses of caffeine.

Phenylpropanolamine: Increases caffeine effect by additive sympathomimetic actions. Reports of manic psychosis with phenylpropanolamine and high caffeine doses. Monitor patient closely; discourage excessive caffeine use.

Theophylline: Decreases theophylline levels with excessive caffeine intake. Monitor theophylline levels; discourage excess caffeine use.

Verapamil: Increases caffeine effects caused by decreased metabolism. Monitor closely.

Herb-herb. *Coffee, cola nut, ephedra, guarana, maté and tea, or ma huang:* May increase stimulant effects of cocoa. Discourage use together.

EFFECTS ON LAB TEST RESULTS
None reported.

CAUTIONS
No studies or reports of women who consumed excessive doses of chocolate during pregnancy are known. Theobromine is teratogenic to animals when given in doses dozens to hundreds of times the equivalent of normal human consumption of chocolate. High dosages of caffeine (that is, more than 300 mg per day) are linked to lower birth weight and higher risk of spontaneous abortion in some studies. Caffeine appears in small amounts in breast milk.

NURSING CONSIDERATIONS
- Explore patient's knowledge of this herb.
- Caffeine may interfere with phenobarbital and uric acid assay.
- Cocoa butter may be allergenic and cause acne.
- Although no chemical interactions are known, the pharmacologic properties of cacao and the potential to exacerbate the intended therapeutic effect of conventional drugs must be considered.
- A link to migraine and tension headache is controversial.
- Use may worsen symptoms of irritable bowel syndrome.
- Chocolate contains relatively low amounts of caffeine compared with other food sources.

PATIENT TEACHING
- Advise patient to consult a health care provider before using an herbal preparation because another treatment may be available.
- Tell patient that when filling a new prescription he should inform pharmacist of any herbal or dietary supplement he's taking.
- Advise pregnant or breast-feeding patients to avoid excessive chocolate consumption.
- Instruct patient to promptly report adverse effects.

---

*Liquid contains alcohol.

• Inform the patient not to delay treatment for an illness that doesn't improve after using this product.

calumba

Jateorhiza palmata, colombo

Common trade names
Calumba Dried Root

AVAILABLE FORMS
Available as the dried root in pieces or powder.

ACTIONS & COMPONENTS
The medicinal components of calumba aren't known.

USES
Used as a bitter tonic to treat GI disorders such as diarrhea, dysentery, flatulence, colic, and GI upset.

DOSAGE & ADMINISTRATION
Not well documented.

ADVERSE REACTIONS
CNS: unconsciousness and paralysis (with very high doses).
GI: vomiting, epigastric pain.

INTERACTIONS
None reported.

EFFECTS ON LAB TEST RESULTS
None reported.

CAUTIONS
Pregnant patients should avoid use because herb's effects on the fetus are unknown.

NURSING CONSIDERATIONS
• Explore patient's knowledge of this herb.
• Very little information is available on calumba.

PATIENT TEACHING
• Advise patient to consult a health care provider before using an herbal preparation because another treatment may be available.
• Tell patient that when filling a new prescription he should inform pharmacist of any herbal or dietary supplement he's taking.
• Warn patient not to treat symptoms of gastric distress with calumba before seeking appropriate medical evaluation because doing so may delay diagnosis of a potentially serious medical condition.
• Inform patient about other herbs and drugs, such as antidiarrheals or antiflatulents, that are more effective in treating GI disorders.
• Discuss dietary habits and fluid intake and their importance for proper bowel function.
• Advise pregnant or breast-feeding patient not to use calumba, and to immediately report planned or suspected pregnancy to her health care provider.
• Tell patient the herb must be kept dry.

Bold italic type indicates that reaction may be life-threatening.

capsicum

Capsicum annuum, C. frutescens, African chilies, bird pepper, capsaicin, cayenne, chili pepper, goat's pod, grains of Paradise, Mexican chilies, red pepper, tabasco pepper, Zanzibar pepper

Common trade names
Topical products: *Capsin (0.025% or 0.075% lotion), Capzasin-P (0.025% cream), Dolorac (0.025% cream in emollient base), No Pain-HP (0.075% roll-on), Pain Doctor (0.025% cream with methyl-salicylate and menthol), Pain-X (0.05% gel), R-Gel (0.025% gel), Zostrix (0.025% cream in emollient base), Zostrix-HP (0.075% cream in emollient base)*
Oral products: *Cajun Seasoning, Capsicool, Cayenne, Cayenne Extra Hot, Cayenne Pepper Capsules, Kidney Blend, Tincture of Capsicum*

AVAILABLE FORMS
Available as cayenne pepper capsules, extract*, and topical preparation.

ACTIONS & COMPONENTS
The active component of capsicum (capsaicin) is isolated from the membrane and seeds of the pepper.

Topically applied capsaicin depletes substance P from peripheral sensory neurons and blocks its synthesis and transport. Substance P is a neurotransmitter involved in transmitting pain and itch sensations from the periphery to the CNS, and may have vasodilating effects. The effects may be similar to cutting or ligating a nerve.

Oral capsicum may interfere with gastric basal acid output and may inhibit platelet aggregation, but it doesn't alter PT or PTT. High-dose capsicum therapy may decrease coagulation (because of higher antithrombin III levels), lower plasma fibrinogen levels, and increase fibrinolytic activity.

Capsaicin also is highly irritating to mucous membranes and eyes.

USES
The FDA has approved topical capsicum for temporary relief from pain caused by rheumatoid arthritis, osteoarthritis, postherpetic neuralgia (shingles), and diabetic neuropathy. The herb is being tested for treatment of psoriasis, intractable pruritus, vitiligo, phantom limb pain, mastectomy pain, Guillain-Barré syndrome, neurogenic bladder, vulvar vestibulitis, apocrine chromhidrosis, and reflex sympathetic dystrophy. It's also used in personal defense sprays.

Oral capsicum is used for various GI complaints, including dyspepsia, flatulence, ulcers, and stomach cramps. It's used to treat hypertension and improve circulation. It's also used in some weight-loss and metabolic-enhancement products.

DOSAGE & ADMINISTRATION
Oral: In adults, up to 3 g P.O. daily, as a spice on food.
Topical: For adults and children age 2 and older, capsicum is applied topically to affected area, not more than t.i.d. or q.i.d. Hands

*Liquid contains alcohol.

should be washed immediately after applying capsicum.

ADVERSE REACTIONS
EENT: eye irritation, corneal abrasion.
GI: oral burning, diarrhea, gingival irritation, bleeding gums.
Respiratory: cough, ***bronchospasm,*** respiratory irritation.
Skin: burning sensation, stinging sensation, erythema, contact dermatitis.

INTERACTIONS
Herb-drug. *ACE inhibitors:* Increases risk of cough when applied topically. Monitor patient closely.
Anticoagulants: May alter anticoagulant effects. Monitor PT and INR closely; advise patient to avoid using herb and drug together.
Antiplatelet drugs, heparin and low-molecular-weight heparin, warfarin: May cause additive effects. Discourage use together. If herb and drug must be used together, monitor patient for bleeding.
Aspirin, salicylic acid compounds: Reduces bioavailability of these drugs. Discourage use together.
Disulfiram: Herbal products prepared with alcohol may cause a disulfiram-like reaction. Discourage use together.
Theophylline: Increases absorption when taken with capsicum. Discourage use together.
Herb-herb. *Feverfew, garlic, ginger, ginkgo, ginseng:* These anticoagulant or antiplatelet herbs may increase the anticoagulant effects of cayenne, thus increasing bleeding tendencies. Discourage use together. If herb and drug must be

used together, monitor patient for bleeding.

EFFECTS ON LAB TEST RESULTS
None reported.

CAUTIONS
Pregnant patients should avoid use because herb's effects on the fetus aren't known. Patients with irritable bowel syndrome shouldn't use herb because of its irritant and peristaltic effects. Breast-feeding patients and those hypersensitive to herb should avoid use.

Patients with asthma who use capsicum may experience bronchospasm.

NURSING CONSIDERATIONS
● Explore patient's knowledge of this herb.
● Alcoholic extracts may be unsuitable for children, alcoholic patients, patients with liver disease, and those taking disulfiram or metronidazole.
● Topical product shouldn't be used on broken or irritated skin or covered with a tight bandage.
● Treat adverse skin reactions to topically applied capsaicin by washing the area thoroughly with soap and water. Soaking the area in vegetable oil after washing provides a slower onset but longer duration of relief than cold water. Vinegar water irrigation is moderately successful. Rubbing alcohol may also help.
● EMLA (a topical emulsion of lidocaine and prilocaine) provides pain relief in about 1 hour to skin that has been severely irritated by capsaicin.

Bold italic type indicates that reaction may be life-threatening.

⚠**ALERT:** Capsicum shouldn't be taken orally for more than 2 days and then shouldn't be used again for 2 weeks.

PATIENT TEACHING
• Advise patient to consult a health care provider before using an herbal preparation because another treatment may be available.
• Tell patient that when filling a new prescription he should inform pharmacist of any herbal or dietary supplement he's taking.
• Advise patient not to take this herb if she is pregnant, breast-feeding, or planning a pregnancy.
• If patient is applying capsicum topically, inform him that it may take 1 to 2 weeks for him to experience maximum pain control.
• If patient is using capsicum topically, instruct him to wash his hands before and immediately after applying it and to avoid contact with eyes. Advise contact lens wearer to wash his hands and to use gloves or an applicator if handling lenses after applying capsicum.
• If patient is using capsicum topically, advise him not to use topical capsicum on broken or irritated skin and instruct him not to tightly bandage any area to which he has applied it.
• Inform patient not to delay treatment for an illness that doesn't improve after taking capsicum. If he is applying it topically, advise him to promptly contact his health care provider if the condition worsens or if symptoms persist for 2 to 4 weeks.

• Tell patient to store capsicum in a tightly sealed container, away from light.

caraway

Carum carvi

Common trade names
Caraway Seed

AVAILABLE FORMS
Available as dried fruit and seed, alcoholic extract*, and tincture*.

ACTIONS & COMPONENTS
Caraway contains a volatile oil that produces a characteristic taste and smell. This oil contains carvole and d-limonene (carvene), which may be active against GI discomfort. Caraway may have weak antispasmodic activity.

USES
Most commonly used as a spice. Also used to treat GI upset, nausea, flatulence, bloating, menstrual discomfort, and incontinence; to promote lactation; and to stimulate appetite.
     Caraway oil is used to make herbal mouthwashes and liqueurs such as Aquavite.

DOSAGE & ADMINISTRATION
Dried fruit: 1.5 to 6 g/day.
Extract: 3 or 4 gtt in liquid t.i.d. to q.i.d.
Seeds: 1 teaspoon chewed t.i.d. to q.i.d.
Tea: Prepared by steeping 1 or 2 teaspoons of freshly crushed fruit in 5 ounces of boiling water for 5 to 10 minutes, and then straining. For adults, 1 cup of tea b.i.d. to

---

*Liquid contains alcohol.

q.i.d. between meals; for children, 1 teaspoon of tea.
Tincture: ½ to 1 teaspoon daily to t.i.d.

ADVERSE REACTIONS
Skin: contact dermatitis.

INTERACTIONS
Herb-drug. *Disulfiram:* Herbal products prepared with alcohol may cause a disulfiram-like reaction. Discourage use together.

EFFECTS ON LAB TEST RESULTS
None reported.

CAUTIONS
Pregnant and breast-feeding patients should avoid using caraway, even in food, because of its antispasmodic effects.

NURSING CONSIDERATIONS
• Explore patient's knowledge of this herb.
• Many tinctures contain between 15% and 90% alcohol and may be unsuitable for children, alcoholic patients, patients with liver disease, and those taking disulfiram or metronidazole.
• Because the active component of caraway isn't water soluble, extracts and tinctures may be more effective than teas.

PATIENT TEACHING
• Advise patient to consult a health care provider before using an herbal preparation because another treatment may be available.
• Tell patient that when filling a new prescription he should inform pharmacist of any herbal or dietary supplement he's taking.

• If patient is pregnant, advise her not to use caraway.
• Inform patient not to delay treatment for an illness that doesn't resolve after taking caraway.
• Instruct patient to promptly report adverse reactions or new signs or symptoms.

cardamom

Elettaria cardamomum, cardamom fruit, cardamom seeds

Common trade names
Cardamom

AVAILABLE FORMS
Available as ground seeds and as a tincture*.

ACTIONS & COMPONENTS
Obtained from the dried, almostripened fruit of *E. cardamomum.* Only the seeds of the fruit and the oils obtained from the seeds are used to prepare supplements.
    The active ingredients of cardamom are believed to be the volatile oils contained within the seeds of the fruit. The volatile oils consist primarily of cineol, alphaterponyl acetate, and linalyl acetate.
    Cardamom also may have antiviral properties.

USES
Used to soothe the stomach and treat dyspepsia. Used for its antispasmodic, antiflatulent, and motility-enhancing effects, making it potentially useful in other GI conditions.

Bold italic type indicates that reaction may be life-threatening.

DOSAGE & ADMINISTRATION
Ground seeds: Average daily dose is 1.5 g.
Tincture: 1 or 2 g/day.

ADVERSE REACTIONS
Hepatic: gallstone colic.

INTERACTIONS
Herb-drug. *Disulfiram:* Herbal products prepared with alcohol may cause a disulfiram-like reaction. Discourage use together.

EFFECTS ON LAB TEST RESULTS
None reported.

CAUTIONS
Patients with gallstones and pregnant and breast-feeding patients should avoid use.

NURSING CONSIDERATIONS
• Explore patient's knowledge of this herb.
• Tinctures may contain a significant amount of alcohol.

PATIENT TEACHING
• Advise patient to consult a health care provider before using an herbal preparation because another treatment may be available.
• Tell patient that when filling a new prescription he should inform pharmacist of any herbal or dietary supplement he's taking.
• Warn patient not to treat symptoms of gastric distress with cardamom before seeking appropriate medical evaluation because doing so may delay diagnosis of a potentially serious medical condition.
• Instruct patient to promptly report adverse reactions and new signs or symptoms.

carline thistle

Carlina acaulis, dwarf carline, ground thistle, southernwood root, stemless carlina root

Common trade names
None known

AVAILABLE FORMS
Obtained from the root of the *C. acaulis* plant, it's used both internally and externally. The dried root is used to prepare tea, wine, and tinctures*.

ACTIONS & COMPONENTS
The medicinal portion of the plant is found in the root. The acetone extract and the essential oils found in the root of carline thistle are believed to possess antibacterial properties that seem to hinder the growth of *Staphylococcus aureus*.

USES
Orally, carline thistle has been used to treat gallbladder disease, digestive problems, and alimentary tract spasms. It may also act as a mild diuretic and cause diaphoresis.

Externally, carline thistle has been used to treat dermatosis, rinse wounds and ulcers and, when used as a gargle, to alleviate symptoms associated with cancer of the tongue.

DOSAGE & ADMINISTRATION
Tea: Prepared by steeping 3 g of finely cut dried root in 5 ounces of boiling water for 5 to 10 minutes, and then straining. Dosage is 3 cups daily.

*Liquid contains alcohol.

Tincture: Prepared by steeping 20 g of chopped root in 80 g of 60% ethanol for 10 days. Dosage is 40 to 50 gtt four to five times daily.

Topical preparation: Prepared by steeping 30 g of dried root in 1 quart of boiling water for 5 to 10 minutes, and then straining.

Wine: Prepared by steeping 50 g of the dried root in 1 quart of white wine for a minimum of 12 days, and then straining. Dosage is one small glass before meals.

ADVERSE REACTIONS
Other: allergic reactions.

INTERACTIONS
Herb-drug. *Disulfiram:* Herbal products prepared with alcohol may cause a disulfiram-like reaction. Discourage use together.

EFFECTS ON LAB TEST RESULTS
None reported.

CAUTIONS
Pregnant and breast-feeding patients should avoid use.

NURSING CONSIDERATIONS
• Explore patient's knowledge of this herb.
• Find out if patient has a history of seasonal allergies. He may be more likely to experience a hypersensitivity reaction.
• Wine and tincture preparations contain significant amounts of alcohol; therefore, these aren't suitable for children, alcoholic patients, and patients with liver disease.

PATIENT TEACHING
• Advise patient to consult a health care provider before using an herbal preparation because another treatment may be available.
• Tell patient that when filling a new prescription he should inform pharmacist of any herbal or dietary supplement he's taking.
• Encourage patient to consider other treatment options because little information about the safety and efficacy of carline thistle exists.
• Advise patient to seek medical attention immediately if he suspects he's having an allergic reaction to the herb.
• Instruct patient to promptly report adverse reactions or new signs and symptoms.

carob

Ceratonia siliqua, locust bean, locust pods, St. John's bread, sugar pods

Common trade names
None known

AVAILABLE FORMS
The fruit and seeds of the *C. siliqua* are used to prepare dry carob extracts.

ACTIONS & COMPONENTS
Believed to act as a dietary binding drug and antidiarrheal; the exact mechanism of action is unknown.

May also have hypoglycemic and hypolipidemic effects, caused by an increase in the viscosity of GI contents.

USES
Used orally to treat acute nutritional disorders, diarrhea, obesity, dyspepsia, enterocolitis, sprue, and celiac disease. It's also used for vomiting in infants and during pregnancy.

Carob can be found in health food products for weight loss and energy and as a chocolate substitute. Carob flour and extracts are used as flavoring agents in foods and beverages.

DOSAGE & ADMINISTRATION
For oral use: 20 to 30 g of carob can be added to water, tea, or milk and can be consumed throughout the day.

ADVERSE REACTIONS
None known.

INTERACTIONS
None reported.

EFFECTS ON LAB TEST RESULTS
• May decrease glucose level.

CAUTIONS
Pregnant or breast-feeding patients should consult health care provider before use.

NURSING CONSIDERATIONS
• Explore patient's knowledge of this herb.
⚠ **ALERT:** Don't confuse carob with carob tree, *Jacaranda procera*, or *Jacaranda caroba*.

PATIENT TEACHING
• Advise patient to consult a health care provider before using an herbal preparation because another treatment may be available.

• Tell patient that when filling a new prescription he should inform pharmacist of any herbal or dietary supplement he's taking.
• Warn patient not to treat vomiting infant with carob before seeking appropriate medical evaluation because doing so may delay diagnosis of a potentially serious medical condition.
• Discuss with patient other options for treating diarrhea or GI complaints.
• Instruct patient to promptly report adverse reactions and new signs and symptoms.

cascara sagrada

Frangula purshiana, Rhamni purshianae cortex, bearberry, bitter bark, California buckthorn, chittem bark, persian bark, purshiana bark, sacred bark, yellow bark

Common trade names
Aromatic Cascara Fluidextract, Cascara Aromatic, Cascara Sagrada, Cascara Sagrada Bark, Vegitabs

AVAILABLE FORMS
Available as cut bark, powder, and dry extracts.

ACTIONS & COMPONENTS
Obtained from the dried bark of *R. purshianae;* the bark must be aged 1 year or heat treated before use. The active ingredients are anthraglycosides or anthraquinones, which consist primarily of cascarosides A and B.

Cascara is a stimulant laxative. When ingested, the herb triggers

*Liquid contains alcohol.

the secretion of water and electrolytes into the small intestine. In the large intestine, the herb inhibits the absorption of these products, allowing the contents of the bowel to grow in volume. This increased volume stimulates peristalsis and advances the bowel contents quickly through the large intestine for evacuation.

Cascara may also have antileukemic properties.

USES

Mainly used as a stimulant laxative to treat constipation; the FDA has approved the herb for this use. Used to make teas, decoctions, elixirs, or for cold maceration. Also used as sunscreens in cosmetic products.

DOSAGE & ADMINISTRATION

For constipation: 20 to 70 mg daily P.O. of hydroxyanthracene derivatives, calculated as cascaroside A, from the cut bark, powder, or dry extract. Tea is prepared by steeping 2 g of finely cut bark in 5 ounces of boiling water for 5 to 10 minutes, and then straining. The correct dose is the smallest necessary to maintain soft stools.

ADVERSE REACTIONS

CV: *arrhythmias (with prolonged use).*
GI: abdominal cramping, abdominal discomfort, bloody diarrhea, colic (from intake of fresh rind).
GU: albuminuria, hematuria, kidney irritation (from intake of fresh rind).
Metabolic: potassium deficiency, weight loss.

INTERACTIONS

Herb-drug. *Cardiac glycosides, digoxin:* Long-term use of cascara may lead to hypokalemia, which may enhance digoxin action. Monitor patient for signs of digoxin toxicity.
Laxatives: Increases the likelihood of diarrhea and fluid or electrolyte disturbances. Advise patient to avoid using herb and drug together.
Potassium-sparing diuretics and corticosteroids: Increases risk of potassium depletion. Discourage use together.
Herb-herb. *Licorice root:* Increases risk of potassium depletion. Advise patient to avoid using herb and root at the same time.

EFFECTS ON LAB TEST RESULTS

• May decrease potassium level.

CAUTIONS

Children younger than age 12, pregnant or breast-feeding patients, and patients with intestinal obstruction, ulcerative colitis, appendicitis, abdominal pain of unknown origin, diarrhea, or acute intestinal inflammation (such as Crohn's disease) should avoid using this herb.

NURSING CONSIDERATIONS

• Explore patient's knowledge of this herb.
• Liquid and solid forms are for oral use only.
• Effects are generally seen within 6 to 8 hours.
• Long-term use may cause hypokalemia that can lead to cardiac problems and muscle weakness.
• Pseudomelanosis coli, a harmless pigmentation of the intestinal mu-

---

Bold italic type indicates that reaction may be life-threatening.

cosa, may develop; it should reverse when patient stops taking the herb.
- Lazy bowel (an inability to move bowels without a laxative) may develop with long-term use of cascara.
- Fresh bark can cause severe vomiting or intestinal cramping.
- Overdose can cause diarrhea and fluid and electrolyte imbalance.

PATIENT TEACHING
- Advise patient to consult a health care provider before using an herbal preparation because another treatment may be available.
- Tell patient that when filling a new prescription he should inform pharmacist of any herbal or dietary supplement he's taking.
- Before patient uses stimulant laxatives such as cascara, encourage patient to use milder methods of relieving constipation, including making dietary changes and using bulk-forming products.
- Tell patient not to begin using cascara if he's experiencing abdominal pain or diarrhea.
- Caution patient that children younger than age 12 and pregnant or breast-feeding patients shouldn't use cascara unless under the supervision of a health care provider.
- Advise patient not to use the fresh rind of the cascara plant because it can cause intestinal spasms, bloody diarrhea, or intestinal irritation.
- Advise patient that cascara isn't intended for long-term use and that he shouldn't use it for longer than 10 days without medical advice.

- Inform patient that if abdominal discomfort develops with cascara use, the discomfort will go away with lower doses. Patient should consult his health care provider.
- Advise patient that herb may discolor urine.

castor bean

Ricinus communis, African coffee tree, bofareira, castor, Mexico seed, Mexico weed, tangantangan oil plant, wonder tree

Common trade names
Castor

AVAILABLE FORMS
Available as a paste for external use.

ACTIONS & COMPONENTS
Contains a constituent called ricin, a protoplasmic poison. Causes cell death after binding to normal cells and disrupting DNA synthesis and protein metabolism. Ricin may have analgesic and antiviral properties.

USES
Used externally as a paste to treat inflammatory skin conditions, boils, carbuncles, abscesses, inflammation of the middle ear, and migraines.

DOSAGE & ADMINISTRATION
Topical use: A paste made from ground seeds can be applied externally to affected areas b.i.d. Treatment may take up to 15 days.

*Liquid contains alcohol.

ADVERSE REACTIONS
Skin: rash.
Other: *toxic reaction,* allergic reaction.

INTERACTIONS
Herb-drug. *Digoxin:* Potassium depletion from herb use can increase body's sensitivity to drug. Discourage use together.

EFFECTS ON LAB TEST RESULTS
● May decrease potassium level if taken orally.

CAUTIONS
Pregnant and breast-feeding patients should avoid using castor beans.

NURSING CONSIDERATIONS
● Explore patient's knowledge of this herb.
⚠ALERT: Castor beans can be toxic when chewed and swallowed; 1 to 2 *chewed* seeds can be lethal to an adult. Leaves of the plants may also be poisonous.
● Signs and symptoms of overdose, or toxicity, include severe stomach pain, nausea, hemoptysis, bloody diarrhea, and burning of the mouth. Seizures, hepatic and renal failure, and death can occur.
● If overdose occurs, provide supportive therapy.
● Castor bean dust can be an inhalant allergen.

PATIENT TEACHING
● Advise patient to consult a health care provider before using an herbal preparation because another treatment may be available.
● Tell patient that when filling a new prescription he should inform

pharmacist of any herbal or dietary supplement he's taking.
● Advise patient not to use on broken or damaged skin.
● Advise patient to discontinue use if he develops a rash after using castor bean.
● Instruct patient to seek medical help immediately if he suspects he has taken an overdose.
● Warn patient to keep all herbal products away from children and pets.

catnip

Nepeta cataria, catmint, catnep, catswort, field balm

Common trade names
Catnip Bulk Tea, Cat Nip, Catnip Herb, Leaves of Catnip

AVAILABLE FORMS
Available as capsules, dried leaf, tea, and tincture*.

ACTIONS & COMPONENTS
The volatile oil (nepetalactone), iridoids, and tannins are the major active ingredients. The essential oil has sedative, carminative, and antispasmodic effects. It's a good source of iron, selenium, potassium, manganese, and chromium.
　Catnip may also have diaphoretic and astringent effects. It may help relieve flatulence and colic.

USES
Used to treat colds, cough, fever, migraines, and hives. Dry leaves are smoked to treat bronchitis and asthma. It's also used internally for menstrual cramps, dyspepsia, and

---

Bold italic type indicates that reaction may be life-threatening.

colic because it helps relax smooth muscles.

This herb has been used for insomnia, diuresis, and diaphoresis, and for children with diarrhea. Topical poultice is used to relieve swelling.

Ether extracts of the plant have been shown to have antimicrobial activity against fungi and gram-positive bacteria.

DOSAGE & ADMINISTRATION

Decoction: 1 or 2 teaspoons of tea steeped in 6 to 8 ounces of boiling water for 10 to 15 minutes. Or 1 or 2 teaspoons of tea boiled in 6 to 8 ounces of water, set to simmer at low heat for 3 to 5 minutes, and then strained.
Infusion: 2 teaspoons of dried herb infused in 8 ounces of boiling water for 10 to 15 minutes. Dosage is 1 cup t.i.d.
Tincture: 2 to 4 ml t.i.d.

ADVERSE REACTIONS

CNS: malaise, headache, sedation.
GI: abdominal discomfort, nausea, vomiting.

INTERACTIONS

Herb-drug. *Benzodiazepines, barbiturates:* May cause additive CNS depression. Discourage use together.
Disulfiram: Herbal products prepared with alcohol may cause a disulfiram-like reaction. Discourage use together.

EFFECTS ON LAB TEST RESULTS

None reported.

CAUTIONS

Pregnant and breast-feeding patients should avoid use.

NURSING CONSIDERATIONS

• Explore patient's knowledge of this herb.
• The leaves and flowering tops and fennel of *N. cataria* are harvested between June and September and are used in the preparation of catnip products.
• Catnip was used for tea in Europe until Chinese tea was introduced.
• Children and elderly patients should start with weak preparations and increase the strength, as needed.
• Catnip abuse involves either smoking the dried leaves similar to smoking marijuana, or making a volatile oil or extract of the herb, soaking the tobacco in the extract, and then smoking the tobacco. If abuse is suspected, watch patient for signs of mood elevation, such as giddiness.
• Monitor any patient using catnip for sedative effects.

PATIENT TEACHING

• Advise patient to consult a health care provider before using an herbal preparation because another treatment may be available.
• Tell patient when filling new prescriptions he should inform pharmacist of any herbal or dietary supplement he's taking.
• Advise patient not to use catnip if she is pregnant or is planning pregnancy.
• Caution patient about potential sedative effects and impairment of cognitive ability.

*Liquid contains alcohol.

- Instruct patient to avoid activities that require mental alertness, such as driving, until CNS effects are known.
- Advise patient that extract may contain alcohol and may be unsuitable for children.
- Instruct patient that the liquid form of catnip needs to be shaken well before each use.
- Warn patient to keep all herbal products and drugs away from children and pets.

cat's claw

Uncaria tomentosa, life-giving vine of Peru, miracle herb from the rain forest of Peru, samento, secondary root, una de gato

Common trade names
Cat's Claw Bark, Cat's Claw Inner Bark, Cat's Claw-Power, Cat's Claw Standardized Extract, Cat's Claw Tea Bags, Cat's Claw (Una de Gato), Devil's Claw, Devil's Claw Root, Garbato, Paraguaya, Peruvian Cat's Claw, Secondary Root, Tambor Hausca, Toron

AVAILABLE FORMS
Available as capsules, dried inner stalk bark or root for decoction, extract*, powdered extract, and tea bags.
Capsules: 175 mg of standardized cat's claw bark extract delivering 7 mg of alkaloids, 3 mg total of oxindole alkaloids
Extract: 250 mg of cat's claw bark extract per milliliter, standardized to contain 3% of oxindole alkaloids; extract contains alcohol. An alcohol-free extract is available.

Powdered extract: Packed in 500-mg capsules

ACTIONS & COMPONENTS
Contains many alkaloids that are pharmacologically active dietary supplements and are produced from inner stalk bark, woody vine, or roots of *U. tomentosa.* It also inhibits urinary bladder contractions and has local anesthetic effects.

Most cat's claw alkaloids have immunostimulant properties, which may stimulate phagocytosis. The major alkaloids dilate peripheral blood vessels, inhibit the sympathetic nervous system, and relax smooth muscles.

Cat's claw may lower cholesterol levels and decrease heart rate.

Cat's claw alkaloids have been shown to have antioxidant and anti-inflammatory properties by inhibiting tumor necrosis factor and prostaglandin production.

USES
Used to treat GI problems—including Crohn's disease, colitis, inflammatory bowel disease, and hemorrhoids—and to enhance immunity. Also used in cancer patients for its antimutagenic effects. It's also used with AZT to stimulate the immune system in those with HIV infection.

Topically, it's used to relieve pain from minor injuries and to treat acne.

This herb has also been used to treat diverticulosis, ulcers, rheumatism, menstrual disorders, osteoarthritis, diabetes, prostate problems, gonorrhea, and cirrhosis, and to prevent pregnancy.

Bold italic type indicates that reaction may be life-threatening.

DOSAGE & ADMINISTRATION

Capsules: 2 capsules (175 mg per capsule) P.O. daily or 3 capsules P.O. t.i.d.; dosage varies by manufacturer.

Decoction: 10 to 30 g inner stalk bark or root in 1 quart of water for 30 to 60 minutes. Dosage is 2 to 3 cups per day.

Extract (alcohol free): 7 to 10 gtt t.i.d.; may increase to 15 gtt five times a day.

Liquid or alcohol extract: 10 to 15 gtt b.i.d. to t.i.d., to 1 to 3 ml t.i.d.

Powdered extract: 1 to 3 capsules (500 mg per capsule) P.O. b.i.d. to q.i.d.

ADVERSE REACTIONS

CV: hypotension.
GU: *acute renal failure.*

INTERACTIONS

Herb-drug. *Antihypertensives:* May potentiate hypotensive effects of conventional drugs. Discourage use together.

Drugs metabolized by cytochrome P-450 3A4, such as alprazolam, atorvastatin, diazepam, sildenafil, and warfarin: May increase levels of drug. Monitor serum levels and effect of drug.

Immunosuppressants: May counteract the therapeutic effects because herb has immunostimulant properties. Discourage use together.

SSRIs: May lead to serotonin syndrome. Discourage use together.
Herb-food. *Any food:* Enhances absorption of herb. Advise patient to take herb with food.

EFFECTS ON LAB TEST RESULTS
None reported.

CAUTIONS

Pregnant and breast-feeding patients, patients who have had transplant surgery, and those with autoimmune disease, multiple sclerosis, or tuberculosis should avoid use.

Patients with a history of peptic ulcer disease or gallstones should use caution when taking this herb because it stimulates stomach acid secretion.

NURSING CONSIDERATIONS

• Explore patient's knowledge of this herb.
• Some liquid extracts contain alcohol and may be unsuitable for children or patients with liver disease.
• This herb and its contents vary from manufacturer to manufacturer; the alkaloid concentration varies from season to season.

PATIENT TEACHING

• Advise patient to consult a health care provider before using an herbal preparation because another treatment may be available.
• Tell patient that when filling a new prescription he should inform pharmacist of any herbal or dietary supplement he's taking.
• This product and its contents may vary among manufacturers, and its alkaloid concentration varies from season to season. Advise patient to purchase cat's claw from the same reputable source.
• Inform patient that herb should be used for no longer than 8 weeks

without a 2- to 3-week rest period from the herb.
• Instruct patient to promptly report adverse reactions and new signs or symptoms.
• Warn patient to keep all herbal products away from children and pets.

cat's foot

Antennariae dioica, cudweed, life everlasting, mountain everlasting

Common trade names
Catsfoot, Cudweed

AVAILABLE FORMS
Available as bulk dried herb.

ACTIONS & COMPONENTS
Cat's foot flower consists of the fresh or dried flowers of *A. dioica.*

Cat's foot stimulates the flow of gastric and pancreatic secretions. It may raise blood pressure, and it may have spasmolytic, choleric, discutient, and astringent effects. Its effects on the GI system may be due to high concentrations of chromium isolated from the plant.

USES
Used to stimulate the flow of bile from the gallbladder to the duodenum and to treat dysentery.

This herb has been used as a diuretic. In Europe, it's also used to cure quinsy and mumps and to treat bites of poisonous reptiles.

DOSAGE & ADMINISTRATION
Infusion: Prepared by steeping 1 teaspoon fresh or dried flowering herb in ½ cup of boiling water for 10 minutes. Dosage is ½ to 1 cup P.O. daily

ADVERSE REACTIONS
None known.

INTERACTIONS
Herb-drug. *Antihypertensives:* Herb may interfere with the intended therapeutic effect of antihypertensives. Advise patient to use with caution.

EFFECTS ON LAB TEST RESULTS
None reported.

CAUTIONS
Pregnant and breast-feeding patients should avoid use.

NURSING CONSIDERATIONS
• Explore patient's knowledge of this herb.
• Therapeutic use of cat's foot isn't recommended.
• Monitor patient's blood pressure when therapy is initiated and regularly thereafter.

PATIENT TEACHING
• Advise patient to consult a health care provider before using an herbal preparation because another treatment may be available.
• Tell patient that when filling a new prescription he should inform pharmacist of any herbal or dietary supplement he's taking.
• Instruct patient to promptly report adverse reactions and new signs or symptoms.

Bold italic type indicates that reaction may be life-threatening.

celandine

Chelidonii herba, Chelidonium majus, celandine herb, greater celandine, jewel weed, pilewort, quick-in-the-hand, schöllkraut, slipperweed, tetterwort, touch-me-not

Common trade names
Celandine, Swallow-Wort

AVAILABLE FORMS
Available as dry plant, dry root, liquid extract*, ointment, and tinctures*. Also available in various combination products.
Liquid extract: 1:1 in 25% alcohol
Tinctures: 1:10 in 45% alcohol

ACTIONS & COMPONENTS
When used topically, celandine has analgesic, antiseptic, and caustic effects.

When taken orally, the herb may have cytostatic activity with nonspecific immune stimulation and may facilitate bile flow in the GI system. It may also have antispasmodic and diuretic effects.

USES
Used orally to treat nonobstructive cholecystitis, jaundice, cholelithiasis, hypercholesterolemia, angina pectoris, asthma, breast lumps, constipation, diffused latent liver complaints, stomach cancer, and gout. May also help manage blood pressure, but such use must be further investigated.

Used topically as an analgesic, antiseptic, and caustic agent for eczema, blister rashes, scabies, scrofulous diseases, and hemorrhoids.

DOSAGE & ADMINISTRATION
Herb decoction, infusion: 2 to 4 g powdered herb, not root, in 1 cup of boiling water t.i.d.
Liquid extract: 1 to 2 ml P.O. t.i.d.
Ointment: Applied to affected area t.i.d. p.r.n., for insect bites or dermatitis.
Root decoction, infusion: Prepared by steeping 1 level teaspoon of rootstock in 1 cup of boiling water for 30 minutes. Dosage is ½ cup daily, consumed when it's cold.
Tincture: 10 to 15 gtt S.L. t.i.d.
Topical juice: Mixed with vinegar and dabbed on no more than 2 or 3 warts at a time, b.i.d. to t.i.d.

ADVERSE REACTIONS
CNS: stupor, *seizures,* drowsiness.
GI: burning in the mouth, abdominal discomfort, nausea, vomiting, bloody diarrhea, salivation.
GU: hematuria.
Hepatic: jaundice, *acute hepatitis, cholestatic hepatitis.*
Skin: contact dermatitis.
Other: allergic response.

INTERACTIONS
Herb-drug. *Disulfiram:* Products prepared with alcohol may cause a disulfiram-like reaction. Discourage use together.

EFFECTS ON LAB TEST RESULTS
• May increase liver function test values, including direct and indirect bilirubin levels.

CAUTIONS
Pregnant and breast-feeding patients and those who have latex or celandine allergy, painful gallstones, acute bilious colic, obstruc-

---

*Liquid contains alcohol.

tive jaundice, or acute viral hepatitis should avoid use.

NURSING CONSIDERATIONS
- Explore patient's knowledge of this herb.
- Dried plant is less active than fresh.
- Patient should use this herb only under the supervision of a health care provider.
- A cross-sensitivity between latex allergy and celandine exists. A patient should carefully weigh the benefits against the risks before taking celandine orally.
- ⚠ALERT: Overdose could be life-threatening. Stem juice overdoses may cause paralysis and death.

PATIENT TEACHING
- Advise patient to consult a health care provider before using an herbal preparation because another treatment may be available.
- Tell patient that when filling a new prescription he should inform pharmacist of any herbal or dietary supplement he's taking.
- Caution patient that he should only use celandine under a health care provider's supervision.
- Advise patient not to use celandine if she is pregnant or is planning pregnancy.
- Encourage patient to alert his health care provider if he's allergic to latex or herbs before starting celandine therapy.
- Warn patient not to exceed the recommended dosage.
- Advise patient to notify his health care provider if herb causes allergic reaction, yellowing of the skin, or sclera, and to immediately

seek medical attention if any of these occur.
- Inform patient that herb isn't recommended for long-term use.

celery, celery seed

Apium graveolens, celery fruit, celery herb, celery root, celery seed oil, garden celery, smallage

Common trade names
Celery, Celery Fruit, Celery Seed

AVAILABLE FORMS
Available as capsules, dried fruits, dried seeds, liquid extract*, tincture, and in combination products for internal use.
Capsules: 450 mg of celery seed extract
Liquid extract:* 1:1 in 50% alcohol

ACTIONS & COMPONENTS
High in minerals, including sodium and chlorine, but a poor source of vitamins. May have antirheumatic, anti-inflammatory, diuretic, sedative, anticonvulsive, fungicidal, and anticarcinogenic effects.
    The juice has antihypertensive effects, and the oil may cause hypoglycemia.

USES
Celery is used to relieve GI gas and colic and to treat bladder and kidney disorders, rheumatic arthritis, gout, and calculosis. Dieters use celery because of its high fiber content.
    Celery oil is used as a spasmolytic and sedative for nervousness and hysteria and as an antiflat-

---

Bold italic type indicates that reaction may be life-threatening.

ulent. It's also used to manage hypertension and blood glucose level and to promote menses. Oil extract from the root is used to restore sexual potency impaired by illness.

Celery seeds are used to treat bronchitis and rheumatism.

DOSAGE & ADMINISTRATION
Capsules: 2 to 3 capsules P.O. b.i.d. to t.i.d.; dosage varies among products.
Decoction: Prepared by boiling ½ teaspoon of seeds in ½ cup of water briefly, and then straining. Taken t.i.d.
Dried fruits: 0.5 to 2 g or by prepared liquid substance 1:5 b.i.d. to t.i.d.
Infusion: Prepared by steeping 1 or 2 teaspoons of freshly crushed seeds in 1 cup of water for 10 to 15 minutes. Taken t.i.d.
Juice: 1 tablespoon b.i.d. to t.i.d. before meals.
Liquid extract (1:1 in 50% alcohol): 0.3 to 1.2 ml t.i.d.
Oil: 6 to 8 gtt in water b.i.d.
Tincture: 1 to 5 ml t.i.d.

ADVERSE REACTIONS
CNS: sedation.
Respiratory: respiratory difficulty.
Skin: dermatitis, urticaria, depigmentation, hyperpigmentation.
Other: *angioedema,* allergic reaction including *anaphylactoid shock.*

INTERACTIONS
Herb-drug. *Diuretics, antihypertensives:* May cause additive hypotensive effects. Discourage use together.

Insulin, oral antidiabetics: May cause additive hypoglycemic effects. Discourage use together.
Warfarin: Using celery with warfarin may increase the risk of bleeding. Monitor patient closely for bleeding.
Herb-lifestyle. *Sun exposure:* Increases risk of photosensitivity reactions. Advise patient to use sunscreen, wear protective clothing, and avoid prolonged exposure to the sun.

EFFECTS ON LAB TEST RESULTS
• May decrease glucose level.

CAUTIONS
Pregnant patients shouldn't use celery seed and shouldn't use more than moderate amount of plant. Patients with kidney infection or insufficiency should avoid this herb.

NURSING CONSIDERATIONS
• Explore patient's knowledge of this herb.
• Ingestion of large amounts of celery oil may cause toxic reaction.
• If patient has diabetes, monitor blood glucose level because celery may cause hypoglycemia.
• If patient is also taking a diuretic or an antihypertensive, check his blood pressure regularly.
• Patients allergic to celery have a greater risk of severe allergic reactions to latex following repeated exposure to latex.

PATIENT TEACHING
• Advise patient to consult a health care provider before using an herbal preparation because another treatment may be available.

- Tell patient that when filling a new prescription he should inform pharmacist of any herbal or dietary supplement he's taking.
- Instruct patient to promptly report adverse reactions and new signs or symptoms.
- If patient has a kidney disease or infection, advise him not to use celery medicinally because the volatile oils can irritate the kidneys.
- If patient is pregnant or is planning pregnancy, advise her not to use celery seed and to be extremely cautious if using celery for therapeutic effects.
- Tell patient that latent yeast infections may grow within the plant when it's stored, causing the furanocoumarin content to rise, which could lead to phototoxicosis.

centaury

Centaurii herba, Centaurium minus, C. umbellatum, Erythraea centaurium, centaury gentian, centory, Christ's ladder, feverwort, red centaury, tausendgüldenkraut

Common trade names
Centaury

AVAILABLE FORMS
Available as the dried flowering tops of common centaury and *E. centaurium,* liquid extract*, powder, tea, and tincture*.

ACTIONS & COMPONENTS
Contains phenolic acids, alkaloids, monoterpenoids, triterpenoids, flavonoids, beta-coumaric, caffeic acids, xanthones, fatty acids, alkanes, and waxes. The major component is gentiopicroside, which has antimalarial effects.

May have antipyretic, diuretic, and stomachic effects. The compounds erythrocentaurin and erytaurin may be responsible for centaury's bitter tonic effects. The phenolic acids may have antipyretic activity.

USES
Mainly used to treat anorexia and dyspepsia.

DOSAGE & ADMINISTRATION
Liquid extract (1:1 in 25% alcohol):* 2 to 4 ml P.O. up to t.i.d.
Powder: Sprinkled on a wafer with honey.
Tea: Prepared by steeping 2 to 3 g in 5 ounces of boiling water for 15 minutes, and then straining.
Tincture (essence of centaury, 27% alcohol):* 2 gtt in water or under tongue, p.r.n.

ADVERSE REACTIONS
None reported.

INTERACTIONS
Herb-drug. *Anticoagulants:* May reduce drug effect. Discourage use together.
Disulfiram: Herbal products prepared with alcohol may cause a disulfiram-like reaction. Discourage use together.

EFFECTS ON LAB TEST RESULTS
None reported.

CAUTIONS
Pregnant and breast-feeding patients, patients sensitive to the herb or its components, and those with

---

Bold italic type indicates that reaction may be life-threatening.

stomach or intestinal ulcers should avoid this herb.

NURSING CONSIDERATIONS
• Explore patient's knowledge of this herb.
• Excessive use of centaury should be avoided because information about safety and toxicity is limited.
• Centaury may interfere with the intended therapeutic effect of conventional drugs.
• If patient is also taking an anticoagulant, monitor him for lack of therapeutic effect.

PATIENT TEACHING
• Advise patient to consult a health care provider before using an herbal preparation because another treatment may be available.
• Tell patient that when filling a new prescription he should inform pharmacist of any herbal or dietary supplement he's taking.
• Encourage patient to promptly report adverse reactions and new signs and symptoms.
• Advise patient to avoid excessive use.
• If patient is taking disulfiram or metronidazole or if he has a history of alcoholism or cirrhosis, inform him that he should avoid centaury liquid extracts and tincture because of their alcohol content.

chamomile

Chamaemelum nobile (English or Roman chamomile), *Chamomillae anthodium, Matricaria* (or *Chamomilla*) *recutita* (genuine, German, or Hungarian chamomile), anthemis nobilis, chamomilla, ground apple, pin heads, whig plant, wild chamomile

Common trade names
Azulon, Chamomile Flowers, Chamomile Tea, Kid Chamomile, Standardized Chamomile Extract, Wild Chamomile

AVAILABLE FORMS
Available as capsules, fresh or dried flowerheads of *M. recutita* and *C. nobile,* liquid extract*, raw herb, tea, and topical cream.
Capsules: 350 to 400 mg/capsule (standardized to contain 1% apigenin and 0.5% essential oil)
Liquid extracts:* The strength of the liquid extracts available is usually 1:1 or 1:1.5. Some liquid extracts contain between 10% and 63% grain alcohol. Nature's Answer makes a liquid extract for children that contains glycerin, not alcohol.
Raw herb: Frontier offers whole German chamomile flowers for making teas or massage oils.
Teas: Made from dried chamomile flowers. Most chamomile teas are organic and caffeine free.

ACTIONS & COMPONENTS
Contains a volatile oil that consists of up to 50% alpha-bisabolol. Bisabolol reduces inflammation and is an antipyretic. It also shortens the

---

*Liquid contains alcohol.

healing times of superficial burns and ulcers and inhibits development of ulcers. The essential oil also has antibacterial and slight antiviral effects.

Chamazulene, a minor component of the oil, has anti-inflammatory and antioxidant effects. The flavonoids apigenin and luteolin also contribute to the anti-inflammatory effect. Unlike the benzodiazepines, apigenin is primarily responsible for the anxiolytic and slight sedative effect through action on the CNS benzodiazepine receptors. Apigenin doesn't produce anticonvulsant effects.

Bisabolol, bisabolol oxides A and B, and the essential oil of chamomile are probably best known for their antispasmodic effects. Other compounds in chamomile that exert antispasmodic effects include apigenin, quercetin, luteolin, and the coumarins umbelliferone and herniarine.

USES

Used orally to treat diarrhea, anxiety, restlessness, stomatitis, hemorrhagic cystitis, flatulence, and motion sickness.

Used topically to stimulate skin metabolism, reduce inflammation, encourage the healing of wounds, and treat cutaneous burns. Also used for its antibacterial and antiviral effects.

Teas are mainly used for sedation or relaxation.

DOSAGE & ADMINISTRATION
Adults: 1:1 or 1:1.5 liquid extract in 10% to 70% alcohol, 1 to 4 ml t.i.d.

Children age 2 and older: 1:4 strength alcohol-free extract, 1 to 4 ml t.i.d.
Children ages 2 to 4: ⅛ to ¼ teaspoon directly or in water or juice b.i.d. to t.i.d.
Children weighing 41 to 54 kg (90 to 119 lb): 1 to 2 teaspoons directly or in water or juice b.i.d. to t.i.d.
Children weighing 27 to 41 kg (60 to 90 lb): ½ to 1 teaspoon directly or in water or juice b.i.d. to t.i.d.
Children weighing 14 to 27 kg (31 to 60 lb): ¼ to ½ teaspoon directly or in water or juice b.i.d. to t.i.d.
Raw herb: Used in massage oils, p.r.n.
Teas: For GI upset, tea is taken t.i.d. to q.i.d. between meals.
Adults and children older than age 6: Prepared by pouring boiling water over 1 tablespoon of chamomile or one chamomile tea bag, covering it for 5 to 10 minutes, and then (if using bulk herbs) straining it. For inflammation of the mucous membranes in the mouth and throat, tea is used as a wash or gargle. For young children, tea should be diluted.
Children ages 5 to 6: 100 to 120 ml daily to q.i.d.
Children ages 3 to 4: 50 to 80 ml daily to q.i.d.
Children ages 1 to 2: 20 to 40 ml daily to q.i.d.
Adults and children: Apply topical cream q.i.d. to affected areas.

ADVERSE REACTIONS
EENT: conjunctivitis, eyelid angioedema.
GI: nausea, vomiting.

Bold italic type indicates that reaction may be life-threatening.

Skin: eczema, contact dermatitis.
Other: *anaphylaxis.*

INTERACTIONS
Herb-drug. *CNS depressants:*
May have additive effects. Discourage use together.
Drugs metabolized by cytochrome P-450 3A4 such as alprazolam, atorvastatin, diazepam, ketoconazole, verapamil: May increase levels of drugs metabolized by cytochrome P-450 3A4 because chamomile is a weak inhibitor of this enzyme. Monitor drug concentrations and effects of using this herb with these drugs.
Warfarin: The coumarin content of chamomile may antagonize or potentiate the effect of an anticoagulant. Discourage use together.

EFFECTS ON LAB TEST RESULTS
None reported.

CAUTIONS
Patients with known or suspected allergy to chamomile or related members of the Compositae family should avoid use because of the potential for anaphylaxis. Pregnant patients should avoid use because chamomile may trigger menstruation or a miscarriage.

Herb shouldn't be used in teething babies and in children younger than age 2.

Safety in breast-feeding patients and those with liver or kidney disorders hasn't been established; therefore, these patients should avoid use.

NURSING CONSIDERATIONS
• Explore patient's knowledge of this herb.

☑**ALERT:** People sensitive to ragweed and chrysanthemums or other Compositae family members (arnica, yarrow, feverfew, tansy, artemisia) may be more susceptible to contact allergies and anaphylaxis. Patients with hay fever or bronchial asthma caused by pollens are more susceptible to anaphylactoid reactions.
• Signs and symptoms of anaphylaxis include shortness of breath, swelling of the tongue, rash, tachycardia, and hypotension.

PATIENT TEACHING
• Advise patient to consult a health care provider before using an herbal preparation because another treatment may be available.
• Tell patient that when filling a new prescription he should inform pharmacist of any herbal or dietary supplement he's taking.
• Advise patients who are pregnant or planning pregnancy not to use chamomile.
• If patient is taking a blood thinner, advise him not to use chamomile because it may thin the blood too much.
• Advise patient that chamomile may enhance an allergic reaction or make existing symptoms worse in susceptible patients.
• Instruct parent not to give chamomile to any child before checking with a knowledgeable practitioner.
• Advise patient to avoid herb if taking CNS depressants.

*Liquid contains alcohol.

chaparral

Larrea tridentata, chaparro, creosote bush, covillea, dwarf evergreen oak, el gobernadora, falsa alcaparra, greasewood, hediondilla, shoegoi, zygophyllaceae

Common trade names
Chaparral Capsules, Chaparral Leaf, Chaparral Liquid, Creosote Herpestate

AVAILABLE FORMS
Available as bulk powder; capsules; the flowers, leaves, and twigs of the *L. tridentata;* liquid extract*, oil infusion; tablet; tea; and tincture*.
Capsules: 500 mg of chaparral leaf/capsule
Liquid extracts:* 1:2.5 to 1:5 dry herb strength in 68% to 75% grain alcohol
Tablets: 500 mg of chaparral leaf/capsule combined with 100 mg of vitamin C, 65 mg of alfalfa, 10 mg of yucca, and 10 mg of zinc

ACTIONS & COMPONENTS
Major constituent is the lignin nordihydroguaiaretic acid (NDGA), which makes up 1.84% of the plant's active compounds. NDGA has potent anti-inflammatory activity because of its ability to block the enzyme lipoxygenase. Lipoxygenase is a precursor to many inflammatory prostaglandins; therefore, by blocking this enzyme, chaparral may help treat certain inflammatory conditions.

Besides inhibiting platelet aggregation in those taking aspirin, NDGA also has some antioxidant effects. Other components of chaparral that add to its antioxidant activity include flavonoids, saponins, and lignins.

The lignins have amoebicidal, antiparasitic, and fungicidal activity. NDGA has also been reported to have antimicrobial activity against certain species of *Penicillium,* streptococci, *Staphylococcus aureus, Bacillus subtilis,* and *Pseudomonas aeruginosa.*

USES
Used orally as supportive therapy for cancer, dyspepsia, venereal disease, tuberculosis, and parasitic infections. Used as an oral rinse to help prevent tooth decay, halitosis, and gum disease.

Used topically as supportive therapy for allergies, dysmenorrhea, intestinal cramping, rheumatoid arthritis, and wound healing.

DOSAGE & ADMINISTRATION
For antimicrobial use: Swished with tea and spit out, or applied directly to minor abrasions.
To treat allergy symptoms: Tea is prepared by steeping 1 teaspoon of leaves and flowers in 1 cup hot water for 10 to 15 minutes; 1 to 3 cups P.O. daily for several days. Or, 20 gtt of tincture of liquid extract P.O. daily to t.i.d. Alcohol content ranges from 68% to 75%.
To treat arthralgia: 1 to 3 cups of tea P.O. daily. Or, 20 gtt of tincture or liquid extract daily to t.i.d. Treatment should be limited to a few days.
To treat autoimmune disease: 20 gtt of tincture P.O. daily to t.i.d.

Bold italic type indicates that reaction may be life-threatening.

To treat dysmenorrhea or intestinal cramps: Infused oil is applied topically to abdomen, p.r.n.

To treat premenstrual syndrome: 1 to 3 cups of tea P.O. daily. Treatment should be limited to a few days. Or, 20 gtt of tincture P.O. daily to t.i.d.

ADVERSE REACTIONS

CNS: fatigue.
GI: anorexia, abdominal pain, nausea, diarrhea, loose stools.
GU: dark urine, induction of cortical and medullary cysts in the kidney.
Hepatic: *hepatotoxicity, acute hepatitis,* jaundice, *cirrhosis, acute fulminant liver failure.*
Metabolic: weight loss.
Skin: pruritus, contact dermatitis.
Other: fever, tumor growth.

INTERACTIONS

Herb-drug. *Anticoagulants, antiplatelet drugs:* NDGA may interfere with platelet adhesion and aggregation in patients taking aspirin. Advise patient not to use the herb.
Disulfiram: Herbal products prepared with alcohol may cause a disulfiram-like reaction. Discourage use together.
MAO inhibitors including phenelzine, tranylcypromine: Excessive doses of chaparral may interfere with MAO inhibitor activity. Discourage use together.

EFFECTS ON LAB TEST RESULTS

• May increase liver function test values.

CAUTIONS

Pregnant and breast-feeding patients and those with a history of liver disease, alcohol abuse, hepatitis, renal insufficiency, preexisting renal disease, or chronic renal failure should avoid use. Because pediatric dosing information isn't available, herb shouldn't be used in children.

NURSING CONSIDERATIONS

• Explore patient's knowledge of this herb.
• Dosages are for adults only.
• Most patients find the very strong taste of chaparral teas and tinctures disagreeable, which limits the amount they can tolerate before feeling nauseated.
• Monitor patient for signs or symptoms of hepatic failure. If patient experiences nausea, fever, fatigue, dark urine, or jaundice, he should stop using the herb.
⚠ **ALERT:** Hepatotoxicity appears as toxic or drug-induced cholestatic hepatitis.
• Gastric lavage may be performed within 60 minutes of a potentially fatal ingestion.
• Activated charcoal may also be used when administered within 1 hour of a potentially fatal ingestion.

PATIENT TEACHING

• Advise patient to consult a health care provider before using an herbal preparation because another treatment may be available.
• Tell patient when filling a new prescription he should inform pharmacist of any herbal or dietary supplement he's taking.
• Warn patient not to postpone seeking appropriate medical evaluation because doing so may delay

*Liquid contains alcohol.

diagnosis of a potentially serious medical condition.
- Instruct patient to stop taking chaparral if he develops nausea, fever, fatigue, dark urine, or jaundice.

chaste tree

Vitex agnus-castus, Abraham's balm, chasteberry, Indian spice, Monk's pepper-tree, safe tree, wild-pepper

Common trade names
Chasteberry Power, Chaste Tree, Chaste Tree Berry Liquid Herbal Extract, Fem-J, Vitex, Vitex Alfalfa Supreme, Vitex Elixir Herbal Extract, Vitex 40 Plus, Vitex 20 to 40 Vegicaps

AVAILABLE FORMS
Available as capsules, elixir*, liquid extract, tablets, tea, and tinctures*. The herb is also contained in various women's multivitamin supplements and combination products used to alleviate menopausal symptoms.
Capsules (Natrol, Nature's Way, Phytopharmica): 150 to 325 mg/capsule (standardized to contain 0.5% agnuside)
Elixir (Gaia): Contains 85% alcohol
Liquid extract (Gaia): 1:1.5 double maceration strength. Contains 65% to 75% vegetable glycerine.
Tablets (Rainbow Light): 500 mg/capsule (standardized to contain 0.5% agnuside)
Teas (Alvita): Caffeine free
Tinctures (Gaia): Contain 40% grain alcohol

ACTIONS & COMPONENTS
Derived from the dried, ripened fruit of *V. agnus-castus*, chaste tree is believed to act directly on the hypothalamic-pituitary axis.

Chaste tree contains the two iridoid glycosides agnuside and aucubin, flavonoids, essential oils, and progestins. The berries exert a progesterogenic effect on women and an antiandrogenic effect on men. By increasing the release of luteinizing hormone, which in turn increases progesterone production in the ovaries, Vitex helps to regulate a woman's cycle. Progestin components include progesterone, testosterone, and androstenedione.

A component in chaste tree has been shown to bind to dopamine receptors, thereby inhibiting the release of prolactin. This is particularly useful in treating premenstrual breast pain associated with excess secretion of prolactin. May also act as a diuretic to reduce water retention before menstruation.

USES
Chaste tree fruit is used to treat menstrual irregularities, such as amenorrhea or excessive menstrual bleeding, and premenstrual complaints, menopausal symptoms, and fibroids.

Chaste tree is also used to increase breast milk production and treat fibrocystic breast disease, infertility in women, and acne.

DOSAGE & ADMINISTRATION
Capsules, tablets: 150 to 325 mg (standardized to contain 0.5% agnuside) P.O. daily or b.i.d.
Liquid extracts, tinctures: German Commission E recommends

Bold italic type indicates that reaction may be life-threatening.

aqueous-alcoholic extracts with 30 to 40 mg of the active herb. Extracts from the crushed fruits, which contain between 50% and 70% alcohol, are taken as liquid or dry extract.

ADVERSE REACTIONS
CNS: headaches.
GI: GI upset.
GU: increased menstrual flow.
Skin: itching, urticaria.

INTERACTIONS
Herb-drug. *Antihypertensives:* May reduce drug effect. Discourage use together.
Beta blockers: May cause hypertensive crisis. Discourage use together.
Dopamine agonists: May reduce drug effects. Discourage use together.

EFFECTS ON LAB TEST RESULTS
None reported.

CAUTIONS
Men, pregnant patients, breast-feeding patients, breast cancer patients, adolescents, patients hypersensitive to chaste tree or its components, patients with active urticaria, and patients who are receiving hormone replacement therapy or taking hormonal contraceptives should avoid use.

NURSING CONSIDERATIONS
• Explore patient's knowledge of this herb.
• Oral use of chaste tree can cause urticaria and itching. If these symptoms occur, patient should discontinue use.

• If patient is using chaste tree orally, monitor him for signs or symptoms of hypersensitivity, including shortness of breath and swelling of the tongue.
• Women with amenorrhea or infertility can use chaste tree for 12 to 18 months.

PATIENT TEACHING
• Advise patient to consult a health care provider before using an herbal preparation because another treatment may be available.
• Tell patient that when filling a new prescription he should inform pharmacist of any herbal or dietary supplement he's taking.
• Advise patients who are pregnant or breast-feeding not to use chaste tree.
• If patient is taking high blood pressure medication (especially a beta blocker), advise him not to use chaste tree because of the potential for a sudden severe rise in blood pressure.
• Caution men against using this herb because of the antiandrogen effects.
• Inform patient that chaste tree may cause rash or itching and that he should stop taking it if either develops.
• Remind patient that the herb isn't fast acting.
• Warn patient to keep all herbal products away from children and pets.

---

*Liquid contains alcohol.

chaulmoogra oil

Taraktogenos kurzii,
chaulmogra, chaulmugra,
hydnocarpus, hydnocarpus oil,
hynocardia oil, kalaw tree oil,
leprosy oil, taraktogenos kurzii

Common trade names
*Chaulmoogra, Gynocardia Oil,
Oleum Chaulmoograe*

AVAILABLE FORMS
Available as oil and ointment.

ACTIONS & COMPONENTS
Topical chaulmoogra oil comes
from the expressed oil of the seeds
of the chaulmoogra tree. The active
ingredient in the oil is chaul-
moogric acid, also known as hyd-
nocarpic acid. The oil may have
antimicrobial activity, especially
against *Mycobacterium leprae.*

Other compounds that have
been isolated from the chaulmoogra tree include palmitic acid,
glycerol, phytosterols, and a mixture of fatty acids.

USES
Used to treat rheumatoid arthritis,
eczema, psoriasis, and tuberculosis
as well as sprains, bruises, or other
inflammation of the skin. Applied
directly to open wounds and sores.

In the past, chaulmoogra oil was
used for its antimicrobial effects as
supportive treatment for leprosy. It
has since been replaced with new-
er, more effective drugs.

DOSAGE & ADMINISTRATION
Oil: 5 to 60 minims applied topically to lesions, p.r.n.

ADVERSE REACTIONS
Skin: irritation.

INTERACTIONS
None reported.

EFFECTS ON LAB TEST RESULTS
None reported.

CAUTIONS
Patients sensitive to chaulmoogra
oil or its components, pregnant and
breast-feeding patients, and children should avoid use.

NURSING CONSIDERATIONS
• Explore patient's knowledge of
this herb.
☑ **ALERT:** Chaulmoogra oil
should never be taken orally because the seeds are poisonous
because of their cyanogenic glycoside content. If accidental ingestion occurs, patient will likely require emergency cardiac and
respiratory treatment.
• Oil may be painful to administer
to open wounds because it's highly
viscous.
• Patients with leprotic wounds
show significant improvement
when they use chaulmoogra oil,
but few data exist regarding chaulmoogra oil's safety and efficacy.

PATIENT TEACHING
• Advise patient to consult a health
care provider before using an
herbal preparation because a standard treatment that has been
proven effective may be available.
• Tell patient when filling a new
prescription he should inform
pharmacist of any herbal or dietary
supplement he's taking.

Bold italic type indicates that reaction may be life-threatening.

- Advise patients who are pregnant or breast-feeding not to use chaulmoogra oil.
- Advise parents not to use the oil for their children.
- Encourage patient with leprosy wounds or ulcers to obtain professional medical treatment and to discuss with his health care provider the possibility of using chaulmoogra oil ointment as an additional treatment.

chickweed

Stellaria media, adder's mouth, mouse ear, passerina, satin flower, starweed, starwort, stitchwort, tongue-grass, winterweed

Common trade names
None known

AVAILABLE FORMS
Available as dry herb, fluidextract*, ointment, tea, and tincture*.

ACTIONS & COMPONENTS
The leaves of chickweed contain potassium, phosphorus, and nitrate salts. Chickweed also contains 150 to 550 mg of vitamin C per 100 g of herb and the flavonoid rutin, which may explain its topical effects in the treatment of rheumatism; rutin is a counterirritant or rubefacient.

USES
Used to treat respiratory problems, such as bronchitis, asthma, cold, flu, cough, and tuberculosis. Also used to treat constipation and blood disorders.

In homeopathic medicine, used to treat rheumatism, gout, blood disorders, eczema, and psoriasis.

DOSAGE & ADMINISTRATION
Dried herb: 1 to 5 g t.i.d.
Fluidextract (1:1 in 25% alcohol): 1 to 5 ml t.i.d.
Ointment (1:5 in a lard or paraffin base): External use only for eczema and psoriasis.
Tea: Made from ½ to 1 teaspoon dried herb.
Tincture (1:5 in 45% alcohol): 2 to 10 ml t.i.d.

ADVERSE REACTIONS
CNS: paralysis (from large amounts).

INTERACTIONS
Herb-drug. *Disulfiram:* Herbal products prepared with alcohol may cause a disulfiram-like reaction. Discourage use together.

EFFECTS ON LAB TEST RESULTS
None reported.

CAUTIONS
Patients sensitive to the herb or its components should avoid use. Patients with chronic renal failure or heart failure and those taking potassium or phosphorus supplements should avoid use because chickweed contains high amounts of potassium and phosphorus.

Pregnant and breast-feeding women should avoid ingesting amounts larger than those found in food.

NURSING CONSIDERATIONS
- Explore patient's knowledge of this herb.

---

*Liquid contains alcohol.

• Consuming excessive amounts of chickweed may cause nitrate poisoning.
• Monitor patient for hypersensitivity reaction.
• If patient is also taking a cardiac drug, monitor his electrolyte levels.

PATIENT TEACHING
• Advise patient to consult a health care provider before using herbal therapy because a treatment that has been proven effective may already be available.
• Tell patient when filling a new prescription he should inform pharmacist of any herbal or dietary supplement he's taking.
• Warn patient not to postpone seeking medical evaluation because doing so may delay diagnosis of a potentially serious medical condition.
• Advise patient to promptly report adverse reactions and new signs or symptoms.
• Advise patient not to consume excessive amounts of chickweed because it may cause nitrate poisoning.

chicory

Cichorium intybus, blue sailor's succory, hendibeh, succory, wild chicory, wild succory

Common trade names
Chicory

AVAILABLE FORMS
Available as fresh and dried leaves, stems, and roots as well as dry root stock.

ACTIONS & COMPONENTS
Choriin, a 6,7 hydroxycoumarin derivative, is a pharmacologically active component. Lactucin, a bitter component, may be responsible for chicory's sedative effects and ability to counteract the effects of caffeine. Other bitter substances—such as intybin, fructose, and inulin—may be responsible for chicory's actions on the GI tract as a digestive tonic. Inulin also has quinidine-like effects.

USES
Used as a sedative, mild diuretic, laxative, and digestive agent to manage indigestion or dyspepsia. Also used as a salad green.

Used in the past to treat cardiac arrhythmias. Being studied for effects in preventing colon cancer.

DOSAGE & ADMINISTRATION
Comminuted drug: 3 to 5 g.
Decoction: Prepared by adding 1 teaspoon rootstock to ½ cup cold water; mixture is then boiled and strained. Dosage is 1 to 1½ cups P.O. daily (1 mouthful at a time).
Infusion, tea: Prepared by steeping 2 to 4 g of whole herb in 7 ounces of boiling water for 10 minutes, and then straining.

ADVERSE REACTIONS
CNS: sedation.
CV: lower heart rate.
Respiratory: asthma.
Skin: contact dermatitis.
Other: allergic toxic reaction.

INTERACTIONS
None reported; however, herb has cardioactive effects and may inter-

---

Bold italic type indicates that reaction may be life-threatening.

act with drugs affecting heart rate, heart rhythm, or blood pressure.

EFFECTS ON LAB TEST RESULTS
• May alter anticoagulation study results.

CAUTIONS
Patients sensitive to chicory and pregnant patients should avoid use.

Patients sensitive to ragweed, chrysanthemums, marigolds, or daisies should use cautiously.

NURSING CONSIDERATIONS
• Explore patient's knowledge of this herb.
🖉**ALERT:** Some commercially prepared chicory products may contain crushed cashew shells, which can cause an allergic reaction similar to poison ivy.
• Chicory is generally recognized as safe. Monitor blood pressure and heart rate in those using it for its therapeutic effects.
• If patient is also taking warfarin, monitor INR.
• Handling chicory can cause contact dermatitis.

PATIENT TEACHING
• Advise patient to consult a health care provider before using an herbal preparation because another treatment may be available.
• Tell patient when filling a new prescription he should inform pharmacist of any herbal or dietary supplement he's taking.
• Advise patient to immediately report any heart abnormalities to his health care provider.

• Advise patient to watch for adverse reactions, especially sedation and skin irritation.
• Warn patient not to perform activities that require mental alertness until he knows how the herb affects his CNS.

Chinese cucumber

Trichosanthes kirilowii, alpha-trichosanthin, Chinese snake gourd, compound Q, GLQ 223, gua louren seed, gualoupi (fruit peel), gualouzi (seed), snakegourd fruit, tian-hua-fen (root)

Common trade names
None known

AVAILABLE FORMS
Available as dry ripe fruit, dry seeds, dry roots, fresh roots, dry fruit peel, and purified trichosanthin.

ACTIONS & COMPONENTS
Chinese cucumber juice contains trichosanthin and karasurin, which are abortifacient proteins. The purified protein alpha-trichosanthin from the root of Chinese cucumber is cytotoxic to some HIV-infected macrophage and monocytes and may increase CD_4 cell counts in AIDS patients. Trichosanthin may be useful in treating lymphomas and leukemias by helping to kill leukemia-lymphoma cells.

The herb may have antitumorigenic and anti-inflammatory effects.

USES
Used to treat invasive moles.

---

*Liquid contains alcohol.

In traditional Chinese medicine, herb is used with other drugs to treat fever, dry and productive cough, mastitis, angina, constipation, lung abscess, and appendicitis.

DOSAGE & ADMINISTRATION
To treat fever, congestion, or constipation: 9 to 15 g of dried fruit.

ADVERSE REACTIONS
CNS: cerebral edema, *cerebral hemorrhage, seizures.*
CV: myocardial damage.
GI: nausea, vomiting.
Hematologic: blood cell damage.
Respiratory: *acute pulmonary edema.*
Other: *fatal anaphylactoid reactions, prolonged anaphylactoid reactions,* including fever, follicular atresia, ovulation changes.

INTERACTIONS
Herb-drug. *Antidiabetics:* Causes additive hypoglycemic effects. Advise diabetic patients to avoid use.

EFFECTS ON LAB TEST RESULTS
• May decrease hormone levels.
• May increase or decrease CBC.

CAUTIONS
Patients sensitive to Chinese cucumber, pregnant patients, and those planning a pregnancy should avoid use.

Cancer patients and those receiving immunosuppressants should use herb cautiously.

NURSING CONSIDERATIONS
• Explore patient's knowledge of this herb.
ALERT: This herb is used by some HIV-positive patients as ad-

junctive treatment. However, the extracts can be extremely toxic and should be used only under the direction of a knowledgeable practitioner.
• Monitor patient closely for hypersensitivity reactions and mental status changes. Effects may occur more than a decade after a trichosanthin injection.
• Monitor CBC closely at regular intervals.
• If patient is receiving an antidiabetic or another herb that could cause hypoglycemic additive effects, monitor blood glucose level.
• Chinese cucumber may interfere with the intended therapeutic effect of conventional drugs.
• The herb is also being studied as a possible treatment for AIDS infections.

PATIENT TEACHING
• Advise patient to consult a health care provider before using an herbal preparation because another treatment may be available.
• Tell patient that when filling a new prescription he should inform pharmacist of any herbal or dietary supplement he's taking.
• If patient is pregnant, advise her to avoid all contact with Chinese cucumber.
• Warn patient that extracts of Chinese cucumber are extremely toxic.
• Advise patient never to ingest this product unless under the supervision of a qualified health care provider.
• Instruct patient to immediately report to his health care provider any shortness of breath or severe headache.

Bold italic type indicates that reaction may be life-threatening.

• Advise patient that he should follow up regularly with his health care provider to evaluate the effectiveness of therapy.

Chinese rhubarb

Rheum officinale, R. palmatum, R. tanguitcum, Canton rhubarb, China rhubarb, chong-gi-huang, da-huang, daio, Himalayan rhubarb, Indian rhubarb, Japanese rhubarb, medicinal rhubarb, racine de rhubarbee, rhabarber, rhubarb, rhubarb root, Russian rhubarb, Shenshi rhubarb, tai huang, Turkey rhubarb

Common trade names
Phytoestrol N
Combination products:
Abdominolon, Certobil, Cholaflux, Colax, Compound Fix Elixir, Dragees Laxatives, Enteroton, Fam-Lax, Herbalax, Herbal Laxative, Neo-Cleanse, New Lax, Plantago Complex, Tisana Arnaldi, Vegebyl

AVAILABLE FORMS
Available as dry roots, stem parts, bark, and powder.

ACTIONS & COMPONENTS
Contains the anthraquinone rhein, so higher doses have a stimulant laxative effect similar to that of cascara and senna. In contrast, lower doses have antidiarrheal effects because tannins in the herb have astringent effects; Chinese rhubarb contains between 5% and 10% tannins. Laxative effects generally occur 6 to 10 hours after ingestion.

May also increase cardiac contractility, with the polysaccharides inhibiting calcium influx in the myocardium, as well as slow the progression of diabetic nephropathy and chronic renal failure. It may lower proteinuria, heal GI bleeding ulcers, and have antiviral, antibacterial, antineoplastic, and diuretic effects. The anthraquinones rhein and emodin may inhibit growth of *Staphylococcus aureus.*

USES
Used to treat jaundice, kidney stones, gout, headache, toothache, renal failure, and skin and mucous membrane inflammation. Also used to heal skin sores and scabs.

German Commission E has approved the herb as a treatment for constipation; lower dosages are used to treat diarrhea.

In traditional Chinese medicine, the herb is used to treat delirium, edema, amenorrhea, and abdominal pain.

DOSAGE & ADMINISTRATION
To treat constipation: 20 to 30 mg of rhein (1.2 g of whole roots and stem of Chinese rhubarb) as a single daily dose for a maximum of 14 days. Or, 1 teaspoon of powdered root boiled in 1 cup of water for 10 minutes, taken 1 tablespoon at a time, up to 1 cup daily. Or, ½ to 1 teaspoon of tincture daily.
To treat diarrhea: ¼ to ½ teaspoon of powdered root boiled in 1 cup of water for 10 minutes, taken 1 tablespoon at a time, up to 1 cup daily. Or, ¼ teaspoon of tincture daily.

*Liquid contains alcohol.

To treat toothache: Tincture is applied by cotton swab directly to the painful tooth.

ADVERSE REACTIONS

GI: abdominal cramping, diarrhea, nausea, vomiting, reduced gastric motility, pigmentation of the intestinal mucosa.

GU: kidney stones, hematuria, discolored urine.

Metabolic: dehydration, hypokalemia, electrolyte imbalance.

Musculoskeletal: weakness.

INTERACTIONS

Herb-drug. *Calcium:* May cause kidney stones. Discourage use together.

Corticosteroids, potassium-wasting diuretics: May increase risk of hypokalemia. Monitor patient and potassium level closely.

Digoxin, other antiarrhythmics: May increase the cardiac toxicity of these drugs as a result of potassium loss and effects on drug absorption. Discourage use together.

Laxatives: May potentiate drug effects. Discourage use together.

Vitamin K: May potentiate the anticoagulant effect by reducing absorption of vitamin K. Discourage use together.

EFFECTS ON LAB TEST RESULTS

• May decrease potassium level.

CAUTIONS

Patients sensitive to the herb or its components, pregnant patients, breast-feeding patients, and children should avoid use. Patients with intestinal obstruction or ileus; appendicitis, chronic intestinal inflammation such as gastric duodenal ulcer, Crohn's disease, or ulcerative colitis; abdominal pain of unknown origin; or a history of kidney stones should also avoid using this herb.

NURSING CONSIDERATIONS

• Explore patient's knowledge of this herb.

• Oral ingestion of Chinese rhubarb may cause hypokalemia. Monitor levels of potassium and other electrolytes carefully.

• Lazy bowel syndrome may develop with prolonged use.

• If patient is also taking digoxin or another antiarrhythmic, monitor ECG results for cardiac toxicity.

• If patient is also taking an anticoagulant, watch his INR closely.

• Patient may experience red or bright yellow discoloration of urine.

• Use of Chinese rhubarb may interfere with diagnostic urine tests.

PATIENT TEACHING

• Advise patient to consult a health care provider before using an herbal preparation because another treatment may be available.

• Tell patient that when filling a new prescription he should inform pharmacist of any herbal or dietary supplement he's taking.

⚠ **ALERT:** Caution patient against using the leaf of Chinese rhubarb because it's extremely toxic.

• If patient has a medical condition such as small bowel disease, a stomach ulcer, or heart disease, advise him not to use Chinese rhubarb.

• If patient is taking digoxin, warfarin, a corticosteroid, or a diuretic, tell him to notify his health care provider before using Chinese rhubarb.

• Although Chinese rhubarb has been used to treat constipation, instruct patient not to take it without medical advice and even then to only use it when needed, to help reduce the chance of low blood levels of potassium.

• Advise patient to use only the smallest possible dose to achieve therapeutic effect.

• Instruct patient not to take Chinese rhubarb for longer than 10 days.

• Warn patient about laxative dependency.

cinnamon

Cinnamomum verum

Common trade names
Ceylon Cinnamon, Cinnamomon, Cinnamon

AVAILABLE FORMS
Available as tea and tincture*, essential oil, bulk herb (bark) and powder.

ACTIONS & COMPONENTS
The medicinal source of the herb is the oil extracted from the bark, the bark of young trees, and the leaf. Cinnamaldehyde accounts for 65% to 80% of the herb. This essential oil possesses analgesic, antifungal, and antidiarrheal effects. Specifically, the essential oils from cinnamon bark are active against *Aspergillus* species and inhibit aflatoxin growth.

USES
Used to treat loss of appetite, GI upset, bloating, flatulence, infections, fever, colds, dysmenorrhea, minor cuts and abrasions, and diarrhea.

DOSAGE & ADMINISTRATION
Essential oil: 0.05 to 0.2 g daily p.r.n.
Tea: Prepared by steeping 0.5 to 1 g of bark into 7 ounces of boiling water for 5 to 10 minutes, and then straining. Dosage is 1 cup of tea P.O.; daily dosage of bark is 2 to 4 g.
Tincture: Prepared by moistening 200 parts cinnamon bark evenly with ethanol and percolate to produce 1,000 parts tincture. Daily dosage of tincture is 2 to 4 ml t.i.d.

ADVERSE REACTIONS
CNS: sedation, sleepiness, depression.
CV: tachycardia.
EENT: oral lesions (with chronic use).
GI: increased intestinal movement, nausea, vomiting, *liver damage.*
GU: *renal damage.*
Respiratory: tachypnea.
Skin: allergic reactions of skin and mucosa, skin irritation, pruritus, increased perspiration.

INTERACTIONS
Herb-drug. *Warfarin:* The oil contains trace amounts of coumarin. If patient is also taking warfarin, monitor him for bleeding. Dosage adjustments may be needed.

EFFECTS ON LAB TEST RESULTS
• May increase PT and INR.

---

*Liquid contains alcohol.

CAUTIONS
Patients allergic to cinnamon or Peruvian balsam, pregnant and breast-feeding patients, and those planning a pregnancy should avoid use. Patients who have GI conditions, including ulcers, should avoid using cinnamon for therapeutic purposes because it may irritate the GI tract.

NURSING CONSIDERATIONS
• Explore patient's knowledge of this herb.
• Cinnamon may cause an allergic skin reaction.

PATIENT TEACHING
• Advise patient to consult a health care provider before using an herbal preparation because another treatment may be available.
• Tell patient when filling a new prescription he should inform pharmacist of any herbal or dietary supplement he's taking.
• If patient is pregnant or is planning pregnancy, advise her not to use cinnamon medicinally.
• If patient is taking warfarin, advise him to check with a health care provider before using cinnamon medicinally.
• Advise patient to stop using cinnamon and to promptly contact his health care provider if he experiences stomach upset, diarrhea, or signs of bleeding.
• Instruct patient to promptly report adverse reactions and new signs or symptoms.

clary

Salvia sclarea

Common trade names
Clarry, Clary Sage, Clear Eye, Essential Oil Clary Sage, Eye Bright, Muscatel Sage, Orvale, See Bright

AVAILABLE FORMS
Available as oil distilled from the flowering tops and leaves of the plant.

ACTIONS & COMPONENTS
Yields an essential oil that is made up largely of alcohols and up to 75% linalyl acetate, linlol, pinene, myrcene, and phellandrene. May have muscle relaxant, analgesic, anxiolytic, and some antiestrogenic effects.

USES
Used to treat mental fatigue, depression, anxiety, tension, and migraine. Used as an astringent, antiinflammatory, and antispasmodic. Also used to help restore hormonal balance and relieve symptoms of premenstrual syndrome or menopause and to treat sore throats, halitosis, and toothaches. Also used as an insect repellent.

The essential oil is used as a decoction, tincture, and topical agent; in aromatherapy it's also used for baths, sprays, diffusers, and massages. Seeds are used in clearing eye of debris. Used rarely in kidney disease.

Bold italic type indicates that reaction may be life-threatening.

DOSAGE & ADMINISTRATION
Atomizer: 8 gtt of the essential oil added to 1 ounce of water in an atomizer.
Bath: 8 gtt of the essential oil blended with 1 tablespoon of unscented bath oil or water and stirred well to disperse oil.
Diffuser: 6 to 10 gtt of the essential oil added to 2 tablespoons water in diffuser bowl.

ADVERSE REACTIONS
None known.

INTERACTIONS
Herb-lifestyle. *Alcohol use:* Use with this essential oil may result in enhanced sedation. Discourage use together.

EFFECTS ON LAB TEST RESULTS
None reported.

CAUTIONS
Pregnant and breast-feeding patients and those planning a pregnancy should avoid use.
Patients who have breast cysts, uterine fibroids, or other estrogen-related disorders should avoid long-term use.

NURSING CONSIDERATIONS
• Explore patient's knowledge of this herb.
• Clary is intended primarily for aromatherapy use.
☑ALERT: This essential oil is for external use only.

PATIENT TEACHING
• Advise patient to consult a health care provider before using an herbal preparation because another treatment may be available.

• Tell patient that when filling a new prescription he should inform pharmacist of any herbal or dietary supplement he's taking.
• Warn patient not to treat migraine, depression, or anxiety with clary before seeking medical evaluation because doing so may delay diagnosis of a potentially serious medical condition.
• Advise patients who are pregnant, planning pregnancy, or are breast-feeding not to use the essential oil.
• If patient is taking estrogen, instruct her to inform her health care provider before using herb.
• Warn patient that the essential oil is for external use only.
• Tell patient not to apply undiluted essential oils to skin.

clove oil

Syzygium aromaticum

Common trade names
Caryophyllus, Clove Buds, Clove Oil

AVAILABLE FORMS
Available for topical use or as a mouthwash or toothpaste. Also in cigarettes.

ACTIONS & COMPONENTS
The medicinal action of clove oil comes from dried, powdered flower buds. The chief components of clove are the volatile oils eugenol (85%), eugenyl acetate, and beta-caryophyllene (5% to 8%).
The eugenyl acetate component has antihistaminic and spasmolytic properties. Eugenol suppresses the pain pathways and may also inhibit

prostaglandin and leukotriene biosynthesis by inhibiting cyclo-oxygenase and lipoxygenase.

Clove oil inhibits gram-positive and gram-negative bacteria and may also have fungistatic, anthelmintic, and larvicidal effects.

USES
Used as a dental analgesic and antiseptic. Also used to inhibit platelet aggregation and as an antipyretic.

Clove oil is used to relieve signs and symptoms of the common cold and to treat coughs, bronchitis, inflammation of the mouth and pharynx, and infections.

DOSAGE & ADMINISTRATION
As mouthwash: Aqueous solutions equal to 1% to 5% essential oil used as a rinse.
As toothpaste: One to three times daily p.r.n.
For toothache: Cotton is dipped into undiluted oil and then applied topically to area of tooth pain.

ADVERSE REACTIONS
CNS: depression.
Hematologic: *DIC.*
Hepatic: *liver failure.*
Respiratory: *pulmonary toxicity*, blood-tinged sputum.
Skin: irritation of skin and mucous membranes.
Other: toxic reaction.

INTERACTIONS
Herb-drug. *Anticoagulants, platelet aggregation inhibitors:* May increase drug effects. Discourage use together.

EFFECTS ON LAB TEST RESULTS
• May increase or decrease electrolyte levels.
• May increase liver function test values.

CAUTIONS
Children shouldn't use clove oil.

NURSING CONSIDERATIONS
• Explore patient's knowledge of this herb.
• Allergic reactions to clove oil are rare.
• Inspect patient's gums and mucous membranes for signs of local irritation.

PATIENT TEACHING
• Advise patient to consult a health care provider before using an herbal preparation because another treatment may be available.
• Tell patient that when filling a new prescription he should inform pharmacist of any herbal or dietary supplement he's taking.
• Warn patient of the risks of using clove oil and of its potential for altering the effects of conventional drugs.
• Tell patient not to use herb if he's also taking blood thinners because bleeding may occur.
• Tell patient that undiluted oil shouldn't be swallowed.
• Instruct patient to stop using clove oil if adverse reactions or local irritation occurs. Discourage use in patient who's allergic to herb.
• Tell patient that clove cigarettes act as a local anesthetic and may numb the throat.

Bold italic type indicates that reaction may be life-threatening.

coffee

Coffea arabica, Arabian coffee, caffea, java

Common trade names
Chock Full O'Nuts, Folgers, Maxwell House

AVAILABLE FORMS
Available as dried, freeze-dried, or ground beans.

ACTIONS & COMPONENTS
Medicinal components of coffee come from the seeds, or beans. The coffee seeds contain 1% to 2% caffeine, 0.25% trigonelline, 3% to 5% tannins, 15% glucose and dextrin, 10% to 13% fatty oil (trioleoyl glycerol and tripalmitoyl glycerol), and 10% to 13% proteins.

Caffeine is the active component of coffee and acts as a CNS stimulant. Caffeine has positive inotropic and chronic effects on the heart, may increase gastric secretions, and may relax smooth muscles of the blood vessels and the bronchioles of the respiratory tract. Caffeine may also increase lowdensity lipoprotein (LDL) and total cholesterol levels in those consuming more than 5 cups of coffee per day.

USES
Used most notably for its stimulant effects and for its ability to relieve malaise and weariness. Also used for its diuretic and antiinflammatory effects. May also be used as a laxative.

Spray-dried crystals are used for instant coffee. Coffee grounds are used in enema form to dilate bile ducts or improve gallbladder function.

DOSAGE & ADMINISTRATION
Oral use: Maximum daily dose shouldn't exceed 1.5 g/day, although nonpregnant adults should limit caffeine intake to less than 250 mg/day. Many health care providers advise pregnant patients to limit coffee intake to 1 cup/day (1 cup brewed coffee contains 100 to 150 mg caffeine).

ADVERSE REACTIONS
CNS: anxiety, insomnia, irritability, nervousness, dizziness, headache.
CV: hypertension, tachycardia, palpitations, irregular heart rate.
GI: ulcers, heartburn, vomiting, diarrhea, loss of appetite, abdominal spasms.
Metabolic: hyperglycemia, increased excretion of calcium.
Musculoskeletal: stiffness, muscle spasms.
Respiratory: tachypnea.

INTERACTIONS
Herb-drug. *Benzodiazepines:* Reduces sedative effects. Discourage use together.
Beta blockers (metoprolol, propranolol): Slightly increases blood pressure. Discourage use together.
Oral drugs: Coffee charcoal compound may interfere with the absorption of other drugs. Monitor patient for lack of therapeutic effect.

---

*Liquid contains alcohol.

Theophylline: May potentiate the adverse effects of drug and increase jitteriness. Monitor patient closely, and advise him to avoid excessive use.

EFFECTS ON LAB TEST RESULTS
• May increase total cholesterol, LDL, and glucose levels. May decrease calcium level.

CAUTIONS
Pregnant patients and breast-feeding patients, those planning a pregnancy, and those with ulcers, chronic digestive disorders, hypertension, or heart disease should avoid coffee.

NURSING CONSIDERATIONS
• Explore patient's knowledge of this herb.
⚡**ALERT:** Although lethal overdose is unlikely, the first signs and symptoms of poisoning are vomiting and abdominal spasms.
• Caffeine is believed to increase the risk of late first- and second-trimester miscarriages.
• Caffeine consumed by a breast-feeding mother can cause sleep disorders in her infant.
• Sustained intake of coffee can lead to physical dependence.
• Withdrawal symptoms include headache and sleep disorders.

PATIENT TEACHING
• Advise patient to consult a health care provider before using an herbal preparation because another treatment may be available.
• Tell patient that when filling a new prescription he should inform pharmacist of any herbal or dietary supplement he's taking.

• Advise patient with risk factors for heart disease (that is, high cholesterol level or high blood pressure) to discuss caffeine consumption with his health care provider.
• Advise patient to inform his health care provider if he experiences sleeping problems or stomach irritation.
• Advise patient who is pregnant, breast-feeding, or planning pregnancy to consider avoiding or limiting her caffeine intake.
• Discuss potential adverse effects with patient and instruct him to promptly report signs and symptoms.
• Tell patient to limit intake of coffee to 4 cups or fewer daily to avoid risk of increasing LDL cholesterol levels.

cola

Sterculia acuminata, bissy nut, cola accuminata, cola nut, cola seeds, guru nut, kola nuts, kola seeds, kola tree

Common trade names
Alert

AVAILABLE FORMS
Available as liquid extract*, cola nut, cola extract, tea, tincture, and wine.

ACTIONS & COMPONENTS
Medicinal properties are found in the plant's seed. Contains theobromine, theophylline, and 0.6% to 3.7% caffeine—all of which are CNS stimulants.
    Cola also has a diuretic effect, stimulates gastric acid production and gastric motility, and has mild

---

Bold italic type indicates that reaction may be life-threatening.

chronotropic activity. Cola may contain potentially carcinogenic primary and secondary amines as well as tannins.

USES
Used as a stimulant to counteract mental and physical fatigue. Cola seeds are chewed to suppress hunger, thirst, morning sickness, and migraines.

DOSAGE & ADMINISTRATION
Cola extract: 0.25 to 0.75 g daily.
Cola nut: 2 to 6 g daily.
Liquid extract: 2.5 to 7.5 g daily.
Tea: 1 to 2 g of cola nut can be taken t.i.d.
Tincture: 10 to 30 g daily.
Wine: 60 to 180 g daily.

ADVERSE REACTIONS
CNS: insomnia, restlessness, nervousness, excitability, paranoia.
CV: tachycardia, palpitations, elevated blood pressure.
GI: gastric irritation.

INTERACTIONS
Herb-drug. *Beta agonists, such as albuterol, metaproterenol, salmeterol, and terbutaline:* Increases cardiac stimulation. Discourage use together.
CNS stimulants, such as pseudoephedrine; decongestants: Increases cardiac and CNS stimulation. Discourage use together.
Diuretics: Enhances diuretic effect. Monitor fluid status to avoid potential dehydration.
Lithium: May increase lithium levels if caffeine intake alters during lithium therapy. Abrupt caffeine withdrawal can increase the risk of lithium toxicity. Recommend consistent intake of caffeine-containing products during lithium therapy.
MAO inhibitors: Excessive amounts of caffeine can trigger hypertensive crisis. Recommend avoiding caffeine-containing products during MAO inhibitor therapy.
Quinolone antibiotics: May decrease caffeine clearance, increasing adverse effects such as elevated blood pressure and heart rate and excessive CNS stimulation. Recommend limiting intake of herb during treatment with a quinolone antibiotic.
Theophylline: Enhances adverse effects. Monitor patient for signs of excessive CNS stimulation and advise him to avoid using drug and herb at the same time.
Herb-food. *Caffeine-containing products:* Enhances adverse effects. Advise patient to limit daily sources of caffeine, particularly if he has a history of CV disease.
Grapefruit juice: May increase caffeine levels, increasing risk of adverse effects. Recommend avoiding grapefruit juice altogether or maintaining a consistent intake.

EFFECTS ON LAB TEST RESULTS
None reported.

CAUTIONS
Patients with underlying cardiac disease or renal insufficiency, geriatric patients, and those with a history of gastric or duodenal ulcers should avoid use. Pregnant and breast-feeding patients should limit use.

---

*Liquid contains alcohol.

Patients with renal dysfunction should use cola cautiously.

NURSING CONSIDERATIONS
- Explore patient's knowledge of this herb.
- Monitor heart rate and blood pressure for increases.
- The diuretic effect of excessive cola may result in dehydration.
- Observe for signs of excess CNS stimulation. Before using a drug to treat symptoms of excitability such as insomnia, check to see if the patient should simply decrease his intake of cola.
- Because some preparations contain significant amounts of alcohol, they should be avoided by children, alcoholic patients, patients with liver disease, patients receiving metronidazole or disulfiram, and pregnant and breast-feeding patients.
- Abrupt discontinuation can sometimes lead to physical withdrawal symptoms, including headaches, irritability, dizziness, and anxiety. Monitor patient for these signs and symptoms.
- Geriatric patients may be especially prone to adverse cardiac and CNS effects.

PATIENT TEACHING
- Advise patient to consult a health care provider before using an herbal preparation because another treatment may be available.
- Tell patient that when filling new prescription he should inform pharmacist of any herbal or dietary supplement he's taking.
- Advise patient to limit his sources of caffeine in order to avoid excessive stimulation of heart and CNS.
- Advise patients to avoid cola preparations if they have high blood pressure or heart disease, or if they are pregnant or breast-feeding.
- Advise patient to consult his health care provider if he experiences palpitations or dyspepsia.
- Tell patient to inform all his health care providers about his use of cola.
- Instruct patient and family to avoid using cola preparations with alcohol in children, those with a history of alcohol abuse or liver disease, and those taking disulfiram or metronidazole.
- Advise patient that yellow staining of the lining of the mouth is associated with chewing cola nuts.

coltsfoot

Tussilago farfara, ass's foot, British tobacco, bullsfoot, butterbur, coughwort, donnhove, farfarae folium, fieldhove, flower velure, foal's-foot, foalswort, hallfoot, horsefoot, horsehoof, kuandong hua

Common trade names
Coltsfoot Leaf, Coltsfoot Tea

AVAILABLE FORMS
Available as bulk leaf, capsules, leaf extract*, tincture*, and tea.
Capsules: 50 to 100 mg of coltsfoot combined with other natural products
Leaf extract: 1:1 strength
Tincture: 1:5 strength

Bold italic type indicates that reaction may be life-threatening.

ACTIONS & COMPONENTS

Contains 5% to 10% mucilage, which may produce a soothing effect by physically coating the irritated mucosa of the mouth and throat. The plant's polysaccharides, flavonoids, and phenolic components may have anti-inflammatory and antibacterial activity. The plant also contains tussilagone, a sesquiterpene thought to have CV and respiratory stimulant properties, and a number of pyrrolizidine alkaloids (primarily senkirkine and senecionine) that are converted to toxic metabolites in the liver and cause liver toxicity.

The dried leaf is most commonly used for medicinal purposes. Although the flower also contains medicinal components, it has higher levels of pyrrolizidine alkaloids.

USES

Used to soothe throat irritation and mild inflammations of the mouth and throat, to alleviate cough, and to treat symptoms of respiratory infections, acute and chronic bronchitis, laryngitis, asthma, colds, and emphysema. Also used as a smoking mixture.

DOSAGE & ADMINISTRATION

Extract: 0.6 to 2 ml t.i.d. Daily dose shouldn't exceed 1 mcg of pyrrolizidine alkaloids with a 1,2 necine structure.
Tea: Prepared by adding 1.5 to 2.5 g of cut leaf to boiling water. Taken P.O. several times a day. Dose shouldn't exceed 6 g/day, or 10 mcg of pyrrolizidine alkaloids with a 1,2 necine structure.
Tincture: 2 to 8 ml t.i.d.

ADVERSE REACTIONS

CNS: lethargy.
GI: anorexia, abdominal pain and swelling, nausea, vomiting, right upper quadrant pain.
Hepatic: *hepatotoxicity,* liver changes, reversible hepatic veno-occlusive disease, jaundice.
Other: allergic reaction, *cancer.*

INTERACTIONS

Herb-drug. *Antihypertensives, cardiac drugs:* Excessive consumption of coltsfoot may interfere with these drug therapies. Discourage use together.
Disulfiram, metronidazole: Herbal products prepared with alcohol may cause a disulfiram-like reaction. Discourage use together.

EFFECTS ON LAB TEST RESULTS

• May increase liver function test values.

CAUTIONS

Pregnant and breast-feeding patients should avoid this herb because of its abortifacient effects. Patients with underlying liver disease should avoid use because of the herb's hepatotoxic effects. Patients with a history of heart disease, circulatory problems, alcohol abuse, or liver disease and those allergic to ragweed or other members of the Asteraceae family should also avoid use.

Patients taking an antihypertensive should use coltsfoot cautiously.

Internal use isn't recommended because of increased incidence of liver damage and cancerous liver tumors.

*Liquid contains alcohol.

This herb shouldn't be used consecutively for longer than 1 month without the advice of a knowledgeable health care provider.

NURSING CONSIDERATIONS
• Explore patient's knowledge of this herb.
• Consider recommending alternative therapies that don't have severe adverse effects, such as OTC lozenges or sprays.
• Many countries have banned the internal use of other herbal products containing pyrrolizidine alkaloids because of the risk of liver toxicity.
• Some extracts may contain up to 45% alcohol, so children, alcoholic patients, those with liver disease, and those receiving metronidazole or disulfiram should avoid them.
• Some of coltsfoot's components may antagonize the effect of antihypertensives on blood pressure.
• Those with an allergy to plants in the Asteraceae family (such as ragweed, marigolds, daisies, and chrysanthemums) may experience hypersensitivity reactions to coltsfoot.
• The active ingredient (mucilage) is destroyed when burned.
• Monitor blood pressure and liver function test results, and watch for signs and symptoms of liver dysfunction, such as right upper quadrant pain, nausea, vomiting, abdominal distention, and jaundice.
• Regardless of the preparation used, therapy should last no longer than 4 to 6 weeks per year, to prevent exposure to large amounts of pyrrolizidine alkaloids.

PATIENT TEACHING
• Advise patient to consult a health care provider before using an herbal preparation because another treatment may be available.
• Tell patient that when filling a new prescription he should inform pharmacist of any herbal or dietary supplement he's taking.
• Caution patients taking metronidazole or disulfiram to avoid using coltsfoot.
• Advise patients who have cancer or are undergoing chemotherapy to avoid using this herb.
• Advise patients who are pregnant, breast-feeding, or planning pregnancy not to use this herb.
• Discuss with patient other OTC products, such as lozenges, that may be safer to use.
• Caution patients that manufacturers don't report the pyrrolizidine alkaloid content of their products, making it difficult to determine the exact dose being ingested.
• Inform patient that coltsfoot shouldn't be used for longer than 4 to 6 weeks per year.
• Warn patient that use in higher doses or for longer than recommended may increase the risk of liver toxicity and malignancy.
• Instruct patient to report any signs or symptoms of liver toxicity, such as nausea, vomiting, right upper quadrant pain, and jaundice.

Bold italic type indicates that reaction may be life-threatening.

comfrey

Symphytum officinale, ass ear, black root, blackwort, boneset, bruisewort, consound, gum plant, healing herb, knitback, knitbone, Russian comfrey, salsify, slippery root, wallwort

Common trade names
Comfree, Comfrey Leaf, Comfrey Root

AVAILABLE FORMS
Available as alcohol-free root extract, capsules, compounded oil, cream, leaf extract*, ointment, and root extract*.
Capsules: 50 mg, 100 mg, and 225 mg, along with other natural products
Compounded oil: Contains multiple herbal components along with comfrey
Cream, ointment: Contains 5% to 20% leaf or root extract, for external use
Leaf extract:* 1:1.5 strength; 25 mg/ml with 35% to 40% grain alcohol

ACTIONS & COMPONENTS
Medicinal products are derived from the fresh or dried root and leaves of *S. officinale.* The leaves and roots from Russian or prickly comfrey (a hybrid between *S. officinale* and *S. asperum)* also are used.
The medicinal effect may result from the allantoin content of this herb, which promotes cell proliferation and enhances wound healing. The roots contain more allantoin (0.6% to 0.7%) than the leaves (0.3%). Other components include

rosmarinic acid—also believed to have anti-inflammatory properties—mucilage, and numerous pyrrolizidine alkaloids. Pyrrolizidine alkaloids are converted in the liver to toxic metabolites that have been linked to hepatotoxicity. The root contains a higher amount of pyrrolizidine alkaloids than the leaves.
Russian comfrey also contains echimidine, which may be the most toxic pyrrolizidine alkaloid found in this herb.

USES
Used to help heal wounds and to treat bruises, sprains, eczema, psoriasis, insect bites, joint inflammation, and swelling.

DOSAGE & ADMINISTRATION
External use: Ointments and other external preparations containing 5% to 20% dried herb should be applied topically to intact skin with the daily dose not exceeding 100 mcg of pyrrolizidine alkaloids with 1,2 unsaturated necine structure.
Note: Internal use has been banned by the FDA.

ADVERSE REACTIONS
GI: *pancreatic islet cell tumors.*
GU: *urinary bladder tumors.*
Hepatic: *hepatotoxicity,* liver damage, veno-occlusive disease.
Other: *cancer.*

INTERACTIONS
Herb-drug. *Disulfiram:* Herbal products prepared with alcohol may cause a disulfiram-like reaction. Discourage use together.

*Liquid contains alcohol.

EFFECTS ON LAB TEST RESULTS
• May increase liver function test values.

CAUTIONS
Pregnant and breast-feeding patients, those planning a pregnancy, and those with a history of alcohol abuse or liver disease should avoid this herb.

NURSING CONSIDERATIONS
• Explore patient's knowledge of this herb.
⚡ALERT: Comfrey preparations have been identified as potentially harmful because of reported liver toxicity, according to several agencies, including the *U. S. Pharmacopoeia*'s expert advisory panel and the American Herbal Products Association. Many countries have banned internal use of comfrey, so such use is highly discouraged. The FDA also has banned internal use.
• Some comfrey preparations may contain significant levels of alcohol, so children, alcoholic patients, those with liver disease, and those receiving metronidazole or disulfiram should avoid them.
• Infants may be more susceptible to hepatic veno-occlusive disease.
• Patients who ingest comfrey should be monitored for signs and symptoms of hepatotoxicity, including abdominal distention, nausea, and abdominal pain, and elevated liver function test values.
• If patient is using comfrey to promote wound healing, monitor the wound being treated. Evaluate the possibility of an infectious cause of cellulitis and inflammation.

• Use of comfrey should be limited to 4 to 6 weeks per year, to prevent exposure to large amounts of pyrrolizidine alkaloids.

PATIENT TEACHING
• Advise patient to consult a health care provider before using an herbal preparation because another treatment may be available.
• Tell patient that when filling a new prescription he should inform pharmacist of any herbal or dietary supplement he's taking.
• Caution patients who are pregnant, breast-feeding, or planning to get pregnant not to use comfrey.
• Advise patient that the internal use of comfrey isn't recommended and should be avoided.
• Inform patient that external preparations shouldn't be applied to broken skin.
⚡ALERT: Advise patient that many comfrey preparations don't indicate the amount of pyrrolizidine alkaloids they contain, making it impossible to determine the dose of toxic alkaloids being ingested. Also, products labeled as comfrey may contain prickly comfrey, which is reported to provide the most toxic pyrrolizidine compounds. Tell patient not to take this herb internally.
• Advise patient that if he experiences any adverse reactions (such as visual disturbances, fast or slow heartbeats, dry skin and mouth), he should discontinue the product and consult his health care provider.
• Warn patient to obtain herbal products from reputable sources to help ensure the product isn't contaminated.

Bold italic type indicates that reaction may be life-threatening.

- Warn patient to keep all herbal products away from children.
- Inform patient that internal use of this product is highly discouraged.

condurango

Marsdenia condurango, condurango bark, condurango blanco, condurango cortex, eagle vine

Common trade names
In many homeopathic preparations

AVAILABLE FORMS
Available as liquid extract*, tincture*, and bark.

ACTIONS & COMPONENTS
Medicinal components of this plant are found in the bark of the branches and trunk of *M. condurango.* Includes numerous glycosides, including condurangin, which stimulates saliva and gastric juice secretion.

USES
Used to stimulate appetite, alleviate dyspepsia, promote diuresis, and treat stomach cancer. Also used to increase peripheral circulation.

Commonly used in South America as an alternative treatment for chronic syphilis.

DOSAGE & ADMINISTRATION
Aqueous extract: 0.2 to 0.5 g daily
Bark: 2 to 4 g daily
Liqueur, tea: Prepared by steeping 50 to 100 g of bark in 1 quart of wine for several days. A cup of the liqueur or tea can be taken 30 minutes before each meal.

Liquid extract, tincture*:* 2 to 5 g p.r.n.

ADVERSE REACTIONS
CNS: vertigo, paralysis.
EENT: visual changes.
Other: *anaphylactoid reaction.*

INTERACTIONS
Herb-drug. *Disulfiram, metronidazole:* Herbal products prepared with alcohol may cause a disulfiram-like reaction. Discourage use together.

EFFECTS ON LAB TEST RESULTS
None reported.

CAUTIONS
Pregnant and breast-feeding patients shouldn't use condurango because it has an alkaloid component that resembles strychnine. Geriatric patients and children shouldn't use this herb.

Patients with severe allergy to natural rubber latex should use herb cautiously because of the potential for cross-sensitivity.

NURSING CONSIDERATIONS
- Explore patient's knowledge of this herb.
⚡ALERT: If patient has a severe allergy to natural rubber latex, monitor him for signs and symptoms of cutaneous reactions or respiratory compromise, such as shortness of breath, hypotension, or tachycardia.
- If patient is taking condurango to alleviate dyspepsia, find out how serious his condition is and whether he has tried other therapies to treat it.

*Liquid contains alcohol.

• If patient is taking condurango to stimulate his appetite, evaluate possible causes of his condition and whether patient has also experienced significant weight loss because this may indicate a more serious condition.

• Patients who also report melena or hematemesis should be referred for further workup.

• Overdose may produce seizures, resulting in paralysis, vertigo, and visual changes. Monitor patient closely for these.

PATIENT TEACHING

• Advise patient to consult a health care provider before using an herbal preparation because another treatment may be available.

• Tell patient that when filling a new prescription he should inform pharmacist of any herbal or dietary supplement he's taking.

• Advise patient not to take condurango if she has a latex allergy or is pregnant or breast-feeding.

• If patient has a history of alcohol abuse or liver disease or is taking disulfiram or metronidazole, advise him to avoid taking preparations that contain alcohol.

• Inform patient that dosing varies according to the preparation used.

• Warn patient to avoid using condurango with other drugs because information regarding interactions with them are lacking.

• Advise patient to report continued weight loss, GI bleeding, or worsening indigestion to his health care provider.

• Teach patient the signs and symptoms of overdose, such as visual disturbances, seizures, and dizziness; tell him to seek medical attention immediately if these occur.

coriander

Coriandrum sativum, Chinese parsley, coriander fruit, coriander seed, koriander

Common trade names
None known

AVAILABLE FORMS
Available as capsules, pure coriander seed, essential oil, powder, liquid extract*, and tea. Also available in natural deodorant products and in curry powder.
Capsules: Contain 83.3 mg coriander, along with other vitamins and natural products

ACTIONS & COMPONENTS
This medicinal seed is used ripe and dried. It contains 0.5% to 1% essential oil. The volatile oil, which consists primarily of linalool, stimulates gastric acid secretion and has spasmolytic properties. It also provides vitamin C, calcium, magnesium, potassium, and iron.

Coriander may have hypoglycemic, hypolipidemic, and antiseptic effects.

USES
Used to enhance appetite and treat dyspepsia, flatulence, diarrhea, and colic. Also used to treat coughs, chest pains, fever, bladder ailments, halitosis, postpartum complications, colic, measles, dysentery, hemorrhoids, and toothaches.

Bold italic type indicates that reaction may be life-threatening.

In aromatherapy, the essential oil is used for its soothing effects and to improve blood circulation.

Coriander is also used as a flavoring agent, culinary spice, and fragrance in bath and beauty products. It also can be used to disguise the unpleasant taste of medicine. It's a component in U.S. cigarettes.

DOSAGE & ADMINISTRATION

Dried seed: 3 g/day.
Powder: 0.3 to 1 g/dose.
Tea: Prepared by pouring 7 ounces of boiling water over 1 to 3 g of crushed coriander seed, steeping for 10 to 15 minutes, and then straining. It's then ingested between meals.
Tincture: 10 to 40 gtt daily after meals.

ADVERSE REACTIONS
Other: *anaphylactoid reaction.*

INTERACTIONS
Herb-lifestyle. *Sun exposure:* Increases risk of photosensitivity reactions. Patient should avoid unprotected exposure to sunlight.

EFFECTS ON LAB TEST RESULTS
None reported.

CAUTIONS
Patients sensitive to herb or its components, pregnant patients, breast-feeding patients, and children should avoid use.

NURSING CONSIDERATIONS
• Explore patient's knowledge of this herb.
• Breathing difficulty, airway tightness, and urticaria may occur in patients with severe allergy to co-

riander. Monitor patient for signs and symptoms of respiratory distress and vital signs closely.
• Some preparations may contain alcohol, so these should be avoided by children, geriatric patients, those with a history of alcohol abuse or liver disease, and those taking disulfiram or metronidazole.
• Assess patient's use of other therapies to manage GI complaints.
• Evaluate patient for complications, such as melena, hematemesis, and significant unintended weight loss.

PATIENT TEACHING
• Advise patient to consult a health care provider before using an herbal preparation because another treatment may be available.
• Tell patient that when filling a new prescription he should inform pharmacist of any herbal or dietary supplement he's taking.
• Advise patient not to use this herb if she's pregnant or breast-feeding, and tell patient not to give it to a child.
• Instruct patient not to take coriander if he's allergic to any of its components.
• Advise patient to seek emergency medical help immediately if he experiences adverse reactions, such as shortness of breath, rapid heart rate, or dizziness.
• Advise patient to wear sunscreen and protective clothing and to avoid exposure to direct sunlight.

---

*Liquid contains alcohol.

corkwood

Duboisia myoporoides,
corkwood tree, pituri

Common trade names
None known

AVAILABLE FORMS
Available as extract, leaves, and
twigs.

ACTIONS & COMPONENTS
Contains alkaloids, including
hyoscyamine, hyoscine, scopolamine, atropine, and butropine,
which have potent anticholinergic
properties and can be fatal in large
doses. Leaves may contain nicotine
and nornicotine.

USES
Used for its stimulant, euphoric,
and hallucinogenic effects. Some
patients chew the leaves and twigs.
   In homeopathy, corkwood is
used to treat eye disorders.
   Corkwood was used as a substitute for atropine and scopolamine
before commercial sources were
readily available.

DOSAGE & ADMINISTRATION
Not well documented.

ADVERSE REACTIONS
CNS: drowsiness, euphoria, exci-
tation, hallucinations, anger, psy-
chosis, other CNS disturbances.
CV: altered heart rate.
EENT: blurred vision, dry mucous
membranes, paralyzed eye mus-
cles.
GI: constipation.
GU: urine retention.
Respiratory: tachypnea.

INTERACTIONS
Herb-drug. *Anticholinergics, such
as atropine and tricyclic antidepressants:* Potentiates the anticholinergic effects of these drugs,
increasing risk of blurred vision,
dry mouth, urine retention, disorientation, and drowsiness. Advise
patient to discontinue use if he experiences these.
Antiparkinsonians: May interfere
with drug effect. Monitor patient,
provide supportive care, and advise
him to stop using corkwood.
Beta blockers, digoxin: Corkwood
can alter heart rate and cardiac
work. Monitor patient closely, and
advise him to avoid using herb and
drug together.

EFFECTS ON LAB TEST RESULTS
None reported.

CAUTIONS
Patients with a history of allergy to
corkwood or its components, atropine, or scopolamine should
avoid using this herb. Pregnant and
breast-feeding patients and patients
with glaucoma, intestinal disease
or obstruction, heart disease, or
myasthenia gravis should also
avoid use.

NURSING CONSIDERATIONS
• Explore patient's knowledge of
this herb.
⚠ALERT: Corkwood contains
scopolamine, which is fatal in
large doses.
• Monitor patient for anticholinergic adverse effects and drug interactions, including rapid heart rate,
decreased salivation, urine retention, psychosis, and constipation.

Bold italic type indicates that reaction may be life-threatening.

• Signs and symptoms of overdose include anticholinergic responses, such as tachycardia, tachypnea, constipation, urine retention, dry mouth, and CNS disturbances.
• Coffee or lemon juice is an antidote of homeopathic tinctures.

PATIENT TEACHING
• Advise patient to consult a health care provider before using an herbal preparation because another treatment may be available.
• Tell patient that when filling a new prescription he should inform pharmacist of any herbal or dietary supplement he's taking.
• Advise patients who are pregnant or breast-feeding not to use corkwood.
• Inform patient that corkwood isn't recommended for medicinal use and can be dangerous or fatal in high doses.

cornflower

Centaurea cyanus, bluebottle, bluebow, blue cap, cyani flos, cyani flowers, hurtsickle

Common trade names
None known

AVAILABLE FORMS
Available as ray flowers, dried ray florets, and tubular florets of the cornflower plant.

ACTIONS & COMPONENTS
Several compounds—including anthocyans, flavonoids, and bitter principles—may be responsible for cornflower's activity. The flowers are generally considered to have tonic, stimulant effects and an ability to stimulate menstruation, with effects similar to blessed thistle.

USES
Used as a diuretic, an expectorant, a laxative, and as a stimulant for liver and gallbladder function. Used to treat cough, fever, menstrual disorders, vaginal candidiasis, and eczema of the scalp. Also used as an eye wash to treat eye inflammation and conjunctivitis, and as a mouthwash and coloring agent in teas.

DOSAGE & ADMINISTRATION
Not well documented.

ADVERSE REACTIONS
Other: allergic reaction.

INTERACTIONS
None reported.

EFFECTS ON LAB TEST RESULTS
None reported.

CAUTIONS
Patients with an allergy to cornflower or its components, geriatric patients, pregnant patients, breast-feeding patients, and children shouldn't use this herb.

NURSING CONSIDERATIONS
• Explore patient's knowledge of this herb.
• This herb shouldn't be used to treat amenorrhea.

PATIENT TEACHING
• Advise patient to consult a health care provider before using an herbal preparation because another treatment may be available.

*Liquid contains alcohol.

- Tell patient that when filling a new prescription he should inform pharmacist of any herbal or dietary supplement he's taking.
- Tell patient that cornflower shouldn't be used by geriatric patients, pregnant patients, breastfeeding patients, or children.
- Warn patient not to treat irregular menstrual periods with cornflower before seeking medical evaluation because doing so may delay diagnosis of an underlying medical condition.

couch grass

Agropyron repens, Elymus repens, Graminis rhizome, cutch, dog-grass, durfa grass, quackgrass, quickgrass, quitch grass, Scotch quelch, triticum, triticum repens, twitch grass, witch grass

Common trade names
Couch Grass Root, Diuplex

AVAILABLE FORMS
Available as capsules, liquid extracts, tablets, decoctions, and teas.
Capsules: 380 mg
Tablets: 60 mg

ACTIONS & COMPONENTS
Contains the carbohydrate triticin, mucilages, sugar alcohols, soluble silicic acid, and volatile oils.

The essential oil has an antimicrobial effect. Couch grass may also have a diuretic effect, probably a result of its sugar content. It increases urine volume and prevents kidney stone formation.

USES
Used to prevent kidney stones and other kidney obstructions, and to treat arthritis, bronchitis, the common cold, constipation, cough, fever, inflammatory diseases of the urinary tract, and premenstrual syndrome. It's also used as a diuretic.

German Commission E has approved couch grass to help treat UTIs.

DOSAGE & ADMINISTRATION
Oral use: 6 to 9 g daily. Diuplex tablets have a recommended dose of 2 or 3 tablets P.O. once daily to b.i.d.
Decoction: 2 to 4 ounces of infusion put into quart of water and reduced to pint by boiling.
Liquid extract*: 2.5 to 5 ml per dose, given in water.

ADVERSE REACTIONS
Metabolic: electrolyte depletion, hyperglycemia because of sugar content of grass.
Skin: rash.

INTERACTIONS
Herb-drug. *Disulfiram, metronidazole:* Herbal products prepared with alcohol may cause a disulfiram-like reaction. Discourage use together.
Insulin, other antidiabetics: Hyperglycemia may develop. Dosage of antidiabetic may need to be increased. Monitor patient closely.

EFFECTS ON LAB TEST RESULTS
- May increase glucose level. May decrease electrolyte levels.

Bold italic type indicates that reaction may be life-threatening.

CAUTIONS
Patients with edema from cardiac or renal insufficiency should avoid using this herb. Pregnant and breast-feeding patients should also avoid couch grass.

NURSING CONSIDERATIONS
• Explore patient's knowledge of this herb.
• Liquid extracts may contain between 12% to 14% alcohol.
• Dietary supplements of couch grass may contain the rhizome, roots, and short stems of the plant.
• Patients using couch grass for urinary tract irrigation should drink plenty of fluids.
• Safety and efficacy of couch grass in geriatric patients and children are unknown.
• Monitor glucose levels in diabetic patients.

PATIENT TEACHING
• Advise patient to consult a health care provider before using an herbal preparation because another treatment may be available.
• Tell patient that when filling a new prescription he should inform pharmacist of any herbal or dietary supplement he's taking.
• Warn patient not to postpone seeking medical evaluation because doing so may delay diagnosis of a potentially serious medical condition.
• Advise patients who are pregnant or breast-feeding to avoid using couch grass.
• Advise parent that couch grass shouldn't be given to children because its effects on them haven't been studied.

• Advise patient to avoid using alcohol preparations of couch grass if he has a history of alcohol abuse or liver disease, or takes metronidazole or disulfiram.
• Advise patient to drink plenty of fluids if he uses couch grass to irrigate the urinary tract.
• Teach diabetic patient the signs of high blood glucose levels and tell him to monitor his glucose levels closely.

cowslip

Primula veris, P. officinalis, arthritica, buckles, butter rose, crewel, cuylippe, fairy caps, herb Peter paigle, key flower, key of heaven, mayflower, our lady's keys, paigle, palsywort, password, peagles, peggle, petty mulleins, plumrocks

Common trade names
None known

AVAILABLE FORMS
Available as flowers and roots of the plant, liquid extract*, and tea.

ACTIONS & COMPONENTS
Contains flavonoids, saponin glycosides, and volatile oil, which may be responsible for its ability to inhibit or dry up secretions.

USES
Used to treat asthma, cardiac insufficiency, dizziness, gout, headache, nervous diseases, neuralgia, tremors, and whooping cough, and to inhibit or dry up secretions.
Used as an antispasmodic, diuretic, expectorant, hypnotic, and sedative.

*Liquid contains alcohol.

DOSAGE & ADMINISTRATION

Dosage varies with herb form.
Dried and powdered flowers: 900
to 1,200 mg in divided doses daily.

ADVERSE REACTIONS

CV: *heart dysfunction.*
GI: nausea, vomiting, diarrhea, irritation of the digestive tract.
Hematologic: destruction of RBCs.
Hepatic: liver damage.
Other: allergic reaction.

INTERACTIONS

Herb-drug. *Antihypertensives:*
Cowslip may potentiate the effects
of antihypertensives. Discourage
use together.
Diuretics: Cowslip may potentiate
electrolyte depletion. Monitor electrolyte levels closely, especially
potassium levels.
Sedatives: Cowslip may potentiate
the effects of sedatives. Advise patients to avoid using the herb and
drug at the same time.

EFFECTS ON LAB TEST RESULTS

• May increase liver function test
values. May decrease RBC count.

CAUTIONS

Patients with an allergy to cowslip
or other member of the primrose
family (such as primrose, *Anagallis
arvensis,* yellow loose-strife, moneywort, water violet, and cyclamen) should avoid this herb. Pregnant and breast-feeding patients,
geriatric patients, and those with
heart failure, heart disease, or renal
insufficiency shouldn't use
cowslip.

NURSING CONSIDERATIONS

• Explore patient's knowledge of
this herb.
• Internal use isn't recommended
because of the toxic effects of
cowslip.
• If patient is also taking a diuretic,
monitor electrolyte levels.
• If patient is using cowslip externally, monitor him for irritation to
the skin and mucous membranes.
• If overdose occurs, perform gastric lavage, and then administer activated charcoal. Provide symptomatic and supportive measures.

PATIENT TEACHING

• Advise patient to consult a health
care provider before using an
herbal preparation because another
treatment may be available.
• Tell patient that when filling a
new prescription he should inform
pharmacist of any herbal or dietary
supplement he's taking.
• Warn patient not to postpone
seeking medical evaluation because doing so may delay diagnosis of a potentially serious medical
condition.
• Advise patients not to use cowslip if they are pregnant, breastfeeding, or taking a diuretic or
blood pressure drug.
• Instruct patient to promptly report adverse reactions and new
signs or symptoms.
• Advise geriatric patient or patient
with heart failure, heart disease, or
kidney problems to avoid herb.

Bold italic type indicates that reaction may be life-threatening.

cranberry

bog cranberry, marsh apple,
mountain cranberry

Common trade names
*Cran-Actin, Cranberry Plus,
Emergen-C Cranberry, Ultra
Cranberry*

AVAILABLE FORMS
Available as capsules and tablets of
concentrated extract, concentrated
liquids*, syrups, tinctures*, tea,
and unsweetened and sweetened
juices.
Capsules: 300 mg to 1,000 mg

ACTIONS & COMPONENTS
Obtained from the juice of the ripe
cranberry fruit. Contains substances called proanthocyanidins
that appear to prevent *Escherichia
coli,* a common pathogen in UTIs,
from adhering to the epithelial
cells lining the bladder wall. Cranberry acidifies urine, which increases hippuric acid levels, leading to an inhospitable environment
for pathogens.

USES
Used to prevent UTIs, particularly
in women prone to recurrent infection. Also used to prevent kidney
stones and scurvy, promote wound
healing, and to treat asthma, fever,
and active UTI.

DOSAGE & ADMINISTRATION
Capsules, tablets: 300 to 500 mg
P.O. b.i.d. to q.i.d.
Cranberry juice, unsweetened: 8 to
16 ounces daily.
Cranberry tincture: 3 to 5 ml t.i.d.
Tea: As needed.

ADVERSE REACTIONS
GI: diarrhea, irritation.

INTERACTIONS
Herb-drug. *Alkaline drugs such
as sodium bicarbonate and
methotrexate:* May increase excretion rate of these drugs. Monitor
patient for lack of therapeutic effect.
Herb-herb. *Uva-ursi:* May reduce
herb's effect. Discourage use together.

EFFECTS ON LAB TEST RESULTS
None reported.

CAUTIONS
Patients allergic to cranberry
should avoid its use. Cranberry
shouldn't be used as a substitute
for an antibiotic in acute infections.

NURSING CONSIDERATIONS
• Explore patient's knowledge of
this herb.
• Tinctures may contain up to 45%
alcohol.
• Contrary to early investigations
focusing on cranberry's ability to
acidify the urine, its ability to prevent bacteria from adhering to the
bladder wall seems to be more important in preventing UTIs.
• Only the unsweetened, un-
processed form of cranberry juice
is effective in preventing bacteria
from adhering to the bladder wall.
• Cranberry is safe for use in pregnant and breast-feeding patients.
• When consumed regularly, cranberry may be effective in reducing
the frequency of bacteriuria with
pyuria in women with recurrent
UTIs.

---

*Liquid contains alcohol.

PATIENT TEACHING

• Advise patient to consult a health care provider before using an herbal preparation because another treatment may be available.

• Tell patient that when filling a new prescription he should inform pharmacist of any herbal or dietary supplement he's taking.

• To prevent UTI, tell patient to use only unsweetened juice and encourage him to drink at least 8 to 10 glasses of water daily to promote urine flow.

• Advise patient that an appropriate antibiotic is usually needed to treat an active UTI.

• If patient is using cranberry to prevent a UTI, advise him to notify his health care provider if signs or symptoms of a UTI appear.

• If patient has diabetes, inform him that cranberry juice contains sugar, but that sugar-free cranberry supplements and juices are available.

cucumber

Cucumis sativus, cowcumber, wild cucumber

Common trade names
Cucumber Cleansing Bar, Sea Cucumber Vegicaps

AVAILABLE FORMS

Available as emollient ointments and lotions.

ACTIONS & COMPONENTS

Cucurbitin and fatty oil, contained in the cucumber seeds, may have mild diuretic properties when ingested and a soothing effect when used topically.

Cucumber flower may be an effective diuretic and may be helpful in treating pulmonary diseases and diseases of the GI and GU systems. Cucumbers are high in potassium.

USES

Used to treat high and low blood pressure, to cool and soothe irritated skin in patients with sunburn, and to provide fragrance in perfumes. Also used as a cooling and beautifying agent.

DOSAGE & ADMINISTRATION

Lotion, cream: Apply topically to affected areas, p.r.n.

ADVERSE REACTIONS

Metabolic: fluid loss, electrolyte imbalances.

INTERACTIONS

Herb-drug. *Diuretics:* Excessive use of cucumber may potentiate the diuretic effect, leading to fluid and electrolyte disturbances. Discourage use together.

EFFECTS ON LAB TEST RESULTS

• May increase sodium level. May decrease potassium level.

CAUTIONS

Pregnant and breast-feeding patients should avoid medicinal use of cucumber.

NURSING CONSIDERATIONS

⚠ **ALERT:** Don't confuse this herb with the sea cucumber (echinoderm).

• Explore patient's knowledge of this herb.

Bold italic type indicates that reaction may be life-threatening.

- Monitor patient for electrolyte imbalances.
- Monitor fluid intake and output.

PATIENT TEACHING
- Advise patient to consult a health care provider before using an herbal preparation because another treatment may be available.
- Tell patient that when filling a new prescription he should inform pharmacist of any herbal or dietary supplement he's taking.
- Warn patient not to treat swelling or fluid buildup with cucumber before seeking medical evaluation because doing so may delay diagnosis of a potentially serious medical condition.
- Advise patient not to use cucumber medicinally if she is pregnant or breast-feeding.
- Advise patient to promptly report adverse reactions to his health care provider.

cumin

Cuminum cyminum, C. odorum

Common Trade Names
Cummin

AVAILABLE FORMS
The applicable part of cumin is the fruit and seed. Available as seeds, ground powder, and fruit.

ACTIONS & COMPONENTS
The fatty oil components of cumin (10% to 15%) and its constituent, cuminaldehyde, have been reported to exhibit strong larvicidal and antibacterial activity. A powder suspension of cumin has shown inhibitory effects on mycelium growth, toxin production, and alfatoxin production in *Aspergillus ochraceus, C. versicolor,* and *C. flavus.*

Cumin has also been shown to influence blood clotting by interfering with arachidonic acid-induced platelet buildup in platelet-rich plasma. Cumin may also have some estrogenic effects.

USES
Traditionally, cumin is used for flatulence, stomach disorders, diarrhea, and colic. It has also been taken for rheumatic ailments. In food and beverages, it's used as a flavoring agent.

It has been used as an abortive and as an emmenagogue. It's also used in India to treat kidney and bladder stones, chronic diarrhea, leprosy, and eye disease. In Indonesia, cumin is used in cases of bloody diarrhea; for headache, a paste is applied to the forehead.

DOSAGE & ADMINISTRATION
Average single dose: 300 to 600 mg P.O. (equivalent to 5 to 10 fruits).

ADVERSE REACTIONS
Skin: phototoxicity.

INTERACTIONS
Herb-drug. *Barbiturates:* May increase or decrease level of barbiturate depending on cumin dose. Monitor barbiturate levels and symptoms of toxicity or exacerbation of disease.

EFFECTS ON LAB TEST RESULTS
- May decrease glucose level.

*Liquid contains alcohol.

CAUTIONS
Pregnant and breast-feeding patients should avoid excessive use (beyond what would be used for food preparation).

NURSING CONSIDERATIONS
• Explore patient's knowledge of this herb.

☑**ALERT:** Don't confuse cumin with certain Indian products such as *Carum carvi* or the fruit of the earth chestnut, *Bunium bulbocastanum.*

• If patient has diabetes, monitor blood glucose level regularly.

PATIENT TEACHING
• Advise patient to consult a health care provider before using an herbal preparation because another treatment may be available.

• Tell patient that when filling a new prescription he should inform pharmacist of any herbal or dietary supplement he is taking.

• Fine grinding of the cumin seed can cause loss of half of the volatile oil, most within 1 hour.

• Advise patients who are pregnant or planning on getting pregnant to avoid amounts beyond what would be used in foods

D

daffodil

Narcissus pseudonarcissus, asphodel, daffodowndilly, daffy-down-dilly, fleur de coucou, goose leek, Lent lily

Common trade names
None known

AVAILABLE FORMS
Available as powder and extract*.

ACTIONS & COMPONENTS
Contains alkaloids such as lycorine and galanthamine.

In small doses, lycorine may cause salivation, vomiting, and diarrhea; in high doses, paralysis and collapse. Galanthamine is an anticholinesterase that also exhibits analgesic activity.

In resting bulbs, daffodil exhibits pilocarpine-like activity; in flowering bulbs, atropine-like activity.

USES
Used as a topical astringent for treating wounds, burns, stiff joints, and strained muscles.

DOSAGE & ADMINISTRATION
Extract: 2 to 3 grains.
Powder: 20 grains to 2 drams.

ADVERSE REACTIONS
CNS: CNS disorders, paralysis, fainting episodes, paresthesia.
CV: *CV collapse.*
EENT: irritation and swelling of the mouth, tongue, and throat; miosis.
GI: vomiting, salivation, diarrhea.
Respiratory: *respiratory collapse.*
Skin: dermatitis.
Other: chills, shivering.

INTERACTIONS
None reported.

EFFECTS ON LAB TEST RESULTS
None reported.

CAUTIONS
Patient shouldn't consume any part of this herb because the flowers and bulbs are poisonous and can lead to rapid death.

NURSING CONSIDERATIONS
● Explore patient's knowledge of this herb.
● Accidental poisoning may result if daffodil bulbs are mistaken for onions and eaten.
☑ALERT: Daffodil may affect the CNS, causing paralysis and possibly death.

PATIENT TEACHING
● Instruct patient not to consume any part of a daffodil; inform him of daffodil's adverse effects.
● Instruct patient to seek immediate emergency medical help if he notices any CNS symptoms, such as numbness or paralysis of arms or legs.
● Warn patient to keep all herbal products away from children and pets.

*Liquid contains alcohol.

daisy

bairnwort, bruisewort, common daisy, day's eye

Common trade names
None known

AVAILABLE FORMS
Available as dried herb, fresh herb, and tincture*.

ACTIONS & COMPONENTS
Derived from the dried flowering herb. May have anti-inflammatory and astringent properties.

USES
Used to treat migraine, neuralgia, rheumatism, GI complaints (such as bloating and anorexia), and liver inflammation. Also used to reduce fevers.

The oil is used internally for rheumatic complaints, joint pain, and dysmenorrhea; externally, for gout, bruises, sprains, and wounds.

As an ointment or salve, daisy is applied directly to the inflammation site.

DOSAGE & ADMINISTRATION
Infusion: 1 teaspoon of dried herb steeped in boiling water for 10 minutes and taken t.i.d.
Tincture: 2 to 4 ml t.i.d.

ADVERSE REACTIONS
None reported.

INTERACTIONS
Herb-drug. *Disulfiram, metronidazole:* May cause a disulfiram-like reaction if herbal preparation contains alcohol. Advise patient to avoid use together.

EFFECTS ON LAB TEST RESULTS
None reported.

CAUTIONS
Components of the volatile oil can vary with the variety of daisy from which the oil is derived. Varieties that have a high thujone content are particularly toxic. Patients shouldn't use this herb internally.

Pregnant and breast-feeding patients shouldn't use this herb.

NURSING CONSIDERATIONS
• Explore patient's knowledge of this herb.
• Monitor patient for adverse reactions and new signs and symptoms.
• Monitor inflammation site for improvement, change, or worsening of inflammation.
• Tinctures and extracts contain 15% to 60% alcohol and may be unsuitable for children, patients with a history of alcoholism or liver disease, or patients taking certain drugs.

PATIENT TEACHING
• Advise patient to consult a health care provider before using an herbal preparation because another treatment may be available.
• Tell patient that when filling a new prescription he should inform pharmacist of any herbal or dietary supplement he's taking.
• If patient has a history of alcoholism or liver disease, inform him that some herbal products contain alcohol.
• Advise patient that daisy has a bitter, pungent taste.

Bold italic type indicates that reaction may be life-threatening.

- Instruct patient to promptly report adverse reactions and new signs and symptoms to his health care provider.
- Discuss with patient other proven medical treatments for his condition.
- Warn patient to keep all herbal products away from children and pets.

damiana

Turnera diffusa, damiana herb, damiana leaf, herba de la pastora, Mexican damiana, old woman's broom

Common trade names
Damiana, Damiana Root

AVAILABLE FORMS
Available as capsules, powder, tea, extract, and tincture*.

ACTIONS & COMPONENTS
The leaf and the stem of the damiana plant are the most commonly used components. Ethanolic extracts have CNS-depressant activity, and the quinone arbutin may be responsible for antibacterial activities.

USES
Used mainly for its aphrodisiac effects and for prophylaxis and treatment of sexual disturbances. Damiana is also used to control bed-wetting, depression, constipation, and nervous dyspepsia; to strengthen and stimulate during exertion; and to boost and maintain mental and physical capacity. It's also boiled in water and the steam inhaled to relieve headaches. There have been some reports of recreational use, with euphoric and hallucinogenic effects.

DOSAGE & ADMINISTRATION
Extract: 2 to 4 ml.
Oral: 2 to 4 g (capsules) P.O. of dried leaf t.i.d. or 1 cup of tea (2 to 4 g) in 5 ounces boiling water, P.O. t.i.d.

ADVERSE REACTIONS
CNS: insomnia, headache, hallucinations.
GU: urethral mucous membrane irritation.
Hepatic: liver injury.

INTERACTIONS
Herb-drug. *Antidiabetics:* May interfere with drug action. Monitor glucose level closely.
Disulfiram, metronidazole: May cause a disulfiram-like reaction if herbal preparation contains alcohol. Advise patient to avoid use together.

EFFECTS ON LAB TEST RESULTS
- May increase liver enzyme levels. May alter glucose level if patient is taking an antidiabetic.

CAUTIONS
Pregnant and breast-feeding patients shouldn't use this herb because the effects on them are unknown.

NURSING CONSIDERATIONS
- Explore patient's knowledge of this herb.
- Tinctures and extracts contain 15% to 60% alcohol and may be unsuitable for children, patients with a history of alcoholism or

*Liquid contains alcohol.

liver disease, or patients taking certain drugs.
● Patient may display tetanus-like seizures and paroxysms when more than 7 ounces of extract is consumed.
● If patient is taking both damiana and an antidiabetic, monitor glucose level closely.
● Monitor liver enzyme levels as needed.
● Evaluate patient for drug use if he claims to have had damiana-induced hallucinations.

PATIENT TEACHING
● Advise patient to consult a health care provider before using an herbal preparation because another treatment may be available.
● Tell patient that when filling a new prescription he should inform pharmacist of any herbal or dietary supplement he's taking.
● Advise pregnant and breast-feeding patients and women of childbearing age to avoid using this herb because information about its safety is lacking.
● Advise patient to use caution when performing activities that require mental alertness until he knows how the herb affects his CNS.
● If patient has diabetes, advise him to check his glucose level regularly and to report changes.
● If patient is taking an antidiabetic, advise him to consult his health care provider before using damiana.
● If patient has a history of alcoholism or liver disease, inform him that some herbal products contain alcohol.

● Tell patient to promptly report adverse reactions or new signs and symptoms to his health care provider.
● Warn patient to keep all herbal products away from children and pets.

dandelion

Taraxacum officinale, blowball, cankerwort, dandelion herb, dandelion root with herb, lion's tooth, priest's crown, swine snout, wild endive

Common trade names
Dandelion Leaf, Dandelion Leaf Tea, Dandelion Root Capsules, Dandelion Root Extract

AVAILABLE FORMS
Available as fresh greens, capsules, fluidextract*, tablets, tea, and tincture*.

ACTIONS & COMPONENTS
Contains sesquiterpenes, triterpenes, fatty acids, flavonoids, minerals (297 mg of potassium, 7.6 mEq/100 mg of leaves), phenolic acids, phytosterols, sugars, vitamins (up to 14,000 units of vitamin A/100 g of leaves), inulin, and taxarin, which makes it bitter. The leaves also contain the coumarins cichorin and aesculin.
  Dandelion has a diuretic effect, probably from the sesquiterpenes and the high potassium content. It may help prevent and treat kidney stones because of its disinfectant and solvent actions on urinary calculi. The inulin component, with its hypoglycemic effects, may affect the glucose level.

Bold italic type indicates that reaction may be life-threatening.

Dandelion may have some immune-modulating effects. It may also stimulate nitric oxide production, which affects immune regulation and defense, and induce the secretion of tumor necrosis factor-alpha in the peritoneal cells.

The enzyme taraxalisin is present in dandelion roots. The bitter effects stimulate the gallbladder to release bile and the upper GI tract and salivary glands to secrete juices.

USES
Traditionally used to treat ailments of the liver, gallbladder, and spleen.

In Germany, the herb with the root is used as an appetite stimulant, a diuretic, a bile stimulator, and a treatment for dyspepsia. The herb without the root is used for loss of appetite and dyspepsia involving flatulence and feelings of fullness. Also used as a mild laxative and an antidiabetic. Dandelion is also used in salads and wines, and the dried roots are used as a coffee substitute.

DOSAGE & ADMINISTRATION
Herb without root. *Fluidextract (1 g/ml of 25% ethanol):* 4 to 10 ml P.O. t.i.d.
Fresh herb: 4 to 10 g cut herb P.O. t.i.d.
Infusion: 4 to 10 g in 5 to 9 ounces water P.O. t.i.d.
Succus: 5 to 10 ml pressed sap from fresh plant P.O. b.i.d.
Tincture (1 g/5 ml of 25% ethanol): 2 to 5 ml P.O. t.i.d.
Herb with root. *Fluidextract (1 g/ml of 25% ethanol):* 3 to 4 ml P.O. t.i.d.

Infusion: 1 tablespoon cut roots and herb in 5 ounces water.
Tincture (1 g/5 ml of 25% ethanol): 10 to 15 gtt P.O. t.i.d.

ADVERSE REACTIONS
GI: GI discomfort, GI or biliary tract blockage, gallbladder inflammation, gallstones.
Skin: contact dermatitis.
Other: allergic reaction.

INTERACTIONS
Herb-drug. *Anticoagulants; antiplatelet drugs, including aspirin, clopidogrel, heparin, ticlopidine, and warfarin; NSAIDs:* Increases risk of bleeding. Advise patient to use caution if using the herb and drug together.
Antidiabetics: May cause potentiated effects, leading to hypoglycemia. Advise patient to avoid use together.
Antihypertensives: May cause additive effects. Advise patient to avoid use together.
Ciprofloxacin: Decreases ciprofloxacin levels. Advise patient to avoid use together.
Disulfiram, metronidazole: May cause a disulfiram-like reaction if herbal preparation contains alcohol. Advise patient to avoid use together.
Fluoroquinolone antibiotics: May cause binding effects because of the herb's rich mineral content. Advise patient to avoid use together.

EFFECTS ON LAB TEST RESULTS
• May increase liver enzyme levels. May decrease glucose level if patient is taking an antidiabetic. May alter potassium level.

---

*Liquid contains alcohol.

• May alter PT, INR, PTT, and platelet count.

CAUTIONS
Patients who are allergic to the herb shouldn't use it, nor should those who have photosensitive dermatitis, allergies to other plants in the Compositae family, empyema, ileus, or bile obstruction.

NURSING CONSIDERATIONS
• Explore patient's knowledge of this herb.
• All parts of the dandelion plant are edible. The stems, leaves, and flowers can be harvested alone, or the whole plant (including the roots) can be used.
• Tinctures and extracts contain 15% to 60% alcohol and may be unsuitable for children, patients with a history of alcoholism or liver disease, or patients taking certain drugs.
• Sesquiterpene lactones are thought to be the allergenic components, but not all people with dandelion dermatitis react to sesquiterpene patch testing.
• A few reports of allergic reactions to ingested bee pollen that contained dandelion pollen have been reported. All patients were sensitive to the pollens of dandelions and other plants in the Compositae family.
• The bitter substances contained in the leaves may cause GI discomfort.
• If patient is also taking an antidiabetic, closely monitor his glucose level.

PATIENT TEACHING
• Advise patient to consult a health care provider before using an herbal preparation because another treatment may be available.
• Tell patient that when filling a new prescription he should inform pharmacist of any herbal or dietary supplement he's taking.
• Warn patient against harvesting dandelions from areas that may have been treated with weed killer or fertilizer.
• If patient has a history of alcoholism or liver disease, inform him that some herbal products contain alcohol.
• Caution patient not to substitute dandelion therapy for a prescribed diuretic.
• If patient is taking a fluoroquinolone antibiotic, advise him not to use dandelion therapy because it may decrease his antibiotic level.
• If patient is taking an antidiabetic, advise him to closely monitor his glucose level and to report changes to his health care provider.
• Advise patient to immediately report any rashes or signs of bleeding to his health care provider.
• Instruct patient to contact his health care provider if signs and symptoms don't improve or if new ones develop.
• Warn patient to keep all herbal products away from children and pets.

Bold italic type indicates that reaction may be life-threatening.

devil's claw

Harpagophytum procumbens, Harpagophyti radix, grapple plant

Common trade names
Devil's Claw, Devil's Claw Root, Devil's Claw Tincture, Devil's Claw Tuber

AVAILABLE FORMS
Available as capsules, extracts*, fresh herb, and tincture*.

ACTIONS & COMPONENTS
The iridoid glycosides harpagoside, harpagide, and procumbide—the chemically active components in devil's claw—and various other glycosides are found in the primary roots and the secondary roots, called tubers. The secondary roots contain more active ingredients. Trace amounts of these glycosides are also found in the leaves.

Devil's claw may have anti-inflammatory, analgesic, hypotensive, and bradycardic effects and may interfere with calcium influx into smooth-muscle cells. However, stomach acid may inactivate the iridoid glycosides, thus decreasing the herb's effectiveness. The herb also affects platelet aggregation.

USES
Used for its anti-inflammatory and analgesic effects. Also used to treat allergies, atherosclerosis, GI disturbances and heartburn, menstrual difficulties, menopausal signs and symptoms, nicotine poisoning, neuralgia, and liver, kidney, and bladder diseases.

In Germany, devil's claw is approved for use as an appetite stimulant and digestive aid.

DOSAGE & ADMINISTRATION
Decoction: 1.5 g in 5 ounces water P.O. t.i.d.
Dried tuber/root: 6 g P.O. once daily.
Fluidextract (1 g/ml): 1.5 ml P.O. t.i.d.
Infusion: Prepared by steeping 4.5 g of herb in 10 ounces boiling water for 8 hours. Dosage is 3 portions P.O. once daily.
Standardized extracts: 600 to 800 mg P.O. t.i.d.; standardized to 2% to 3% iridoid glycosides or 1% to 2% harpagoside.
For loss of appetite: 0.5 g decoction in 5 ounces water P.O. t.i.d. Or 0.5 ml fluidextract (1g/ml) P.O. t.i.d. Or 1.5 g freshly cut tuber P.O. once daily.

ADVERSE REACTIONS
CNS: headache.
CV: *bradycardia,* hypotension.
EENT: tinnitus.
GI: anorexia.
Other: allergic reaction.

INTERACTIONS
Herb-drug. *Disulfiram, metronidazole:* May cause a disulfiram-like reaction if herbal preparation contains alcohol. Advise patient to avoid use together.

EFFECTS ON LAB TEST RESULTS
• May alter PT and PTT.

CAUTIONS
Patients with a gastric or duodenal ulcer shouldn't use the herb because it increases production of

*Liquid contains alcohol.

stomach acid. Patients with active bleeding should avoid the herb as well.

Patients who have a history of bleeding or who are taking an NSAID, warfarin, aspirin, or an antiplatelet drug should use caution when using the herb. Patients taking a beta blocker, a calcium channel blocker, an antihypertensive, or an antiarrhythmic also should use caution because the herb may have hypotensive, bradycardic, and antiarrhythmic effects. Patients with heart failure should use the herb cautiously because it may have negative inotropic effects at high doses.

NURSING CONSIDERATIONS
• Explore patient's knowledge of this herb.
• Devil's claw may increase the intended therapeutic effect of conventional drugs.
• Tinctures and extracts contain 15% to 60% alcohol and may be unsuitable for children, patients with a history of alcoholism or liver disease, or patients taking certain drugs.

PATIENT TEACHING
• Advise patient to consult a health care provider before using an herbal preparation because another treatment may be available.
• Tell patient that when filling a new prescription he should inform pharmacist of any herbal or dietary supplement he's taking.
• If patient has a chronic illness, advise him not to put off seeking appropriate medical evaluation, because doing so may delay diagnosis of a potentially serious medical condition.
• If patient has a history of alcoholism or liver disease, inform him that some herbal products contain alcohol.
• If patient is taking a drug for his heart or his blood pressure, advise him to promptly report any lightheadedness, dizziness, abnormal heartbeats, or swelling.
• Instruct patient to seek medical attention if signs and symptoms don't improve.
• Tell patient to stop taking herb at least 14 days before a dental or surgical procedure.
• Warn patient to keep all herbal products away from children and pets.

dill

Anethum graveolens, dill herb, dill seed, dillweed

Common trade names
Dill Seed, Dill Weed

AVAILABLE FORMS
Available as fresh greens, dried greens, dried seeds, or tincture*.

ACTIONS & COMPONENTS
The dried seeds contain an essential oil (carvone) that may have an effect on smooth- and skeletal-muscle response.

USES
Dill is used to prevent and treat diseases affecting the GI and urinary tracts and kidneys as well as to treat sleep disorders and spasms.

Dill seed is used as an antispasmodic and bacteriostatic. It's also

---

used to treat dyspepsia. The upper stem and seeds of the plant are used, either fresh or dried, as a flavoring agent and a garnish.

DOSAGE & ADMINISTRATION
Oil of dill: 0.1 to 0.3 g, or 2 to 6 gtt.
Tea: Prepared by steeping 2 teaspoons of mashed seeds in 1 cup of boiling water for 10 minutes. Dosage is 3 cups P.O. once daily.
Tincture: ½ to 1 teaspoon up to t.i.d.

ADVERSE REACTIONS
Other: allergic reaction.

INTERACTIONS
Herb-drug. *Disulfiram, metronidazole:* May cause a disulfiram-like reaction if herbal preparation contains alcohol. Advise patient to avoid use together.
Herb-lifestyle. *Sun exposure:* Contact with the juice from the fresh dill plant may cause skin to react badly when exposed to sunlight. Advise patient to take precautions to avoid this.

EFFECTS ON LAB TEST RESULTS
• May increase sodium level.

CAUTIONS
Patients allergic to the herb shouldn't use it.

NURSING CONSIDERATIONS
• Explore patient's knowledge of this herb.
• Dill weed is high in sodium. If patient has a condition that requires sodium restriction, such as heart failure or renal failure, use should be kept to a minimum.

• Tinctures and extracts contain 15% to 60% alcohol and may be unsuitable for children, patients with a history of alcoholism or liver disease, or patients taking certain drugs.
• Monitor patient's response to therapy, including improvement of signs and symptoms and adverse reactions.

PATIENT TEACHING
• Advise patient to consult a health care provider before using an herbal preparation because another treatment may be available.
• Tell patient that when filling a new prescription he should inform pharmacist of any herbal or dietary supplement he's taking.
• If patient has an allergy to dill, advise him to avoid using dill products.
• If patient has a chronic illness, advise him not to put off seeking appropriate medical evaluation, because doing so may delay diagnosis of a potentially serious medical condition.
• If patient has a history of alcoholism or liver disease, inform him that some herbal products contain alcohol.
• Instruct patient to promptly report adverse reactions and new signs or symptoms.
• Warn patient to keep all herbal products away from children and pets.

*Liquid contains alcohol.

dong quai

Angelica sinensis, Chinese angelica, dang-gui, tang-kuei

Common trade names
Dong Kwai, Dong Quai Capsules, Dong Quai Fluidextract, Dong Quai Root
Combination products: *Dong Quai and Royal Jelly, Menopausal Formula, Nature's Fingerprint, PMS Formula, Rejuvex*

AVAILABLE FORMS
Available as capsules and extract*.
Capsules: 200 mg, 250 mg, 500 mg
Extract in vegetable glycerin: 565 mg

ACTIONS & COMPONENTS
Dong quai dietary supplements are obtained from the roots of *A. sinensis.*

Dong quai extracts contain at least six coumarin derivatives (including bergapten, osthol, oxypeucedanin, and psoralen) and two furocoumadin derivatives, sen-byak-angelicole and 7-demethylsuberosin. Coumarin derivatives have anticoagulant, vasodilating, and antispasmodic activity. Also, osthol may have CNS stimulant activity.

Other components found in the essential oil include *n*-butylphthalide, cadinene, isosafrole, and safrole. Safrole may be carcinogenic, so ingestion should be avoided.

Root extracts may contain various lactones and vitamins A, E, and B_{12}. Dong quai is rich in phytoestrogens. Extracts may have a modulatory effect on endogenous estrogens.

USES
Used to treat anemia, hepatitis, hypertension, migraines, neuralgia, rhinitis, and gynecologic disorders, including irregular menstruation, dysmenorrhea, premenstrual syndrome, and menopausal signs and symptoms.

DOSAGE & ADMINISTRATION
Capsules: 500 mg P.O., or 1 to 2 capsules t.i.d.
Liquid extract: 1 or 2 gtt t.i.d.

ADVERSE REACTIONS
CNS: fever.
EENT: bleeding gums.
GI: diarrhea, bloody stools.
GU: hematuria.
Hematologic: bleeding.
Skin: photosensitivity reactions.
Other: *cancer.*

INTERACTIONS
Herb-drug. *Estrogens:* May potentiate drugs' effects. Advise patient to use caution if using the herb and drug together.
Disulfiram, metronidazole: May cause a disulfiram-like reaction if herbal preparation contains alcohol. Advise patient to avoid use together.
Warfarin and other anticoagulants: May potentiate anticoagulant effects. Advise patient to avoid use together.
Herb-lifestyle. *Sun exposure:* Increases risk of photosensitivity. Advise patient to wear protective clothing and sunscreen outdoors and to limit exposure to direct sunlight.

Bold italic type indicates that reaction may be life-threatening.

EFFECTS ON LAB TEST RESULTS
• May increase PT, INR, and PTT.

CAUTIONS
Patients who are taking an anticoagulant or who have a history of bleeding shouldn't use the herb. Use is contraindicated in those with bleeding.

Because of potential effects on uterine contractions and unknown direct effects on the developing fetus, pregnant patients shouldn't use the herb, nor should breast-feeding patients.

Patients who are taking an antihypertensive or who have a history of heart disease and might not be able to tolerate hypotension should use caution when using the herb. Patients with a history of breast or endometrial cancer should use caution as well.

NURSING CONSIDERATIONS
• Explore patient's knowledge of this herb.
• Monitor patient for signs of easy bruising or bleeding.
• Tinctures and extracts contain 15% to 60% alcohol and may be unsuitable for children, patients with a history of alcoholism or liver disease, or patients taking certain drugs.
• If dong quai must be used with another anticoagulant, closely monitor PT and INR.
• Monitor patient for photosensitivity reactions.

PATIENT TEACHING
• Advise patient to consult a health care provider before using an herbal preparation because another treatment may be available.
• Tell patient that when filling a new prescription he should inform pharmacist of any herbal or dietary supplement he's taking.
• If patient is pregnant or breast-feeding, advise her not to use the herb.
• If patient is taking a blood thinner, advise him to avoid taking the herb, unless otherwise instructed by his health care provider.
• If patient has a history of alcoholism or liver disease, inform him that some herbal products contain alcohol.
⚡ ALERT: If patient is scheduled for a dental or surgical procedure, advise him to stop taking herb at least 14 days beforehand.
• Caution patient to avoid prolonged exposure to the sun.
• Warn patient to keep all herbal products away from children and pets.

*Liquid contains alcohol.

E

echinacea

Echinacea angustifolia, E. pallida, E. purpurea, American coneflower, black sampson, black susans, cockup hat, comb flower, hedgehog, Indian head, Missouri snakeroot, narrow-leaved purple coneflower, purple coneflower, purple Kansas coneflower, red sunflower, rudbeckia, scurvy root, snakeroot

Common trade names
Coneflower Extract, EchinaCare Liquid, Echinacea, Echinacea Angustifolia Herb, Echinacea Extract, Echinacea Fresh Freeze Dried, Echinacea Glycerite, Echinacea Herbal Comfort, Echinacea Red Root Supreme, Echinacea Root Complex, Echinacea Root Extract, Echinacea Xtra, Echina Fresh, EchinaGuard Liquid, EchinaGuard Pro, Echinex, Enhanced Echinacea, Standardized Echinacea Extract

AVAILABLE FORMS
Available as capsules, glycerite, expressed juice*, hydroalcoholic extract*, lozenges, tablets, tea, tinctures (1:5, 15% to 90% alcohol)*, and whole dried root.
Capsules: 125 mg, 250 mg, 355 mg, 500 mg
Hydroalcoholic extracts: (50%)
Tablets: 335 mg

ACTIONS & COMPONENTS
Obtained from the dried rhizomes and roots of *E. angustifolia* and *E. pallida* and the roots or above-ground parts of *E. purpurea.* Extracts of echinacea contain numerous components, including alkylamides, caffeic acid derivatives, polysaccharides, essential oils, chicoric acids, flavonoids, and glycoproteins.

Echinacea—most notably the lipophilic fraction in the roots and leaves—may enhance immune system function. When taken internally, echinacea may increase the number of circulating leukocytes, enhance phagocytosis, stimulate cytokine production, and trigger the alternate complement pathway. In vitro, some components are directly bacteriostatic and exhibit antiviral activity. Applied topically, echinacea can exert local anesthetic, antimicrobial, and anti-inflammatory activity, and it can stimulate fibroblasts.

Echinacea's effects on cytokines may result in antitumorigenic activity.

USES
Used to stimulate the immune system and to treat acute and chronic upper respiratory tract infections and UTIs. Used also to heal wounds, including abscesses, burns, eczema, and skin ulcers. May be used as an adjunct to a conventional antineoplastic and may provide prophylaxis against upper respiratory tract infections and the common cold.

Bold italic type indicates that reaction may be life-threatening.

DOSAGE & ADMINISTRATION

Capsules containing powdered E. pallida root extract: Equivalent to 300 mg P.O. t.i.d.

Expressed juice of E. purpurea (2.5:1, 22% alcohol): 6 to 9 ml P.O. daily. When used externally, juice should be used for no longer than 8 weeks.

Hydroalcoholic tincture (15% to 90% alcohol): 3 to 4 ml P.O. t.i.d.

Tea: Prepared by simmering ½ teaspoon of coarsely powdered herb in 1 cup of boiling water for 10 minutes. For colds, the dosage is 1 cup of freshly made tea taken several times daily.

Whole dried root: 1 to 2 g P.O. t.i.d.

ADVERSE REACTIONS

CNS: fever.
EENT: taste perversion.
GI: nausea, vomiting, minor GI complaints.
Skin: diuresis.
Other: allergic reaction, *tachyphylaxis.*

INTERACTIONS

Herb-drug. *Amprenavir, other protease inhibitors:* May cause exacerbation of HIV or AIDS (because the herb depresses CD4$^+$ cells and increases HIV replication). Advise patient to avoid use together.

Disulfiram, metronidazole: May cause a disulfiram-like reaction if herbal preparation contains alcohol. Advise patient to avoid use together.

Immunosuppressants such as cyclosporine, corticosteroids, and methotrexate: Decreases drug effectiveness. Advise patient to avoid use together.

Prednisone: May interfere with drug's immunosuppressive effect. Monitor patient for therapeutic effect. Advise patient to avoid use together.

Herb-lifestyle. *Alcohol use:* May enhance CNS depression (if herbal preparation contains alcohol). Advise patient to avoid use together.

EFFECTS ON LAB TEST RESULTS
None reported.

CAUTIONS
Patients with HIV infection, AIDS, tuberculosis, collagen disease, multiple sclerosis, or another autoimmune disease shouldn't use this herb; nor should patients who are pregnant or breast-feeding.

NURSING CONSIDERATIONS
• Explore patient's knowledge of this herb.
• Daily dose depends on the preparation and potency, but patient shouldn't take the herb for more than 8 weeks. Consult specific manufacturer's instructions for parenteral administration, if applicable.
• Echinacea is considered supportive treatment for infection; it shouldn't be used in place of antibiotic therapy.
• Tinctures and extracts contain 15% to 60% alcohol and may be unsuitable for children, patients with a history of alcoholism or liver disease, or patients taking certain drugs.
• Some active components may be water-insoluble.

---

*Liquid contains alcohol.

- Echinacea is usually taken at the first sign of illness and continued for up to 14 days. Prolonged use isn't recommended.
- Herbalists recommend using liquid preparations because they believe echinacea functions in the mouth and should come in direct contact with the lymph tissues at the back of the throat.

PATIENT TEACHING
- Advise patient to consult a health care provider before using an herbal preparation because another treatment may be available.
- Tell patient that when filling a new prescription he should inform pharmacist of any herbal or dietary supplement he's taking.
- If patient has a chronic illness, advise him not to put off seeking appropriate medical evaluation, because doing so may delay diagnosis of a potentially serious medical condition.
- If patient has a history of alcoholism or liver disease, inform him that some herbal products contain alcohol.
- Advise patient that prolonged use can result in either overstimulation or suppression of the immune system. Echinacea shouldn't be used for more than 14 days as supportive treatment of infection.
- Inform patient that the herb should be stored away from direct light.
- Warn patients to keep all herbal products away from children and pets.

elderberry

Sambucus canadensis, S. ebulus, S. nigra, black-berried alder, black elder, blood elder, blood hilder, boretree, common elder, danewort, dwarf elder, elder, ellanwood, ellhorn, European alder

Common trade names
Elderberry, Elderberry Flowers, Elderberry Powder

AVAILABLE FORMS
Available as aqueous solution, berries, extract*, flowers, oil, and wine*.

ACTIONS & COMPONENTS
Extracts of the berries and flowers contain an essential oil that is made up of free fatty acids, such as palmitic acid, alkanes, triterpenes, ursolic acid, oleanic acid, betulin, and betulic acid. Other components found in the leaves include the cyanogenic glycoside sambunigrin, flavonoids, and caffeic acids. Anthocyanin glycosides, a component of elderberry juice, may exhibit pro-oxidant activity. Elderberry extracts also inhibit the replication of certain strains of the human influenza virus and decrease inflammatory cytokines. The component sambuculin A may protect the liver.

USES
Extracts are used to treat asthma, bronchitis, cough, epilepsy, fever, fungal infection, gout, headache, hepatic dysfunction, neuralgia, rheumatic disease, and toothache.

Bold italic type indicates that reaction may be life-threatening.

They're also used as diuretics, insect repellents, and laxatives.

DOSAGE & ADMINISTRATION
Infusion: Prepared by adding 3 to 4 g of elderberry flowers to 5 ounces of simmering water. The dosage is 1 to 2 cups P.O. taken several times daily.

ADVERSE REACTIONS
GI: diarrhea, nausea, vomiting.
Other: *cyanide-like poisoning.*

INTERACTIONS
None reported.

EFFECTS ON LAB TEST RESULTS
• May alter electrolyte levels. May alter digoxin and lithium levels with long-term or high-dose therapy.

CAUTIONS
Patients who are pregnant or breast-feeding shouldn't use this herb. All patients should avoid consuming berries from the dwarf elder (*S. ebulus*) because it can contain an especially high content of cyanide-like compounds.
    Patients taking a diuretic should use caution when using the herb.

NURSING CONSIDERATIONS
• Explore patient's knowledge of this herb.
• Leaves and stems shouldn't be crushed when making elderberry juice because of potential for cyanide toxicity.
• Elderberry may interfere with the intended therapeutic effect of conventional drugs.
• Elderberry (especially *S. ebulus*) can cause cyanide-like poisoning

characterized by diarrhea, vomiting, vertigo, numbness, and stupor, particularly if patient consumes uncooked portions. The herb can also cause a toxic reaction in children who use elderberry stems for peashooters.
• Uncooked elderberries are more likely to cause nausea than other parts of the herb.
• Monitor patients for nausea and vomiting.
• Tinctures and extracts contain 15% to 60% alcohol and may be unsuitable for children, patients with a history of alcoholism or liver disease, or patients taking certain drugs.

PATIENT TEACHING
• Advise patient to consult a health care provider before using an herbal preparation because another treatment may be available.
• Tell patient that when filling a new prescription he should inform pharmacist of any herbal or dietary supplement he's taking.
• Warn patient not to treat signs and symptoms of asthma, infection, or liver disease with elderberry before seeking appropriate medical evaluation, because doing so may delay diagnosis of a potentially serious medical condition.
• If patient has a history of alcoholism or liver disease, inform him that some herbal products contain alcohol.
• Inform patient of the toxic potential of certain varieties of elderberry.
• Warn patients to keep all herbal products away from children and pets.

* Liquid contains alcohol.

elecampane

Inula helenium, elf dock, elfwort, horse-elder, horseheal, scabwort, velvet dock, wild sunflower

Common trade names
None known

AVAILABLE FORMS
Available as fluidextract and in powdered root preparations.

ACTIONS & COMPONENTS
Obtained from the dried cut root and rhizomes of *I. helenium.* Extracts generally contain a volatile oil whose chief components are alantolactone; isoalantolactone; 11,13-dihydroisoalantolactone; 11,13-dihydroalanlantolactone; and other sesquiterpene lactones. These compounds may exhibit various antiseptic, antibacterial, antifungal, diuretic, expectorant, and hypotensive activities.

USES
Used to treat diseases of the respiratory tract, such as bronchitis, asthma, and cough; diabetes; hypertension; diseases of the GI tract; and diseases of the kidney and lower urinary tract. Also used to stimulate appetite and bile production, to treat dyspepsia and menstrual complaints, and to promote diuresis.

DOSAGE & ADMINISTRATION
Dried root: 2 to 3 g P.O. t.i.d.
Fresh root: 1 to 2 tablespoons P.O. t.i.d.
Tea: Prepared by steeping 1 g of ground herb in boiling water for 10 to 15 minutes and then straining (1 teaspoon is equivalent to 4 g of drug). Dosage is 1 cup t.i.d. to q.i.d. as an expectorant.

ADVERSE REACTIONS
CNS: paralysis with larger doses.
EENT: mucous membrane irritation.
GI: nausea, vomiting, diarrhea, and cramps with larger doses.
Skin: allergic contact dermatitis.
Other: allergic reaction.

INTERACTIONS
None reported.

EFFECTS ON LAB TEST RESULTS
None reported.

CAUTIONS
Patients with a history of sensitivity or contact dermatitis shouldn't use this herb, nor should those who are pregnant or breast-feeding.

NURSING CONSIDERATIONS
• Explore patient's knowledge of this herb.
• Elecampane may interfere with the intended therapeutic effect of conventional drugs.
• Monitor patient for signs and symptoms of allergic reaction, especially dermatologic reactions.
• The alantolactone component can irritate mucous membranes.
• If overdose occurs, perform gastric lavage and administer activated charcoal.

PATIENT TEACHING
• Advise patient to consult a health care provider before using an herbal preparation because another treatment may be available.

Bold italic type indicates that reaction may be life-threatening.

• Tell patient that when filling a new prescription he should inform pharmacist of any herbal or dietary supplement he's taking.

• Advise patient that little evidence supports the therapeutic use of elecampane and that the herb can cause an allergic reaction.

• Instruct patient not to store the herb in a plastic container.

• Warn patient to keep all herbal products away from children and pets.

ephedra

Ephedra sinica, Brigham tea, cao ma huang (Chinese ephedra), desert herb, desert tea, ephedrine, epitonin, joint fir, ma huang, mahuuanggen (root), Mexican tea, Mormon tea, muzei mu huang (Mongolian ephedra), popotillo, sea grape, squaw tea, teamster's tea, yellow astringent, yellow horse, zhong ma huang

Common trade names
Combination products:
ChromeMate, Escalation, Excel, Herbal Ecstasy, Herbal Fen-Phen, Herbalife, Metabolife, Power Trim, Up Your Gas

AVAILABLE FORMS
Available as crude extracts of root and aerial parts of *E. sinica* and *E. shennungiana;* other forms include *E. nevadensis, E. trifurca, E. equisetina,* and *E. distachya.* Available also as capsules, tablets, teas, and tinctures*.

ACTIONS & COMPONENTS
The primary active ingredient of ephedra extract is ephedrine, although extracts generally contain between 0.5% and 2.5% of alkaloids of the 2-aminophenylpropane type, including ephedrine, methylephedrine, pseudoephedrine, norephedrine, and norpseudoephedrine.

Similar to the structurally related drug amphetamine, ephedrine acts by directly stimulating the sympathomimetic system and the CNS (alpha and beta agonists), possibly increasing heart rate, myocardial contraction, peripheral vasoconstriction with associated elevations in blood pressure, bronchodilation, and mydriasis. Ephedrine is active when given orally, parenterally, or ophthalmically.

Other components in ephedra extracts include volatile oils, catechins, gallic acid, tannins, flavonoids, inulin, dextrin, starch, and pectin.

USES
Used to treat respiratory tract diseases with mild bronchospasm. Allopathic practitioners have used it since the 1930s to treat asthma, but the herb has become less popular as more specific beta agonists have become available.

Also used as a CV stimulant. Pseudoephedrine remains a common ingredient in many OTC cough and cold preparations. Ephedrine is used to treat various other conditions, including chills, coughs, colds, flu, fever, headaches, edema, and nasal congestion; it's also used as an appetite suppressant. The alkaloid-free

---

*Liquid contains alcohol.

North American species is used to treat venereal disease.

DOSAGE & ADMINISTRATION
Extract: 1 to 3 ml P.O. t.i.d.
Oral use: For adults, 15 to 30 mg total alkaloid, calculated as ephedrine, taken q 6 to 8 hours for a total maximum daily dose of 300 mg. For children older than age 6, the dose is 0.5 mg total alkaloid/kg. The usual daily dose is 2 mg.
Tea: 1 to 4 g P.O. t.i.d.
Tincture (1:1): Average single dose is 5 g P.O.
Tincture (1:4): 6 to 8 ml P.O. t.i.d.

ADVERSE REACTIONS
CNS: anxiety, confusion, dependency, dizziness, fainting, headache, insomnia, irritability, mania, motor restlessness, nervousness, psychosis, *seizures.*
CV: *arrhythmias, cardiac arrest,* hypertension, hypotension, *MI,* palpitations, tachycardia, chest pain.
GI: nausea.
GU: uterine contractions, urinary disorders.
Metabolic: hyperglycemia, *hypoglycemia.*
Respiratory: shortness of breath.
Skin: dermatitis.

INTERACTIONS
Herb-drug. *Beta blockers such as propranolol:* May cause enhanced sympathomimetic effects on vasculature from unopposed alpha-agonist effects, thus increasing risk of hypertensive effects. Advise patient to avoid use together.
Cardiac glycosides, halothane: May cause disturbed heart rhythm.
Advise patient to avoid use together.
CNS stimulants such as dextroamphetamine: May result in additive pharmacodynamic effects. Advise patient to avoid use together.
Disulfiram, metronidazole: May cause a disulfiram-like reaction if herbal preparation contains alcohol. Advise patient to avoid use together.
Drugs containing pseudoephedrine: May increase risk of adverse effects of the drug or herb. Advise patient to avoid use together.
Guanethidine: Causes increased sympathomimetic effect. Advise patient to avoid use together.
MAO inhibitors: May cause hypertensive crisis. Advise patient to avoid use together.
Oxytocin, secale alkaloid derivatives: Causes increased blood pressure. Advise patient to avoid use together.
Phenelzine: May cause severe reactions, including hypertensive crisis. Advise patient to avoid use together.
Theophylline: May increase risk of adverse GI and CNS effects. Advise patient to avoid use together.
Herb-food. *Caffeine:* Causes additive sympathomimetic and CNS stimulation. Advise patient to stop using the herb or to reduce caffeine consumption.
Herb-herb. *Yohimbe:* Causes additive sympathomimetic and CNS stimulation. Advise patient to avoid using the herbs together.

EFFECTS ON LAB TEST RESULTS
• May alter glucose level.

Bold italic type indicates that reaction may be life-threatening.

CAUTIONS

Pregnant patients shouldn't use this herb because it may induce uterine contractions, and its effects on the fetus are unknown. Patients who have glaucoma, pheochromocytoma, thyrotoxicosis or any other thyroid problem, underlying CV disease, or a history of cerebrovascular disease shouldn't use this herb. Diabetic patients shouldn't use it because of potential hyperglycemic effects.

Patients with a sleep, mood, anxiety, prostate, or psychotic disorder should use caution when using the herb.

NURSING CONSIDERATIONS

• Explore patient's knowledge of this herb.
• Ephedra compounds have been linked to several deaths and more than 800 adverse effects, many of which appear to be dose related.
• Monitor patient's pulse and blood pressure.
• Ephedra shouldn't be used for more than 7 consecutive days because of the risk of tachyphylaxis and dependence.
• Patients with eating disorders may abuse this herb.
• Tinctures and extracts contain 15% to 60% alcohol and may be unsuitable for children, patients with a history of alcoholism or liver disease, or patients taking certain drugs.
⚡ALERT: Pills containing ephedra have been combined with other stimulants, such as caffeine, and sold as "natural" stimulants in weight-loss products. Deaths from overstimulation have been reported.

⚡ALERT: Dosages high enough to produce psychoactive or hallucinogenic effects are toxic to the heart.
• Signs and symptoms of a toxic reaction include diaphoresis, dilated pupils, muscle spasms, fever, and cardiac and respiratory failure.
• If overdose occurs, perform gastric lavage and administer activated charcoal. Treat spasms with diazepam, replace electrolytes with I.V. fluids, and prevent acidosis with sodium bicarbonate infusions.

PATIENT TEACHING

• Advise patient to consult a health care provider before using an herbal preparation because another treatment may be available.
• Tell patient that when filling a new prescription he should inform pharmacist of any herbal or dietary supplement he's taking.
• Remind patient that the herb isn't a substitute for medical evaluation, especially if he has a chronic illness.
• Advise patient not to use ephedra if he has thyroid disease, high blood pressure, cerebrovascular disease, or diabetes.
• If patient has a valid need for ephedrine or pseudoephedrine, recommend a standard pharmaceutical formulation because preparations may differ in ephedrine alkaloid content by as much as 130%.
• Tell patient not to take this herb along with other drugs containing pseudoephedrine.
• If patient has a history of alcoholism or liver disease, inform

---

*Liquid contains alcohol.

him that some herbal products contain alcohol.

• Instruct patient not to use ephedra-containing products for more than 7 consecutive days.

• Advise patient not to use ephedra at dosages that are said to produce psychoactive or hallucinogenic effects because such amounts could be toxic to the heart.

• Advise patient to watch for adverse reactions, particularly chest pain, shortness of breath, palpitations, dizziness, and fainting.

• Instruct patient to store ephedra away from direct light.

• Warn patient to keep all herbal products away from children and pets.

eucalyptus

Eucalyptus globulus, blue gum tree, eucalyptol, fevertree, gum tree, red gum, stringy bark tree

Common trade names
Eucalyptamint, Eucalyptus Oil, Eucalyptus Rub

AVAILABLE FORMS
Available as dried herb, eucalyptus leaf, essential oil, tincture*, and tea bags.

ACTIONS & COMPONENTS
The primary component of eucalyptus oil is the volatile substance 1,8-cineol (cineole). Oil preparations are standardized to contain 80% to 90% cineole.

The effectiveness of the herb as an expectorant is attributed to the local irritant action of the volatile oil.

USES
Used internally and externally as an expectorant. Used to treat nasal congestion. Also used topically to treat sore muscles and rheumatism.

The essential oil (external use only) can be used in massage blends for sore, aching muscles and in foot baths or saunas, steam inhalations, chest rubs, room sprays, bath blends, and air diffusions.

DOSAGE & ADMINISTRATION
Leaf: Average dosage is 4 to 6 g P.O. daily, divided q 3 to 4 hours.
Oil: For internal use, average dosage is 0.3 to 0.6 g P.O. daily. For external use, oil with 5% to 20% concentration or a semisolid preparation with 5% to 10% concentration.
Tea: Prepared using one of two methods: For the infusion method, 6 ounces of dried herb is steeped in boiling water for 2 to 3 minutes and then strained; for the decoction method, 6 to 8 ounces of dried herb is placed in boiling water, boiled for 3 to 5 minutes, and then strained.
Tincture: 3 to 4 g P.O. daily.

ADVERSE REACTIONS
CNS: dizziness.
GI: nausea, vomiting, diarrhea.
Respiratory: *bronchospasm.*

INTERACTIONS
Herb-drug. *Antidiabetics:* Causes enhanced effects. Advise patient to avoid use together unless under the direct supervision of a health care provider.
Disulfiram, metronidazole: May cause a disulfiram-like reaction if

---

Bold italic type indicates that reaction may be life-threatening.

herbal preparation contains alcohol. Advise patient to avoid use together.
Drugs metabolized by the liver:
May alter drug effects. (Eucalyptus oil induces detoxification of the liver's enzyme systems.) Monitor patient for drug effectiveness and toxic reaction.
Herb-herb. *Herbs that cause hypoglycemia (basil, glucomannan, Queen Anne's lace):* Results in decreased glucose level. Monitor patient for this effect.

EFFECTS ON LAB TEST RESULTS
• May decrease glucose level.

CAUTIONS
Patients who are allergic to eucalyptus or its vapors, who are pregnant or breast-feeding, or who have liver disease or intestinal tract inflammation shouldn't use this herb.

Essential oil preparations shouldn't be applied to an infant's or a child's face because of the risk of severe bronchospasm.

NURSING CONSIDERATIONS
• Explore patient's knowledge of this herb.
• Eucalyptus oil, also known as eucalyptol, is steam-distilled from the twigs and long leathery leaves of the eucalyptus tree. Eucalyptus folium contains the dried leaves of older *E. globulus* trees. The leaves are collected after the tree has been cut down and allowed to dry in the shade.
• Monitor patient for allergic reaction.
• Tinctures and extracts contain 15% to 60% alcohol and may be

unsuitable for children, patients with a history of alcoholism or liver disease, or patients taking certain drugs.
• In susceptible patients, particularly infants and children, applying eucalyptus preparations to the face or inhaling vapors can cause asthma-like attacks.
• If patient is diabetic, monitor glucose level.
• Oral administration may cause nausea, vomiting, and diarrhea.
⚠ALERT: The oil has been taken internally after it has been diluted. A few drops of oil for children and 4 to 5 ml of oil for adults can cause poisoning. Signs of poisoning include hypotension, circulatory dysfunction, and cardiac and respiratory failure.
• If poisoning or overdose occurs, don't induce vomiting because of risk of aspiration. Administer activated charcoal, and treat symptomatically.
• If patient is taking any drug that's metabolized in the liver, monitor its effectiveness.

PATIENT TEACHING
• Advise patient to consult a health care provider before using an herbal preparation because another treatment may be available.
• Tell patient that when filling a new prescription he should inform pharmacist of any herbal or dietary supplement he's taking.
• If patient has trouble breathing or develops hives or a rash, advise him to immediately stop taking the herb and to check with his health care provider.
• Inform patient of the herb's adverse effects.

*Liquid contains alcohol.

• If patient has a history of alcoholism or liver disease, inform him that some herbal products contain alcohol.

• Advise patient with diabetes that glucose level may be affected.

• Advise patient to use caution when performing activities that require mental alertness until he knows how the herb affects his CNS.

• Instruct caregiver not to apply eucalyptus preparations to the face of a child or infant, especially around the nose.

• Warn patient to keep all herbal products away from children and pets.

evening primrose oil

Oenothera biennis, evening primrose, fever plant, king's-cure-all, night willow-herb, rock-rose, sand lily, scabish, sun-drop

Common trade names
Evening Primrose Oil Capsules, Mega Primrose Oil, Royal Brittany Evening Primrose Oil

AVAILABLE FORMS
Available as capsules, liquid, oil, and tablets (evening primrose complex).
Capsules: 50 mg, 500 mg, 1,300 mg
Gelcaps: 500 mg, 1,300 mg
Liquid, oil: 2 ounces, 4 ounces

ACTIONS & COMPONENTS
Contains the amino acid tryptophan and a high concentration of essential fatty acids, in particular *cis*-linoleic acid (CLA) and gamma-linoleic acid (GLA). The variety of evening primrose grown for commercial purposes produces oil with 72% CLA and 9% GLA. These fatty acids are prostaglandin precursors.

Conversion of the prostaglandin precursors into prostaglandins is the basis for using this oil to stimulate cervical ripening, prevent heart disease, and reduce signs and symptoms of rheumatoid arthritis. Its efficacy in other clinical conditions may result from its supply of fatty acids.

USES
Primarily used to treat mastalgia and premenstrual syndrome. Used by midwives to stimulate cervical ripening during pregnancy at or near term and to ease childbirth. Also used to manage cyclic mastitis and neurodermatitis. Used as a dietary stimulant.

In Europe, used to treat eczema and diabetic neuropathy, although recent evidence doesn't support its use for these conditions. Also used to treat hypercholesterolemia, rheumatoid arthritis, inflammatory bowel disease, Raynaud's disease, Sjögren's syndrome, chronic fatigue syndrome, endometriosis, obesity, prostate disease, hyperactivity in children, and asthma.

DOSAGE & ADMINISTRATION
Cyclic mastitis: 3 g P.O. daily in two or three divided doses.
Diabetic neuropathy: 4 to 6 g P.O. daily.
Eczema in children: 2 to 4 g P.O. daily.

Bold italic type indicates that reaction may be life-threatening.

Oral use: The usual dose is based on GLA content. Typical dose is 1 to 2 capsules (0.5 to 1 g) t.i.d.
Rheumatoid arthritis: 5 to 10 g daily.

ADVERSE REACTIONS
CNS: headache.
GI: nausea, diarrhea, bloating, vomiting, flatulence.
Other: allergic reaction (including breathing problems, hives, itchy or swollen skin, and rash).

INTERACTIONS
Herb-drug. *Drugs that lower the seizure threshold, such as phenothiazines and TCAs:* May cause additive or synergistic effect, thus lowering the seizure threshold and increasing the risk of seizures. Advise patient to avoid use together.

EFFECTS ON LAB TEST RESULTS
None reported.

CAUTIONS
Patients who are allergic to evening primrose oil or who are pregnant or breast-feeding shouldn't use this herb, nor should those who have a history of epilepsy or are taking a TCA, a phenothiazine, or another drug that lowers the seizure threshold.

NURSING CONSIDERATIONS
• Explore patient's knowledge of this herb.
• The fatty oil, extracted from the seeds of the evening primrose plant by a cold-extraction process, is available with a standardized fatty acid content.
⚠ **ALERT:** The oil may unmask previously undiagnosed seizures, especially when taken with a drug that treats depression or schizophrenia.
• Drug effects may be delayed 4 to 6 weeks (with maximum benefit in 4 to 8 months) for cyclic mastitis and premenstrual syndrome, 3 to 4 months for eczema and decreased pruritus, and 3 to 6 months for diabetic neuropathy.
• Vitamin E may be given with evening primrose oil to prevent toxic metabolites from forming.
• Drug should be taken with food to decrease adverse GI reactions.

PATIENT TEACHING
• Advise patient to consult a health care provider before using an herbal preparation because another treatment may be available.
• Tell patient that when filling a new prescription he should inform pharmacist of any herbal or dietary supplement he's taking.
• Tell patient to discontinue the herb if he has signs or symptoms of an allergic reaction, such as breathing problems, hives, itchy or swollen skin, or rash.
• If patient is pregnant or breast-feeding, advise her to consult her health care provider before using the herb.
• Advise patient to take herb with food to minimize adverse GI reactions.
• Warn patient to keep all herbal products away from children and pets.

eyebright

Euphrasia officinalis, euphrasia

Common trade names
Eyebright

AVAILABLE FORMS
Available as capsules, dried herb, liquid extract*, tablets, and tincture*.
Capsules, tablets: 150 mg of eyebright combined with other herbs

ACTIONS & COMPONENTS
Major components include a glycoside (aucuboside), a tannin (aucubin), caffeic and ferulic acids, sterols, choline, basic compounds, and a volatile oil. Also contains vitamins A and C.

USES
Used topically—in the form of lotions, poultices, and eye baths—to treat ophthalmic disorders, including blepharitis, conjunctivitis, styes, and eye fatigue. Also used internally for coughs, hoarseness, and respiratory tract infections.

Many believe that eyebright has antibacterial and astringent properties, although none of the chemical components has been associated with a significant therapeutic effect. German Commission E doesn't recommend using eyebright for therapeutic purposes.

DOSAGE & ADMINISTRATION
Capsules, tablets: 1 to 2 capsules or tablets P.O. t.i.d.
Liquid extract (alcohol free): 1 to 2 ml (28 to 56 gtt) P.O. t.i.d.
Liquid extract (25% alcohol): 2 to 4 ml (40 to 80 gtt) P.O. t.i.d.

Tea: Prepared using one of two methods: For infusion, 1 to 2 teaspoons of finely cut herb are steeped in 6 ounces of boiling water for 5 to 10 minutes and then strained; for decoction, 1 to 2 teaspoons of finely cut herb are placed in 6 to 8 ounces of boiling water, boiled for 3 to 5 minutes, and then strained. Although the 2% decoction may be used t.i.d. to q.i.d. for eye rinses, such use is strongly discouraged. Maximum dosage is t.i.d. P.O.
Tincture (45% alcohol): 2 to 6 ml P.O. t.i.d.

ADVERSE REACTIONS
CNS: confusion, headache, insomnia, weakness.
EENT: intense pressure in eyes, with tearing, itching, redness, swelling, photophobia, and changes in vision; sneezing; hoarseness.
GI: dyspepsia.
GU: polyuria.
Respiratory: cough, dyspnea.
Skin: diaphoresis, hives, rash, itchy or swollen skin.
Other: toothache, yawning.

INTERACTIONS
Herb-drug. *Disulfiram, metronidazole:* May cause a disulfiram-like reaction if herbal preparation contains alcohol. Advise patient to avoid use together.
Herb-lifestyle. *Alcohol use:* Enhances CNS effects if herbal preparation contains alcohol. Advise patient to avoid use together.

EFFECTS ON LAB TEST RESULTS
None reported.

Bold italic type indicates that reaction may be life-threatening.

CAUTIONS

Patients who are pregnant or breast-feeding or who have an ophthalmic disease such as glaucoma shouldn't use eyebright. Children also shouldn't use the herb. Ophthalmic use is strongly discouraged.

NURSING CONSIDERATIONS

• Explore patient's knowledge of this herb.
• Warn patient not to treat signs and symptoms of an ophthalmic disorder with eyebright before seeking medical evaluation, because doing so can delay diagnosis of a potentially serious medical condition.
• Herbal products containing eyebright are prepared from the above-ground parts of the plant *E. officinalis.*
• Tinctures and extracts contain 15% to 60% alcohol and may be unsuitable for children, patients with a history of alcoholism or liver disease, or patients taking certain drugs.
• Topical ophthalmic use is a risk to the patient for hygienic reasons.

PATIENT TEACHING

• Advise patient to consult a health care provider before using an herbal preparation because another treatment may be available.
• Tell patient that when filling a new prescription he should inform pharmacist of any herbal or dietary supplement he's taking.
• If patient has a history of alcoholism or liver disease, inform him that some herbal products contain alcohol.

• Caution patient not to apply eyebright directly to his eye because the product's sterility can't be guaranteed.
• Tell patient that if he has trouble breathing or develops hives, a rash, or itchy or swollen skin, he should stop taking this herb and contact his health care provider immediately.
• Warn patient to keep all herbal products away from children and pets.

* Liquid contains alcohol.

F

false unicorn root

Chamaelirium luteum, blazing star, devil's bit, drooping starwort, fairy-wand, false unicorn, helonias root, rattlesnake

Common trade names
False Unicorn

AVAILABLE FORMS
Available as dried root or rhizome, liquid extract*, and tincture*.

ACTIONS & COMPONENTS
The root, which is derived from *C. luteum,* contains the steroid saponin mixture chamaelirin. Other components that have been isolated from the root extract are oleic, linoleic, and stearic acids. Chamaelirin is believed to be responsible for the oxytocic, diuretic, and anthelmintic effects of the herb. Although the root probably has no direct effect on uterine tissue, it may increase human chorionic gonadotropin release.

USES
Used to treat dysmenorrhea, amenorrhea, and morning sickness and used as an appetite stimulant, anthelmintic, diuretic, emetic, and insecticide. Also used as a uterine tonic during pregnancy to prevent miscarriage.

DOSAGE & ADMINISTRATION
Dried root or rhizome: As a tea P.O. t.i.d.

Liquid extract (45% alcohol): 1 to 2 ml (20 to 40 gtt) P.O. t.i.d.
Tincture (45% alcohol): 2 to 5 ml P.O. t.i.d.

ADVERSE REACTIONS
GI: gastric upset, vomiting.

INTERACTIONS
Herb-drug. *Ciprofloxacin, levofloxacin, moxifloxacin, ofloxacin:* May reduce drug levels and drug effectiveness. Advise patient to avoid using the herb and drug together or to separate administration times by at least 2 hours.
Disulfiram, metronidazole: May cause a disulfiram-like reaction if herbal preparation contains alcohol. Advise patient to avoid using the herb and drug together.
Estrogen, progesterone: May alter action of the hormones that affect the uterus. If patient is pregnant, monitor her closely.

EFFECTS ON LAB TEST RESULTS
• May increase human chorionic gonadotropin level.

CAUTIONS
Patients who are pregnant or breast-feeding shouldn't use this herb.

NURSING CONSIDERATIONS
• Explore patient's knowledge of this herb.
• Tinctures and extracts contain between 15% and 60% alcohol and may be unsuitable for children, patients with a history of

---

Bold italic type indicates that reaction may be life-threatening.

alcoholism or liver disease, or patients taking certain drugs.

• High doses may cause stomach upset and vomiting.

PATIENT TEACHING

• Advise patient to consult a health care provider before using an herbal preparation because another treatment may be available.

• Tell patient that when filling a new prescription he should inform pharmacist of any herbal or dietary supplement he's taking.

• Advise patient not to use false unicorn root without consulting her health care provider, especially if patient is pregnant or breast-feeding.

• If patient has a chronic illness, advise him not to delay medical evaluation, because doing so can delay diagnosis of a potentially serious medical condition.

• Inform patients with a history of alcoholism or liver disease to be aware that some products may contain alcohol.

• Tell patient that false unicorn root produces vomiting if used at high doses.

• Instruct patient to stop taking this herb and to contact a health care provider immediately if he experiences difficulty breathing, hives, itchy or swollen skin, or a rash.

• Warn patient to keep all herbal products away from children and pets.

fennel

Foeniculum vulgare, fenkel, large fennel, sweet or bitter fennel, wild fennel

Common trade names
Fennel, Fennel Herb Tea, Fennel Seed

AVAILABLE FORMS
Available as essential oil, honey syrup, and seeds.

ACTIONS & COMPONENTS
Fennel oil is obtained from the ripe or dried seeds of either sweet or bitter fennel. The composition of the oil varies slightly, depending on the source.

Fennel oil extracted from bitter fennel is made up of 50% to 75% trans-anetholes, 12% to 33% fenchone, and 2% to 5% estragole; fennel oil extracted from sweet fennel, 80% to 90% trans-anetholes, 1% to 10% fenchone, and 3% to 10% estragole. Additional components are present in smaller quantities. Fennel oil stimulates GI motility, and at high levels it has antispasmodic activity. The anethole and fenchone components have a secretolytic effect on the respiratory tract, probably because of fennel's local irritant effects on the respiratory tract.

USES
Used as an expectorant to manage cough and bronchitis. Also used to treat mild, spastic disorders of the GI tract, feelings of fullness, and flatulence. Fennel syrup has been used to treat upper respiratory tract signs and symptoms in children.

*Liquid contains alcohol.

DOSAGE & ADMINISTRATION
Essential oil: 0.1 to 0.6 ml P.O. daily (equivalent to 0.1 to 0.6 g of fennel).
Honey syrup with 0.5 g fennel oil/kg: 10 to 20 g P.O. daily.
Seeds: Crushed or ground; used for teas, tealike products, and internal use. Daily dose is 5 to 7 g.

ADVERSE REACTIONS
CNS: *seizures,* hallucinations.
GI: nausea, vomiting.
Respiratory: *pulmonary edema.*
Skin: photosensitivity reactions, contact dermatitis.
Other: allergic reaction.

INTERACTIONS
Herb-drug. *Anticonvulsants, drugs that lower the seizure threshold:* Increases risk of seizures. Monitor patient closely.
Herb-lifestyle. *Sun exposure:* Increases risk of photosensitivity. Advise patient to wear protective clothing and sunscreen and to limit exposure to direct sunlight.

EFFECTS ON LAB TEST RESULTS
None reported.

CAUTIONS
Patients with sensitivity to fennel, celery, or similar foods and herbs should avoid use, as should pregnant patients and those with a history of seizures. The herb shouldn't be used for small children.

Diabetic patients should use caution when using honey syrup because of the sugar content.

NURSING CONSIDERATIONS
• Explore patient's knowledge of this herb.

• Verify that patient isn't allergic to celery, fennel, or similar spices and herbs.
⚠**ALERT:** Don't confuse fennel with poison hemlock. Hemlock can cause vomiting, paralysis, and death.
• If patient decides to take the herb while undergoing anticonvulsant therapy, monitor him closely.
• Most adverse reactions are caused by fennel oil.

PATIENT TEACHING
• Advise patient to consult a health care provider before using an herbal preparation because another treatment may be available.
• Tell patient that when filling a new prescription he should inform pharmacist of any herbal or dietary supplement he's taking.
• If patient is taking an anticonvulsant, advise him to avoid using this herb.
• If patient has diabetes, make sure he's aware of the sugar content of the product.
⚠**ALERT:** Advise patient that he shouldn't take the herb for longer than 2 weeks.
• Tell patient to stop taking this herb and to contact health care provider immediately if he experiences difficulty breathing, hives, or a rash.
• Warn patient to keep all herbal products away from children and pets.

Bold italic type indicates that reaction may be life-threatening.

fenugreek

Foeniculum vulgare, Trigonella foenum-graecum, bird's foot, bockshornsamen, fenugreek seed, foenugraeci semen, Greek hay seed

Common trade names
Fenugreek, Fenugrene

AVAILABLE FORMS
Available as capsules, paste, powder, ripe seeds, dried seeds, and as a spice.

ACTIONS & COMPONENTS
Active components in fenugreek include mucilages, proteins, steroid saponins, flavonoids, and volatile oils. Trigonelline, an alkaloid found in fenugreek, is degraded to nicotinic acid (niacin), which may partially explain its ability to lower cholesterol levels. Steroid saponins may also lower glucose and glucagon levels and enhance food consumption and appetite.

The seeds contain up to 50% mucilaginous fiber and are thus commonly used to treat diarrhea and constipation. The seeds also contain coumarin compounds.

USES
Used to treat GI complaints and to relieve upper respiratory tract congestion and allergies. Used to lower cholesterol, glucose, insulin, and hemoglobin A_{1C} levels and to improve glucose tolerance. Also used to stimulate appetite.

Topically, it's used to treat skin inflammation, muscle pain, and gout, and to help heal wounds and skin ulcers.

DOSAGE & ADMINISTRATION
External: Poultice is prepared by mixing 50 g of powdered fenugreek with 1 quart of water. The mixture is then applied topically to affected area as needed.
Internal: Dosage is 1 to 6 g P.O., or a cup of tea taken several times a day. Infusion is prepared by steeping 0.5 g of fenugreek in cold water for 3 hours and then straining. Honey may be used to sweeten the infusion.

ADVERSE REACTIONS
EENT: watery eyes.
GU: maple-syrup odor to urine.
Hepatic: *hepatotoxicity* (including jaundice, nausea, vomiting, and increased bilirubin level).
Metabolic: *hypoglycemia.*
Respiratory: wheezing.
Skin: contact dermatitis, rash, flushing.
Other: numbness, *angioedema.*

INTERACTIONS
Herb-drug. *Adrenergic blockers:* Causes additive vasodilating effect, possibly leading to hypotension. Monitor blood pressure closely.
Anticoagulants such as aspirin, heparin, low-molecular-weight heparin, NSAIDs, warfarin: Increases PT and INR and potentiates risk of abnormal bleeding. Monitor PT and INR.
Antidiabetics, insulin: Decreases glucose level. Monitor glucose level.
Probenecid, sulfinpyrazone: Decreases uricosuric effect. Monitor patient for therapeutic effect.
Other drugs: May alter drug absorption because of the herb's binding effects. Instruct patient to

*Liquid contains alcohol.

separate administration times by at least 2 hours.

EFFECTS ON LAB TEST RESULTS
• May increase liver enzyme levels. May decrease glucose level.
• May alter PT, PTT, and INR.

CAUTIONS
Patients who have had an allergic reaction to the herb or to nicotinic acid shouldn't use fenugreek, nor should breast-feeding patients. Pregnant patients shouldn't use it because of its potential abortifacient properties; alcohol and water extracts of the herb may stimulate uterine activity. Those with liver disease, peptic ulcers, or severe hypotension shouldn't use it because of the formation of nicotinic acid.

Those taking an anticoagulant—such as warfarin, heparin, aspirin, or an NSAID—should use caution when using the herb.

NURSING CONSIDERATIONS
• Explore patient's knowledge of this herb.
• If patient is taking an anticoagulant, monitor INR, PTT, and PT. Observe patient for abnormal bleeding.
• If patient is taking a uricosuric drug, monitor him for therapeutic effect.
• Appearance of rash or contact dermatitis may indicate sensitivity to fenugreek.
⚠ALERT: Nausea, vomiting, jaundice, or elevated bilirubin level may indicate liver damage and hepatotoxicity from nicotinic acid. If patient develops these signs or symptoms, he should immediately stop using the herb.

PATIENT TEACHING
• Advise patient to consult a health care provider before using an herbal preparation because another treatment may be available.
• Tell patient that when filling a new prescription he should inform pharmacist of any herbal or dietary supplement he's taking.
• If patient is pregnant or breast-feeding, or planning to become pregnant, advise her to avoid using the herb.
• Tell patient to avoid using herb if he's taking a uricosuric or an antidiabetic.
• Caution patient that a rash or abnormal skin change may indicate an allergy to fenugreek and that nausea, vomiting, and skin color changes may indicate liver damage. Tell patient to discontinue use if such signs and symptoms appear.
• Remind patient not to take fenugreek at the same time as other drugs and to separate administration times by 2 hours.
• Warn patient to keep all herbal products away from children and pets.

feverfew

Chrysanthemum parthenium,
Tanacetum parthenium,
altamisa, bachelor's button, chamomile grande, featherfew, featherfoil, feather-fully, febrifuge plant, flirtroot, grande chamomile, midsummer daisy, mutterkraut, nose bleed, Santa Maria, tanacetum, vetter-voo, wild chamomile, wild quinine

---

Bold italic type indicates that reaction may be life-threatening.

Common trade names
*Feverfew, Feverfew Extract,
Feverfew Extract Complex,
Feverfew Leaf, Feverfew Leaf and
Flower, Feverfew LF and FL-GBE,
Feverfew Power, Fresh Freeze-
Dried Feverfew, Migracare
Feverfew Extract, Migracin,
MigraSpray, MygraFew, Partenelle,
Tanacet*

AVAILABLE FORMS
Available as capsules, dried leaves,
liquid, powder, seeds, and tablets.
Capsules containing leaf extract:
250 mg
Capsules containing pure leaf:
380 mg

ACTIONS & COMPONENTS
Has more than 35 chemical components. Of these, sesquiterpene
lactones are the most well known
and studied, and parthenolide, a
germacranolide, is the most abundant of them. Monoterpenes, such
as camphor; flavonoids, such as
luteolin and apigenin; and volatile
oils, including angelate, costic
acid, and pinene are also found in
feverfew. Traces of melatonin appear in pure leaves and commercial
preparations of the herb.
  Parthenolide is thought to be the
major component responsible for
the pharmacologic effects of feverfew. It inhibits prostaglandin synthesis, platelet aggregation, serotonin release from platelets, release
of granules from polymorphonuclear leukocytes, histamine release
from mast cells, and phagocytosis.
Parthenolide may have thrombo-
lytic, cytotoxic, and antibacterial
activity and may cause contraction

and relaxation of vascular smooth
muscle.
  Monoterpenes, and possibly
melatonin, may be responsible for
feverfew's sedative and mild tran-
quilizing effects.

USES
Used most commonly to prevent or
treat migraine headaches and to
treat rheumatoid arthritis. Used to
treat asthma, psoriasis, menstrual
cramps, digestion problems, and
intestinal parasites; to debride
wounds; and to promote menstrual
flow. Also used as a mouthwash after tooth extraction, a tranquilizer,
an abortifacient, and an external
antiseptic and insecticide.

DOSAGE & ADMINISTRATION
Infusion: Prepared by steeping
2 teaspoons of feverfew in a cup
of water for 15 minutes. For a
stronger infusion, double the
amount of feverfew, and allow it to
steep for 25 minutes. Infusion dose
is 1 cup t.i.d.; stronger infusions
are used for washes.
Migraines: 125 mg of dried leaf
preparation daily; *T. parthenium*
content should be standardized to
contain at least 0.2% parthenolide,
equivalent to 250 mcg of feverfew.
Powder: Recommended daily dose
is 50 mg to 1.2 g.

ADVERSE REACTIONS
CNS: dizziness.
CV: tachycardia.
EENT: mouth ulcerations (from
chewing fresh leaf).
GI: GI upset.
Skin: contact dermatitis, rash, ab-
normal change in the skin.

---

*Liquid contains alcohol.

INTERACTIONS

Herb-drug. *Anticoagulants, antiplatelet drugs including aspirin, and thrombolytics:* Inhibits prostaglandin synthesis and platelet aggregation, thus increasing risk of bleeding. Monitor patient for abnormal bleeding.

Iron: May decrease iron absorption. Instruct patient to separate administration times by at least 2 hours.

EFFECTS ON LAB TEST RESULTS
● May increase PT, INR, and PTT.

CAUTIONS
Pregnant women shouldn't use this herb because of its potential abortifacient properties, nor should patients who are breast-feeding. Patients allergic to members of the daisy, or Asteraceae, family— including yarrow, southernwood, wormwood, chamomile, marigold, goldenrod, coltsfoot, and dandelion—and patients who have had previous reactions to feverfew— shouldn't take it internally. The herb shouldn't be used in children younger than age 2.

Patients taking an anticoagulant, such as warfarin or heparin, should use caution when using the herb.

NURSING CONSIDERATIONS
● Explore patient's knowledge of this herb.
● If patient is taking an anticoagulant, monitor appropriate coagulation values—such as INR, PTT, and PT. Observe patient for abnormal bleeding.
● Rash or contact dermatitis may indicate sensitivity to feverfew. Patient should discontinue use immediately.
● Abruptly stopping the herb may cause postfeverfew syndrome, which is characterized by tension headaches, insomnia, joint stiffness and pain, and lethargy.

PATIENT TEACHING
● Advise patient to consult a health care provider before using an herbal preparation because another treatment may be available.
● Tell patient that when filling a new prescription he should inform pharmacist of any herbal or dietary supplement he's taking.
● If patient is pregnant or breast-feeding, or planning to become pregnant, advise her not to use this herb.
● Inform patient that combining the herb with an anticoagulant, such as warfarin or heparin, or an antiplatelet, such as aspirin or another NSAID, can increase the risk of abnormal bleeding.
● Caution patient that a rash or an abnormal change in the skin may indicate an allergy to feverfew. Instruct patient to stop taking the herb if a rash appears.
● Advise patient not to stop taking herb abruptly.
● Warn patient to keep all herbal products away from children and pets.

Bold italic type indicates that reaction may be life-threatening.

figwort

Scrophularia nodosa,
carpenter's square, heal-all
scrofula plant, kernelwort,
rosenoble, throatwort

Common trade names
None known

AVAILABLE FORMS
Available as dried herb and root,
liquid extract*, and tincture*.

ACTIONS & COMPONENTS
Contains iridoids, flavonoids, tannins, and phenolic acids. Iridoid
and phenylethanoid glycosides
have also been isolated from the
aerial parts of the plant. Two of
these glycosides, harpagoside
and harpagide, may have heart-
strengthening and anti-inflammatory properties.

USES
Used externally to treat skin conditions, such as eczema and psoriasis. May also help heal wounds,
ulcers, burns, and hemorrhoids.
   Used internally for its mild laxative effect and its mild diuretic and
heart-strengthening properties.
   In homeopathic medicine, used
to treat decreased resistance, tonsillitis, and lymph edema.

DOSAGE & ADMINISTRATION
*Liquid extract (1:1 preparation in
25% alcohol USP):* 2 to 8 ml P.O.
t.i.d.
Tea: Prepared by steeping 2 to 8 g
of dried leaves and stems in 5
ounces of boiling water for 5 to 10
minutes. Dosage is t.i.d.

*Tincture (1:10 preparation in 45%
alcohol USP):* 2 to 4 ml P.O. t.i.d.

ADVERSE REACTIONS
CV: irregular pulse, ***bradycardia.***
GI: nausea, vomiting, diarrhea.

INTERACTIONS
Herb-drug. *Antiarrhythmics,
digoxin:* May increase risk of adverse reactions because of the
herb's cardiac glycoside content.
Monitor patient for adverse reactions.
*Antidiabetics such as insulin, met-
formin, sulfonylureas:* May increase glucose level, thus decreasing drug effectiveness. Monitor
glucose level.
Disulfiram, metronidazole: May
cause a disulfiram-like reaction.
Advise patient to avoid using the
herb and drug together.
Herb-herb. *Cardiac glycoside–
containing herbs such as black
hellebore, digitalis leaf, lily of the
valley, motherwort, oleander leaf,
pheasant's eye, pleurisy root,
uzara:* Increases cardiac effects.
Advise patient to avoid using these
herbs together.

EFFECTS ON LAB TEST RESULTS
• May increase glucose level.

CAUTIONS
Patients with preexisting cardiac
abnormalities including arrhythmias or conduction disturbances
shouldn't use this herb, nor should
pregnant or breast-feeding patients.

NURSING CONSIDERATIONS
• Explore patient's knowledge of
this herb.

---

*Liquid contains alcohol.

• Figwort may interfere with the intended therapeutic effect of conventional drugs.

• Monitor patient for cardiac abnormalities.

• If patient has diabetes, monitor him for fluctuations in glucose level because herb may cause hyperglycemia.

• Tinctures and extracts contain between 15% and 60% alcohol and may be unsuitable for children, patients with a history of alcoholism or liver disease, or patients taking certain drugs.

• Advise patient to avoid using figwort with other herbs that have cardiac glycoside effects.

PATIENT TEACHING

• Advise patient to consult a health care provider before using an herbal preparation because another treatment may be available.

• Tell patient that when filling a new prescription he should inform pharmacist of any herbal or dietary supplement he's taking.

• If patient is pregnant or breastfeeding or planning to become pregnant, advise her not to use figwort.

• If patient has a history of alcoholism or liver disease, inform him that some herbal products contain alcohol.

• Inform patient about the potential for heart problems. If patient experiences any heart disturbances while taking figwort, instruct him to stop taking it and to immediately report his signs and symptoms to his health care provider.

• Instruct diabetic patient to monitor glucose level frequently and to watch for abnormal fluctuations.

• Warn patient to keep all herbal products away from children and pets.

flax

Linum usitatissimum, flaxseed, leinsamen, lini semen, linseed, lint bells, linum, winterlien

Common trade names
Dakota Flax Gold, Flax Seed Oil, Flax Seed Whole

AVAILABLE FORMS
Available as capsules, flour, fresh flowering plant, oil, and whole seeds. Also, many cereals, pancake and muffin mixes, and eggs contain flax.
Capsules: 1,000 mg; 1,300 mg

ACTIONS & COMPONENTS
Contains mucilages, cyanogenic glycosides, 10% to 25% linoleic acid, oleic acid proteins (albumin), xylose, galactose, rhamnose, and galacturonic acid. Cyanogenic acids, with the activity of a certain enzyme, have the potential to release cyanide. Linolenic, linoleic, and oleic acids are classified as omega fatty acids.

The mucilaginous fiber absorbs and expands. The omega fatty acid component may decrease total cholesterol and low-density lipoprotein levels and may decrease platelet aggregation.

USES
Used internally to treat diarrhea, constipation, diverticulitis, irritable bowel, colons damaged by laxative abuse, gastritis, enteritis, and bladder inflammation. It may help to

remove heavy metals from the body.

Used externally to remove foreign objects from the eye. Also used as a poultice for skin inflammation.

DOSAGE & ADMINISTRATION

For gastritis, enteritis: 1 tablespoon of the whole or bruised seed, not ground, mixed with 5 ounces of liquid and taken b.i.d. or t.i.d. Or, 5 to 10 g of whole seed soaked in cold water for 30 minutes; liquid is then discarded, the seeds are ground, and 2 to 4 tablespoons are used as linseed gruel.
Ophthalmic: A single moistened flaxseed is placed under the eyelid until the foreign object sticks to the mucous secretion from the seed.
Topical: 30 to 50 g of the flour is used for a hot poultice or compress.

ADVERSE REACTIONS

GI: *intestinal obstruction,* diarrhea, flatulence, nausea.

INTERACTIONS

Herb-drug. *Oral drugs:* Alters or blocks drug absorption, resulting from the herb's fibrous content and binding potential. Instruct patient to separate administration times by at least 2 hours.

EFFECTS ON LAB TEST RESULTS

None reported.

CAUTIONS

Patients with an ileus, an esophageal stricture, or an acute inflammatory illness of the GI tract shouldn't use this herb, nor should patients who are pregnant, breast-

feeding, or planning to become pregnant.

NURSING CONSIDERATIONS

●Explore patient's knowledge of this herb.
●When flax is used internally, it should be taken with more than 5 ounces of liquid per tablespoon of flaxseed.
●Cyanogenic glycosides may release cyanide; however, the body only metabolizes these to a certain extent. At therapeutic doses, flax doesn't elevate cyanide ion level.
●Even though flax may decrease a patient's cholesterol level or increase bleeding time, it's unnecessary to monitor cholesterol level or platelet aggregation.

PATIENT TEACHING

●Advise patient to consult a health care provider before using an herbal preparation because another treatment may be available.
●Tell patient that when filling a new prescription he should inform pharmacist of any herbal or dietary supplement he's taking.
●Warn patient not to treat chronic constipation or other GI disturbances or eye injury with flax before seeking medical evaluation, because doing so can delay diagnosis of a potentially serious medical condition.
●If patient is pregnant or breastfeeding or planning to become pregnant, advise her not to use flax.
●Instruct patient to drink plenty of water when taking flaxseed.
●Instruct patient not to take any drug for at least 2 hours after taking flax.

---

*Liquid contains alcohol.

- Tell patient to refrigerate flax oil and protect flaxseeds from light.
- Warn patient to keep all herbal products away from children and pets.

fumitory

Fumaria officinalis, beggary, common fumitory, earth smoke, fumitory wax dolls

Common trade names
None known

AVAILABLE FORMS
Available as leaves, liquid extract*, powder, and tincture*.

ACTIONS & COMPONENTS
The above-ground parts of the dried or fresh flowering plant are used medicinally. Active components include isoquinoline alkaloids such as scoulerine, protopine, fumaricine, fumariline, fumaritine, flavonoids such as rutin, fumaric acid, and hydroxycinnamic acid derivatives.

Isoquinolone alkaloids may contribute to the herb's antispasmodic effects on the gallbladder, bile ducts, and GI tract. Cinnamic acid has a choleretic effect. Fumaric acid works as an antioxidant, a flavoring agent, and a chelating agent. Flavonoids and their derivatives may improve capillary function by decreasing abnormal leakage.

USES
Used to relieve liver, gallbladder, and GI complaints and to treat cystitis, atherosclerosis, rheumatism, arthritis, hypoglycemia, and infections. Also used as a blood purifier.

Fumitory has been used to treat skin diseases such as chronic eczema and psoriasis.

DOSAGE & ADMINISTRATION
For gallbladder complaints: Infusion is prepared by pouring boiling water over 2 to 3 g of fumitory, and then straining after 20 minutes. Dosage is 1 cup warmed and taken before meals.
Internal use: 2 to 4 g P.O. or 1 cup of tea several times a day.
Liquid extract (1:1 preparation in 25% alcohol USP): 2 to 4 ml P.O. t.i.d.
Tincture (1:5 preparation in 45% alcohol USP): 1 to 4 ml P.O. t.i.d.

ADVERSE REACTIONS
CNS: *seizures* (with high doses).
CV: hypotension, ***bradycardia.***
EENT: increased intraocular pressure.
GU: *acute renal failure.*

INTERACTIONS
Herb-drug. *Antiglaucoma drugs:* May increase intraocular pressure and reverse drug effect. Advise patient to use caution if using the herb and drug together.
Antihypertensives: Increases hypotension. Carefully monitor blood pressure.
Disulfiram, metronidazole: May cause a disulfiram-like reaction if herbal preparation contains alcohol. Advise patient to avoid using the herb and drug together.
Oral drugs: Alters or blocks drug absorption, resulting from the herb's chelating properties. Advise

---

Bold italic type indicates that reaction may be life-threatening.

patient to avoid using the herb and drug together.

Herb-lifestyle. *Alcohol use:* Increases CNS effects. Advise patient to avoid using the herb and alcohol together.

EFFECTS ON LAB TEST RESULTS
• May increase BUN and creatinine levels.

CAUTIONS
Patients with glaucoma shouldn't use this herb, nor should patients who are pregnant or breast-feeding. Because fumaric acid may cause renal failure, those with renal dysfunction should also avoid use.

Patients taking an antihypertensive should use caution when using the herb because it may increase the risk of hypotension.

NURSING CONSIDERATIONS
• Explore patient's knowledge of this herb.
• Monitor patient for renal dysfunction (BUN and creatinine levels) because fumaric acid may cause renal failure.
• Monitor blood pressure and heart rate.
• Because tinctures and extracts contain between 15% and 60% alcohol, they may be unsuitable for children, alcoholics, those with a previous history of alcohol abuse, those with preexisting liver disease, and those taking disulfiram or metronidazole.

PATIENT TEACHING
• Advise patient to consult a health care provider before using an herbal preparation because another treatment may be available.
• Tell patient that when filling a new prescription he should inform pharmacist of any herbal or dietary supplement he's taking.
• If patient is pregnant or breast-feeding or is planning to become pregnant, advise her not to use the herb.
• If patient has a history of alcoholism or liver disease, inform him that some herbal products contain alcohol.
• If patient is also taking blood pressure medication, inform him of the possibility of low blood pressure. Instruct him to report feelings of weakness, dizziness, or light-headedness to his health care provider.
• Instruct patient not to take any drug for at least 2 hours after taking fumitory.
• Caution patient not to use fumitory with alcohol.
• Instruct patient to report feelings of increased eye pressure or pain and to stop taking the herb immediately if he experiences such symptoms.
• Warn patient to keep all herbal products away from children and pets.

---

*Liquid contains alcohol.

G

galangal

Alpinia officinarum, catarrh root, China root, Chinese galangal, Chinese ginger, colic root, East India catarrh root, East India root, galanga, gargaut, greater galangal, India root, lesser galangal

Common trade names
None known

AVAILABLE FORMS
Available as dried powder, fluidextract*, tincture*, oil, rhizome, and tea.

ACTIONS & COMPONENTS
A dioxyflavanol whose rhizome contains a volatile oil, resin, galangol, kaempferid, galangin, and alpinin. The volatile oil may play a role in the herb's active medicinal properties, including its calming effect on the stomach.

USES
Used to relieve flatulence, dyspepsia, nausea, vomiting, loss of appetite, and motion sickness. Used to treat fevers, colds, cough, sore throat, bronchitis, infection, rheumatism, and liver and gallbladder complaints. Used to inhibit prostaglandin synthesis. Used as an antibacterial and antispasmodic. Also used as perfume and as a spice because of its pungent and spicy flavor.

Used in homeopathic medicine as a stimulant.

DOSAGE & ADMINISTRATION
Infusion: Prepared by pouring boiling water over 0.5 to 1 g of galangal and then straining after 10 minutes. Dosage is 1 cup 30 minutes before meals.
Tincture or rhizome: 2 to 4 g P.O. daily.

ADVERSE REACTIONS
CNS: hallucinations.

INTERACTIONS
Herb-drug. *Disulfiram, metronidazole:* May cause a disulfiram-like reaction if herbal preparation contains alcohol. Advise patient to avoid use together.

EFFECTS ON LAB TEST RESULTS
None reported.

CAUTIONS
Patients who are pregnant or breast-feeding shouldn't use this herb.

NURSING CONSIDERATIONS
• Explore patient's knowledge of this herb.
• Galangal isn't widely used in the United States and may be difficult to obtain. Patient should be careful when using products with an unknown origin.
• Tinctures and extracts contain 15% to 60% alcohol and may be unsuitable for children, patients with a history of alcoholism or liver disease, or patients taking certain drugs.

Bold italic type indicates that reaction may be life-threatening.

• This herb may interfere with the intended therapeutic effect of conventional drugs.

PATIENT TEACHING
• Advise patient to consult a health care provider before using an herbal preparation because another treatment may be available.
• Tell patient that when filling a new prescription he should inform pharmacist of any herbal or dietary supplement he's taking.
• If patient has a history of alcoholism or liver disease, inform him that some herbal products contain alcohol.
• Tell patient that galangal may be hard to get in the United States, and advise him to buy it only from a reputable, known source.
• Inform patient that dosing may be difficult if he's using galangal powder that is made for cooking. Tell him to consult a health care provider with a background in natural medicine before use.
• Caution patient that this herb may cause hallucinations.
• Warn patient to keep all herbal products away from children and pets.

garlic

Allium sativum, clove garlic, poor man's treacle, rustic treacle, stinking rose

Common trade names
Garlicin, Garlic Powermax, Garlinase 4000, GarliPure, Garlique, Garlitrin 4000, Kwai, Kyolic Liquid, Sapec, Wellness GarliCell

AVAILABLE FORMS
Available as aqueous extract (1:1), capsules, fermented garlic, fresh cloves, garlic oil maceration (1:1), powdered cloves, softgel capsules, solid garlic extract*, and tablets.

ACTIONS & COMPONENTS
Medicinal ingredients of garlic are obtained from the bulb of the *A. sativum* plant. The aroma, flavor, and medicinal properties of garlic are primarily the result of sulfur compounds, including alliin, ajoens, and allicin. Also found in garlic are vitamins, minerals, and the trace elements germanium and selenium.

Garlic inhibits lipid synthesis, thus decreasing cholesterol and triglyceride levels. Works as an anticoagulant by inhibiting platelet aggregation, which is probably the work of allicin and ajoens. Lowers blood pressure. Lowers the glucose level by increasing the body's circulating insulin level and glycogen storage in the liver. As an antibacterial, garlic acts against both gram-positive and gram-negative organisms, including *Helicobacter pylori* (the causative organism in many peptic ulcers and in certain gastric cancers). May also have antifungal and antitumorigenic effects.

USES
Used most commonly to decrease total cholesterol and triglyceride levels and to increase the high-density-lipoprotein level. Also used to help prevent atherosclerosis because of its effect on blood pressure and platelet aggregation. Used to decrease the risk of cancer,

*Liquid contains alcohol.

especially cancer of the GI tract; to decrease the risk of stroke and heart attack; and to treat cough, colds, fevers, and sore throats.

Used orally and topically to fight infection through its antibacterial and antifungal effects.

DOSAGE & ADMINISTRATION

Cholesterol reduction: 900 mg of dried power, 2 to 5 mg of allicin, or 2 to 5 g of fresh clove. Average dose is 4 g of fresh garlic or 8 mg of essential oil daily.

ADVERSE REACTIONS

CNS: headache, insomnia, fatigue, vertigo.
CV: tachycardia, orthostatic hypotension
EENT: bad breath.
GI: heartburn, flatulence, nausea, vomiting, bloating, diarrhea.
Metabolic: hypothyroidism.
Respiratory: asthma, shortness of breath.
Skin: contact dermatitis, burns.
Other: hypersensitivity reactions, facial flushing, body odor.

INTERACTIONS

Herb-drug. *Acetaminophen, other drugs metabolized by the enzyme CYP2E1 (a member of the CYP450 system):* Causes decreased drug metabolism. Monitor patient for drug effectiveness and toxic reaction.
Anticoagulants, NSAIDs, prostacy-clin: May cause increased bleeding time. Advise patient to avoid use together.
Antidiabetics: Causes decreased glucose level. Advise patient to use caution if using the herb and drug

together. Monitor patient's glucose level.
Disulfiram, metronidazole: May cause a disulfiram-like reaction if herbal preparation contains alcohol. Advise patient to avoid use together.
Ritonavir: May cause severe GI toxicity. Advise patient to avoid use together.
Herb-herb. *Herbs that exert anticoagulant effects, such as feverfew and ginkgo:* Results in increased bleeding time. Advise patient to avoid use together.
Herbs that exert antihyperglycemic effects, such as glucomannan: Causes decreased glucose level. Advise patient to use caution if using these herbs together. Monitor patient's glucose level.

EFFECTS ON LAB TEST RESULTS

• May decrease glucose, cholesterol, and triglyceride levels.
• May increase PT, INR, and PTT.

CAUTIONS

Patients who are allergic to garlic shouldn't use this herb. Patients who are pregnant or breast-feeding shouldn't use it in amounts greater than those used in cooking.

Patients with severe hepatic or renal disease should use caution when using garlic, as should those using garlic for young children.

NURSING CONSIDERATIONS

• Explore patient's knowledge of this herb.
• Garlic isn't recommended for patients with diabetes, insomnia, pemphigus, organ transplants, or rheumatoid arthritis or for postsurgical patients.

Bold italic type indicates that reaction may be life-threatening.

• Tinctures and extracts contain 15% to 60% alcohol and may be unsuitable for children, patients with a history of alcoholism or liver disease, or patients taking certain drugs.
• Consuming excessive amounts of raw garlic increases the risk of adverse reactions.
• Monitor patient for signs and symptoms of bleeding.
• Garlic may lower glucose level. If patient is taking an antidiabetic, watch for signs and symptoms of hypoglycemia, and monitor glucose level.
⚡**ALERT:** Garlic oil shouldn't be used to treat inner ear infections in children.

PATIENT TEACHING
• Advise patient to consult a health care provider before using an herbal preparation because another treatment may be available.
• Tell patient that when filling a new prescription he should inform pharmacist of any herbal or dietary supplement he's taking.
• If patient has a chronic illness, advise him not to put off seeking medical evaluation, because doing so may delay diagnosis of a potentially serious medical condition.
• If patient has a history of alcoholism or liver disease, inform him that some herbal products contain alcohol.
• Advise patient to consume garlic in moderation to minimize the risk of adverse reactions.
• If patient is scheduled for upcoming surgery, advise him to use garlic only in moderation.
• If patient is using garlic to lower his cholesterol levels, advise him

to notify his health care provider and to have his cholesterol levels monitored.
• If patient is diabetic, advise him to carefully monitor his glucose level.
• If patient is taking an anticoagulant, inform him that using garlic may increase his risk of bleeding.
• If patient is using garlic as a topical anesthetic, advise him to avoid prolonged use because it could burn the skin surface.
• Warn patient to keep all herbal products away from children and pets.

gentian

Gentiana lutea, bitter root, feltwort, pale gentian, stemless gentian, yellow gentian

Common trade names
Gentian Root

AVAILABLE FORMS
Available as dried rhizome, bitter tonic*, dried powder, dried root, extract*, tincture*, and tea.

ACTIONS & COMPONENTS
The medicinal components of gentian are derived from the roots and rhizome of the *G. lutea* plant. They includes amarogentin, gentiopicrin, gentiopicroside, swertiamarin, the alkaloids gentianine and gentialutine, xanthones, carbohydrates, pectin, tannins, triterpenes, and volatile oils.
Gentian may stimulate gastric secretions. Because the herb is usually administered with alcohol, it's difficult to determine whether

---

*Liquid contains alcohol.

the gentian or the alcohol produces the gastric effects.

USES
Used to stimulate appetite and to aid in digestion by stimulating gastric juices. May have some anti-inflammatory effects.

DOSAGE & ADMINISTRATION
Dried rhizome or root: 2 to 4 g P.O. daily.
Liquid extract: 2 to 4 g P.O. daily.
Tea: Prepared by steeping 1 to 2 g of the herb in boiling water for 5 to 10 minutes.
Tincture: 1 to 4 ml P.O. t.i.d. The average dosage is 1 to 3 g daily.

ADVERSE REACTIONS
CNS: headache.
GI: dyspepsia, nausea, vomiting.

INTERACTIONS
Herb-drug. *Barbiturates, benzodiazepines:* Causes increased sedation if herbal preparation contains alcohol. Advise patient to avoid use together.
Cephalosporins, disulfiram, metronidazole: May cause a disulfiram-like reaction if herbal preparation contains alcohol. Advise patient to avoid use together.
Herb-lifestyle. *Alcohol use:* May increase CNS effects. Advise patient to avoid use together.

EFFECTS ON LAB TEST RESULTS
None reported.

CAUTIONS
Patients with a stomach or duodenal ulcer or excessive acid production shouldn't use this herb, nor should patients who are pregnant or breast-feeding.
Patients with a GI disorder, such as peptic ulcer disease or Zollinger-Ellison syndrome, and those with hypertension should use caution if using the herb and drug together.

NURSING CONSIDERATIONS
• Explore patient's knowledge of this herb.
⚠ **ALERT:** Don't confuse gentian with gentian violet, also known as crystal violet; they have different uses.
• Tinctures and extracts contain 15% to 60% alcohol and may be unsuitable for children, patients with a history of alcoholism or liver disease, or patients taking certain drugs.

PATIENT TEACHING
• Advise patient to consult a health care provider before using an herbal preparation because another treatment may be available.
• Tell patient that when filling a new prescription he should inform pharmacist of any herbal or dietary supplement he's taking.
• Tell patient to stop using gentian if stomach upset occurs.
• If patient has a history of alcoholism or liver disease, advise him that the tincture form contains alcohol.
• Advise patient to keep product out of direct light.
• Warn patient to keep all herbal products away from children and pets.

Bold italic type indicates that reaction may be life-threatening.

ginger

Zingiber officinale, zingiber

Common trade names
*Alcohol-Free Ginger Root,
Caffeine-Free Ginger Root, Ginger
Aid Tea, Ginger Kid, GingerMax,
Ginger Powder, Ginger Root,
Quanterra Stomach Comfort,
Zintona*

AVAILABLE FORMS
Available as candied ginger root,
fresh root, oil, powdered spice,
syrup, tablet, tea, and tincture*.
Capsules: 250 mg, 410 mg,
550 mg

ACTIONS & COMPONENTS
Ginger's medicinal components
are derived from the rhizome or
root of the plant *Z. officinale.* Its
pungent properties also contribute
to its pharmacologic activities.
Ginger contains cardiotonic compounds known as gingerols,
volatile oils, and other compounds, such as (6)-, (8)-, and
(10)-shogaol, (6)- and (10)-
dehydrogingerdione, (6)- and
(10)-gingerdione, zingerone, and
zingibain.

The root has antiemetic effects,
resulting from its carminative and
absorbent properties and from its
ability to enhance GI motility. In
large doses, the root has positive
inotropic effects on the CV system.
Ginger's ability to inhibit prostaglandin, thromboxane, and
leukotriene biosynthesis may have
an anti-inflammatory effect; its
ability to inhibit prostaglandins
and thromboxane, an antimigraine
effect; its ability to inhibit platelet
aggregation, antithrombotic effects. The volatile oil may have
antimicrobial effects.

USES
Used most commonly as an antiemetic in those with motion sickness, morning sickness, or generalized nausea. Used to treat colic,
flatulence, and indigestion. Used
to treat hypercholesterolemia, burns,
ulcers, depression, impotence, and
liver toxicity. Used as an anti-
inflammatory for those with arthritis and as an antispasmodic. Also
used for its antitumorigenic activity in patients with cancer.

DOSAGE & ADMINISTRATION
As an antiemetic: 2 g of fresh powder P.O. taken with some liquid.
Total daily recommended dose is 2
to 4 g of dried rhizome powder.
For arthritis: 1 to 2 g daily.
*For migraine headache or arthri-
tis:* Up to 2 g daily.
For motion sickness: 1 g P.O. 30
minutes before travel, then 0.5 to
1 g q 4 hours; may also begin treatment 1 to 2 days before trip.
*For nausea associated with chemo-
therapy:* 1 g before chemotherapy.
Infusion: Prepared by steeping
0.5 to 1 g of herb in boiling water
and then straining after 5 minutes
(1 teaspoon is equivalent to 3 g of
drug).

ADVERSE REACTIONS
CNS: CNS depression.
CV: *arrhythmias*.
GI: heartburn.

INTERACTIONS
Herb-drug. *Anticoagulants, other
drugs that can increase bleeding*

*Liquid contains alcohol.

time: May further increase bleeding time. Advise patient to avoid use together.

Disulfiram, metronidazole: May cause a disulfiram-like reaction if herbal preparation contains alcohol. Advise patient to avoid use together.

Herb-herb. *Herbs that may increase bleeding time:* May further increase bleeding time. Advise patient to avoid use together.

EFFECTS ON LAB TEST RESULTS
• May increase bleeding time with large doses.

CAUTIONS
Patients with gallstones or an allergy to ginger shouldn't use it. Patients who are pregnant or who have a bleeding disorder shouldn't use large amounts of the herb.

Patients taking a CNS depressant or an antiarrhythmic should use caution when using the herb and drug together.

NURSING CONSIDERATIONS
• Explore patient's knowledge of this herb.
• Adverse reactions are uncommon.
• Tinctures and extracts contain 15% to 60% alcohol and may be unsuitable for children, patients with a history of alcoholism or liver disease, or patients taking certain drugs.
• Monitor patient for signs and symptoms of bleeding. If patient is taking an anticoagulant, monitor PTT, PT, and INR closely.
• Use in pregnant patients is questionable, although small amounts used in cooking are safe. It's un-

known if ginger appears in breast milk.
• Ginger may interfere with the intended therapeutic effect of conventional drugs.
• If overdose occurs, monitor patient for arrhythmias and CNS depression.

PATIENT TEACHING
• Advise patient to consult a health care provider before using an herbal preparation because another treatment may be available.
• Tell patient that when filling a new prescription he should inform pharmacist of any herbal or dietary supplement he's taking.
• If patient has a history of alcoholism or liver disease, inform him that some herbal products contain alcohol.
• If patient is pregnant, advise her to consult with a knowledgeable practitioner before using ginger medicinally.
• Instruct patient to look for signs and symptoms of bleeding, such as nosebleeds or excessive bruising.
• Warn patient to keep all herbal products away from children and pets.

ginkgo

Ginkgo biloba, ginkgo nut, kew tree, maidenhair tree, yinhsing

Common trade names
Bioginkgo, Gincosan, Ginkgo Go!, Ginkgo Liquid Extract, Ginkgo Power, Ginko Capsules, Ginkyo, Quanterra Mental Sharpness

---

Bold italic type indicates that reaction may be life-threatening.

AVAILABLE FORMS
Available as tablets, capsules, and liquid preparations*.

ACTIONS & COMPONENTS
Medicinal parts include dried or fresh leaves and the seeds separated from the fleshy outer layer. The flavonoids and terpenoids of ginkgo extracts are considered antioxidants that serve as free radical scavengers. Other suggested mechanisms of action include arterial vasodilation, increased tissue perfusion, increased cerebral blood flow, decreased arterial spasm, decreased blood viscosity, and decreased platelet aggregation.

Ginkgo may be effective in managing cerebral insufficiency, dementia, and circulatory disorders.

USES
Primarily used to manage cerebral insufficiency, dementia, and circulatory disorders such as intermittent claudication. Also used to treat headaches, asthma, colitis, impotence, depression, altitude sickness, tinnitus, cochlear deafness, vertigo, premenstrual syndrome, macular degeneration, diabetic retinopathy, and allergies.

Used as an adjunctive treatment for pancreatic cancer and schizophrenia. Also used with physical therapy to decrease pain during ambulation in Fontaine stage IIb peripheral arterial disease (with at least 6 weeks of treatment).

In Germany, standardized ginkgo extracts are required to contain 22% to 27% ginkgo flavonoids and 5% to 7% terpenoids.

DOSAGE & ADMINISTRATION
Tablets and capsules: 40 to 80 mg P.O. t.i.d.
Tincture (1:5 tincture of crude ginkgo leaf): 0.5 ml P.O. t.i.d.

ADVERSE REACTIONS
CNS: headaches, dizziness, **subarachnoid hemorrhage.**
CV: palpitations.
GI: nausea, vomiting, flatulence, diarrhea.
Hematologic: *bleeding.*
Other: allergic reaction.

INTERACTIONS
Herb-drug. *Anticoagulants, antiplatelet drugs, high doses of vitamin E:* May increase risk of bleeding. Advise patient to avoid use together.
Carbamazepine, phenobarbital, phenytoin: May decrease drug effectiveness. Advise patient to avoid use together.
Disulfiram, metronidazole: May cause a disulfiram-like reaction if herbal preparation contains alcohol. Advise patient to avoid use together.
Drugs that lower seizure threshold, such as bupropion; TCAs: May further decrease the seizure threshold. Advise patient to avoid use together.
MAO inhibitors: May potentiate drug activity. Advise patient to use caution if using the herb and drug together.
SSRIs: May reverse the sexual dysfunction associated with these drugs. Advise patient to consult health care provider before taking herb for sexual dysfunction resulting from SSRI use.

*Liquid contains alcohol.

Trazodone: May cause coma (can occur after only four doses of ginkgo). Advise patient to avoid use together.
Herb-herb. *Garlic, other herbs that increase bleeding time:* May potentiate anticoagulant effects. Advise patient to use caution if using the herb and drug together.

EFFECTS ON LAB TEST RESULTS
None reported.

CAUTIONS
Patients with a history of an allergic reaction to ginkgo or its components or with risk factors for intracranial hemorrhage (such as hypertension or diabetes) shouldn't use ginkgo, nor should patients receiving an antiplatelet drug or an anticoagulant, because of the increased risk of bleeding.

The neurotoxin ginkgo toxin is present in leaf and seeds; patients prone to seizures also should avoid using the herb.

Ginkgo shouldn't be used in the perioperative period or before childbirth.

NURSING CONSIDERATIONS
● Explore patient's knowledge of this herb.
● Ginkgo extracts are considered standardized if they contain 24% ginkgo flavonoids and 6% terpenids.
● Tinctures and extracts contain 15% to 60% alcohol and may be unsuitable for children, patients with a history of alcoholism or liver disease, or patients taking certain drugs.

● Treatment should continue for at least 6 weeks, but for no more than 3 months.
⚠ **ALERT:** Seizures have been reported in children who ate more than 50 seeds.
● Patients must be monitored for possible adverse reactions, such as GI problems, headaches, dizziness, allergic reactions, and serious bleeding.
● Toxicity may cause atonia and adynamia.

PATIENT TEACHING
● Advise patient to consult a health care provider before using an herbal preparation because another treatment may be available.
● Tell patient that when filling a new prescription he should inform pharmacist of any herbal or dietary supplement he's taking.
● If patient has a history of alcoholism or liver disease, inform him that some herbal products contain alcohol.
● Inform patient that the therapeutic and toxic components of ginkgo can vary significantly from product to product. Advise him to obtain his ginkgo from a reliable source.
● If patient is scheduled for upcoming surgery, advise him to stop using ginkgo at least 2 weeks beforehand.
● Warn patient to keep all herbal products away from children and pets.

Bold italic type indicates that reaction may be life-threatening.

ginseng

Panax ginseng, P. quinquefolius, American ginseng, Asian ginseng, chikusetsu ginseng, Chinese ginseng, dwarf ginseng, five-fingers, Himalayan ginseng, Korean ginseng, Manchurian ginseng, Oriental ginseng, Sanchiginseng, zhuzishen

Common trade names
American Ginseng, American Ginseng Root, Centrum Ginseng, Chinese Red Panax Ginseng, Concentrated Ginseng Extract, Gin-Action, Ginsai, Ginsana, Ginseng Concentrate, Ginseng Natural, Ginseng Power Max 4X, Ginseng Solution, Ginseng Up, Korean Ginseng Power-Herb, Korean Ginseng Root, Korean White Ginseng, Lynae Ginse-Cool

AVAILABLE FORMS
Available as powdered root, tablets, capsules, and tea.

ACTIONS & COMPONENTS
The dried root is medicinal. It contains triterpenoid saponins called ginsenosides that appear to be the active ingredients responsible for the plant's immunomodulatory effects. Ginsenosides seem to increase natural-killer cell activity, stimulate interferon production, accelerate nuclear RNA synthesis, and increase motor activity.

Ginsenosides also have been found to protect against stress ulcers, to decrease the glucose level, to increase the high-density-lipoprotein level, and to affect CNS activity by acting as a depressant, anticonvulsant, analgesic, and antipsychotic.

USES
Used to manage fatigue and lack of concentration and to treat atherosclerosis, bleeding disorders, colitis, diabetes, depression, and cancer. Also used to help recover health and strength after sickness or weakness.

DOSAGE & ADMINISTRATION
Powdered root: For a healthy patient, 0.5 to 1 g of the root P.O. daily in two divided doses for 15 to 20 days. The morning dose is usually taken 1 to 2 hours before breakfast; the evening dose, 2 hours after dinner. If a second course of therapy is desired, patient must wait at least 2 weeks before starting ginseng again.

For a geriatric or sick patient, 0.4 to 0.8 g of the root P.O. daily taken continuously.
Solid extracts in tablets and capsules: 100 to 300 mg P.O. t.i.d.
Tea: 1 cup daily to t.i.d. for 3 to 4 weeks. Prepared by steeping 3 g of the herb in a cup of boiling water for 5 to 10 minutes.

ADVERSE REACTIONS
CNS: headache, insomnia, dizziness, restlessness, nervousness.
CV: hypertension, hypotension.
GI: diarrhea, vomiting.
GU: estrogenic-like effects, such as vaginal bleeding and mastalgia.
Other: ginseng abuse syndrome (including increased motor and cognitive activity combined with significant diarrhea, nervousness, insomnia, hypertension, edema, and skin eruptions).

---

*Liquid contains alcohol.

INTERACTIONS

Herb-drug. *Anticoagulants, antiplatelet drugs:* May decrease drug effects. Monitor PT and INR.
Antidiabetics, insulin: Increases hypoglycemic effects. Monitor glucose level.
CNS stimulants, corticosteroids: May cause excessive CNS stimulation. Monitor patient, and advise him not to take these drugs near bedtime.
Drugs metabolized by CYP3A4: May result in inhibition of this enzyme system. Monitor patient for effects and toxicity.
Estrogen: May cause additive estrogenic effect. Monitor patient.
Furosemide: May decrease diuretic effect. Advise patient to avoid use together; otherwise, furosemide dosage may need to be reduced.
Ibuprofen: May increase risk of bleeding from decreased platelet aggregation. Advise patient to avoid using herb and drug together. If patient uses them together, monitor him for signs of unusual bleeding or bruising.
Phenelzine and other MAO inhibitors: May cause headache, irritability, and visual hallucinations. Advise patient to avoid using herb and drug together.

EFFECTS ON LAB TEST RESULTS
● May decrease glucose level.
● May decrease PT and INR.

CAUTIONS
Patients with a history of an allergic reaction to ginseng or its components shouldn't use it, nor should patients taking an MAO inhibitor.

Patients receiving an anticoagulant or an antiplatelet drug and those with a manic-depressive disorder, psychosis, diabetes, or a CV disorder should use caution if using the herb.

NURSING CONSIDERATIONS
● Explore patient's knowledge of this herb.
● The German Commission E doesn't recommend using ginseng for more than 3 months.
● Ginseng is believed to strengthen the body and increase resistance to disease.
⚡**ALERT:** Reports have circulated of a severe reaction known as ginseng abuse syndrome in patients taking large doses (more than 3 g daily for up to 2 years). Patients experiencing this syndrome report a feeling of increased motor and cognitive activity combined with significant diarrhea, nervousness, insomnia, hypertension, edema, and skin eruptions.

PATIENT TEACHING
● Advise patient to consult a health care provider before using an herbal preparation because another treatment may be available.
● Tell patient that when filling a new prescription he should inform pharmacist of any herbal or dietary supplement he's taking.
● Inform patient that the therapeutic and toxic components of ginseng can vary significantly from product to product. Advise him to obtain his ginseng from a reliable source.

Bold italic type indicates that reaction may be life-threatening.

• Warn patient to keep all herbal products away from children and pets.

ginseng, Siberian

Acanthopanax senticosus, Eleutherococcus senticosus, devil's shrub, shigoka, spiny ginseng, wild pepper

Common trade names
Eleuthero Ginseng, Eleuthero Ginseng Root, Siberian Ginseng Power Herb, Siberian Ginseng Root

AVAILABLE FORMS
Available as dried roots, rhizome, pulverized root rinds, tablets, capsules, liquid (ethanol extract)*, and tea.

ACTIONS & COMPONENTS
The dried root is medicinal. Eleutherosides appear to be the active ingredient responsible for the plant's immunomodulatory effects. They may also affect the pituitary-adrenocortical system and may increase T-lymphocyte counts in healthy people. Siberian ginseng is believed to strengthen the body and increase resistance to disease.

USES
Used to manage fatigue and difficulty concentrating. Also used to treat hypotension, diabetes, cancer, and infertility.

DOSAGE & ADMINISTRATION
Capsules: 1 g of powdered root in capsule P.O. daily.

Dry root: 2 to 3 g P.O. daily for up to 1 month.
Ethanol extract: 2 to 16 ml P.O. daily to t.i.d. for up to 2 months. If a second course of therapy is desired, patient must wait 2 to 3 weeks before restarting Siberian ginseng.

For someone in poor health, 0.5 to 6 ml P.O. daily to t.i.d. for 35 days. If a second course of therapy is desired, patient must wait 2 to 3 weeks before restarting Siberian ginseng.
Root decoction: 35 ml P.O. b.i.d.

ADVERSE REACTIONS
CNS: drowsiness, anxiety, insomnia.
CV: tachycardia, hypertension, pericardial pain.
Musculoskeletal: muscle spasm.

INTERACTIONS
Herb-drug. *Anticoagulants, antiplatelet drugs:* May decrease effectiveness of these drugs. Monitor PT and INR.
Barbiturates: May cause decreased metabolism of these drugs, leading to additive adverse effects. Advise patient to use caution if using the herb and drug together.
Digoxin: May result in increased digoxin levels and possibly other effects. Monitor digoxin level.
Disulfiram, metronidazole: May cause a disulfiram-like reaction if herbal preparation contains alcohol. Advise patient to avoid use together.

EFFECTS ON LAB TEST RESULTS
• May increase BUN, creatinine, alkaline phosphatase, and glu-

*Liquid contains alcohol.

tamyltransferase levels. May decrease glucose and triglyceride levels. May alter digoxin levels.
• May decrease PT and INR.

CAUTIONS
Patients with a history of allergic reactions to Siberian ginseng or its components shouldn't use the herb, nor should patients with underlying hypertension.

Patients receiving an anticoagulant or an antiplatelet drug should use caution when using the herb and drug together.

NURSING CONSIDERATIONS
• Explore patient's knowledge of this herb.
• Tinctures and extracts contain 15% to 60% alcohol and may be unsuitable for children, patients with a history of alcoholism or liver disease, or patients taking certain drugs.
• The German Commission E doesn't recommend using Siberian ginseng for more than 3 months.
 ALERT: Adulterating ginseng with other herbs and caffeine is dangerous. Ginseng products contaminated with germanium may cause nephrotoxicity.
• Monitor patient for adverse reactions, such as tachycardia, hypertension, pericardial pain, drowsiness, anxiety, muscle spasm, and insomnia.
• Monitor patient's laboratory results, as needed.

PATIENT TEACHING
• Advise patient to consult a health care provider before using an herbal preparation because another treatment may be available.

• Tell patient that when filling a new prescription he should inform pharmacist of any herbal or dietary supplement he's taking.
• If patient has a history of alcoholism or liver disease, inform him that some herbal products contain alcohol.
• Inform patient that the therapeutic and toxic components of Siberian ginseng can vary significantly from product to product. Advise him to obtain his ginseng from a reliable source.
• Warn patient to keep all herbal products away from children and pets.

glucomannan

Amorphophallus konjac Koch, konjac, konjac mannan

Common trade names
Glucomannan

AVAILABLE FORMS
Available as tablets, capsules, liquid, powder, and hydrophilic gum.

ACTIONS & COMPONENTS
Glucomannan is a polysaccharide derived from the underground stems of *A. konjac*. This herb absorbs water, promoting hydration of stool and thus helping to relieve constipation. It may increase the viscosity of intestinal contents, decrease gastric emptying time, act as a barrier to diffusion, delay the absorption of glucose from the intestines, and decrease the need for antidiabetics in diabetic patients. May also inhibit the active transport of cholesterol in the jejunum and prevent the absorption of bile

---

Bold italic type indicates that reaction may be life-threatening.

acids in the ileum. Reduces intestinal flora.

USES
Used to manage constipation, diabetes, obesity, hypercholesterolemia, and hyperlipidemia. Also used to induce weight loss and inhibit cancer.

DOSAGE & ADMINISTRATION
Diabetes: 3.6 to 7.2 g P.O. daily.
Hyperlipidemia: 3.9 g P.O. daily.
Weight loss: 1 g P.O. t.i.d. 2 hours before each meal.

ADVERSE REACTIONS
GI: esophageal or lower-GI obstruction, flatulence, diarrhea.
Metabolic: *hypoglycemia.*

INTERACTIONS
Herb-drug. *Insulin, oral antidiabetics:* May cause significant hypoglycemia. Advise patient to use caution if using the herb and drug together. Monitor patient's glucose level. Antidiabetic dosage may need to be reduced.
Oral drugs: May cause impaired drug absorption because of herb's fiber content. Instruct patient to separate administration times by at least 2 hours.

EFFECTS ON LAB TEST RESULTS
• May decrease glucose level.

CAUTIONS
Patients with a history of allergic reaction to glucomannan or any of its components shouldn't use the herb.

Patients who have GI dysfunction or diabetes and those who are prone to hypoglycemia should use caution when using the herb.

NURSING CONSIDERATIONS
• Explore patient's knowledge of this herb.
• Consuming glucomannan may result in a feeling of fullness, thereby decreasing the appetite.
• Monitor patient for adverse reactions, such as esophageal or lower-GI obstruction, flatulence, diarrhea, and hypoglycemia.
• Monitor patient's weight and cholesterol and glucose levels.

PATIENT TEACHING
• Advise patient to consult a health care provider before using an herbal preparation because another treatment may be available.
• Tell patient that when filling a new prescription he should inform pharmacist of any herbal or dietary supplement he's taking.
• Advise patient to avoid using tablet form because it increases risk of esophageal obstruction.
• Inform patient that the therapeutic and toxic components of glucomannan can vary significantly from product to product. Advise him to obtain glucomannan from a reliable source.
• Warn patient to keep all herbal products away from children and pets.

*Liquid contains alcohol.

goat's rue

Galega officinalis, French honeysuckle, French lilac, Italian fitch

Common trade names
Goat's Rue

AVAILABLE FORMS
Available as dried leaves.

ACTIONS & COMPONENTS
Consists of the dried, above-ground parts of *G. officinalis,* which include the stalk, leaves, and flowers; the leaves are collected at the beginning of the flowering season. Contains lectins, flavonoids, and the alkaloids galegine and 4-hydroxygalegine. May have diuretic and hypoglycemic activity and may also promote weight loss. Its effect on glucose level has been attributed to the galegine component.

USES
Used to promote diuresis and milk production in breast-feeding patients. Also used to reduce hyperglycemia and to treat plague, fever, and snakebites.

DOSAGE & ADMINISTRATION
Extract: Prepared by steeping 1 teaspoon of dried leaves in 1 cup of boiling water for 10 to 15 minutes. The fluidextract is taken P.O. b.i.d.

ADVERSE REACTIONS
CNS: headache, weakness, nervousness.

INTERACTIONS
Herb-drug. *Antidiabetics:* May cause additive hypoglycemic effects. Advise patient of this interaction. Tell him to consult health care provider before using together.

EFFECTS ON LAB TEST RESULTS
• May decrease glucose level.

CAUTIONS
Pregnant or breast-feeding patients and children shouldn't use this herb.

NURSING CONSIDERATIONS
• Explore patient's knowledge of this herb.
• If patient has diabetes, he should be evaluated by his health care provider before using goat's rue.
• Goat's rue may affect the intended therapeutic effect of conventional drugs.
• Fatal poisoning has occurred in animals grazing on the herb. Signs and symptoms of toxicity in animals include salivation, labored breathing, spasms, and paralysis as well as asphyxiation leading to death.

PATIENT TEACHING
• Advise patient to consult a health care provider before using an herbal preparation because another treatment may be available.
• Tell patient that when filling a new prescription he should inform pharmacist of any herbal or dietary supplement he's taking.
• If patient has diabetes, inform him that he shouldn't use goat's rue to manage his condition. In-

---

Bold italic type indicates that reaction may be life-threatening.

stead he should consult a health care provider for diabetes care.
- If patient is pregnant or breast-feeding, advise her not to use this herb.
- Warn patient to keep all herbal products away from children and pets.

goldenrod

Solidago canadensis, S. gigantea, S. virgaurea, Aaron's rod, blue mountain tea, European goldenrod, sweet goldenrod, woundwort

Common trade names
Golden Rod

AVAILABLE FORMS
Available as ethanol extracts and aqueous extracts*.

ACTIONS & COMPONENTS
Consists of the aboveground parts of *S. virgaurea,* gathered during the flowering season. The active medicinal ingredients identified include flavonoids, saponins, tannins, diterpenes, and carotenoids. The herb also contains phenol glucosides and caffeic acid derivatives.

Flavonoids and saponins exert a diuretic action on the kidneys. Astringent properties are derived from tannins. The herb also has anti-inflammatory activity.

USES
Used to treat and prevent the formation of kidney stones and to treat inflammatory diseases of the urinary tract.

German Commission E has approved goldenrod for use as a diuretic, an anti-inflammatory, and a mild antispasmodic.

DOSAGE & ADMINISTRATION
Daily dose: 6 to 12 g of herb, as recommended by German Commission E.
Infusion: Prepared by steeping 1 to 2 tablespoons of dried herb in 5 to 9 ounces of boiling water and then straining after 15 minutes. Dosage is b.i.d. to q.i.d. between meals.
Liquid extract (1:1 in 25% ethanol): 0.5 to 2 ml P.O. b.i.d. to t.i.d.
Tincture (1:5 in 45% ethanol): 0.5 to 1 ml P.O. b.i.d. to t.i.d.

ADVERSE REACTIONS
GI: vomiting after ingesting dried plant.
Respiratory: asthma, hay fever, rapid breathing after ingesting dried plant.
Other: allergic reaction; ***poisoning*** (resulting from parasites, fungus, and rust in the dried plant may lead to weight loss, leg and abdominal edema, enlarged spleen, and GI hemorrhage).

INTERACTIONS
Herb-drug. *Cephalosporins, disulfiram, metronidazole:* May cause a disulfiram-like reaction if herbal preparation contains alcohol. Advise patient to avoid use together.
Diuretics: May increase sodium retention and interfere with diuretic therapy. Monitor patient closely.
Other CNS depressants including barbiturates and benzodiazepines: Increases CNS depression. Advise

---

*Liquid contains alcohol.

patient to use caution if using the herb and drug together.

EFFECTS ON LAB TEST RESULTS
● May increase sodium level.

CAUTIONS
Pregnant patients shouldn't use goldenrod because of risk of miscarriage. Patients with edema from impaired cardiac or renal function should avoid use.

Patients allergic to marigolds, ragweed, daisies, or chrysanthemums may be prone to developing allergic reactions to goldenrod.

NURSING CONSIDERATIONS
● Explore patient's knowledge of this herb.
● If patient is using goldenrod to treat hypertension or kidney stones, he should consult his health care provider for evaluation and treatment.
● Tinctures and extracts contain 15% to 60% alcohol and may be unsuitable for children, patients with a history of alcoholism or liver disease, or patients taking certain drugs.

PATIENT TEACHING
● Advise patient to consult a health care provider before using an herbal preparation because another treatment may be available.
● Tell patient that when filling a new prescription he should inform pharmacist of any herbal or dietary supplement he's taking.
● If patient has a history of alcoholism or liver disease, inform him that some herbal products contain alcohol.

● If patient is using goldenrod as a diuretic or as treatment for high blood pressure or kidney stones, recommend that he seek medical supervision.
● If patient is pregnant or planning pregnancy, advise her not to use goldenrod.
● If patient has allergies, advise him not to use this herb.
● Encourage patient to drink at least 2 quarts of fluids per day when taking this herb.
● Tell patient to store the herb away from light and moisture.
● Warn patient to keep all herbal products away from children and pets.

goldenseal

Hydrastis canadensis, eye balm, eye root, golden root, ground raspberry, Indian dye, Indian turmeric, jaundice root, orange root, sceau d'or, turmeric root, yellow Indian paint, yellow puccoon, yellow root

Common trade names
Golden Seal Extract, Golden Seal Extract 4:1, Golden Seal Power, Golden Seal Root, Nu Veg Golden Seal Herb, Nu Veg Golden Seal Root

AVAILABLE FORMS
Available as capsules, dried ground root powder, cream, tablets, tea, tincture*, and water ethanol extracts*.
Capsules, tablets: 250 mg, 350 mg, 400 mg, 404 mg, 470 mg, 500 mg, 535 mg, 540 mg

---

Bold italic type indicates that reaction may be life-threatening.

ACTIONS & COMPONENTS

Consists of the rhizome and roots of *H. canadensis*. Principal chemical components are the alkaloids hydrastine and berberine. Also contains other alkaloids, volatile oils, chlorogenic acid, phytosterols, and resins.

May have anti-inflammatory, antihemorrhagic, immunomodulatory, and muscle relaxant properties. Decreases hyperphagia and polydipsia associated with streptozocin diabetes in mice. Exhibits inconsistent uterine hemostatic properties. Hydrastine causes peripheral vasoconstriction. Berberine can decrease the anticoagulant effect of heparin; it stimulates bile secretion and exhibits some antineoplastic and antibacterial activity. Berberine also can stimulate cardiac function in lower doses or inhibit it at higher doses.

USES

Used to treat postpartum hemorrhage and to improve bile secretion. Also used to treat UTIs, dysmenorrhea, hemorrhoids, constipation, and flatulence. Also used as a digestive aid and expectorant. Used topically on wounds and genital herpes lesions.

DOSAGE & ADMINISTRATION

Alcohol and water extract: 250 mg P.O. t.i.d.
Dried rhizome: 0.5 to 1 g in 1 cup of water t.i.d.
Expectorant: 250 to 500 mg P.O. t.i.d.
For symptomatic relief of mouth sores and sore throat: 2 to 4 ml of tincture (1:10 in 60% ethanol) swished or gargled t.i.d.

Topical use: Small amount of cream, ointment, or powder applied to wound once daily. Wound should be cleaned at least once daily.

ADVERSE REACTIONS

CNS: sedation, reduced mental alertness, hallucinations, delirium, paresthesia, paralysis.
CV: hypotension, hypertension, *asystole, heart block.*
EENT: mouth ulceration.
GI: nausea, vomiting, diarrhea, abdominal cramps.
Hematologic: megaloblastic anemia from decreased vitamin B absorption, *leukopenia.*
Respiratory: *respiratory depression.*
Skin: contact dermatitis.

INTERACTIONS

Herb-drug. *Acid-reducing drugs, such as H_2 antagonists, antacids, and proton pump inhibitors:* May increase stomach acid and thus interfere with drug action. Advise patient to avoid use together.
Anticoagulants: May cause decreased anticoagulant effect. Advise patient to avoid use together.
Antidiabetics, insulin: May increase hypoglycemic effect. Advise patient to use caution if using the herb and drug together.
Antihypertensives: May increase or decrease hypotensive effect. Advise patient to avoid use together.
Beta blockers, calcium channel blockers, digoxin: May increase or decrease cardiac effect. Advise patient to avoid use together.
Cephalosporins, disulfiram, metronidazole: May cause a disulfiram-like reaction if herbal

*Liquid contains alcohol.

preparation contains alcohol. Advise patient to avoid use together. *CNS depressants such as benzodiazepines:* May increase sedative effects. Advise patient to avoid use together.

Herb-lifestyle. *Alcohol use:* May increase sedative effects. Advise patient to avoid use together.

EFFECTS ON LAB TEST RESULTS
• May decrease bilirubin level.
• May decrease PTT.

CAUTIONS
Patients with hypertension, heart failure, or an arrhythmia shouldn't use this herb, nor should patients who are pregnant or breast-feeding or who have severe renal or hepatic disease. The herb shouldn't be given to infants because it increases their bilirubin levels.

NURSING CONSIDERATIONS
• Explore patient's knowledge of this herb.
• Tinctures and extracts contain 15% to 60% alcohol and may be unsuitable for children, patients with a history of alcoholism or liver disease, or patients taking certain drugs.
• German Commission E hasn't endorsed the use of goldenseal for any condition because of the potential toxicity and lack of well-documented efficacy.
• Goldenseal is less effective than ergot alkaloids in treating postpartum hemorrhage.
• Berberine can decrease the duration of diarrhea caused by various pathogens such as *Vibrio cholerae, Shigella, Salmonella, Giardia,* and some Enterobacteriaceae.

• Monitor patient for signs and symptoms of vitamin B deficiency, such as megaloblastic anemia, paresthesia, seizures, cheilosis, glossitis, and seborrheic dermatitis.
• Monitor patient for adverse CV, respiratory, and neurologic effects. If patient has a toxic reaction, induce vomiting and perform gastric lavage. After lavage, administer activated charcoal and treat symptoms.

PATIENT TEACHING
• Advise patient to consult a health care provider before using an herbal preparation because another treatment may be available.
• Tell patient that when filling a new prescription he should inform pharmacist of any herbal or dietary supplement he's taking.
• If patient has a history of alcoholism or liver disease, inform him that some herbal products contain alcohol.
• Advise patient not to use goldenseal because of its toxicity and lack of documented efficacy, especially if he has CV disease.
• ☑**ALERT:** High doses may lead to vomiting, slowed heart rate, high blood pressure, respiratory depression, exaggerated reflexes, seizures, and death.
• Advise patient to avoid performing activities that require mental alertness until he knows how the drug affects his CNS.
• Warn patient to keep all herbal products away from children and pets.

Bold italic type indicates that reaction may be life-threatening.

gossypol

Gossypium herbaceum, G. hirsutum, American upland cotton, common cotton, cotton root, upland cotton, wild cotton

Common trade names
Cotton Seed Oil

AVAILABLE FORMS
Available as liquid extracts* and tinctures*.

ACTIONS & COMPONENTS
Derived from the stems, roots, and seeds of plants from the Malvaceae family. The cotton plant (*Gossypium* species) is the most common source. Gossypol is the active ingredient found in seeds and other parts of the plant; however, content varies significantly from species to species.

Exerts antifertility action by inhibiting sperm production and motility. Possesses antitumorigenic activity and may also have anti-HIV properties.

USES
Used in China as an oral male contraceptive. Also used topically by women as a spermicide.

DOSAGE & ADMINISTRATION
Contraceptive use: 20 mg P.O. daily for 2 to 3 months until sperm count is decreased to less than 4 million/ml. Maintenance dosage then reduced to 50 mg weekly to 75 to 100 mg twice a month.

ADVERSE REACTIONS
CNS: paralysis.

CV: circulatory problems, ***heart failure.***
GI: diarrhea, malnutrition, decreased appetite.
GU: *nephrotoxicity.*
Metabolic: hypokalemia.
Musculoskeletal: muscle fatigue, muscular weakness.
Other: hair discoloration.

INTERACTIONS
Herb-drug. *Digoxin:* May increase risk of digoxin toxicity because of herb's potassium-depleting effects. Monitor digoxin levels closely.
Disulfiram, metronidazole: May cause a disulfiram-like reaction if herbal preparation contains alcohol. Advise patient to avoid use together.
Nephrotoxic drugs: May increase risk of nephrotoxicity. Advise patient to avoid use together.
NSAIDs: May increase risk of adverse GI effects. Advise patient to avoid use together.
Potassium-wasting diuretics: May cause hypokalemia. Advise patient to avoid use together.

EFFECTS ON LAB TEST RESULTS
• May decrease potassium level.

CAUTIONS
Patients who are pregnant or breast-feeding shouldn't use this herb.

Patients with renal insufficiency should use caution when using the herb.

NURSING CONSIDERATIONS
• Explore patient's knowledge of this herb.

*Liquid contains alcohol.

• The contraceptive effect of gossypol in men is higher than 99%. Fertility usually returns to normal within 3 months after patient stops using the herb; however, in up to 20% of men, inhibition of spermatogenesis may persist for up to 2 years and may be irreversible.

⚡**ALERT:** Gossypol may be cytotoxic to endometrial cells.

• Monitor electrolyte levels, especially potassium, as well as creatinine and BUN levels.

• Monitor patient for muscle weakness and fatigue.

• Tinctures and extracts contain 15% to 60% alcohol and may be unsuitable for children, patients with a history of alcoholism or liver disease, or patients taking certain drugs.

PATIENT TEACHING

• Advise patient to consult a health care provider before using an herbal preparation because another treatment may be available.

• Tell patient that when filling a new prescription he should inform pharmacist of any herbal or dietary supplement he's taking.

• If patient is pregnant or breastfeeding, advise her not to use the herb.

• If patient has a history of alcoholism or liver disease, inform him that some herbal products contain alcohol.

• Inform men of the potential for permanent sterility after taking the herb orally.

• Advise women who are considering using gossypol as a topical spermicide that information on the safety and efficacy of the herb is lacking. Inform them of alternative, safe, and effective contraceptive methods.

• Warn patient to keep all herbal products away from children and pets.

gotu kola

Centella asiatica, C. coriacea, brahma-buti, brahma-manduki, gotu cola, hydrocotyle, Indian pennywort, Indian water navelwort, marsh penny, talepetrako, TECA, thick-leaved pennywort, white rot

Common trade names
Centelase, Centasium, Emdecassol, Gotu Kola Gold Extract, Gotu Kola Herb, Madecassol

AVAILABLE FORMS
Available as ampules, capsules, ointment, powder, tablets, tinctures*, and extract.
Ampule: 10 mg/ml
Capsules: 221 mg, 250 mg, 435 mg, 439 mg, 441 mg
Ointment: 1%
Powder: 2%

ACTIONS & COMPONENTS
Derived from the leaves, stem, and aerial parts of *C. asiatica*. Contains madecassol, madecassic acid, asiatic acid, asiaticentoic acid, centellic acid, centoic acid, isothankuniside, flavonoids (including quercetin and kaempferol), and various terpenoids (such as asiaticoside, brahminoside, brahmoside, centelloside, and madecasoside). Also contains fatty acids, amino acids, phytosterols, and tannin.

Bold italic type indicates that reaction may be life-threatening.

Asiaticoside promotes wound healing, brahminoside and brahmoside possess sedative properties, and madecassoid exerts anti-inflammatory action.

USES
Used for its anticarcinogenic, anti-fertility, and antihypertensive effects. Also used to treat chronic venous insufficiency, chronic hypertension, and chronic hepatic disorders. Used topically to treat psoriasis and burns and to promote wound healing in patients with chronic lesions, such as cutaneous ulcers, leprosy sores, fistulas, and surgical and gynecologic wounds.

DOSAGE & ADMINISTRATION
Capsules: 450 mg once daily.
Creams, ointments: Applied to affected area daily to b.i.d.
Dried leaves: 0.6 g of dried leaves or infusion P.O. t.i.d.
Standardized extract (40% asiaticoside; 29% to 30% asiatic acid and madecassic acid, respectively; and 1% to 2% madecasoside): 20 to 40 mg P.O. t.i.d.

ADVERSE REACTIONS
CNS: sedation.
CV: hypertension.
Metabolic: hypercholesterolemia, hyperglycemia.
Skin: contact dermatitis, burning, pruritus, photosensitivity reactions.

INTERACTIONS
Herb-drug. *Antidiabetics, cholesterol-lowering drugs:* May interfere with drug effect (with large doses). Advise patient to avoid use together.

CNS depressants: May cause additive effects. Advise patient to avoid use together.
Disulfiram, metronidazole: May cause a disulfiram-like reaction if herbal preparation contains alcohol. Advise patient to avoid use together.

EFFECTS ON LAB TEST RESULTS
• May increase glucose and cholesterol levels.

CAUTIONS
Patients who are pregnant or breast-feeding or who have severe renal or hepatic disease shouldn't use this herb. Young children also shouldn't use it.

Patients with a history of contact dermatitis should use caution when using the herb.

NURSING CONSIDERATIONS
• Explore patient's knowledge of this herb.
• Tinctures and extracts contain 15% to 60% alcohol and may be unsuitable for children, patients with a history of alcoholism or liver disease, or patients taking certain drugs.
• Monitor patient for signs of CNS depression, including drowsiness and increased sleep time.
• Monitor glucose and cholesterol levels.

PATIENT TEACHING
• Advise patient to consult a health care provider before using an herbal preparation because another treatment may be available.
• Tell patient that when filling a new prescription he should inform

*Liquid contains alcohol.

pharmacist of any herbal or dietary supplement he's taking.
- If patient has a history of alcoholism or liver disease, inform him that some herbal products contain alcohol.
- Warn patient about the potential for sedation. Advise him to use caution when performing activities that require mental alertness until he knows how the herb affects his CNS.
- If patient is using the herb for contraception, recommend another method.
- Tell patient not to use the herb for longer than 6 weeks at a time.
- Tell patient to take capsules with meals.
- Advise patient to notify her health care provider before using the herb if she suspects or knows that she's pregnant or if she plans to become pregnant.
- Warn patient to keep all herbal products away from children and pets.

grapeseed

Vitis coignetiae, V. vinifera, grapeseed extract, grapeseed oil, muskat

Common trade names
Antistax, Grape Seed Extract, Mega Juice, NutraPack

AVAILABLE FORMS
Available as tablets, capsules, drops, cream, and grape liquid concentrate.

ACTIONS & COMPONENTS
Obtained by grinding the seeds of red grapes. Grapeseed extract contains procyanidins, also called proanthocyanidins, or flavonoids, which are free radical scavengers. The procyanidins inhibit proteolytic enzymes, including hyaluronidase, collagenase, elastase, and beta-glucuronidase. By this mechanism, they help stabilize collagen.

Grapeseed oil contains essential fatty acids and vitamin E. Its antioxidant properties are said to be greater than those of vitamin C or E.

Grapeseed extract also has anticarcinogenic effects. It prevents oxidative damage to cholesterol and may lower the cholesterol level. It protects collagen lining the walls of the arteries and stabilizes the vasculature. It also protects the eyes against oxidative damage and prevents diabetic retinopathy and macular degeneration.

Grapeseed may also prevent dental caries by inhibiting *Streptococcus mutans* and glucan formation from sugar.

USES
Used to prevent CV disease and cancer through its antioxidant properties. Also used to treat venous insufficiency, bruising, edema, and allergic rhinitis.

DOSAGE & ADMINISTRATION
Capsules or tablets: Initially, 75 to 300 mg P.O. daily for 3 weeks, then 40 to 80 mg daily.
Liquid concentrate: 1 tablespoon mixed in 1 cup of water P.O.

Bold italic type indicates that reaction may be life-threatening.

ADVERSE REACTIONS
Hepatic: *hepatotoxicity.*

INTERACTIONS
Herb-drug. *Warfarin:* May increase bleeding potential. Advise patient to avoid use together.

EFFECTS ON LAB TEST RESULTS
• May increase liver enzyme levels. May decrease cholesterol levels.

CAUTIONS
Patients with liver dysfunction should use caution when using the herb.

NURSING CONSIDERATIONS
• Explore patient's knowledge of this herb.
• If patient has liver dysfunction, monitor liver enzyme test results.
• Grapeseed may interfere with the intended therapeutic effect of conventional drugs.
• Grapeseed extract may have antiplatelet effects. If a patient is scheduled for surgery, it may be wise that he stop the supplement 2 to 3 days beforehand. Monitor PT and INR.

PATIENT TEACHING
• Advise patient to consult a health care provider before using an herbal preparation because another treatment may be available.
• Tell patient that when filling a new prescription he should inform pharmacist of any herbal or dietary supplement he's taking.
• Warn patient not to use grapeseed to treat signs and symptoms of venous insufficiency or a circulatory disorder before seeking medical evaluation, because doing so may delay diagnosis of a potentially serious medical condition.
• Warn patient to keep all herbal products away from children and pets.

green tea

Camellia sinensis, C. thea, C. theifera, Thea bohea, T. sinensis, T. viridis, Chinese tea, Matsucha

Common trade names
Chinese Green Tea Bags, Green Tea Extract, Green Tea Power, Green Tea Power Caffeine Free, Standardized Green Tea Extract

AVAILABLE FORMS
Available as capsules, dried extract, liquid, tablets, and teas.
Capsules: 100 mg, 150 mg, 175 mg, 333 mg, 383 mg, 500 mg
Tablets: 100 mg

ACTIONS & COMPONENTS
Prepared from the steamed and dried leaves of *C. sinensis.* Contains the polyphenols epigallocatechin and epigallocatechin-3-gallate, two of the most potent anticarcinogenic substances found in nature.

Green tea's anticarcinogenic effects are attributed to its antioxidant activity and its ability to inhibit cell proliferation and induce apoptosis. The caffeine may stimulate the CNS. The tannins have astringent properties, which provide an antidiarrheal effect.

Green tea may also decrease cholesterol levels and have antibacterial properties.

*Liquid contains alcohol.

USES
Used to prevent cancer, hyperlipidemia, atherosclerosis, dental caries, and headaches and to treat wounds, skin disorders, stomach disorders, and infectious diarrhea. Also used as a CNS stimulant, a mild diuretic, an antibacterial and, topically, an astringent.

DOSAGE & ADMINISTRATION
Oral use: Typically 300 to 400 mg of polyphenols daily (3 cups of green tea contain 240 to 320 mg of polyphenols).

ADVERSE REACTIONS
CNS: nervousness, insomnia.
CV: tachycardia.
GI: hyperacidity, GI irritation, decreased appetite, constipation, diarrhea.
Respiratory: asthma.
Other: allergic reactions.

INTERACTIONS
Herb-drug. *Anticoagulants, antiplatelet drugs:* May increase bleeding potential. Monitor patient closely.
Beta agonists: May potentiate cardiac inotropic effects because of the caffeine component. Advise patient to avoid use together.
Cimetidine: May decrease caffeine clearance (by 30% to 50%). Advise patient to avoid use together.
Ephedrine, other stimulant drugs: Increases stimulatory effects because of the caffeine component. Advise patient to avoid use together.
Hormonal contraceptives: May cause decreased caffeine clearance. Advise patient to avoid use together.

Lithium: Lithium levels increase significantly with abrupt withdrawal of caffeine. Tell patient not to stop drinking the tea abruptly.
MAO inhibitors: May cause hypertensive crisis because of the caffeine component. Advise patient to avoid use together.
Theophylline: May cause decreased theophylline clearance and, thus, increased theophylline levels. Advise patient to avoid use together.

EFFECTS ON LAB TEST RESULTS
• May increase glucose, cholesterol, urine creatine, urine catecholamine, 5-hydroxyindoleacetic acid, vanillylmandelic acid, and theophylline levels.
• May cause false-positive results for urate tests and tests for pheochromocytoma and neuroblastoma. May alter anticoagulant test results.

CAUTIONS
Patients who are allergic to green tea or are breast-feeding shouldn't use green tea. Green tea shouldn't be given to infants or small children. Pregnant women should avoid or minimize use because of the caffeine.

Patients with CV or renal disease, hyperthyroidism, or a nervous disorder should use caution when using the herb.

NURSING CONSIDERATIONS
• Explore patient's knowledge of this herb.
• Look for products standardized to 80% polyphenol and 55% epigallocatechin-3-gallate.

Bold italic type indicates that reaction may be life-threatening.

• Daily consumption should be limited to 4 cups, or the equivalent of 300 mg of caffeine, to avoid the adverse effects of caffeine.

• Prolonged high caffeine intake may cause restlessness, irritability, insomnia, palpitations, vertigo, headache, and adverse GI effects. Monitor patient's intake.

• The adverse GI effects of chlorogenic acid and tannin can be avoided by adding milk to the tea mixture.

• The tannin content in tea increases the longer the tea is left to brew; a high tannin content increases the tea's antidiarrheal properties.

• Administering green tea with an iron supplement or a multivitamin with iron inhibits the body from absorbing the iron, especially in children.

• The first signs of a toxic reaction are vomiting and abdominal spasm.

PATIENT TEACHING

• Advise patient to consult a health care provider before using an herbal preparation because another treatment may be available.

• Tell patient that when filling a new prescription he should inform pharmacist of any herbal or dietary supplement he's taking.

• Instruct patient not to drink more than 4 cups a day to avoid or minimize the adverse effects of caffeine.

• Inform patient that heavy tea consumption may be associated with esophageal cancer as a result of the tannin content.

• Tell patient that the first indications of a toxic reaction are vomiting and abdominal spasm.

• Warn patient to keep all herbal products away from children and pets.

ground ivy

Glechoma hederacea, alehoof, cat's-foot, creeping Charlie, gill-go-by-the-hedge, gill-go-over-the-ground, haymaids, hedgemaids, lizzy-run-up-the-hedge, robin-run-in-the-hedge, tun-hoof, turnhoof

Common trade names
None known

AVAILABLE FORMS
Available as a tea of leaves and flowers, liquid extract*, and tincture*.

ACTIONS & COMPONENTS
Contains the volatile oil pulegone, which has abortifacient, hepatotoxic, and irritant properties.

USES
Used to dry secretions, to treat poorly healing wounds, and to treat upper-respiratory-tract complaints, including problems with the ears, nose, and throat. Used as a decongestant, an anti-inflammatory, and an astringent. May also help with problems in the GI tract, including diarrhea, gastritis, and hemorrhoids.

In Chinese medicine, ground ivy is used to treat irregular periods, lower abdominal pain, scabies, carbuncles, dysentery, and jaundice.

DOSAGE & ADMINISTRATION
Dried drug: 2 to 4 g P.O. daily.

---

*Liquid contains alcohol.

Fluidextract (1:1, 25% ethanol):
14 to 28 grains P.O. t.i.d.
Topical: Crushed leaves are applied to affected area.

ADVERSE REACTIONS
GI: mucosal irritation (with high oral doses)

INTERACTIONS
Herb-drug. *Disulfiram, metronidazole:* May cause a disulfiram-like reaction if herbal preparation contains alcohol. Advise patient to avoid use together.

EFFECTS ON LAB TEST RESULTS
None reported.

CAUTIONS
Children, women who are pregnant or breast-feeding, and those with renal or hepatic impairment shouldn't use the herb.

NURSING CONSIDERATIONS
• Explore patient's knowledge of this herb.
• Ground ivy may interfere with the intended therapeutic effects of conventional drugs.
• Tinctures and extracts contain 15% to 60% alcohol and may be unsuitable for children, patients with a history of alcoholism or liver disease, or patients taking certain drugs.
• Horses grazing on this plant have experienced cyanosis, lung congestion, sweating, salivation, pupil dilation, and death.

PATIENT TEACHING
• Advise patient to consult a health care provider before using an herbal preparation because another treatment may be available.
• Tell patient that when filling a new prescription he should inform pharmacist of any herbal or dietary supplement he's taking.
• If patient has a history of alcoholism or liver disease, inform him that some herbal products contain alcohol.
• Warn patient to keep all herbal products away from children and pets.

guarana

Paullinia cupana, P. sorbilis,
Brazilian cocoa, guarana bread,
guarana gum, guarana paste,
guarana seed, guarana seed
paste, paullinia, zoom

Common trade names
*Guarana Plus, Guarana Rush,
Superguarana*

AVAILABLE FORMS
Available as alcoholic extracts*, capsules, elixirs, syrups, tablets, and teas. Also available in various soft drinks, weight-loss products, energy drinks, and vitamin supplements.

ACTIONS & COMPONENTS
Guarana is the dried paste made from the peeled, dried, roasted, and crushed seeds of *P. cupana.* Contains 3% to 7% caffeine (whereas coffee contains 1% to 2% caffeine); tannins, which provide an astringent taste; and theophylline and theobromine, which are alkaloids that are similar to caffeine.
  Primarily used for its caffeine content. Stimulates the CNS, sup-

presses the appetite, and inhibits platelet aggregation. Also induces diuresis and relaxes bronchial smooth muscle.

USES
Used to promote weight loss, to enhance athletic performance, to protect against malaria and dysentery, and to treat headaches, painful menstruation, and digestion problems. Used as a stimulant similar to coffee or tea, an aphrodisiac, and a tonic to quiet hunger or thirst. Also used as a flavoring agent and a source of caffeine in soft drinks.

DOSAGE & ADMINISTRATION
Capsules: 1 to 2 capsules contain 200 to 800 mg of guarana extract. Dosage shouldn't exceed 3 g daily.

ADVERSE REACTIONS
CNS: insomnia, irritation, nervousness, anxiety, headache, *seizures.*
CV: rapid heart rate, *arrhythmias.*
EENT: tinnitus.
GI: abdominal spasms, vomiting.
GU: diuresis, painful urination
Hematologic: inhibited platelet aggregation.
Other: fibrocystic breast disease.

INTERACTIONS
Herb-drug. *Adenosine:* Causes decreased antiarrhythmic effect. Patient may require additional doses or another drug.
Anticoagulants, antiplatelet drugs: May increase bleeding tendency. Monitor PT and INR.
Caffeine-containing drugs such as NoDoz, Vivarin, and some analgesics: May potentiate effects of caffeine. Advise patient to avoid use together.
Cimetidine: May cause decreased clearance of caffeine from the body, thus increasing its effects. Monitor patient for toxic reaction.
Ciprofloxacin: May cause decreased clearance of caffeine from the body, thus increasing its effects. Advise patient to use caution if using the herb and drug together.
Disulfiram, metronidazole: May cause a disulfiram-like reaction if herbal preparation contains alcohol. Advise patient to avoid use together.
Ephedrine, phenylpropanolamine: Causes increased stimulant effects and possibly increased blood pressure. Advise patient to avoid use together.
Theophylline: May cause increased drug effects (with large amounts of guarana and caffeine). Monitor patient for toxic reaction.
Herb-herb. *Green tea, black tea, yerba maté:* May cause additive effects. Advise patient to avoid use together.
Herb-food. *Products containing caffeine, including coffee and cola beverages:* Cause additive effects. Advise patient to avoid use together.

EFFECTS ON LAB TEST RESULTS
- May increase urate levels.
- May cause false-positive test results for pheochromocytoma and neuroblastoma. May increase bleeding time.

CAUTIONS
Patients who are pregnant or breast-feeding or who have a car-

---

*Liquid contains alcohol.

diac arrhythmia shouldn't use the herb.

Patients sensitive to caffeine and patients with CV or renal disease, hyperthyroidism, or a nervous disorder such as panic attacks or anxiety should use caution when using the herb.

NURSING CONSIDERATIONS
• Explore patient's knowledge of this herb.
• High doses may cause caffeine-like adverse reactions.
• Tinctures and extracts contain 15% to 60% alcohol and may be unsuitable for children, patients with a history of alcoholism or liver disease, or patients taking certain drugs.
• If patient is sensitive to caffeine, monitor blood pressure and heart rate.
• If patient is taking an anticoagulant or an antiplatelet drug, monitor PT and INR.
• The first indications of a toxic reaction are dysuria, vomiting, and abdominal spasms.

PATIENT TEACHING
• Advise patient to consult a health care provider before using an herbal preparation because another treatment may be available.
• Tell patient that when filling a new prescription he should inform pharmacist of any herbal or dietary supplement he's taking.
• If patient has a history of alcoholism or liver disease, inform him that some herbal products contain alcohol.
• If patient is pregnant or is planning to become pregnant, advise her not to use the herb.

• Tell patient that herb may increase blood pressure, cause abnormal heart rhythms, and aggravate hiatal hernia, peptic ulcer disease, gastroesophageal reflux disease, and anxiety or depressive disorders.
• Inform patient that caffeine content in guarana is higher than in coffee.
• Warn patient to keep all herbal products away from children and pets.

guggul

Commiphora mukul, guggal, guggal gum, guggal gum resin, guggalsterones, gugulipid, gum guggulu

Common trade names
Doctor's Best Ultra Guggulow , Guggul Raj, Gugulmax, GugulPlus

AVAILABLE FORMS
Available as capsules and tablets.

ACTIONS & COMPONENTS
An extract of the plant containing gugulipid and guggulsterone is used medicinally. It may lower cholesterol levels by 24% and triglyceride levels by 23% by increasing the hepatic binding of low-density lipoproteins. The herb may also alter the high-density-lipoprotein level. Guggulsterone stimulates the thyroid gland, has anti-inflammatory properties, may help in weight reduction, and protects against myocardial necrosis resulting from drug toxicity.

Bold italic type indicates that reaction may be life-threatening.

USES

Used primarily for its ability to decrease cholesterol levels. Also used to treat atherosclerosis and high cholesterol and triglyceride levels.

In Ayurvedic medicine, guggul is used to treat arthritis and to aid in weight loss.

DOSAGE & ADMINISTRATION

Oral use: Daily dose of guggulsterone is 25 mg t.i.d. This is provided in a 500-mg tablet standardized to contain 5% guggulsterone.

ADVERSE REACTIONS

CNS: headaches.
GI: diarrhea, anorexia, abdominal pain.
Respiratory: hiccups.
Skin: rash.

INTERACTIONS

Herb-drug. *Thyroid drugs:* Causes altered effects because of herb's stimulation of the thyroid gland. Advise patient to avoid use together.
Herb-herb. *Garlic:* Increases lipid-lowering effect, which is a therapeutic effect.

EFFECTS ON LAB TEST RESULTS

• May decrease LDL and total cholesterol and triglyceride levels.

CAUTIONS

Package inserts of products sold in India recommend against using guggul in patients with liver or kidney disease. Patients who are pregnant or breast-feeding also shouldn't use the herb.

NURSING CONSIDERATIONS

• Explore patient's knowledge of this herb.
• Monitor patient who has thyroid disease or takes a thyroid supplement because guggul stimulates the thyroid gland.
• Guggul may interfere with the intended therapeutic effects of conventional drugs.
• Only preparations with standardized amounts of guggulsterone should be used.
• Use should be limited to 12 to 24 weeks.
• Monitor patient's cholesterol level.

PATIENT TEACHING

• Advise patient to consult a health care provider before using an herbal preparation because another treatment may be available.
• Tell patient that when filling a new prescription he should inform pharmacist of any herbal or dietary supplement he's taking.
• If patient is pregnant, breast-feeding, or planning to become pregnant, advise her not to use this herb.
• Tell patient that herb isn't a substitute for healthy eating and exercise.
• Warn patient to keep all herbal products away from children and pets.

H

hawthorn

Crataegus laevigata, C. monogyna, English hawthorn, haw, may, maybush

Common trade names
Hawthorne Berry, Hawthorne Extract, Hawthorne Formula, Hawthorne Power

AVAILABLE FORMS
Available as dried leaves, liquid extract*, and tincture*.

ACTIONS & COMPONENTS
The active compounds of hawthorn are obtained from the berries, flowers, and leaves of the *Crataegus* species, most commonly from *C. laevigata* or *C. monogyna.* The primary ingredients responsible for the pharmacologic effects of hawthorn include flavonoids and procyanidins.

The hawthorn flavonoids increase myocardial contraction by dilating coronary blood vessels, reducing peripheral resistance, and reducing oxygen consumption. They also lower blood pressure by inhibiting angiotensin-converting enzymes. The procyanidins slow the heart rate, lengthening the refractory period, and also have mild CNS depressant effects. Hawthorn's pharmacologic effects usually develop slowly.

USES
Used to regulate blood pressure and heart rate and to treat atherosclerosis. Used as a cardiotonic and as a sedative for sleep. Used in mild cardiac insufficiency, heart conditions not requiring digoxin, mild stable forms of angina pectoris, and mild forms of bradycardia and palpitations.

DOSAGE & ADMINISTRATION
Dried fruit: 300 to 1,000 mg P.O. t.i.d. after meals.
Liquid extract (1:1 in 25% alcohol): 0.5 to 1 ml P.O. t.i.d.
Oral use: Average daily dose is 5 g or 160 to 900 mg of extract.
Tincture (1:5 in 45% alcohol): 1 to 2 ml P.O. t.i.d.

ADVERSE REACTIONS
CNS: agitation, dizziness, fatigue, headache, insomnia, sedation.
CV: circulatory disturbances, palpitations, chest pain.
GI: GI complaints, nausea.
Respiratory: shortness of breath.
Skin: diaphoresis, rash on hands.

INTERACTIONS
Herb-drug. *Antiarrhythmics:* May increase antiarrhythmic action. (Herb's action is similar to that of a class III antiarrhythmic.) Advise patient to avoid use together.
Antihypertensives, nitrates: Increases risk of hypotension. Advise patient to avoid use together.
Cardiac glycosides: Increases risk of cardiac toxicity. Advise patient to avoid use together. If used together, monitor digoxin level.
CNS depressants: Causes additive depressant effects. Monitor patient closely.

Bold italic type indicates that reaction may be life-threatening.

Disulfiram, metronidazole: May cause a disulfiram-like reaction if herbal preparation contains alcohol. Advise patient to avoid use together.

EFFECTS ON LAB TEST RESULTS
• May increase digoxin level.

CAUTIONS
Patients who are sensitive to hawthorn or have severe renal or hepatic impairment shouldn't use this herb, nor should children or patients who are pregnant or breast-feeding.

NURSING CONSIDERATIONS
• Explore patient's knowledge of this herb.
• Tinctures and extracts contain 15% to 60% alcohol and may be unsuitable for children, patients with a history of alcoholism or liver disease, or patients taking certain drugs.
• High doses may cause hypotension and sedation. Monitor patient for adverse CNS reactions, and monitor blood pressure.
• This herb may interfere with digoxin's effects or blood levels.
• If patient has heart failure, he should use hawthorn only under close medical supervision and in combination with other standard treatments, as directed.
• Observe patient closely for adverse reactions, especially CNS reactions.

PATIENT TEACHING
• Advise patient to consult a health care provider before using an herbal preparation because another treatment may be available.

• Tell patient that when filling a new prescription he should inform pharmacist of any herbal or dietary supplement he's taking.
• Warn patient not to treat cardiac signs and symptoms, such as swelling and angina, before seeking medical evaluation, because doing so may delay diagnosis of a potentially serious medical condition.
• If patient has a history of alcoholism or liver disease, inform him that some herbal products contain alcohol.
• Advise patient to use hawthorn only under medical supervision.
• Advise patient to use caution when performing activities that require mental alertness until he knows how the herb affects his CNS.
• Warn patient that hawthorn won't stop an angina attack.
• Instruct patient to notify his health care provider if he experiences dizziness, excessive sedation, irregular heartbeats, or any other adverse reaction.
• Instruct patient to seek emergency medical help if he experiences shortness of breath or chest pain.
• Warn patient to keep all herbal products away from children and pets.

*Liquid contains alcohol.

hellebore, American

Veratrum viride, bear's foot, bugbane, devil's bite, Earth gall, false hellebore, green hellebore, Indian poke, itch-weed, swamp hellebore, tickleweed, white hellebore

Common trade names
Cryptenamine

AVAILABLE FORMS
Available as liquid extract*, powder, and tincture*.

ACTIONS & COMPONENTS
The active ingredients of American hellebore are steroid ester alkaloids, which are obtained from the dried rhizome and roots of *Veratrum viride.* They exert their physiologic effects by lowering arterial blood pressure and heart and respiratory rates. They also inhibit inactivation of sodium-ion channels in excitable cells, thus increasing nerve and muscle excitability, especially in the cardiac muscles.

USES
Used to depress the action of the heart and reduce blood pressure. Also used as a diuretic, an antispasmodic, an antipyretic, and a sedative.

DOSAGE & ADMINISTRATION
Tincture (1:10): 0.3 to 2 ml P.O. daily.

ADVERSE REACTIONS
CNS: *seizures,* syncope, sedation, paralysis.
CV: *arrhythmias, bradycardia,* ECG changes, hypertension, hypotension.
EENT: blindness, burning sensation in the mouth and pharynx, lacrimation, salivation, sneezing.
GI: abdominal pain and distention, diarrhea, nausea, vomiting.
Musculoskeletal: muscular weakness.
Respiratory: *respiratory depression.*

INTERACTIONS
Herb-drug. *Cardiac drugs, including antiarrhythmics, antihypertensives, cardiac glycosides, and nitrates:* May cause increased or decreased drug effects. Monitor patient closely if used together.
CNS depressants: Causes increased sedation and respiratory depression. Advise patient to use caution if using the herb and drug together.
Disulfiram, metronidazole: May cause a disulfiram-like reaction if herbal preparation contains alcohol. Advise patient to avoid use together.
H_2 blockers, proton-pump inhibitors: May increase infectious GI inflammatory conditions because of herb's ability to irritate GI tract. Advise patient to avoid use together.

EFFECTS ON LAB TEST RESULTS
• May alter digoxin level.

CAUTIONS
Medicinal use isn't recommended because of the herb's narrow therapeutic index and highly toxic adverse effects.

Bold·italic type indicates that reaction may be life-threatening.

NURSING CONSIDERATIONS
• Explore patient's knowledge of this herb.
• The herb shouldn't be used in allopathic medicine because of the high risk of a toxic reaction.
• Tinctures and extracts contain 15% to 60% alcohol and may be unsuitable for children, patients with a history of alcoholism or liver disease, or patients taking certain drugs.

⚡ALERT: Signs and symptoms of a toxic reaction include burning of mouth and throat, inability to swallow, abdominal pain, cardiac abnormalities, seizures, impaired vision, nausea, shortness of breath, loss of consciousness, and paralysis. Monitor patient closely for adverse reactions.
• If overdose occurs, perform gastric lavage and administer activated charcoal, I.V. diazepam to treat spasms, and sodium bicarbonate to counteract acidosis. Patient may need respiratory support with mechanical ventilation.

PATIENT TEACHING
• If patient has a chronic illness, advise him not to put off seeking medical evaluation, because doing so may delay diagnosis of a potentially serious medical condition.
• If patient has a history of alcoholism or liver disease, inform him that some herbal products contain alcohol.
• Advise patient not to use the herb because of toxic adverse effects and narrow therapeutic index.
• Warn patient to keep all herbal products away from children and pets.

hellebore, black

Helleborus niger, Christe herbe, Christmas rose, melampode

Common trade names
None known

AVAILABLE FORMS
Available as liquid extract*, powder, and solid extract.

ACTIONS & COMPONENTS
The active ingredients are obtained from the rhizome and root of the *H. niger* plant. The whole black hellebore plant is considered poisonous. Black hellebore root contains glycosides with cardioactive properties similar to digitalis. It also contains saponins that can irritate the mucous membranes. Topical application of the herb may cause serious skin irritation.

USES
Used to treat nausea, worm infestations, amenorrhea, and anxiety. Also used as a laxative and an abortifacient. Because of its possible immunostimulatory effects, black hellebore is used as adjuvant therapy in cancer patients.

Used in homeopathy to treat eclampsia, epilepsy, meningitis, encephalitis, and mental disorders.

DOSAGE & ADMINISTRATION
Powder (medicine content 10%):
The average daily dose in one source is 0.05 g, with a maximum single dose of 0.2 g.

ADVERSE REACTIONS
CNS: dizziness.

*Liquid contains alcohol.

CV: *arrhythmias, bradycardia,* irregular pulse.
EENT: burning sensation in the mouth and pharynx, increased salivation, sneezing.
GI: abdominal pain, diarrhea, nausea, vomiting.
Respiratory: shortness of breath, *respiratory failure.*
Skin: irritation or inflammation.

INTERACTIONS
Herb-drug. *Cardiac drugs, including antiarrhythmics, beta blockers, and cardiac glycosides:* May cause increased or decreased drug effects. Monitor patient closely if he's using the herb and drug together.
CNS depressants: May cause increased sedation and respiratory depression. Advise patient to use caution if using the herb and drug together.
Disulfiram, metronidazole: May cause a disulfiram-like reaction if herbal preparation contains alcohol. Advise patient to avoid use together.

EFFECTS ON LAB TEST RESULTS
• May alter digoxin level.

CAUTIONS
Medicinal use isn't recommended because of the plant's poisonous nature and its highly toxic adverse effects.

NURSING CONSIDERATIONS
• Explore patient's knowledge of this herb.
• Herb is considered dangerous in allopathic doses.

⚡**ALERT:** Signs and symptoms of poisoning include a scratchy throat or mouth, excessive salivation, dizziness, abdominal cramps, shortness of breath, and asphyxiation.
• Monitor patient closely for a toxic reaction.
• Tinctures and extracts contain 15% to 60% alcohol and may be unsuitable for children, patients with a history of alcoholism or liver disease, or patients taking certain drugs.

PATIENT TEACHING
• Advise patient that black hellebore may interfere with the therapeutic effects of conventional drugs.
• If patient has a history of alcoholism or liver disease, inform him that some herbal products contain alcohol.
• If patient has a chronic illness, advise him not to put off seeking medical evaluation, because doing so can delay diagnosis of a potentially serious medical condition.
⚡**ALERT:** Caution patient that black hellebore is unsafe for use because it's extremely narcotic. It can cause death by seizures and heart failure.
• Warn patient to keep all herbal products away from children and pets.

Bold italic type indicates that reaction may be life-threatening.

hops

Humulus lupulus, common
hops, European hops, lupulin

Common trade names
Ez, RE-X, Stress Free

AVAILABLE FORMS
Available as liquid extract*, tea
preparation, and tincture*.

ACTIONS & COMPONENTS
The medicinal parts include the
glandular hairs separated from the
flowers, the fresh cones, and the
fresh or dried female flowers.

The active ingredient, 2-methyl-
3-butene-2-ol, has sedative-
hypnotic properties. The bitter
acid constituents lupulone and
humulone inhibit the growth of
gram-positive organisms by disrupting the primary membrane of
the bacteria. The flavonoglucosides
have diuretic and antispasmodic
activities. Estrogenic or hormone
activities in hops haven't been
proven in recent studies.

USES
Used to treat neuralgia, nervous
tension, restlessness, intestinal
spasms, anxiety, mood disturbances, sleep disturbances such as
insomnia, and digestive tract disorders involving spasms of the
smooth muscle. Used as a mild
diuretic, an appetite stimulant, a
digestive aid, and an aphrodisiac.
Topically, used as a mild antibacterial. Also used to preserve beer.

DOSAGE & ADMINISTRATION
As a sedative: 500 to 1,000 mg of
dried herb P.O. as a single dose. Or
as tea, prepared by brewing dried
herb in 5 ounces of boiling water
for 5 to 10 minutes and then straining.
*Liquid extract (1:1 preparation in
45% alcohol):* 0.5 to 2 ml P.O. as a
single dose.
*Tincture (1:5 preparation in 60%
alcohol):* 1 to 2 ml P.O. as a single
dose.

ADVERSE REACTIONS
CNS: sedation, depression.
Respiratory: bronchial irritation
and bronchitis after inhalation.
Skin: contact dermatitis.
Other: *anaphylaxis,* allergic reac-
tion.

INTERACTIONS
Herb-drug. *Antidepressants:* May
counteract drug action. Advise patient to avoid use together.
CNS depressants: May cause additive effects. Advise patient to avoid
using the herb and drug together.
Disulfiram, metronidazole: May
cause a disulfiram-like reaction if
herbal preparation contains alcohol. Advise patient to avoid use
together.
Phenothiazine-type antipsychotics:
May increase hyperthermia. Advise patient to avoid use together.

EFFECTS ON LAB TEST RESULTS
None reported.

CAUTIONS
Patients with sensitivity to hops
and patients with estrogenic-
dependent tumors, such as breast,
uterine, or cervical cancer should
avoid use because of possible estrogenic effects.

*Liquid contains alcohol.

Patients taking a CNS depressant or an antipsychotic should use extreme caution if using the herb and drug together.

NURSING CONSIDERATIONS
● Explore patient's knowledge of this herb.
● Tinctures and extracts contain 15% to 60% alcohol and may be unsuitable for children, patients with a history of alcoholism or liver disease, or patients taking certain drugs.
● Monitor patient for adverse reactions, such as increased sedation and respiratory difficulties.
● Patient shouldn't inhale smoke from the plant.

PATIENT TEACHING
● Advise patient to consult a health care provider before using an herbal preparation because another treatment may be available.
● Tell patient that when filling a new prescription he should inform pharmacist of any herbal or dietary supplement he's taking.
● Warn patient not to treat digestive problems or mood disturbances with hops before seeking medical evaluation, because doing so may delay diagnosis of a potentially serious medical condition.
● If patient has a history of alcoholism or liver disease, inform him that some herbal products contain alcohol.
● Although hops is botanically related to marijuana, smoking the plant as a substitute may be dangerous because of the herb's adverse effects.
● Advise patient to use caution when performing activities that require mental alertness until he knows how the herb affects his CNS.
● Advise patient to notify health care provider immediately if he develops a rash, shortness of breath, wheezing, or itching.
● Warn patient to keep all herbal products away from children and pets.

horehound

Marrubium vulgare, common horehound, hoarhound, houndsbane, marrubium, white horehound

Common trade names
Horehound Herb, Horehound Tea

AVAILABLE FORMS
Available as dried herb, liquid extract*, lozenges, powder, syrup, and tea.

ACTIONS & COMPONENTS
The active ingredients are obtained from the leaves and flowers of *M. vulgare.* Horehound's active compound, marrubiin, stimulates secretions in the bronchioles and works as an expectorant. It also contains antiarrhythmic properties but is of limited use because large doses can also cause arrhythmias. Marrubin acid, derived from marrubiin, stimulates bile secretion. An aqueous extract from horehound may have antagonistic activities toward serotonin. The horehound extract has hypoglycemic effects.

USES
Used to treat acute or chronic bronchitis, whooping cough, and

---

Bold italic type indicates that reaction may be life-threatening.

sore throat. Used as an expectorant for treating nonproductive coughs and as a digestive aid. Horehound also may be used for its transient bile secretion-stimulant properties.

DOSAGE & ADMINISTRATION

Dried herbs: 1 to 2 g P.O. t.i.d. as an infusion. Prepared by pouring boiling water over 1 to 2 g of the herb and straining after 10 minutes.

Liquid extract (1:1 preparation in 20% alcohol): 2 to 4 ml P.O. t.i.d.

Oral use: Average daily dose is 4.5 g of the herb; 30 to 60 ml of the pressed juice.

ADVERSE REACTIONS

CV: *arrhythmias.*
GI: dyspepsia, diarrhea.
Metabolic: *hypoglycemia.*
Skin: contact dermatitis.

INTERACTIONS

Herb-drug. *Antiarrhythmics, some antidepressants, antiemetics, and antimigraine drugs:* May potentiate serotonergic effects. Advise patient to use caution if using the herb and drug together.

Antidiabetics, insulin: Causes increased hypoglycemic effects. Monitor glucose level.

Disulfiram, metronidazole: May cause a disulfiram-like reaction if herbal preparation contains alcohol. Advise patient to avoid use together.

EFFECTS ON LAB TEST RESULTS

• May decrease glucose level.

CAUTIONS

Patients with arrhythmias or diabetes mellitus and pregnant or breast-feeding patients shouldn't use this herb.

Patients with CV disease should use caution if using the herb and drug together.

NURSING CONSIDERATIONS

• Explore patient's knowledge of this herb.
• Medicinal use isn't recommended. The FDA banned the use of this herb in OTC cough remedies because of unconvincing evidence to support its effectiveness; however, horehound is still available in products made to treat sore throats.
• Herb may interfere with the intended therapeutic effects of conventional drugs.
• Tinctures and extracts contain between 15% and 60% alcohol and may be unsuitable for children, patients with a history of alcoholism or liver disease, or patients taking certain drugs.
• Monitor patient's glucose level and heart rate and rhythm.
• Monitor patient for changes in his bowel habits.

PATIENT TEACHING

• Advise patient to consult a health care provider before using an herbal preparation because another treatment may be available.
• Tell patient that when filling a new prescription he should inform pharmacist of any herbal or dietary supplement he's taking.
• Warn patient not to treat chronic cough or indigestion with horehound before seeking medical evaluation, because doing so may delay diagnosis of a potentially serious medical condition.

---

*Liquid contains alcohol.

- If patient has a history of alcoholism or liver disease, inform him that some herbal products contain alcohol.
- If patient has diabetes or a cardiac problem, advise him not to use this herb.
- If patient experiences upset stomach or diarrhea after using the herb, advise him to stop using it or to use less of it.
- Advise patient to seek medical help if cough doesn't improve significantly in 2 weeks or if a cough produces brown, black, or bloody phlegm.
- Warn patient to keep all herbal products away from children and pets.

horse chestnut

Aesculus hippocastanum, A. californicum, buckeye, California buckeye, chestnut, Ohio buckeye, Spanish chestnut

Common trade names
Horse Chestnut, Venastat
Combination products: *Arthro-Therapy, Cellu-Var Cream, VariCare, Varicosin, VenoCare*

AVAILABLE FORMS
Available as capsules and as creams made from an aescin–cholesterol complex.
Capsules (extract standardized for an aescin content of 16% to 21%): 250 mg/300 mg

ACTIONS & COMPONENTS
Derived from the seeds and bark of the Aesculus tree. Aescin seems to provide some weak diuretic activity and may decrease the permeability of venous capillaries. Also, it has a tonic effect on the veins and prevents collagen breakdown by inhibiting glycosaminoglycan hydrolases. Sterol content may have some anti-inflammatory activity. The toxic glycoside aesculin is a hydroxycoumarin with potential antithrombotic activity. However, aesculin is removed during preparation.

USES
Used to treat chronic venous insufficiency, varicose veins, leg pain and cramps, tiredness, tension, and leg swelling and edema. Extract is used as a conjunctive treatment for lymphedema, hemorrhoids, and enlarged prostate.

Horse chestnut has been used as an analgesic, anticoagulant, antipyretic, astringent, expectorant, and tonic. It has also been used to treat skin ulcers, phlebitis, cough, and diarrhea.

DOSAGE & ADMINISTRATION
For symptomatic treatment of chronic venous insufficiency:
250 mg P.O. daily to t.i.d. Some sources recommend taking 450 to 750 mg daily to decrease signs and symptoms and then decreasing dose to 175 to 350 mg daily.
Tincture formulation: 1 to 4 ml P.O. t.i.d.

ADVERSE REACTIONS
GI: GI irritation, especially with immediate-release product.
GU: *nephrotoxicity.*
Hepatic: *hepatotoxicity.*
Musculoskeletal: calf cramps.

Bold italic type indicates that reaction may be life-threatening.

Skin: itching, skin cancer (topical skin cleansers).
Other: *anaphylaxis,* increased potential for bleeding or bruising.

INTERACTIONS
Herb-drug. *Anticoagulants:* May increase anticoagulant effects, resulting in increased bleeding and bruising. Monitor PT and INR.
Antidiabetics, insulin: Causes increased hypoglycemic effects. Monitor glucose level.
Drugs that are highly protein-bound: May cause drug displacement from aescin binding to plasma proteins. Monitor patient for drug effectiveness and toxicity.
Herb-herb. *Herbs with anticoagulant or antiplatelet potential such as feverfew, garlic, ginkgo, and ginseng:* May increase anticoagulant effects, resulting in increased bleeding and bruising. Advise patient to use caution if using the herb and drug together.
Herbs with hypoglycemic potential, such as aconite, dong quai, and gotu kola: Causes increased hypoglycemic effects. Monitor glucose level.

EFFECTS ON LAB TEST RESULTS
• May increase liver enzyme levels. May decrease glucose level.
• May increase PT and INR.

CAUTIONS
The FDA considers this herb unsafe. Patients who have severe renal or hepatic impairment or diabetes or who are taking an anticoagulant shouldn't take this herb, nor should pregnant or breast-feeding patients. Patients with infectious or inflammatory GI conditions shouldn't use the herb because of the potential for GI tract irritation.

NURSING CONSIDERATIONS
• Explore patient's knowledge of this herb.
• The nuts, seeds, twigs, sprouts, and leaves of horse chestnut are poisonous. Standardized formulations remove most of the toxins and standardize the amount of aescin.
⚡**ALERT:** High doses and non-standardized forms of horse chestnut can be lethal.
• Signs and symptoms of toxicity include loss of coordination, salivation, hemolysis, headache, dilated pupils, muscle twitching, seizures, vomiting, diarrhea, depression, paralysis, respiratory and cardiac failure, and death.
• Monitor patient for signs and symptoms of toxicity, and instruct him to stop using the herb immediately if any occur.
• If patient is taking an antidiabetic for hypoglycemia, monitor his glucose level.

PATIENT TEACHING
⚡**ALERT:** Inform patient that the FDA considers this herb unsafe and that patients have died after using it.
• Advise patient to use only a standardized extract containing 16% to 21% aescin, at recommended doses, and to discontinue use if he experiences signs or symptoms of a toxic reaction.
• Tell patient that the herb is only symptomatic treatment for chronic venous insufficiency and not a cure.

*Liquid contains alcohol.

• Advise patient not to confuse horse chestnut with sweet chestnut, which is a food.

✒ALERT: Advise patient to keep the herb away from children. Consumption of leaves, twigs, and seeds in amounts equaling 1% of a child's weight may be lethal.

• Warn patient to keep all herbal products away from children and pets.

horseradish

Armoracia rusticana, great raifort, mountain radish, pepperrot, red cole

Common trade names
Horseradish

AVAILABLE FORMS
Available as fresh or dried root, ointment with 2% mustard oil from pressed root, and tincture*.

ACTIONS & COMPONENTS
Topically, the mustard content irritates the skin and stimulates local blood flow, thus relieving minor muscle aches and inflamed joints or tissues. Both the mustard oil and the glucosinolate composition give the root its characteristic pungency, helping to decrease congestion and inflammation of the respiratory tract. Horseradish may also have some antimicrobial activity against both gram-negative and gram-positive bacteria.

USES
Used orally to decrease sinus congestion, to relieve cough from congestion, and to treat edematous conditions; used as an adjunct to treat UTIs and kidney stones. Used topically for respiratory congestion and minor muscle aches. Also used in foods as a flavoring agent.

DOSAGE & ADMINISTRATION
Oral use: Typical dosage ranges from 6 to 20 g of the root daily or an equivalent preparation.
Topical use: Ointments contain a maximum of 2% mustard oil and are applied as needed.

ADVERSE REACTIONS
EENT: mucous membrane inflammation.
GI: GI irritation, abdominal pain, diarrhea; bloody vomit and diarrhea (with large doses).
Metabolic: decreased thyroid function.
Skin: skin irritation and blistering, topical allergic reaction.

INTERACTIONS
Herb-drug. *Anticoagulants, antiplatelet drugs:* Increases bleeding tendencies. Monitor PT and INR.
Disulfiram, metronidazole: May cause a disulfiram-like reaction if herbal preparation contains alcohol. Advise patient to avoid use together.
Levothyroxine, thyroid hormones: Causes further decrease in thyroid function. Monitor T_4 and thyroid-stimulating hormone, and adjust drug dosage as needed.
NSAIDs: May increase frequency of GI irritation. Advise patient to use caution if using the herb and drug together.

Bold italic type indicates that reaction may be life-threatening.

EFFECTS ON LAB TEST RESULTS
• May increase PT and INR. May decrease thyroid function test values.

CAUTIONS
Patients with kidney inflammation shouldn't use this herb because of its diuretic effect. Patients with an infectious or inflammatory GI condition or a stomach or intestinal ulcer shouldn't take this herb. Children younger than age 4 also shouldn't take it.

Pregnant patients should avoid taking large oral doses because of the toxic and irritating mustard oil components. Patients who have a thyroid condition or are taking an anticoagulant or an NSAID should use caution when using this herb.

NURSING CONSIDERATIONS
• Explore patient's knowledge of this herb.
• Tinctures and extracts contain 15% to 60% alcohol and may be unsuitable for children, patients with a history of alcoholism or liver disease, or patients taking certain drugs.
• Large doses of tincture taken regularly may have abortifacient effects.
• Before applying horseradish topically to a large area, the patient should test it on a small area first to see how he responds.

PATIENT TEACHING
• Advise patient to consult a health care provider before using an herbal preparation because another treatment may be available.
• Tell patient that when filling a new prescription he should inform pharmacist of any herbal or dietary supplement he's taking.
• If patient has a history of alcoholism or liver disease, inform him that some herbal products contain alcohol.
• If patient has hypothyroid disease, warn him about possible interactions with horseradish and any other plants from the cabbage family.
• Advise patient to stay within the recommended dosage of 20 g daily and to take the herb with meals to minimize GI irritation and upset.
• Tell patient to stop taking the herb if he experiences adverse reactions, such as GI irritation and abdominal pain.
• Warn patient to keep all herbal products away from children and pets.

horsetail

Equisetum arvense, bottlebrush, corn horsetail, Dutch rushes, field horsetail, horsetail grass, paddock-pipes, pewterwort, shave grass, toadpipe

Common trade names
Alcohol Free Horsetail Herb, Horsetail Grass, Springtime Horsetail

AVAILABLE FORMS
Available as dried extract in powdered form, dried or fresh stem of horsetail plant, infusion, liquid extract (1:1 in 25% alcohol)*, and tea.

ACTIONS & COMPONENTS
Horsetail's mild diuretic action is probably the result of the equise-

---

* Liquid contains alcohol.

tonin and flavonoid glycoside constituents. Horsetail also contains small amounts of pharmacologically active nicotine and inorganic silica components.

USES
Used orally to treat diuresis, edema, and general disturbances of the kidney and bladder. Used topically as supportive treatment for burns and wounds.

The herb has also been used to treat brittle fingernails, rheumatic diseases, gout, frostbite, and profuse menstruation.

DOSAGE & ADMINISTRATION
Diuresis: 6 g of the dried stem P.O. daily with plenty of fluids; or 1 cup of tea made from the dried stem taken several times daily between meals; or 1 to 4 ml of liquid extract P.O. t.i.d.
Infusion: Prepared by placing 1.5 g of dried stem in 1 cup of water. Typical dosage ranges from 2 to 4 g P.O. daily.
Tea: Prepared by pouring boiling water over 2 to 3 g of the herb, boiling for 5 minutes, and then straining after 10 to 15 minutes. Tea should be consumed several times daily between meals.
Topically for burns or wounds: Compress containing 10 g of stem/L of water.

ADVERSE REACTIONS
Metabolic: electrolyte imbalance.
Skin: irritation (topical use).
Other: thiamine deficiency (long-term use), signs and symptoms of nicotine poisoning and toxicity, including nausea and vomiting, muscle weakness, abnormal pulse rate, fever, and ataxia.

INTERACTIONS
Herb-drug. *Benzodiazepines, disulfiram, metronidazole:* May cause a disulfiram-like reaction if herbal preparation contains alcohol. Advise patient to avoid use together.
Digoxin: May cause increased digitalis toxicity as a result of potassium loss with diuretic effect. Advise patient to avoid use together.
Potassium-wasting drugs, including corticosteroids, diuretics, and laxative stimulants: May increase risk of hypokalemia. Advise patient to use caution if using the herb and drug together.
Herb-herb. *Licorice:* May increase potassium depletion and risk of cardiac toxicity (with overuse of herb). Advise patient to avoid overuse of these herbs.
Herb-lifestyle. *Alcohol use:* May cause thiamine deficiency (with excessive use of alcohol). Advise patient to avoid excessive alcohol use.

EFFECTS ON LAB TEST RESULTS
• May decrease thiamine level. May alter digoxin and electrolyte levels.

CAUTIONS
Women who are pregnant or breast-feeding shouldn't use this herb, nor should those who have impaired heart or kidney function, liver problems, or a history or risk of thiamine deficiency (for example, alcoholic patients). Those who are taking a cardiac glycoside also should avoid using horsetail.

Bold italic type indicates that reaction may be life-threatening.

NURSING CONSIDERATIONS
- Explore patient's knowledge of this herb.
- The liquid extract contains 25% alcohol and shouldn't be used with disulfiram, metronidazole, or a benzodiazepine.

⚡ **ALERT:** Dosage varies with the formulation. The FDA lists horsetail on its "undetermined safety" list. Large amounts may cause a toxic reaction.

- The dried extract in the powdered form is more concentrated than the stem alone.
- Monitor potassium level.
- Assess patient for signs and symptoms of hypokalemia, including weakness, muscle flaccidity, and abnormal ECG results.
- Herb should be used only for short-term effects because of potential for toxic reaction and thiamine depletion.

PATIENT TEACHING
- Advise patient to consult a health care provider before using an herbal preparation because another treatment may be available.
- Tell patient that when filling a new prescription he should inform pharmacist of any herbal or dietary supplement he's taking.
- Tell patient that horsetail is for short-term use only.
- If patient has a history of alcoholism or liver disease, inform him that some herbal products contain alcohol.
- Instruct patient to stop taking the herb immediately if he experiences signs or symptoms of nicotine toxicity (including muscle weakness, abnormal pulse rate, fever, ataxia, and cold extremities)

or of potassium depletion (including muscle cramping, irritability, or weakness).
- If patient is pregnant or breast-feeding or is taking a potassium-wasting diuretic, a cardiac glycoside, a corticosteroid, or licorice, advise her not to use this herb.
- Warn patient to keep all herbal products away from children and pets. Poisonings have occurred when stems of horsetail have been used as blow guns or whistles.

hyssop

Hyssopus officinalis

Common trade names
Hyssop Herb

AVAILABLE FORMS
Available as capsules and extracts*.
Capsules: 445 mg
Extract: 0.03% dried plant

ACTIONS & COMPONENTS
Obtained from the dried above-ground parts, including leaves and flowering tops, of *H. officinalis.* The oil used in flavorings and extracts is also made from the aboveground parts of the plant.

The plant contains numerous components that make up the essential oil. One of the glycoside components, marrubiin, stimulates bronchiole secretions. Hyssop has strong antiviral effects, probably because of the caffeic acid, tannin, and high-molecular-weight components present. It may have some activity against HIV-1 replication and herpes simplex virus.

---

*Liquid contains alcohol.

USES
Used orally to treat upset stomach, liver and gallbladder complaints, indigestion, colds, fevers, respiratory and chest ailments, sore throat, asthma, urinary tract inflammation, gas, and colic. Also used as an expectorant and as an appetite and circulation stimulant.

Used topically in a salve or compress to treat skin irritations, burns, bruises, and frostbite. The oil is used as fragrance in soaps and perfumes.

Used in other foods and extracts and as a flavoring in alcoholic beverages, at a maximum level of 0.06% dried herb and 0.004% volatile oil. Also used in soaps and cosmetics.

DOSAGE & ADMINISTRATION
Capsules: Two 445-mg capsules P.O. t.i.d.
Extract: 10 to 15 gtt in water P.O. b.i.d. to t.i.d.
Tea: To be gargled or consumed t.i.d. Prepared by steeping 1 to 2 teaspoons dried hyssop tops in 5 ounces boiling water.

ADVERSE REACTIONS
CNS: *tonic-clonic seizures, neurotoxicity.*
GU: uterine stimulation.

INTERACTIONS
Herb-drug. *Anticonvulsants:* May counteract antiseizure effects. Advise patient to avoid use together. *Disulfiram, metronidazole:* May cause a disulfiram-like reaction if herbal preparation contains alcohol. Advise patient to avoid use together.

EFFECTS ON LAB TEST RESULTS
None reported.

CAUTIONS
Pregnant patients shouldn't use this herb because it may stimulate the uterus, leading to miscarriage and hemorrhage. Patients with a seizure disorder shouldn't use the herb because of reports that 2 or 3 gtt of volatile oil over several days may cause tonic-clonic seizures. Children also shouldn't use the herb.

NURSING CONSIDERATIONS
• Explore patient's knowledge of this herb.
• Tinctures and extracts contain 15% to 60% alcohol and may be unsuitable for children, patients with a history of alcoholism or liver disease, or patients taking certain drugs.
• Only standardized dose forms should be used.
• Internal use of oil may cause seizures or neurotoxicity.
• Herb may alter the intended therapeutic effects of conventional drugs.

PATIENT TEACHING
• Advise patient to consult a health care provider before using an herbal preparation because another treatment may be available.
• Tell patient that when filling a new prescription he should inform pharmacist of any herbal or dietary supplement he's taking.
• If patient has a history of alcoholism or liver disease, inform him that some herbal products contain alcohol.

Bold italic type indicates that reaction may be life-threatening.

• If patient is pregnant, planning to become pregnant, or breast-feeding, advise her not to use this herb.

• Advise patient to use this herb only at the recommended dosages and to avoid long-term use. Warn him that this herb's effectiveness is still undetermined.

• Inform patient that although several other plants have variations of the name "hyssop," they aren't related to the genus *Hyssopus*.

• Warn patient to keep all herbal products away from children and pets.

*Liquid contains alcohol.

Iceland moss

Cetraria islandica, eryngo-leaved liverwort, Iceland lichen, lichen

Common trade names
Iceland Moss

AVAILABLE FORMS
Available as dried whole plant of *C. islandica* and as powdered herb extracts*.

ACTIONS & COMPONENTS
The mucilage components lichenin and isolichenin may have soothing effects on the oral and pharyngeal membranes. The bitter organic components may stimulate the appetite and promote gastric secretion.

USES
Used to soothe oral and pharyngeal membranes, to relieve dry cough, to stimulate appetite, and to prevent infection, the common cold, dyspeptic complaints, and fevers.

The alcoholic extract is used as a flavoring agent in alcoholic beverages.

DOSAGE & ADMINISTRATION
For cough and sore throat: Tea is prepared by simmering 1.5 to 3 g dried plant in 5 ounces of boiling water and then straining.

Maximum dose of the extract is 4 to 6 g daily because of potential lead contamination.

ADVERSE REACTIONS
GI: GI distress.

INTERACTIONS
Herb-drug. *Aspirin, NSAIDs:* May increase irritation of the gastric mucosa. Advise patient to use caution if using the herb and drug together.
Disulfiram, metronidazole: May cause a disulfiram-like reaction if herbal preparation contains alcohol. Advise patient to avoid use together.
Oral drugs: May cause impaired absorption of oral drugs from the fiber in the herb. Instruct patient to separate administration times by at least 2 hours.

EFFECTS ON LAB TEST RESULTS
None reported.

CAUTIONS
Patients with gastroduodenal ulcers or GI distress or disease shouldn't use this herb because it may irritate the gastric mucosa. Patients who are pregnant or breastfeeding shouldn't use it because it can cause lead contamination. Children also shouldn't use it.

NURSING CONSIDERATIONS
• Explore patient's knowledge of this herb.
• Tinctures and extracts contain 15% to 60% alcohol and may be unsuitable for children, patients with a history of alcoholism or liver disease, or patients taking certain drugs.

Bold italic type indicates that reaction may be life-threatening.

• Warn patient not to treat signs and symptoms of respiratory tract infection with Iceland moss before seeking medical evaluation, because doing so may delay diagnosis of a potentially serious medical condition.

PATIENT TEACHING
• Advise patient to consult a health care provider before using an herbal preparation because another treatment may be available.
• Tell patient that when filling a new prescription he should inform pharmacist of any herbal or dietary supplement he's taking.
• If patient has a history of alcoholism or liver disease, inform him that some herbal products contain alcohol.
• Tell patient to take only the recommended dosage and to stop taking the herb if he experiences GI distress.
• Advise patient to take this herb at least 1 hour before or 2 hours after other drugs.
• Inform patient that taking herb with food may help prevent GI upset.
• Advise patient not to put off seeking medical evaluation if the herb doesn't adequately treat his illness.
• Warn patient to keep all herbal products away from children and pets.

indigo

common indigo, Indian indigo, pigmentum indicum

Common trade names
None known

AVAILABLE FORMS
Available as the blue dye that's extracted from the leaves and branches of numerous species of *Indigofera* (for example, *I. tinctoria, I. suffruticosa, I. aspalathoides, I. spicata,* and *I. enneaphylla*).

ACTIONS & COMPONENTS
During fermentation of the leaves, indigo is derived from indican, a glucoside constituent of several *Indigofera* species. Little is known about the pharmacologic effects of the herb. Indigo has emetic, anti-inflammatory, and antipyretic properties.

USES
Used as an emetic. *I. tinctoria,* in particular, is used to treat nematodal infections and cancer of the ovaries or stomach.

In traditional Chinese medicine, indigo is used to detoxify the liver and the blood, reduce inflammation and fever, and relieve pain. Throughout the world, indigo is still used commercially for dyeing wool and cotton.

DOSAGE & ADMINISTRATION
Not well documented.

ADVERSE REACTIONS
EENT: mild ocular irritation.
GI: nausea, vomiting, diarrhea.
Hepatic: *hepatotoxicity.*

---

*Liquid contains alcohol.

INTERACTIONS
None reported.

EFFECTS ON LAB TEST RESULTS
• May increase liver enzyme levels. May alter electrolyte levels.

CAUTIONS
Pregnant patients shouldn't use this herb because some *Indigofera* species have teratogenic effects. Breast-feeding patients should also avoid using it.

All patients should use caution when using the herb because data on its effects are lacking.

NURSING CONSIDERATIONS
• Explore patient's knowledge of this herb.
• With the exception of *I. tinctoria*, many *Indigofera* species are hepatotoxic. *I. spicata* has caused cleft palate and embryonic death.
⚠ **ALERT:** Don't confuse this herb with false, wild, or bastard indigo (*Baptisia tinctoria*).

PATIENT TEACHING
• Advise patient to consult a health care provider before using an herbal preparation because another treatment may be available.
• Tell patient that when filling a new prescription he should inform pharmacist of any herbal or dietary supplement he's taking.
• If patient is pregnant or breast-feeding, advise her not to use this herb.
• Advise patient to use caution when using this herb because it may cause liver toxicity.
• Warn patient to keep all herbal products away from children and pets.

Irish moss

Chondrus crispus, carrageenan, carragheen, carrahan, chondrus extract

Common trade names
None known

AVAILABLE FORMS
Available as dried jellied fruit, jellies, puddings, raw leaves, and teas.

ACTIONS & COMPONENTS
Irish moss is obtained from the dried thallus of *C. crispus.* Considered to be a seaweed and consists of polysaccharides, vitamins, minerals, and iodine. The extract is known as carrageenin, a starchlike substance. This extract can be further differentiated into two types, k-carrageenin and l-carrageenan. The former type is the gelling fraction; the latter, the nongelling component.

The herb has expectorant, demulcent, anti-inflammatory, anticoagulant, antihypertensive, immunosuppressive, and antidiarrheal properties. Irish moss also interferes with the absorption of food; it may reduce cholesterol and have some antiviral activity.

USES
Used to soothe irritating coughs that result from various respiratory tract infections and to produce bulky stools in patients with chronic diarrhea. Because of its demulcent properties, this herb is also used to treat gastritis and peptic ulcer disease. Used as a nutritional supplement to facilitate recuperation in those with debilitating dis-

---

Bold italic type indicates that reaction may be life-threatening.

eases. Irish moss can also be found as an ingredient in weight-loss products.

Used topically to treat anorectal signs and symptoms. Used as a skin softener in commercial cosmetic products and lotions.

In manufacturing, Irish moss can be used as a binder, emulsifier, thickener, and stabilizer in drugs, foods, and toothpaste.

DOSAGE & ADMINISTRATION

Decoction: Prepared by boiling 1 ounce of dried plant in 1 to 1½ pints of water for 10 to 15 minutes, and then straining. Dosage is 1 cup b.i.d. to t.i.d. Lemon, honey, ginger, or cinnamon may be added to enhance the flavor.

ADVERSE REACTIONS

CV: hypotension.
GI: cramps, diarrhea.
Other: infection.

INTERACTIONS

Herb-drug. *Anticoagulants:* Increases risk of bleeding. Advise patient to avoid use together.
Antihypertensives: Potentiates hypotensive effects. Advise patient to use together cautiously.
Other drugs: May decrease drug absorption. Advise patient to separate administration times by at least 2 hours.

EFFECTS ON LAB TEST RESULTS

• May decrease drug and cholesterol levels.
• May increase PT and INR.

CAUTIONS

Pregnant or breast-feeding patients should avoid using Irish moss. In-

fants shouldn't be given this herb because it may suppress the immune system.

Patients with underlying bleeding disorders or hypotension should use caution when using this herb.

NURSING CONSIDERATIONS

• Explore patient's knowledge of this herb.
• Monitor blood pressure regularly during the course of therapy.
• If patient is receiving warfarin, closely monitor PT and INR.

PATIENT TEACHING

• Advise patient to consult a health care provider before using an herbal preparation because another treatment may be available.
• Tell patient that when filling a new prescription he should inform pharmacist of any herbal or dietary supplement he's taking.
• If patient is pregnant or breast-feeding, advise her not to use this herb.
• Tell patient to avoid taking Irish moss within 2 hours of any drug.
• If patient is also taking a drug to lower high blood pressure, instruct him to notify his health care provider if he experiences dizziness, light-headedness, or fainting.
• If patient is using this herb to treat diarrhea, advise him to consult his health care provider if the diarrhea persists for more than 4 days.
• Warn patient to keep all herbal products out of the reach of children and pets.

---

*Liquid contains alcohol.

J

jaborandi

Pilocarpus jaborandi, P. microphyllus, arruda brava, arruda do mato, jamguarandi, juarandi, maranhao jaborandi

Common trade names
None known

AVAILABLE FORMS
Obtained from dried leaves of *P. jaborandi* or *P. microphyllus.*

ACTIONS & COMPONENTS
Contains volatile oils and three alkaloids: pilocarpine, isopilocarpine, and pilocarpidine. Pilocarpine, a parasympathomimetic, is the primary constituent and contributes to the herb's cholinergic effects, including salivation, perspiration, miosis, and increased GI tract motility.

USES
Previously used to induce sweating and diarrhea. Currently used to produce pilocarpine. The herb is FDA-approved for treating glaucoma.

DOSAGE & ADMINISTRATION
Oral use of jaborandi is unsafe. Pilocarpine, a jaborandi component, is commercially available by prescription as an ophthalmic solution in various strengths.

ADVERSE REACTIONS
CNS: *seizures.*
CV: *bradycardia, cardiac arrest,* hypotension.
EENT: miosis.
GI: nausea, vomiting, diarrhea.
Respiratory: *bronchospasm,* dyspnea.
Other: increased sweating, hypersalivation.

INTERACTIONS
None reported.

EFFECTS ON LAB TEST RESULTS
None reported.

CAUTIONS
Patients who are pregnant or breast-feeding shouldn't use the herb because it has teratogenic effects and promotes uterine stimulation.

NURSING CONSIDERATIONS
• Explore patient's knowledge of this herb.
• Patients with cardiac or circulatory diseases are particularly sensitive to adverse CV reactions.
• Because of potential toxicity, jaborandi isn't recommended for oral or topical use. Signs and symptoms of toxicity can develop after ingesting 60 mg or more of jaborandi, which is equivalent to 5 to 10 mg of pilocarpine.
☑**ALERT:** Contact the health care provider if patient shows signs or symptoms of toxicity, including bradycardia, bronchospasm, cardiac arrest, seizures, hypotension, dyspnea, nausea, vomiting, diarrhea, increased sweating, and hypersalivation. If toxicity develops, prepare for gastric lavage followed by administration of activated

---

Bold italic type indicates that reaction may be life-threatening.

charcoal and atropine. Expect to give diazepam if seizures develop. Give I.V. fluids as directed if hypotension occurs. Patient also may undergo hemodialysis.
⚠ALERT: Don't confuse this herb with *Pernambuco jaborandi* or *Paraguay jaborandi*.

PATIENT TEACHING
• If patient has a chronic illness, advise him not to put off seeking medical evaluation, because doing so may delay diagnosis of a potentially serious medical condition.
• Warn patient to avoid using jaborandi because of the risk of toxicity.
• If patient is pregnant or breast-feeding, advise her to avoid using this herb.
• Warn patient to keep all herbal products away from children and pets.

Jamaican dogwood

Piscidia piscipula, P. erythrina, dogwood, fishfuddle, fish poison bark, fish poison tree, Jamaica dogwood, West Indian dogwood

Common trade names
None known

AVAILABLE FORMS
Available as dried bark and liquid extract.

ACTIONS & COMPONENTS
Obtained from the root bark of *P. piscipula* or *P. communis*. Jamaican dogwood contains isoflavones, organic acids, ichthynone, rote-

nones, and tannins. Both rotenone and ichthynone can produce toxic effects; rotenone may be carcinogenic. The liquid extract possesses sedative, hypnotic, antitussive, antipyretic, anti-inflammatory, and antispasmodic properties.

USES
Used for anxiety, neuralgia, migraines, insomnia, and dysmenorrhea.

DOSAGE & ADMINISTRATION
Because of its rotenone and ichthynone components, this herb is toxic and should be avoided. Root bark and liquid extract are no longer used.

ADVERSE REACTIONS
CNS: numbness, tremors.
GI: excessive salivation.
Skin: diaphoresis.

INTERACTIONS
Herb-drug. *CNS depressants:* May increase sedative effects. Advise patient to avoid use together.
Herb-herb. *Herbs with sedative properties, such as calamus, calendula, California poppy, capsicum, catnip, celery, couch grass, elecampane, goldenseal, gotu kola, hops, kava, lemon balm, sage, sassafras, shepherd's purse, Siberian ginseng, skullcap, St. John's wort, valerian, wild lettuce, and yerba maté:* May increase sedative effects. Advise patient to avoid use together.

EFFECTS ON LAB TEST RESULTS
None reported.

*Liquid contains alcohol.

CAUTIONS
Patients who are pregnant or breast-feeding shouldn't use this herb. It also shouldn't be given to children because neuromuscular depressant effects are potentiated in this age-group.

NURSING CONSIDERATIONS
• Explore patient's knowledge of this herb.

⚡ALERT: Patients should avoid using the herb because it's toxic, and data supporting its efficacy are lacking. If patient complains of numbness, tremors, salivation, or sweating, suspect toxicity and contact a health care provider.

• Geriatric patients are more sensitive to the herb's toxic effects.

• Don't confuse this herbal product with American dogwood (*Cornus florida*).

PATIENT TEACHING
• Advise patient to avoid using this herb because of the risk of toxicity.

• Warn patient not to take herb for anxiety, migraine, or insomnia before seeking medical attention, because doing so may delay diagnosis of a potentially serious medical condition.

• Warn patient to keep all herbal products away from children and pets.

jambolan

Syzygium cumini, S. cumini semen (seed), jambul, jamum, java plum, rose apple

Common trade names
None known

AVAILABLE FORMS
Available as dried bark, powdered seeds, and liquid extract.

ACTIONS & COMPONENTS
Derived from dried bark and seeds of *S. cumini* or *S. jambolana*. Bark contains gallic and ellagic acid derivatives, flavonoids, and tannins. Tannins in the bark cause astringent effects. Bark also has antibacterial, hypoglycemic, and sedative activity. Seeds contain fatty oils and tannins and possess hypoglycemic, anti-inflammatory, antipyretic, antispasmodic, sedative, tonic, antidepressant, and aphrodisiac properties.

USES
The bark is taken orally for nonspecific acute diarrhea. It's also applied to the skin, mouth, or pharynx to decrease mild inflammation. The bark has been used orally to treat bronchitis, asthma, and dysentery and topically to treat ulcers.

The seeds are used for diabetes, flatulence, constipation, pancreatic and gastric disorders, muscle spasms, fatigue, depression, and anxiety. The seeds are also used as an aphrodisiac or a diuretic. In India, they're used to manage diabetes-induced polydipsia.

Bold italic type indicates that reaction may be life-threatening.

DOSAGE & ADMINISTRATION
Dried bark: 3 to 6 g P.O. daily.
Liquid extract containing jambolan seed: 4 to 8 ml P.O. daily.
Powdered seeds: 0.3 to 2 g P.O. daily.
Tea: Prepared by simmering 1 to 2 teaspoons of dried bark in 5 ounces of boiling water for 5 to 10 minutes and then straining before use.
Topical: A warm compress is made from jambolan bark tea.

ADVERSE REACTIONS
CNS: sedation.
Metabolic: *hypoglycemia.*

INTERACTIONS
Herb-drug. *Antidiabetics, insulin:* May cause increased hypoglycemic effects. Monitor glucose level closely.

EFFECTS ON LAB TEST RESULTS
• May decrease glucose level.

CAUTIONS
Patients who are pregnant or breast-feeding shouldn't use this herb because its effects are unknown. Diabetic patients should use caution when using jambolan seed because no data exist to support its use.

NURSING CONSIDERATIONS
• Explore patient's knowledge of this herb.
• Although no chemical interactions have been reported in clinical studies, caution patient that the herb may interfere with the therapeutic effects of conventional drugs.

• If patient has diabetes and is using jambolan seeds, monitor his glucose level closely because the seeds may cause hypoglycemia.

PATIENT TEACHING
• Advise patient to consult a health care provider before using an herbal preparation because another treatment may be available.
• Tell patient that when filling a new prescription he should inform pharmacist of any herbal or dietary supplement he's taking.
• Warn patient not to take herb for a GI disorder before seeking medical attention, because doing so may delay diagnosis of a potentially serious medical condition.
• If the patient is using the herb to treat diarrhea, advise him to consult his health care provider if it persists for more than 4 days.
• If patient is using jambolan seeds to treat diabetes, inform him that safer, more effective drugs are available. Also, instruct him to routinely monitor his glucose level.
• If patient is pregnant or breast-feeding, advise her to avoid using this herb.
• Warn patient to keep all herbal products away from children and pets.

*Liquid contains alcohol.

jimsonweed

Datura stramonium, apple of Peru, datura, devil's apple, devil's trumpet, Jamestown weed, mad apple, nightshade, stinkweed, stinkwort, stramonium, thorn apple

Common trade names
None known

AVAILABLE FORMS
Most commonly available as dried leaves, with or without tips of flowering branches. Can be smoked in cigarettes or burned in powder and inhaled. Also available as ripe seeds and flowers without leaves. Seeds—which are small, long, flat, and dark yellow to brown—are the most toxic part. Jimsonweed comes in oral and rectal forms as well.

ACTIONS & COMPONENTS
Primary action is anticholinergic, caused by 0.1% to 0.6% atropine, hyoscyamine, and scopolamine. All parts of the plant contain these compounds, but the highest levels are in the seeds. Anticholinergic levels in other plant parts vary from year to year and from plant to plant. The alkaloids are readily absorbed across GI mucous membranes and the respiratory tract. Anticholinergic effects usually occur within 30 to 60 minutes and may last 24 to 48 hours because of impaired GI motility.

USES
Used to treat asthma and cough from bronchitis or influenza, usually by smoking cigarettes made from the leaves. Also used to treat disorders of the autonomic nervous system. Little data exist to support routine therapeutic use of jimsonweed.

Illicitly, the seeds have been chewed, the leaves smoked as cigarettes, and a tea brewed and ingested to cause hallucinations and euphoria.

DOSAGE & ADMINISTRATION
Not well documented.

ADVERSE REACTIONS
CNS: headache, confusion, hallucinations, agitation, emotional lability, motor incoordination, restlessness, *seizures,* loss of consciousness, hyperthermia.
CV: tachycardia, hypertension leading to hypotension, *arrhythmias.*
EENT: dilated pupils, blurred vision, photophobia, dry mucous membranes.
GI: nausea, vomiting, decreased GI tract motility, excessive thirst.
GU: urine retention.
Respiratory: tachypnea, *respiratory depression, respiratory arrest.*
Skin: dry, flushed skin.

INTERACTIONS
Herb-drug. *Anticholinergics, such as amantadine; antihistamines, such as diphenhydramine; atropine; phenothiazines, such as prochlorperazine and promethazine; TCAs, such as amitriptyline and imipramine; scopolamine:* May cause additive effects. Advise patient to avoid use together.
Herb-herb. *Deadly nightshade:* May cause additive anticholinergic

---

Bold italic type indicates that reaction may be life-threatening.

toxicity. Advise patient to avoid use together.

EFFECTS ON LAB TEST RESULTS
None reported.

CAUTIONS
Patients who are pregnant or breast-feeding shouldn't use this herb, nor should patients who have glaucoma, BPH, urine retention, tachycardia or other cardiac problems, or sensitivity to the herb.

NURSING CONSIDERATIONS
• Explore patient's knowledge of this herb.
• The FDA considers this herb unsafe; therefore, it's use isn't recommended.
☑**ALERT:** Fatal poisonings resulting from respiratory depression and circulatory collapse have been reported from adult doses equal to 10 mg of atropine (15 to 100 g of dried leaves or about 100 [15 to 25 g] seeds). Fatal doses in children may be much smaller.
☑**ALERT:** Don't confuse this herb with deadly nightshade *(Atropa belladonna),* which has similar effects.
• Although no chemical interactions have been reported in clinical studies, caution patient that jimsonweed may interfere with the therapeutic effects of conventional drugs.
• Monitor patient for signs and symptoms of anticholinergic toxicity: mydriasis, blurred vision, photophobia, tachycardia, hypertension or hypotension, confusion, agitation, hallucinations, and motor incoordination.

• If patient develops toxicity, avoid using a sedative or a phenothiazine to treat it because these drugs may produce additive anticholinergic effects.
• The antidote for anticholinergic toxicity is physostigmine. To avoid profound cholinergic effects, use this drug only for severe toxicity characterized by seizures, severe hypertension, severe hallucinations, arrhythmias, or life-threatening respiratory depression.

PATIENT TEACHING
• Warn patient that this herb isn't recommended for routine therapeutic use and is considered illegal for OTC use in the United States.
☑**ALERT:** Tell patient to report signs and symptoms of anticholinergic toxicity, which include dilated pupils, impaired vision, dry mouth, palpitations, dizziness, confusion, hallucinations, and incoordination. Warn him that death can occur as a result of using the drug.
• Warn patient to keep all herbal products away from children and pets.

jojoba

Simmondsia californica, S. chinesis, deernut, goatnut, pignut

Common trade names
None known

AVAILABLE FORMS
Available as soap, shampoo, conditioner, and other skin-care products.

---

*Liquid contains alcohol.

Shampoos and conditioners: 1%
or 2%
Skin care products: 5% to 10%
Soaps: 0.5% to 3%

ACTIONS & COMPONENTS
Wax (commonly called oil) from
the seeds is odorless and colorless
to light yellow. It readily penetrates
the skin. Taken orally, it's absorbed,
not digested, and stored in intestinal and liver cells. The oil contains
14% erucic acid, which in higher
doses has been reported to cause
myocardial fibrosis. Seeds are dark
brown, about the size of coffee
beans or peanuts.

USES
Used topically to treat acne, psoriasis, and sunburn. Also used to un-
clog hair follicles in the scalp, preventing buildup of sebum, which is
believed to contribute to hair loss.
   Commonly used in shampoos,
conditioners, cosmetics, lotions,
sunscreens, and cleaning products.
Used as an industrial lubricant because it doesn't break down at high
temperatures.

DOSAGE & ADMINISTRATION
Not well documented.

ADVERSE REACTIONS
Skin: contact dermatitis (with use
of shampoos, hair conditioners, or
pure oil).

INTERACTIONS
None reported.

EFFECTS ON LAB TEST RESULTS
None reported.

CAUTIONS
Patients who are sensitive to the
herb shouldn't use it.

NURSING CONSIDERATIONS
• Explore patient's knowledge of
this herb.
• Minimal toxicity has been reported, particularly after topical
application.
• Signs and symptoms of contact
dermatitis include itching, erythema, and occasional vesicle formation.
• Herb shouldn't be taken orally
because of the lack of information
regarding its internal use.
• No routine monitoring is needed
after topical application.

PATIENT TEACHING
• Advise patient to consult a health
care provider before using an
herbal preparation because another
treatment may be available.
• Tell patient that when filling a
new prescription he should inform
pharmacist of any herbal or dietary supplement he's taking.
• Warn patient to avoid taking jojoba orally.
• Tell patient to report any skin irritation from products containing
jojoba.
• Teach patient proper skin care for
the prevention of acne.
• Advise patient to avoid excessive
sun exposure.
• Warn patient to keep all herbal
products away from children and
pets.

Bold italic type indicates that reaction may be life-threatening.

juniper

*Baccae juniperi, Juniperi
fructus, Juniperus communis,*
enebro, Genievre, ginepro,
juniper berry, wacholder, zimbro

Common trade names
Juniper, Juniper Berry

AVAILABLE FORMS
Available as fresh or dried ripe
berry, also called *berry-like cones*
or *mature female cones*. Also available as powder, tea, tincture*, oil*,
or liquid extract*. Immature
berries are green, taking 2 to 3
years to ripen to a purplish blue-
black.

ACTIONS & COMPONENTS
Active component is a volatile oil,
which is 0.2% to 3.4% of the
berry. Diuresis, the best described
effect, is caused by terpinene-4-ol,
which directly irritates the kidneys,
leading to increased GFR.

Other reported effects of juniper
are hypoglycemia, hypotension or
hypertension, anti-inflammatory
and antiseptic effects, and uterine
stimulation, leading to decreased
implantation and increased abortifacient effects.

USES
Used to treat UTIs and renal calculi. Also used as a carminative
and for multiple nonspecific GI
tract disorders, including dyspepsia, flatulence, colic, heartburn,
anorexia, and inflammatory GI disorders.

The herb is applied topically to
treat small wounds and relieve
muscle and joint pain caused by
rheumatism. It's inhaled as steam
to treat bronchitis. The oil is used
as a fragrance in many soaps and
cosmetics. It's the principal flavoring agent in gin as well as some
bitters and liqueurs.

As a food, maximum flavoring
concentrations are 0.01% of the
extract or 0.006% of the volatile
oil. At these concentrations, neither therapeutic nor adverse effects
should be experienced.

DOSAGE & ADMINISTRATION
Dried ripe berries: 1 to 2 g P.O.
t.i.d. Maximum dosage is 10 g
dried berry daily, equaling 20 to
100 mg essential oil.
*Liquid extract (1:1 in 25% alco-
hol):* 2 to 4 ml P.O. t.i.d.
Oil (1:5 in 45% alcohol): 0.03 to
0.2 ml P.O. t.i.d.
Tea: Prepared by placing 1 tablespoon crushed berries in 5 ounces
boiling water, steeping 10 minutes,
and then straining. It's typically
taken t.i.d.
Tincture (1:5 in 45% alcohol): 1 to
2 ml P.O. t.i.d.
For hypoglycemic effects: 250 to
500 mg/kg/day.

ADVERSE REACTIONS
CNS: *seizures.*
GI: diarrhea.
GU: *renal failure.*
Skin: local irritation, vesicles.

INTERACTIONS
Herb-drug. *Antidiabetics, such as
insulin, chlorpropamide, glipizide,
and glyburide:* May potentiate hypoglycemic effects. Monitor patient closely.

*Liquid contains alcohol.

Antihypertensives: May interfere with blood pressure. Monitor patient closely.

Disulfiram, metronidazole: May cause a disulfiram-like reaction if herbal preparation contains alcohol. Advise patient to avoid use together.

Diuretics: May potentiate diuretic effects, leading to additive hypokalemia. Monitor potassium levels frequently.

Herb-herb. *Herbs that cause diuresis, such as cowslip, cucumber, dandelion, and horsetail:* May cause additive effects. Monitor patient closely.

Herbs that lower the glucose level, such as Asian and Siberian ginseng, dandelion, and fenugreek: May cause additive hypoglycemic effects. Monitor glucose level closely.

Herb-lifestyle. *Alcohol use:* May cause additive effects (if herbal preparation contains alcohol). Advise patient to avoid use together.

EFFECTS ON LAB TEST RESULTS
- May increase BUN and creatinine levels. May decrease glucose and potassium levels.
- May cause blood and protein to appear in urine.

CAUTIONS
Patients who are pregnant or breast-feeding shouldn't use this herb because of its uterine stimulant and abortifacient properties. Patients who have renal insufficiency, an inflammatory disorder of the GI tract (such as Crohn's disease), a seizure disorder, or known sensitivity to the herb also shouldn't use it. Because the herb may cause local irritation, it shouldn't be used topically on large ulcers or wounds.

NURSING CONSIDERATIONS
- Explore patient's knowledge of this herb.
- Tinctures and extracts contain 15% to 60% alcohol and may be unsuitable for children, patients with a history of alcoholism or liver disease, or patients taking certain drugs.
- **ALERT:** Renal damage may occur in patients taking juniper for longer than 4 weeks. This effect may stem from prolonged kidney irritation caused by terpinene-4-ol or by turpentine oil contamination of juniper products.
- Overdose may cause seizures, tachycardia, hypertension, and renal failure with albuminuria, hematuria, and purplish urine. Monitor blood pressure and potassium, BUN, creatinine, and glucose levels.
- **ALERT:** Don't confuse juniper with cade oil, which is derived from juniper wood.

PATIENT TEACHING
- Advise patient to consult a health care provider before using an herbal preparation because another treatment may be available.
- Tell patient that when filling a new prescription he should inform pharmacist of any herbal or dietary supplement he's taking.
- Recommend that patient seek a medical diagnosis before taking juniper. Unadvised use of juniper could worsen urinary problems, GI disorders, and other conditions if

---

Bold italic type indicates that reaction may be life-threatening.

medical diagnosis and treatment are delayed.

• If patient has a history of alcoholism or liver disease, inform him that some herbal products contain alcohol.

• If patient suspects she is, or is planning to become, pregnant, advise her to check with her health care provider before using this herb.

• Warn patient not to use herb for more than 4 weeks.

• Inform patient that urine may turn purplish with higher doses.

• Tell patient to avoid applying the herb to large ulcers or wounds because local irritation (burning, blistering, redness, and swelling) may occur.

• Caution patient against using alcohol while taking this herb.

• Warn patient to keep all herbal products away from children and pets.

*Liquid contains alcohol.

K

karaya gum

*Sterculia tragacanth, S. urens,
S. villosa, Bassora tragacanth,*
Indian tragacanth, kadaya,
karaya, kullo, mucara, Sterculia
gum

Common trade names
None known

AVAILABLE FORMS
Available as a dry powder or paste.

ACTIONS & COMPONENTS
Karaya gum is obtained from *Sterculia,* a softwood tree cultivated in India and Pakistan. It absorbs more than 100 times its weight in water. Forms a viscous solution in low concentrations in water and a gel or paste in higher concentrations. When taken orally, it isn't digested or systemically absorbed. In the GI tract, it acts as a bulk-forming laxative to stimulate peristalsis.

Dried bark may have astringent properties. Paste is reputedly antibacterial when applied topically to wounds.

USES
Used orally as bulk-forming laxative akin to psyllium. Applied topically as powder or paste to treat pressure sores or care for ileostomies or colostomies. Used industrially as a thickener in pharmaceuticals, cosmetics, hair sprays, lotions, and denture adhesives. Used also as a binder or stabilizer in foods and beverages.

DOSAGE & ADMINISTRATION
Not well documented.

ADVERSE REACTIONS
GI: constipation, distention, bloating, diarrhea.

INTERACTIONS
Herb-drug. *Oral drugs:* May decrease drug absorption. Instruct patient to separate administration times by at least 2 hours.

EFFECTS ON LAB TEST RESULTS
• May decrease glucose and lipid levels.

CAUTIONS
Patients with bowel obstruction shouldn't use karaya gum or any other bulk-forming laxative.

NURSING CONSIDERATIONS
• Explore patient's knowledge of this herb.
• Herb is generally recognized as safe for ingestion as a food additive.
• No information is available regarding use in pregnant or breast-feeding women.
• Like other bulk-forming laxatives, karaya gum may decrease drug absorption when taken together. This effect should be insignificant with amounts found in food and pharmaceuticals.
• To maximize laxative effect, patient should drink plenty of fluids.
• The herb may cause pain when applied topically to wounds.

Bold italic type indicates that reaction may be life-threatening.

PATIENT TEACHING
• Advise patient to consult a health care provider before using an herbal preparation because another treatment may be available.
• Tell patient that when filling a new prescription he should inform pharmacist of any herbal or dietary supplement he's taking.
• Advise patient to increase fiber in his diet and drink plenty of fluids.
• Warn patient to keep all herbal products away from children and pets.

kava

Piper methysticum, ava, awa, kava-kava, kew, sakau, tonga, yagona

Common trade names
Combination products: *Alcohol-Free Kava-Kava, Kavacin, Kava Plus, Kava Kava Root, Kava Tone, St. John's Wort Plus, Standardized Kava Extract, Veggie Capsules*

AVAILABLE FORMS
Available as capsules, soft gel caps, liquid spray, and tea bags.

ACTIONS & COMPONENTS
Obtained from dried rhizome and root of *P. methysticum,* a member of the black pepper family (Piperaceae). Kava contains seven major and several minor kava lactones, both aqueous and lipid soluble. Pharmacologic effects result from lipid-soluble lactones. Their mechanism of action differs from that of benzodiazepines and opiate-agonists. Kava affects the limbic system, modulating emotional processes to produce anxiolytic effects. Kava lactones inhibit MAO type B, producing psychotropic effects. They also inhibit voltage-gated calcium and sodium channels, producing anticonvulsant and skeletal muscle relaxant effects. The kava lactone kawain inhibits cyclo-oxygenase and thromboxane synthase, producing antithrombotic effects on human platelets.

USES
Used to treat anxiety, stress, and restlessness. Used orally to produce sedation, to promote wound healing, and to treat headaches, seizure disorders, the common cold, respiratory tract infection, tuberculosis, and rheumatism. Also used to treat urogenital infections, including chronic cystitis, venereal disease, uterine inflammation, menstrual problems, and vaginal prolapse. Some herbal practitioners consider kava an aphrodisiac. Kava juice is used to treat skin diseases, including leprosy, and as a poultice for intestinal problems, otitis, and abscesses.

DOSAGE & ADMINISTRATION
Anxiety: 50 to 70 mg purified kava lactones t.i.d., equivalent to 100 to 250 mg of dried kava root extract per dose. (By comparison, the traditional bowl of raw kava beverage contains about 250 mg of kava lactones.) Other sources cite 60 to 120 mg of kava lactones daily as a conservative dose.
Restlessness: 180 to 210 mg of kava lactones taken as a tea 1 hour before bedtime. The typical dose in this form is 1 cup t.i.d. Prepared by simmering 2 to 4 g of the root in

*Liquid contains alcohol.

5 ounces boiling water for 5 to 10 minutes and then straining.

ADVERSE REACTIONS

CNS: mild euphoric changes characterized by feelings of happiness, fluent and lively speech, and increased sensitivity to sounds; morning fatigue; headache.

EENT: visual accommodation disorders, pupil dilation, disorders of oculomotor equilibrium, initial numbing or astringent effect (with use of beverage).

GI: mild GI disturbances, mouth numbness.

GU: hematuria.

Hepatic: *hepatitis, cirrhosis, fatal liver failure.*

Respiratory: pulmonary hypertension.

Skin: scaly rash.

INTERACTIONS

Herb-drug. *Antiplatelet drugs, MAO type B inhibitors:* May cause additive effects. Monitor patient closely.

Barbiturates, benzodiazepines: May potentiate CNS depressant effects, leading to toxicity. Advise patient to avoid use together.

Levodopa: May reduce drug effectiveness in patients with Parkinson's disease because of dopamine antagonism. Advise patient to use caution if using the herb and drug together.

Hepatotoxic drugs: Causes additive effects. Advise patient to avoid use together.

Herb-herb. *Calamus, calendula, California poppy, capsicum, catnip, celery, couchgrass, elecampane, German chamomile, goldenseal, gotu kola, hops, Jamaican dogwood, lemon balm, sage, sassafras, shepherd's purse, Siberian ginseng, skullcap, stinging nettle, St. John's wort, valerian, wild lettuce, yerba maté:* Causes additive sedative effects. Monitor patient closely.

Herb-lifestyle. *Alcohol use:* Increases risk of CNS depression and liver damage. Warn patient to avoid use together.

EFFECTS ON LAB TEST RESULTS

• May increase liver enzyme and high-density-lipoprotein levels. May decrease albumin, total protein, bilirubin, and urea levels.

• May increase RBCs in urine. May decrease platelet and lymphocyte counts.

CAUTIONS

The FDA warns that several patients who used kava developed cirrhosis, hepatitis, and liver failure, in some cases requiring transplantation. Patients with liver disease shouldn't use the herb; others should use caution when using it and be alert for signs of liver damage.

Patients sensitive to kava or its components shouldn't use the herb, nor should those who have Parkinson's disease or who are breast-feeding. Depressed or bipolar patients shouldn't use it because of possible sedative activity; those with endogenous depression, because of possibly increased risk of suicide; and pregnant women, because of possible loss of uterine tone. Also, the herb shouldn't be given to children younger than age 12.

Bold italic type indicates that reaction may be life-threatening.

NURSING CONSIDERATIONS

• Explore patient's knowledge of this herb.

• Patient shouldn't use kava with conventional sedative-hypnotics, anxiolytics, MAO inhibitors, other psychotropic drugs, levodopa, or antiplatelet drugs without first consulting a health care provider.

• Adverse effects of kava are mild at suggested dosages. They may occur at start of therapy but are transient.

• Oral use is probably safe for up to 3 months, but using the herb for longer than that may be habit forming.

• Kava can cause drowsiness and may impair motor reflexes.

• Patients should avoid taking herb with alcohol because of increased risk of CNS depression and liver damage.

• Periodic monitoring of liver enzyme levels and CBC may be needed.

• Patients who regularly use high doses of kava are more likely to complain of poor health: 20% are underweight with decreased levels of albumin, total protein, bilirubin, and urea; decreased platelet and lymphocyte counts; increased HDL levels and RBC counts; hematuria; puffy faces; scaly rashes; and some evidence of pulmonary hypertension. However, these signs and symptoms resolve several weeks after the herb is stopped. Toxic doses can cause progressive ataxia, muscle weakness, and ascending paralysis, all of which usually resolve when herb is stopped. Extreme use (more than 300 g per week) may increase GGT levels.

PATIENT TEACHING

• Advise patient to consult a health care provider before using an herbal preparation because another treatment may be available.

• Tell patient that when filling a new prescription he should inform pharmacist of any herbal or dietary supplement he's taking.

• Encourage patient to seek medical diagnosis before taking kava.

⚡**ALERT:** Tell patient that if he experiences any signs or symptoms of liver damage—such as jaundice, nausea, vomiting, or abdominal pain—he should immediately stop taking the herb and report them to his health care provider.

• Because usual doses can affect motor function, advise patient to use caution when performing activities that require mental alertness until he knows how the herb affects his CNS.

• Tell patient that oral use is probably safe for up to 3 months but that using the herb for longer than that may be habit forming.

⚡**ALERT:** Caution patient that kava should never be used above the recommended dosage and that it should be used only under the supervision of a qualified health care provider.

• Warn patient to avoid taking the herb with alcohol because of increased risk of CNS depression and liver damage.

• Warn patient to keep all herbal products away from children and pets.

---

*Liquid contains alcohol.

kelp

Laminariae stipites, seaweed, tangleweed

Common trade names
Kelp, Kelp Liquid, Kelp Norwegian
Combination products: *Many, including Activex 40 Plus, Cellbloc, Fat-Solv, Herbal Diuretic Complex, Kelp Plus 3, Plantiodine Plus, PMT Complex, Vitaforce 21-Plus, and Vitaforce Forti-Plus*

AVAILABLE FORMS
Available as a dried preparation of various species of seaweed. It's also an ingredient of several dietary supplements and herbal preparations.

ACTIONS & COMPONENTS
Not well defined, but kelp is rich in iodine.

USES
Used for regulating thyroid function and for treating goiter, hypertension, and obesity. Also used as a bulk laxative and a source of iodine.

DOSAGE & ADMINISTRATION
Not well documented.

ADVERSE REACTIONS
CNS: restlessness, insomnia.
CV: palpitations.
Metabolic: hyperthyroidism, hypothyroidism.
Skin: acne.
Other: allergic reaction.

INTERACTIONS
Herb-drug. *Amiodarone:* May increase iodine level. (Each tablet contains 75 mg of iodine.) Advise patient to avoid use together.
Diuretics: May decrease drug effectiveness because of herb's high sodium content. Monitor drug response closely.
Iron: May decrease iron absorption with prolonged herb use. Monitor patient closely.
Lithium: May increase hypothyroid activity because of the herb's high iodine content. Monitor patient for hypothyroidism.
Thyroid hormone: May interfere with thyroid hormone replacement therapy. Monitor patient for evidence of hypothyroidism.
Herb-food. *Foods high in iron:* May decrease iron absorption with prolonged herb use. Advise patient that iron replacement may be needed.

EFFECTS ON LAB TEST RESULTS
• May increase sodium and iron levels. May alter T_4 and thyroid-stimulating-hormone levels.
• May decrease hemoglobin.

CAUTIONS
Patients sensitive to kelp or its components, including iodine, shouldn't use it, nor should patients who are pregnant or breast-feeding. The herb also shouldn't be given to children.
    Patients who have hyperthyroidism or iron-deficiency anemia or who need to restrict their sodium intake should use caution when using this herb.

NURSING CONSIDERATIONS
• Explore patient's knowledge of this herb.

Bold italic type indicates that reaction may be life-threatening.

• Kelp can worsen hyperthyroidism and acne. Its high sodium content can worsen conditions that require sodium restriction. Because kelp inhibits iron absorption, it can also worsen iron-deficiency anemia.

• Use of kelp has been linked to heavy-metal poisoning.

• Toxicity can cause various reactions, including palpitations, restlessness, and insomnia.

PATIENT TEACHING

• Advise patient to consult a health care provider before using an herbal preparation because another treatment may be available.

• Tell patient that when filling a new prescription he should inform pharmacist of any herbal or dietary supplement he's taking.

• If patient has a chronic illness, advise him not to delay seeking medical evaluation, because doing so may delay diagnosis of a potentially serious medical condition.

• Advise patient to notify her health care provider before using the herb if she suspects or knows that she's pregnant or if she plans to become pregnant.

• Caution patient who takes a diuretic, amiodarone, lithium, a thyroid hormone, or an iron supplement not to use kelp.

• Warn patient to keep all herbal products away from children and pets.

kelpware

Fucus vesiculosus, Quercus marina, black-tang, bladder fucus, bladderwrack, blasentang, cutweed, fucus, rockweed, rockwrack, seawrack, tang

Common trade names
Combination products:
Advantage, Aqua Greens, Atkins Dieters Better Living Multi Vitamins, Daily Essentials, Doctor's Choice, Osteosupport

AVAILABLE FORMS
Available as dried brown algae plant, liquid extract*, tablets, capsules, and soft gel caps.

ACTIONS & COMPONENTS
Limited information is available, but pharmacologic activities are recognized for the individual components and other brown seaweed species. Kelpware contains more than 600 mcg of iodine per gram of seaweed. The algin component has bulk-laxative and soothing effects. An isolated fraction, fucoidin, has 40% to 50% of the anticoagulant activity of heparin. Live *Fucus* can concentrate heavy metals from seawater.

USES
Used to treat thyroid disorders, iodine deficiency, lymphadenoid goiter, myxedema, obesity, arthritis, and rheumatism. Also used for arteriosclerosis, digestive disorders, blood cleansing, constipation, bronchitis, emphysema, GU disorders, anxiety, skin diseases, burns, and insect bites.

*Liquid contains alcohol.

DOSAGE & ADMINISTRATION
Dried plant: Usual dose is 5 to 10 g P.O. t.i.d.
Liquid extract (1:1): Typically 4 to 8 ml P.O. t.i.d.
Tea: Prepared by soaking 5 to 10 g in 5 ounces of boiling water for 5 to 10 minutes and then straining. Tea is taken t.i.d.

ADVERSE REACTIONS
CNS: restlessness, insomnia.
CV: palpitations.
Hematologic: anemia.
Metabolic: hypothyroidism, hyperthyroidism, thyrotoxicosis.
Skin: acne.
Other: allergic reaction.

INTERACTIONS
Herb-drug. *Amiodarone:* May increase iodine levels. (Tablets contain 75 mg iodine.) Advise patient to avoid use together.
Disulfiram, metronidazole: May cause a disulfiram-like reaction if herbal preparation contains alcohol. Advise patient to avoid use together.
Diuretics: May cause decreased drug effectiveness because of herb's high sodium content. Monitor drug response closely.
Heparin, low-molecular-weight heparin, warfarin: Increases risk of bleeding. Monitor PT, INR, and PTT closely.
Iron preparations: May decrease iron absorption with prolonged herb use. Monitor patient closely.
Lithium: May increase hypothyroid activity because of herb's high iodine content. Monitor patient for signs and symptoms of hypothyroidism.

Thyroid hormone: May interfere with thyroid hormone replacement therapy because of herb's high iodine content. Monitor patient for signs and symptoms of hypothyroidism.
Herb-food. *Foods high in iron:* May decrease iron absorption with prolonged herb use. Inform patient that iron replacement may be needed.

EFFECTS ON LAB TEST RESULTS
● May increase creatinine, urine glucose, and urine protein levels. May decrease iron level. May alter thyroid-stimulating-hormone and T_4 levels.
● May alter results of thyroid function tests that use radioactive iodine uptake. May decrease hemoglobin.

CAUTIONS
Patients sensitive to kelpware or its components, including iodine, shouldn't use this herb.

Kelpware should be used cautiously by patients with hyperthyroidism or hypothyroidism due to iodine deficiency, those who need sodium restriction, and those with iron deficiency anemia. Children and women who are pregnant or breast-feeding should avoid using kelpware.

Patients with kidney disorders should avoid using kelpware because of report of nephrotoxicity thought to be related to arsenic content.

NURSING CONSIDERATIONS
● Explore patient's knowledge of this herb.

Bold italic type indicates that reaction may be life-threatening.

• Tinctures and extracts contain 15% to 60% alcohol and may be unsuitable for children, patients with a history of alcoholism or liver disease, or patients taking certain drugs.

• A case of heavy-metal (arsenic) poisoning has been reported from ingestion of contaminated kelpware.

☑ALERT: Signs and symptoms of toxicity include palpitations, restlessness, and insomnia.

☑ALERT: Don't confuse bladderwrack (kelpware) with bladderwort *(Utricularia)*, a freshwater pond plant.

PATIENT TEACHING
• Advise patient to consult a health care provider before using an herbal preparation because another treatment may be available.

• Tell patient that when filling a new prescription he should inform pharmacist of any herbal or dietary supplement he's taking.

• If patient has a history of alcoholism or liver disease, inform him that some herbal products contain alcohol.

• If patient has a chronic illness, advise him not to delay seeking medical evaluation, because doing so may delay diagnosis of a potentially serious medical condition.

• Advise patient to notify her health care provider before using the herb if she suspects or knows that she's pregnant or if she plans to become pregnant.

• Caution patient to avoid using kelpware if he takes a diuretic, amiodarone, lithium, a thyroid replacement hormone, or an iron supplement.

khat

Catha edulis, Abyssinian tea, Arabian tea, chat, gat, kat, Kus-es-Salahin, qat, Somali tea, tohai, tschat

Common trade names
None known

AVAILABLE FORMS
Available as leaves wrapped in plastic, damp paper, or false banana leaves to avoid wilting and drying. Khat is a tree *(C. edulis)* cultivated in southwestern Arabia and eastern Africa.

ACTIONS & COMPONENTS
Contains mainly the sympathomimetic alkaloids cathinone and cathine (norpseudoephedrine). Cathinone and cathine antagonize the actions of physostigmine, but not those of tubocurarine. Chewing khat causes psychotropic effects from amphetamine-like compounds, which interact with the dopaminergic pathway. Both cathinone and cathine decrease appetite and increase locomotor activity. Fresh leaves contain the most cathinone.

USES
The leaf is used to treat depression, fatigue, obesity, and gastric ulcers. The leaf and stem are chewed by some people in East Africa and the Arabian countries as a euphoriant or appetite suppressant.

DOSAGE & ADMINISTRATION
The leaves are usually chewed and the juice swallowed; the residues are kept in the cheek for up to 2

---

*Liquid contains alcohol.

hours and then expectorated. Sometimes the chewed leaves are also swallowed. Occasionally, khat is brewed as a tea or crushed and mixed with honey to make a paste.

ADVERSE REACTIONS
CNS: insomnia (with long-term use), hyperthermia, euphoria, increased alertness, garrulousness, hyperactivity, excitement, aggressiveness, anxiety, manic symptoms, insomnia, malaise, lack of concentration, psychosis, migraine, psychological dependence, *cerebral hemorrhage.*
CV: hypertension in young adults (with long-term use), tachycardia, palpitations, hypertension, *MI.*
EENT: pupil dilation and decreased intraocular pressure.
GI: stomatitis, esophagitis, gastritis, constipation, anorexia, dry mouth, possible oral cancers, periodontal disease, keratosis of the buccal mucosa.
Hepatic: *cirrhosis.*
Musculoskeletal: temporomandibular joint dysfunction.
Respiratory: increased respiratory rate, pulmonary edema.
Skin: diaphoresis.
Other: increased libido in men, followed by loss of sexual drive, spermatorrhea, and impotence; increased sexual desire and improved performance in women; disturbed circadian rhythms and increased susceptibility to infection (long-term use).

INTERACTIONS
Herb-drug. *Other amphetamine-like drugs:* May potentiate effects. Advise patient to avoid use together.

EFFECTS ON LAB TEST RESULTS
• May increase liver enzyme and glucose levels. May decrease testosterone level.

CAUTIONS
Patients who are sensitive to khat or its components shouldn't use it. Pregnant women shouldn't use it because it may reduce birth weight. Breast-feeding women also shouldn't use it because it contains norpseudoephedrine, which appears in breast milk.

Patients with diabetes, hypertension, tachyarrhythmias, glaucoma, migraines, a GI disorder, or an underlying psychotic disorder should use caution when using the herb.

NURSING CONSIDERATIONS
• Explore patient's knowledge of this herb.
• Although khat doesn't cause physical dependence, it causes psychological dependence, which can lead to serious physical and psychological adverse effects.
• Khat suppresses the appetite, causing users to skip meals, decrease adherence to dietary advice, and increase consumption of sweetened beverages, potentially leading to hyperglycemia.

PATIENT TEACHING
• Advise patient to consult a health care provider before using an herbal preparation because another treatment may be available.
• Tell patient that when filling a new prescription he should inform pharmacist of any herbal or dietary supplement he's taking.
• Inform patient that although the leaf isn't physically addictive, it

---

Bold italic type indicates that reaction may be life-threatening.

can cause psychological dependence.

• If patient is a young adult, inform him that long-term use may cause high blood pressure.

• Advise patient to notify her health care provider before using the herb if she suspects or knows that she's pregnant or if she plans to become pregnant.

• Warn patient to keep all herbal products away from children and pets.

khella

Ammi visnaga, A. daucoides, Ammi visnaga fruits, bishop's weed, greater Ammi, khella fruits, visnaga

Common trade names
Doctor's Choice for Heart Health

AVAILABLE FORMS
Available as capsules, tablets, extract, and tea. One standardized form contains a minimum of 10% gamma-pyrones, calculated as 100 mg of khellin.

ACTIONS & COMPONENTS
Derived from fruits and seeds of *A. visnaga,* a member of the carrot family. The visnadin component acts as a mild positive inotrope by dilating coronary vessels and increasing coronary and myocardial circulation. Another component, khellin, is commercially available and used as a vasodilator in treating bronchial asthma and angina pectoris.

USES
Used orally for angina pectoris, cardiac insufficiency, paroxysmal tachycardia, extrasystoles, hypertonia, asthma, whooping cough, and cramplike complaints. Extracts are used topically for psoriasis.

DOSAGE & ADMINISTRATION
Capsules or tablets: Average daily dose is 20 mg of gamma-pyrones P.O.
Tea: Rarely used as a tea, but prepared by pouring boiling water over the powdered fruits, soaking for 10 to 15 minutes, and then straining.

ADVERSE REACTIONS
CNS: dizziness, headache, insomnia, vertigo.
GI: nausea, constipation, anorexia.
Hepatic: cholestatic jaundice.
Skin: phototoxicity, skin cancer (with topical use), pruritus

INTERACTIONS
Herb-drug. *Anticoagulants, antihypertensives:* May cause potentiated effects. Advise patient to avoid use together.
Hepatotoxic drugs: May cause additive effects. Advise patient to avoid use together.
Herb-herb. *St. John's wort:* Increases photosensitivity risk. Advise patient to wear protective clothing and sunscreen outdoors and to limit exposure to direct sunlight.
Herb-lifestyle. *Alcohol use:* May cause hepatotoxicity. Advise patient to avoid use together.
Sun exposure: May cause photosensitivity. Advise patient to wear protective clothing and sunscreen

---

*Liquid contains alcohol.

outdoors and to limit exposure to direct sunlight.

EFFECTS ON LAB TEST RESULTS
• May increase liver enzyme levels.
• May increase bleeding time, PT, and PTT.

CAUTIONS
Patients sensitive to khella or its components shouldn't use this herb, nor should patients who are pregnant or breast-feeding, have liver disease, or are prone to skin cancer.

NURSING CONSIDERATIONS
• Explore patient's knowledge of this herb.
• Oral use may increase liver enzyme levels. Monitor these levels carefully.

PATIENT TEACHING
• Advise patient to consult a health care provider before using an herbal preparation because another treatment may be available.
• Tell patient that when filling a new prescription he should inform pharmacist of any herbal or dietary supplement he's taking.
• Although chemical interactions haven't been reported in clinical studies, tell patient that herb may interfere with therapeutic effect of conventional drugs.
• Warn patient not to take herb for heart failure before seeking medical evaluation, because doing so may delay diagnosis of a potentially serious medical condition.
• Warn patient not to take the herb with alcohol or a hepatotoxic drug.

• Advise patient to notify her health care provider before using the herb if she suspects or knows that she's pregnant or if she plans to become pregnant.
• Warn patient to keep all herbal products away from children and pets.

kudzu

Pueraria montana var. *lobata, P. montana* var. *thomsonii, P. lobata, P. mirifica, P. pseudohirsuta, P. thomsonii, P. thunbergiana, P. tuberosa, Dolichos lobatus,* ge-gen, Japanese arrowroot, kudsu, kudzu vine, kwaao khruea, mealy kudzu, Pueraria root, Radix Puerariae

Common trade names
Fen Ke, Fenge, Gange, Yege

AVAILABLE FORMS
The useable parts of kudzu are the root and flower. Available as capsules, tablets, and extract.
Capsules: 150 mg

ACTIONS & COMPONENTS
It was originally thought that isoflavone constituents of kudzu (daidzin, daidzein, and puerarin) were reversible inhibitors of alcohol and aldehyde dehydrogenase; however, recent findings have disputed this claim.
    Kudzu extract, daidzein, and daidzin have been shown to decrease alcohol consumption, lower peak blood alcohol levels, and shorten alcohol-induced sleep in alcohol-dependent animal models.

Bold italic type indicates that reaction may be life-threatening.

Preliminary evidence shows puerarin might decrease heart rate, plasma renin activity, capillary permeability, and platelet aggregation. Puerarin has also demonstrated hypoglycemic, hypocholesterolemic, antiarrhythmic, antipyretic, and antioxidant activity.

Kudzu root extract dilates coronary and cerebral blood vessels and increases myocardial and cerebral blood flow, decreasing vascular resistance, myocardial oxygen demand, and lactic acid production in anaerobic myocardial tissues and increasing blood oxygen supply.

USES
In general, kudzu is used alone or in combination with other products for signs and symptoms of alcohol hangover, such as headache, upset stomach, dizziness, and vomiting.

In traditional Chinese medicine, kudzu has been used for managing alcoholism and drunkenness, myalgia, measles, dysentery, gastritis, fever, diarrhea, thirst, cold, flu, and neck stiffness; it has also been used as a diaphoretic.

In more recent years, kudzu has been used for hypertension, angina pectoris, arrhythmias, migraine, deafness, diabetes, traumatic injuries, sinusitis, urticaria, pruritus, and psoriasis.

DOSAGE & ADMINISTRATION
Kudzu root: 9 to 15 g daily.
Kudzu root extract: 150 to 300 mg t.i.d. or 300 mg once daily.
Kudzu root tablets: 30 to 120 mg daily (depending on the product).

ADVERSE REACTIONS
None reported.

INTERACTIONS
Herb-drug. *Anticoagulants:* May potentiate drug effects. Advise patient to avoid use together.
Antidiabetics: May cause additive hypoglycemic effects. Advise patient to avoid use together.
Aspirin: May cause increased hypoglycemic effect of kudzu. Advise patient to avoid use together.
Cardiovascular drugs: May interfere with cardiovascular therapies. Advise patient to avoid use together.

EFFECTS ON LAB TEST RESULTS
• May decrease glucose and cholesterol levels.
• May increase clotting time, including PT and INR.

CAUTIONS
Because of the lack of available data, patients who are pregnant or breast-feeding shouldn't use the herb, nor should patients who have a clotting disorder, cardiovascular disease, or diabetes. Those who are taking an anticoagulant or aspirin shouldn't use this herb.

NURSING CONSIDERATIONS
• Explore patient's knowledge of this herb.
• Monitor vital signs, PT, and INR as needed.
• If patient has diabetes, monitor glucose levels regularly.
• Some commercial kudzu products are standardized for daidzin content.

---

*Liquid contains alcohol.

PATIENT TEACHING
• Advise patient to consult a health care provider before using an herbal preparation because another treatment may be available.
• Tell patient that when filling a new prescription he should inform pharmacist of any herbal or dietary supplement he's taking.
• Warn patient to keep all herbal products away from children and pets.

L

lady's mantle

Alchemilla vulgaris, bear's foot, dewcup, leontopodium, lion's foot, nine hooks, stellaria

Common trade names
None known

AVAILABLE FORMS
Available as tea, tablets, tincture*, and ointment.

ACTIONS & COMPONENTS
Obtained from stem, seeds, leaves, and flowers of A. vulgaris. Above-ground parts of Alchemilla contain tannins, mainly ellagic acid glycosides (6% to 8%); various flavonoids, such as quercitrin; and salicylic acid in trace amounts.

Tannins impart a mild topical astringent action for use as a styptic and in treating mild diarrhea. The amount of salicylic acid isn't enough to provide any therapeutic effect. Lady's mantle is an aquaretic herb, which causes loss of water rather than electrolytes.

USES
Used as a topical astringent or as a styptic for wounds. Also used as a tea to control mild diarrhea and in women to reduce uterine bleeding, ease menstrual cramps, and regulate the menstrual cycle.

DOSAGE & ADMINISTRATION
Ointment: Applied to wounds daily or b.i.d.
Tablets: 1 tablet P.O. q 30 to 60 minutes for acute diarrhea or one

to three times P.O. daily for chronic diarrhea.
Tea: 2 to 4 g of dried herb added to 5 ounces of boiling water and steeped for 10 minutes; prepared daily. Tea is divided and taken t.i.d.
Tincture: 5 gtt of tincture P.O. q 30 to 60 minutes for acute diarrhea or one to three times P.O. daily for chronic diarrhea.

ADVERSE REACTIONS
Hepatic: liver damage.

INTERACTIONS
None reported.

EFFECTS ON LAB TEST RESULTS
• May increase liver enzyme levels.

CAUTIONS
Because safety hasn't been determined, patients who are pregnant or breast-feeding shouldn't use the herb, nor should patients with liver dysfunction.

NURSING CONSIDERATIONS
• Explore patient's knowledge of this herb.
• Long-term use may lead to liver dysfunction. Monitor patient's liver enzyme levels.
• Because clinical and safety data are lacking, use of this herb can't be recommended.
• Tinctures and extracts contain 15% to 60% alcohol and may be unsuitable for children, patients with a history of alcoholism or liver disease, or patients taking certain drugs.

---

*Liquid contains alcohol.

⚠ ALERT: Don't confuse this herb with Alpine lady's mantle *(Alchemilla alpina)*, which is unapproved by the German Commission E because of lack of documented effectiveness and safety.

PATIENT TEACHING
● Advise patient to consult a health care provider before using an herbal preparation because another treatment may be available.
● Tell patient that when filling a new prescription he should inform pharmacist of any herbal or dietary supplement he's taking.
● Warn patient that little data exist to support this herb's use or safety.
● If patient has a history of alcoholism or liver disease, inform him that some herbal products contain alcohol.
● Warn patient not to take herb for a GI disturbance before seeking medical attention, because doing so may delay diagnosis of a potentially serious medical condition.
● If patient is using the herb to treat mild diarrhea, advise him not to take it for more than 4 days. Tell him to consult his health care provider if diarrhea persists or worsens.
● Warn patient to stop taking herb and notify his health care provider if he experiences signs and symptoms of liver dysfunction, such as jaundice, nausea, vomiting, and abdominal pain.
● Warn patient to keep all herbal products away from children and pets.

lady's slipper

Cypripedium calceolus, American valerian, bleeding heart, golden slipper, lady's slipper root, moccasin flower, monkey flower, nerve root, Noah's ark, venus's shoe, whippoorwill's shoe, yellow Indian shoe, yellows

Common trade names
None known

AVAILABLE FORMS
Obtained from *C. calceolus,* a member of the Orchid family. Because this species may be protected, collecting native specimens may be forbidden. It's usually available in combination with other herbs, especially valerian, and as liquid extract*, powdered root, dried root, tea, and tincture*.

ACTIONS & COMPONENTS
Not reported. Some *Cypripedium* species contain allergens and phenanthrene quinones, which are skin irritants.

USES
Used as a tea for nervousness, headaches (especially stress-related headaches), and emotional tension. It's a mild sedative, a mild hypnotic, and a GI antispasmodic.

DOSAGE & ADMINISTRATION
Dried root: 2 to 4 g P.O. t.i.d.
Extract (1:1 water or 1:45% ethanol): 2 to 4 ml P.O. t.i.d.

Bold italic type indicates that reaction may be life-threatening.

ADVERSE REACTIONS
CNS: sedation, giddiness, headache, hallucinations, restlessness.
Skin: contact dermatitis.

INTERACTIONS
Herb-drug. *Disulfiram, metronidazole:* May cause a disulfiram-like reaction if herbal preparation contains alcohol. Advise patient to avoid use together.
Dopamine agonists: Increases risk of hallucinations. Advise patient to avoid use together.

EFFECTS ON LAB TEST RESULTS
None reported.

CAUTIONS
Patients who are allergic to members of the Orchid family or who have a history of other plant allergies shouldn't use this herb. Patients prone to headaches or mental illness shouldn't use the herb unless they're under medical supervision. Patients who are pregnant or breast-feeding also should avoid using the herb.

NURSING CONSIDERATIONS
• Explore patient's knowledge of this herb.
• Tinctures and extracts contain 15% to 60% alcohol and may be unsuitable for children, patients with a history of alcoholism or liver disease, or patients taking certain drugs.
• Monitor patient for psychotic behavior and headaches.
• Because clinical and safety data are lacking, use of this herb can't be recommended.

PATIENT TEACHING
• Advise patient to consult a health care provider before using an herbal preparation because another treatment may be available.
• Tell patient that when filling a new prescription he should inform pharmacist of any herbal or dietary supplement he's taking.
• Warn patient that little data exist to support this herb's use or safety.
• If patient has a history of alcoholism or liver disease, inform him that some herbal products contain alcohol.
• Warn patient not to take herb for headaches or anxiety before seeking medical evaluation, because doing so may delay diagnosis of a potentially serious medical condition.
• Although no chemical interactions have been reported in clinical studies, caution patient that herb may interfere with therapeutic effects of conventional drugs.
• Because sedation is possible, advise patient to use caution when performing activities that require mental alertness until he knows how the herb affects his CNS.
• Tell patient to inform his health care provider if he develops signs or symptoms of contact dermatitis.
• Warn patient to keep all herbal products away from children and pets.

*Liquid contains alcohol.

lavender

Lavandula angustifolia, L. officinalis, aspic, English lavender, French lavender, garden lavender, lavandin, spike lavender, true lavender

Common trade names
Lavender Liquid Extract, Lavender Flowers

AVAILABLE FORMS
Available as a volatile oil distilled from flowers of *L. officinalis* and other species, collected just before they open. Also available as dried, unopened flowers, tincture*, and lavender spirits.

ACTIONS & COMPONENTS
Volatile oil of lavender (1% to 5%) contains more than 100 monoterpene components, up to 30% to 40% linalyl acetate and linalool and less than 1% camphor. Several coumarins, ursolic acid, flavonoids, and tannins are also found in the plant. Monoterpenes account for reported antiseptic actions of the oil—cineole and linalool for the hypotensive action, and linalool and linalyl acetate for CNS depression. Lavender oil's sedative effects have been recorded from oral, topical, and inhaled doses. Lavender may have lipid-lowering activity, may lower EEG potentials, and may prolong sleeping time.

True lavender oil *(L. officinalis)* isn't toxic at oral doses of up to 5 g/kg; it's rarely toxic dermally and seldom causes sensitization. Spike lavender oil *(L. stoechas)* is neurotoxic because of its high camphor content (15% to 30%). Lavendin, an oil from the hybrid *L. intermedia,* may be toxic because of its 5% to 15% camphor content.

USES
The oil is applied topically as an antiseptic to treat psoriasis, minor scrapes, cuts, and burns. The herb is used orally, topically, or by inhalation for its calming, mild sedative effect. Oil is added to warm baths as a relaxation aid. The flowers have been used orally as a tea to calm a "nervous stomach."

DOSAGE & ADMINISTRATION
Dried flowers: 20 to 100 g added to bath.
Oil: 1 to 4 gtt P.O. on a sugar cube, or diluted in a carrier oil (2% to 5%) as a topical massage, or a few drops added to bath for psoriasis, wounds, or burns.
Tea: Prepared by adding 1 to 2 teaspoons of dried flowers to 5 ounces hot water.

ADVERSE REACTIONS
CNS: CNS depression, confusion, dizziness, syncope, drowsiness, headache, *neurotoxicity.*
CV: hypotension.
GI: nausea, vomiting, constipation.
Respiratory: *respiratory depression.*
Skin: contact dermatitis.

INTERACTIONS
Herb-drug. *CNS depressants:* May potentiate drug effects (with the oil). Monitor patient closely for oversedation.
Disulfiram, metronidazole: May cause a disulfiram-like reaction if

---

Bold italic type indicates that reaction may be life-threatening.

herbal preparation contains alcohol. Advise patient to avoid use together.

Herb-lifestyle. *Alcohol use:* May potentiate CNS depressant effects of alcohol (with the oil). Advise patient to avoid use together.

EFFECTS ON LAB TEST RESULTS
• May decrease lipid levels.

CAUTIONS
Patients who are pregnant or breast-feeding or who are sensitive to lavender shouldn't use this herb.

NURSING CONSIDERATIONS
• Explore patient's knowledge of this herb.
• Tinctures and extracts contain 15% to 60% alcohol and may be unsuitable for children, patients with a history of alcoholism or liver disease, or patients taking certain drugs.
• Massaging with diluted oil is unlikely to be toxic.
• Some people may be allergic to lavender-containing perfumes, although the herb's allergenic potential is low.
⚠ **ALERT:** Don't confuse true lavender oil with lavandin or spike lavender oil; the latter two contain high enough levels of camphor to elicit neurotoxicity.

PATIENT TEACHING
• Advise patient to consult a health care provider before using an herbal preparation because another treatment may be available.
• Tell patient that when filling a new prescription he should inform

pharmacist of any herbal or dietary supplement he's taking.
• If patient has a history of alcoholism or liver disease, inform him that some herbal products contain alcohol.
• Although no chemical interactions have been reported in clinical studies, advise patient that lavender may interfere with therapeutic effects of conventional drugs.
• Advise patient that excessive inhalation of the oil may lead to dizziness, nausea, and fainting.
• Teach patient that oil should be purchased in dropper-tipped amber glass bottles and stored away from light, heat, and small children.
• Advise patient to avoid performing activities that require mental alertness until he knows how the drug affects his CNS.
• Warn patient to keep all herbal products away from children and pets.

lemon

Citrus limonum, limone

Common trade names
None known

AVAILABLE FORMS
Available as fruit, fruit juice, expressed peel oil, dried peel, and lemon peel tincture*.

ACTIONS & COMPONENTS
Expressed oil makes up 2.5% of the peel and consists mainly of monoterpenes (up to 70% limonene); some sesquiterpenes, such as bisabolol; several coumarins and furanocoumarins; and citrus

*Liquid contains alcohol.

bioflavonoids, such as hesperidan, rutin, naringoside. The juice contains bioflavonoids plus vitamin C. Pectin is mainly found in the white endocarp of the peel. The bioflavonoids are used to treat vascular insufficiency and problems with capillary fragility by decreasing porosity. Bisabolol possesses some anti-inflammatory activity. The coumarins and furanocoumarins are photodermatotoxic. Various monoterpenes produce antispasmodic (1,8-cineole), antimutagenic (limonene), antitumorigenic or chemopreventive (limonene), antioxidant (myrcene), irritant (terpinene-4-ol), and antiviral (α-pinene) actions.

USES
Lemon oil is used as a carminative and as a mild anti-inflammatory and diuretic. Nutritionally, the juice and pulp are a good source of vitamin C, potassium, and bioflavonoids. Lemon is used as a food and a flavor. The oil is used as a scenting agent in many soaps, cleaners, and cosmetics.

DOSAGE & ADMINISTRATION
Lemon is taken internally as an oil, as a tincture, or as fresh fruit.

ADVERSE REACTIONS
Skin: phototoxicity from expressed oil.

INTERACTIONS
Herb-drug. *Disulfiram, metronidazole:* May cause a disulfiram-like reaction if herbal preparation contains alcohol. Advise patient to avoid use together.

Herb-lifestyle. *Sun exposure:* Using the oil as a tanning substance may cause skin damage. Advise patient not to use herb as a tanning agent.

EFFECTS ON LAB TEST RESULTS
None reported.

CAUTIONS
Oral ingestion of expressed oil isn't recommended for pregnant or breast-feeding patients because of the toxicity of its furanocoumarin constituents. Patients sensitive to members of the citrus family should avoid lemon preparations as well.

NURSING CONSIDERATIONS
• Explore patient's knowledge of this herb.
• Tinctures and extracts contain 15% to 60% alcohol and may be unsuitable for children, patients with a history of alcoholism or liver disease, or patients taking certain drugs.
• Patient should avoid applying expressed oil to skin or mucous membranes because of its irritant qualities.
• Direct application of the oil to skin exposed to sunlight can cause phototoxicity. Products for topical application should contain no more than 2% expressed oil because it contains phototoxic furanocoumarins. Distilled lemon oils have an unpleasant odor and aren't phototoxic.
• Advise patient not to substitute lemon petitgrain oil, the distilled oil from lemon leaf, for lemon peel oil.

Bold italic type indicates that reaction may be life-threatening.

PATIENT TEACHING
- Advise patient to consult a health care provider before using an herbal preparation because another treatment may be available.
- Tell patient that when filling a new prescription he should inform pharmacist of any herbal or dietary supplement he's taking.
- If patient has a history of alcoholism or liver disease, inform him that some herbal products contain alcohol.
- If patient is pregnant or breastfeeding, caution her not to consume the expressed oil.
- Warn patient not to apply expressed oil to the skin or mucous membranes.
- If patient uses the oil, recommend appropriate precautions against prolonged or unprotected sun exposure.
- Advise patient to discontinue use if skin reactions occur.
- Warn patient to keep all herbal products away from children and pets.

lemon balm

Melissa officinalis, balm, common balm, cure-all, dropsy plant, honey plant, Melissa, sweet balm, sweet Mary

Common trade names
Melissa Lemon Balm Herb, Quanterra Sleep

AVAILABLE FORMS
Available as leaf or powder, capsules, creams, volatile oil, liquid extract*, or "Spirits of Melissa"
(75% alcohol). Often combined with other sedative herbs.

ACTIONS & COMPONENTS
Action results from volatile oil consisting of 0.1% to 0.2% citral-a (geranial) and citral-b (neral), limonene, small amounts of flavonoids, tannins, protocatechuic and caffeic acids, and ursolic and pomolic acids. The latter, along with the distinctly lemon-scented volatile oil, may account for its use as a carminative to settle the stomach. The volatile oil components also account for the herb's diaphoretic actions. Limonene, oleanolic acid, and geranial have demonstrated sedative actions. Citronellal, a terpene, may be the primary sedating constituent. Citral has an estrogenic effect. Rosmarinic acid has antiviral actions.

Lemon balm has shown antiviral activity against *Herpes simplex* when applied topically. Minor beneficial effects in treating some psychiatric disorders have been reported. Lemon balm also exerts antithyroid effects by inhibiting thyroid-stimulating hormone and the enzyme iodothyronine deiodinase in vitro. Several components of the volatile oil cause skin sensitization, and some are teratogenic.

USES
Used as a sedative, usually with other herbal sedatives, to treat nervous sleeping disorders. Also used for nervous GI complaints, chronic bronchial catarrh, palpitations related to anxiety or nervousness, vomiting, migraine, headache, and

---

* Liquid contains alcohol.

high blood pressure. Herbal compresses are used to relieve stiff neck, nerve pain, and rheumatism.

DOSAGE & ADMINISTRATION
Tea: 1.5 to 4.5 g of the herb per cup of tea as needed, or the equivalent in other preparations.

ADVERSE REACTIONS
None reported.

INTERACTIONS
Herb-drug. *Disulfiram, metronidazole:* May cause a disulfiram-like reaction if herbal preparation contains alcohol. Advise patient to avoid use together.

EFFECTS ON LAB TEST RESULTS
None reported.

CAUTIONS
Patients who have glaucoma or who are sensitive to lemon balm shouldn't use this herb, nor should patients who are pregnant.

Patients who are breast-feeding or who have BPH, a thyroid disorder, or an allergy to lemon- or citrus-scented perfumes should use caution when using the herb because of the activity of the volatile oil components.

NURSING CONSIDERATIONS
• Explore patient's knowledge of this herb.
• Tinctures and extracts contain 15% to 60% alcohol and may be unsuitable for children, patients with a history of alcoholism or liver disease, or patients taking certain drugs.

• Besides using caution when using the herb, patients with a thyroid disorder should also have their thyroid-stimulating hormone levels monitored as needed.
• Oral use of the volatile oil isn't recommended.

PATIENT TEACHING
• Advise patient to consult a health care provider before using an herbal preparation because another treatment may be available.
• Tell patient that when filling a new prescription he should inform pharmacist of any herbal or dietary supplement he's taking.
• Although no chemical interactions have been reported in clinical studies, advise patient that herb may interfere with therapeutic effects of conventional drugs.
• If patient has a history of alcoholism or liver disease, inform him that some herbal products contain alcohol.
• Advise patient not to take herb for anxiety or a sleep disorder before seeking medical attention, because doing so may delay diagnosis of a potentially serious medical condition.
• Urge patient to stop using the herb if he develops ocular pain or rash.
• Tell patient not to use herb if he's allergic to lemon-scented perfumes or products.
• Caution patient against oral use of lemon balm oil. If needed, mention that brewed tea is usually well tolerated.
• Warn patient to take precautions until the sedative effect of the herb on him is known.

Bold italic type indicates that reaction may be life-threatening.

• Warn patient to keep all herbal products away from children and pets.

lemongrass

Cymbopogon citratus, capim-cidrao, citronella, fevergrass, Indian melissa, Indian verbena

Common trade names
Carmol (lemongrass oil)

AVAILABLE FORMS
Available as leaves and oil.

ACTIONS & COMPONENTS
Lemongrass contains alkaloids, a saponin fraction, and cymbopogonol. Fresh leaves contain 0.4% to 0.5% volatile oil, which contains citral, myrcene, geranial, and several other fragrant compounds. Myrcene may have some peripheral analgesic activity similar to peripherally acting opiates that directly downregulate sensitized receptors.

USES
Leaves are used as an antispasmodic, an analgesic, and a treatment for nervous and GI disorders. Crushed leaves are used topically as a mosquito repellent. Essential oil is used as a food additive and in perfumes.

DOSAGE & ADMINISTRATION
Oil: Applied topically for pain, arthritis, or ringworm.
Tea: 2 to 4 g of fresh or dried leaves boiled in 5 ounces water.

ADVERSE REACTIONS
GI: dry mouth.

GU: polyuria.
Skin: contact dermatitis.

INTERACTIONS
None reported.

EFFECTS ON LAB TEST RESULTS
None reported.

CAUTIONS
Patients who are pregnant or sensitive to the herb shouldn't use it.

NURSING CONSIDERATIONS
• Explore patient's knowledge of this herb.
• Lemongrass may increase the frequency of urination.

PATIENT TEACHING
• Advise patient to consult a health care provider before using an herbal preparation because another treatment may be available.
• Tell patient that when filling a new prescription he should inform pharmacist of any herbal or dietary supplement he's taking.
• Inform patient that animal and human studies haven't supported claimed uses for this herb.
• Caution patient not to take herb at bedtime because it may increase the frequency of urination.
• Warn patient to keep all herbal products away from children and pets.

*Liquid contains alcohol.

licorice

Glycyrrhiza glabra, Chinese licorice, licorice root, Persian licorice, Russian licorice, Spanish licorice, sweet root, sweet wood, sweet wort

Common trade names
Herbal Booster, Herbal Laxative, Herbal Nerve, Honey and Molasses, Licorice Power, Lightning Cough Remedy, Phyto Power, Standardized Licorice, Wild Countryside Licorice Root

AVAILABLE FORMS
Available as liquid and capsules.
Capsules: 100 mg, 200 mg, 400 mg, 444 mg, 445 mg, 450 mg, 500 mg, 520 mg

ACTIONS & COMPONENTS
Obtained from dried, unpeeled roots of *G. glabra.* Licorice contains 7% to 10% glycyrrhizin (glycyrrhizic acid), as well as natural sugars, glucose, mannose, sucrose, flavonoids, isoflavonoids, and sterols (beta-sitosterol and stigmasterol). Glycyrrhizin is a glycoside that is 50 times sweeter than sugar, which helps to mask the bitter taste of quinine and similar drugs. The active ingredient for treating stomach ulcers is carbenoxolone, a semisynthetic ester of glycyrrhetic acid.

Licorice has shown antarthritic and anti-inflammatory effects by inhibiting prostaglandin activity. This activity may make it useful in treating pain and inflammation from arthritis.

The active ingredient, glycyrrhetinic acid, inhibits 11-beta-hydroxy-steroid-dehydrogenase, an enzyme that prevents cortisol from acting as a mineralocorticoid. Inhibiting this enzyme allows increased mineralocorticoid, or aldosterone-like, activity, leading to sodium and water retention and potassium excretion. There have been many reports of severe toxicity caused by these effects.

USES
Licorice is used as a remedy for stomach ulcers and as an expectorant. It's also used in sweets, soft drinks, chewing tobacco, and drugs.

DOSAGE & ADMINISTRATION
Capsules: Doses range from 5 to 15 g/day of licorice root (200 to 600 mg glycyrrhizin). Daily intake of more than 50 g of the herb is considered toxic.

ADVERSE REACTIONS
CNS: paresthesia, paralysis, fatigue, weakness.
CV: hypertension, *heart failure, arrhythmias.*
Metabolic: hypernatremia, hypokalemia.
Musculoskeletal: myopathy, muscle cramps.
Other: swelling.

INTERACTIONS
Herb-drug. *Antiarrhythmics, such as procainamide and quinidine:* Causes hypokalemia and torsades de pointes. Advise patient to avoid use together.
Antihypertensives: May decrease drug effectiveness. Monitor blood pressure closely.

Bold italic type indicates that reaction may be life-threatening.

Corticosteroids: May cause additive effects because of the herb's glycyrrhizin component or interfere with the drug's immunosuppressive effect because of the herb's stimulation of interferon production. Advise patient to avoid use together.

Digoxin: Increases risk of digoxin toxicity. (Hypokalemia increases the risk.) Advise patient to avoid use together.

Diuretics: May worsen hypokalemia. Advise patient to avoid use together.

Herb-lifestyle. *Smoking:* May cause reduced herb metabolism because of reported licorice toxicity. Monitor patient closely.

EFFECTS ON LAB TEST RESULTS
• May increase sodium and 17-hydroxyprogesterone levels. May decrease potassium and testosterone levels.

CAUTIONS
Patients who are pregnant or sensitive to the herb or who have arrhythmias, diabetes, glaucoma, CVA, or renal, hepatic, or cardiac disease shouldn't use this herb.

NURSING CONSIDERATIONS
• Explore patient's knowledge of this herb.
• Toxicity can occur with long-term use or with single large doses of licorice. Licorice shouldn't be used for more than 4 weeks at a time.
• Monitor patient for signs and symptoms of hypokalemia or hypernatremia.
• Assess patient's drug profile for use of diuretics, antihypertensives, antiarrhythmics, corticosteroids, or digoxin.
• Monitor patient's blood pressure closely.

PATIENT TEACHING
• Advise patient to consult a health care provider before using an herbal preparation because another treatment may be available.
• Tell patient that when filling a new prescription he should inform pharmacist of any herbal or dietary supplement he's taking.
• If patient has a chronic illness, advise him not to delay seeking medical evaluation, because doing so may delay diagnosis of a potentially serious medical condition.
• Caution patient not to take large doses of licorice or use it for more than 4 weeks at a time because of the risk of toxicity.
• Tell patient to notify his health care provider if he develops swelling, muscle cramps, tiredness, or weakness.
• Warn patient to keep all herbal products away from children and pets.

lily of the valley

Convallaria majalis, convall-lily, Jacob's ladder, ladder to heaven, lily constancy, maiblume, maiglöckchen, may bells, may lily, muguet, Our Lady's tears

Common trade names
None known

AVAILABLE FORMS
Available as capsules, drops, tablets, and powder.

ACTIONS & COMPONENTS
Obtained from all parts of the of
C. majalis plant. Lily of the valley
has a positive inotropic effect on
the heart through natural cardioactive glycosides, including convalla-
toxin, convalloside, and convalla-
toxol.

USES
Used for mild exertional failure,
age-related cardiac complaints,
and chronic cor pulmonale.

DOSAGE & ADMINISTRATION
No dosage is recommended because of plant's toxic potential. A
dose of 0.6 g of standardized lily-
of-the-valley powder contains
0.2% to 0.3% cardioactive glycosides.

ADVERSE REACTIONS
CNS: headache.
CV: *arrhythmias.*
EENT: visual color disturbances.
GI: nausea, vomiting, abdominal
pain or cramps, diarrhea.
Metabolic: hyperkalemia.
Musculoskeletal: muscle cramps.

INTERACTIONS
Herb-drug. *Beta blockers, calcium channel blockers:* Increases
risk of bradycardia or heart block.
Advise patient to avoid use together.
*Calcium salts, digoxin, glucocorti-
coids, laxatives, quinidine:* May
cause additive effects and increase
risk of adverse reactions. Advise
patient to avoid use together.

EFFECTS ON LAB TEST RESULTS
• May increase potassium level.

CAUTIONS
This herb isn't recommended for
use.

NURSING CONSIDERATIONS
⚠**ALERT:** The FDA considers
lily of the valley an unsafe and poisonous plant because of the level
of toxins.
• Explore patient's knowledge of
this herb.
• Monitor patient for serious adverse reactions, such as increased
potassium levels and cardiac arrhythmias.

PATIENT TEACHING
⚠**ALERT:** Discourage the patient
from using this herb. Warn him
that it's considered poisonous and
that the FDA has deemed it unsafe.
• Inform patient about the herb's
serious adverse effects, especially
when used with digoxin, a beta
blocker, or a calcium channel
blocker.
• Tell patient to notify his health
care provider if he develops nausea, vomiting, muscle cramps, or a
change in heartbeat—all of which
may warn of serious adverse reactions.
• Warn patient to keep all herbal
products away from children and
pets.

linden

*Tilia cordata, T. platyphyllos,
T. tomentosa,* basswood,
European linden, lime flower,
lime tree

Common trade names
Linden Capsules

Bold italic type indicates that reaction may be life-threatening.

AVAILABLE FORMS
Available as liquid extract*.

ACTIONS & COMPONENTS
Obtained from fresh and dried flowers and leaves of *Tilia* trees. Linden extract contains flavonoid compounds, including kaempferol and quercitin; p-coumaric, caffeic, and chlorogenic acids; and amino acids. The plant contains 0.02% to 0.1% volatile oils, including citral, eugenol, and limonene. The ratio of tannins to mucilage polysaccharides contained in various *Tilia* species accounts for differences in the flavor of teas made from this herb. Quercitin, *p*-coumaric acid, and kaempferol may cause diaphoretic action.

USES
Used to induce sweating and to treat various nervous disorders, feverish colds, throat irritation, nasal congestion, infections, and cold-related cough.

DOSAGE & ADMINISTRATION
Liquid extract: 2 to 4 ml of 1:1 preparation with 25% alcohol.
Tea: 2 to 4 g/day.

ADVERSE REACTIONS
CNS: drowsiness.
Skin: contact dermatitis.

INTERACTIONS
Herb-drug. *Disulfiram, metronidazole:* May cause a disulfiram-like reaction if herbal preparation contains alcohol. Advise patient to avoid use together.
Herb-lifestyle. *Alcohol use:* May cause additive effects. Advise patient to avoid use together.

EFFECTS ON LAB TEST RESULTS
None reported.

CAUTIONS
Patients sensitive to herb and those with a history of heart disease shouldn't use herb.

NURSING CONSIDERATIONS
• Explore patient's knowledge of this herb.
• Tinctures and extracts contain 15% to 60% alcohol and may be unsuitable for children, patients with a history of alcoholism or liver disease, or patients taking certain drugs.
• Although no chemical interactions have been reported in clinical studies, the herb may interfere with therapeutic effects of conventional drugs.
• Some patients may be allergic to linden. If signs or symptoms develop, patient should discontinue herb and consult a health care provider.

PATIENT TEACHING
• Advise patient to consult a health care provider before using an herbal preparation because another treatment may be available.
• Tell patient that when filling a new prescription he should inform pharmacist of any herbal or dietary supplement he's taking.
• If patient has a history of alcoholism or liver disease, inform him that some herbal products contain alcohol.
• If patient has a chronic illness, advise him not to delay seeking appropriate medical evaluation, because doing so may delay diagnosis of a potentially serious medical condition.

*Liquid contains alcohol.

- Caution patients with a history of heart disease not to use linden. Frequent use may damage heart tissue.
- Warn patient to contact a health care provider if he develops a rash, swelling, or trouble breathing.
- Advise patient to use caution when performing activities that require mental alertness until he knows how the herb affects his CNS.
- Warn patient to keep all herbal products away from children and pets.

lobelia

Lobelia inflata, asthma weed, bladderpod, cardinal flower, emetic herb, emetic weed, eyebright, gagroot, Indian pink, Indian tobacco, pukeweed, vomitroot, vomitwort, wild tobacco

Common trade names
Lobelia Compound, Lobelia Extract

AVAILABLE FORMS
Available as tablets and tincture*.

ACTIONS & COMPONENTS
Obtained from the dried leaves of *L. inflata.* Contains 6% alkaloids. Lobeline accounts for most of the herb's effects. Lobelanine, lobelanidine, norlobelanine, and isolobinine are also present. Lobelia acts like nicotine and interacts at the nicotine receptor, stimulating the respiratory and emetic centers of the brain.

USES
Used as an antasthmatic, an emetic, and a smoking cessation aid.

DOSAGE & ADMINISTRATION
Lobelia is used as a component of some homeopathic preparations. Doses of 600 to 1,000 mg of the leaves are considered toxic. Some sources consider a dose of lobeline sulfate above 20 mg daily to be toxic. Others warn that a 4-g dose may be fatal.

ADVERSE REACTIONS
CNS: anxiety, dizziness, headache, paresthesia, *seizures.*
CV: increased heart rate or ***bradycardia,*** hypertension or hypotension.
GI: dry mouth, mouth irritation, abdominal pain, diarrhea, nausea, vomiting.
GU: burning of the urinary tract.
Respiratory: cough, tickling or choking sensation, ***paralysis of the respiratory center*** (with overdose).
Skin: diaphoresis, contact dermatitis.
Other: chills.

INTERACTIONS
Herb-drug. *Disulfiram, metronidazole:* May cause a disulfiram-like reaction if herbal preparation contains alcohol. Advise patient to avoid use together.
GI or respiratory irritants, nicotine products: May cause additive toxicity. Advise patient to avoid use together.
Herb-lifestyle. *Smoking:* May increase nicotine effects. Advise patient to avoid smoking while using the herb.

EFFECTS ON LAB TEST RESULTS
None reported.

Bold italic type indicates that reaction may be life-threatening.

CAUTIONS
Patients with heart disease or sensitivity to tobacco or lobelia should avoid using this herb. Women who are pregnant or breast-feeding should also avoid it.

NURSING CONSIDERATIONS
• Explore patient's knowledge of this herb.
• Tinctures and extracts contain 15% to 60% alcohol and may be unsuitable for children, patients with a history of alcoholism or liver disease, or patients taking certain drugs.
• Several studies of lobeline, the active ingredient in lobelia, for smoking cessation have found little evidence to support its efficacy.
• Lobelia shouldn't be used for more than 6 weeks.
• Antacids may decrease the adverse GI effects of lobelia.
• Monitor patient's blood pressure, heart rate, and respirations.

PATIENT TEACHING
• Advise patient to consult a health care provider before using an herbal preparation because another treatment may be available.
• Tell patient that when filling a new prescription he should inform pharmacist of any herbal or dietary supplement he's taking.
• If patient has a history of alcoholism or liver disease, inform him that some herbal products contain alcohol.
• Warn patient not to use lobelia for more than 6 weeks.
• Tell patient not to take lobelia while smoking or chewing tobacco. Offer other smoking-cessation options.

• Inform patient that antacids may decrease adverse GI effects.
• Warn patient to keep all herbal products away from children and pets.

lovage

Aetheroleum levistici, Angelica levisticum, Hipposelinum levisticum, Levisticum officinale, L. radix, lavose, maggi plant, sea parsley, smellage

Common trade names
None known

AVAILABLE FORMS
Available as a tea.

ACTIONS & COMPONENTS
Obtained from roots and seeds of *L. officinale* and *L. radix.* The root contains several compounds that contribute to its aromatic odor and flavor, including butylidenephthalide, butylthalide, and ligustilide; coumarins; terpenoids; and volatile acids, such as caffeic and benzoic acids. Other compounds include camphene, bergapten, and psoralen. Lovage exerts weak diuretic, spasmolytic, and sedative effects; it also stimulates salivation and gastric secretion.

USES
Used for its diuretic properties in treating pedal edema. In Germany, it's approved for irrigation in urinary tract inflammation and for renal calculus prophylaxis. Also used as a spasmolytic, a sedative, a mucolytic, a carminative (to relieve gastric discomfort and flatulence),

*Liquid contains alcohol.

and a remedy for menstrual complaints.

DOSAGE & ADMINISTRATION
Tea: Prepared by pouring 1 cup boiling water over 1.5 to 3 g of finely cut root and draining after 15 minutes. Dosage is 4 to 8 g P.O. daily, taken between meals.

ADVERSE REACTIONS
Skin: photosensitivity reaction, dermatitis.

INTERACTIONS
Herb-drug. *Warfarin and other anticoagulants:* May cause potentiated effects. Advise patient to avoid use together.
Herb-lifestyle. *Sun exposure:* May cause photosensitivity. Advise patient to wear protective clothing and sunscreen outdoors and to limit exposure to direct sunlight.

EFFECTS ON LAB TEST RESULTS
• May increase PT and INR.

CAUTIONS
Patients with acute renal inflammation or dysfunction shouldn't use this herb, nor should pregnant or breast-feeding women.

NURSING CONSIDERATIONS
• Explore patient's knowledge of this herb.
• Patients with a history of photosensitivity reactions and those with plant allergies should use caution when using the herb.
• Monitor electrolyte, BUN, and creatinine levels periodically while patient is taking the herb.
• Make sure patient drinks plenty of fluids.

• Monitor patient for prolonged INR and PT if he also takes an anticoagulant.

PATIENT TEACHING
• Advise patient to consult a health care provider before using an herbal preparation because another treatment may be available.
• Tell patient that when filling a new prescription he should inform pharmacist of any herbal or dietary supplement he's taking.
• If patient takes lovage for swollen feet, recommend a complete medical evaluation by a health care provider. Explain that swollen feet may indicate a serious underlying cardiovascular or kidney disorder that needs medical treatment.
• Discuss other proven diuretics currently available.
• Tell patient to notify health care provider about any skin changes or photosensitivity reactions. Emphasize need to avoid prolonged exposure to sunlight while using the herb.
• Warn patient to keep all herbal products away from children and pets.

lungwort

Pulmonaria officinalis,
Jerusalem cowslip, lung moss, sage of Jerusalem, spotted comfrey

Common trade names
Lungwort Compound

AVAILABLE FORMS
Available as tablets, syrup, juice, drops, and extracts.

Bold italic type indicates that reaction may be life-threatening.

ACTIONS & COMPONENTS
Lungwort leaves contain allantoin, which may contribute to its emollient action. Tannins and flavonoids in the plant may exert astringent and anti-inflammatory action, and mucilage may act as an antitussive. Other components include ascorbic acid, saponins, potassium and iron salts, and salicylic acid.

USES
Used as an antitussive, expectorant, and anti-irritant in bronchitis, cough, influenza, and tuberculosis. Also used for its astringent properties in treating diarrhea, hemorrhoids, GI ulceration, kidney and urinary tract conditions, and excessive menstrual flow. Used topically to encourage wound healing.

DOSAGE & ADMINISTRATION
Infusion: 1.5 g of finely cut dried herb placed in cold water and brought to a rapid boil, or herb steeped in boiling water for 5 to 10 minutes, then taken t.i.d.
Tincture: 1 to 4 ml P.O. t.i.d.

ADVERSE REACTIONS
GI: nausea.
Hematologic: prolonged bleeding time.
Skin: contact dermatitis.

INTERACTIONS
Herb-drug. *Warfarin and other anticoagulants:* May potentiate effects. Advise patient to avoid use together.

EFFECTS ON LAB TEST RESULTS
• May increase PT and INR.

CAUTIONS
Patients who have a history of contact allergies, who take an anticoagulant, or who are pregnant or breast-feeding shouldn't use this herb.

NURSING CONSIDERATIONS
• Explore patient's knowledge of this herb.
• Monitor patient's INR and PT, as needed, because herb may prolong bleeding time.
• Monitor patient for occult blood.

PATIENT TEACHING
• Advise patient to consult a health care provider before using an herbal preparation because another treatment may be available.
• Tell patient that when filling a new prescription he should inform pharmacist of any herbal or dietary supplement he's taking.
• If patient has a respiratory disorder, tell him to discuss conventional medical treatments with a health care provider before using the herb.
• Inform patient that insufficient data exist to support therapeutic use of this herb.
• Tell patient to notify a health care provider about signs and symptoms of increased bleeding time, such as bruising, bleeding gums, or dark stools.
• Warn patient to keep all herbal products away from children and pets.

---

*Liquid contains alcohol.

madder

Rubia tinctorum, Dyer's madder, madder root, robbia

Common trade names
Madder Whole Root

AVAILABLE FORMS
Available as dried root, extract, and capsules.

ACTIONS & COMPONENTS
Contains 2% to 4% anthraquinone derivatives and glycosides. Principal components are ruberythric acid, alizarin, pseudopurpurin, rubiadin, lucidin, and lucidin 3-O-primeveroside. Mechanism of action stems from the Ca^{2+} chelating properties of anthraquinones. Herb may also be mutagenic and carcinogenic because of the lucidin component.

USES
Used as an antispasmodic, a diuretic, and a prophylactic and as treatment for kidney stones. Also added to foods as a colorant.

DOSAGE & ADMINISTRATION
Capsules: 1 capsule P.O. t.i.d. for up to 2 months.
Extract: 20 gtt P.O. t.i.d. for up to 2 months.
Infusion: 1 to 2 g P.O. q.i.d. for up to 2 months.

ADVERSE REACTIONS
Skin: contact dermatitis.

Other: *cancer,* red discoloration of perspiration, saliva, tears, urine, and bones.

INTERACTIONS
None known.

EFFECTS ON LAB TEST RESULTS
None reported.

CAUTIONS
Because of the risk of toxicity, no one should take madder. Patients who do take it should do so only under the supervision of a knowledgeable health care provider. Pregnant and breast-feeding patients shouldn't use the herb because it may have mutagenic and carcinogenic effects. Patients sensitive to madder should avoid it as well.

NURSING CONSIDERATIONS
• Explore patient's knowledge of this herb.

PATIENT TEACHING
• Warn patient about madder's potential mutagenic and carcinogenic effects.
• If patient suspects or knows he has kidney stones, tell him to discuss conventional treatments with his health care provider before using this herb.
• Advise pregnant and breast-feeding patients and women of childbearing age to avoid using this herb.
• Advise patient to notify her health care provider before continuing to use the herb if she suspects

---

or knows that she's pregnant or if she plans to become pregnant.

• Inform patient that madder may discolor body fluids, bone, and items he touches, such as contact lenses.

• Warn patient to keep all herbal products away from children and pets.

male fern

Dryopteris filix-mas, bear's paw root, knotty brake, male shield fern, marginal fern, sweet brake, wurmfarn

Common trade names
Aspidium Oleoresin, Bontanifuge, Extractum Filicis, Extractum Filicis Aethereum, Extractum Filicis Maris Tenue, Male Fern Oleoresin, Paraway Plus

AVAILABLE FORMS
Available as extract (1.5% to 22% filicin), draught (4 g of male fern extract), and capsules.

ACTIONS & COMPONENTS
Filicic and flavaspidic acids are the main active components responsible for herb's anthelmintic properties. Other components include volatile oils, tannin, paraspidin, and desaspidin. Desaspidin and aspidin may have antitumorigenic activity.

USES
Long used as an anthelmintic against pork tapeworm *(Taenia solium),* beef tapeworm *(T. saginata),* and fish tapeworm *(Diphyllobothrium latum).* Also applied topically for muscle pain, arthritis, sciatica, neuralgia, earache, and toothache.

DOSAGE & ADMINISTRATION
Draught: 50 ml given by duodenal tube. Treatment may be repeated in 7 to 10 days, p.r.n.
Extract: For adults, 3 to 6 ml P.O. after fasting. For children older than age 4, 0.25 to 0.5 ml P.O. per year of age. Maximum, 4 ml P.O. in divided doses.

ADVERSE REACTIONS
CNS: headache, *seizures,* queasiness, psychosis, paralysis, *coma.*
CV: *heart failure.*
EENT: optic neuritis, permanent visual disorders.
GI: severe abdominal cramps or pain, diarrhea, nausea, vomiting.
Hepatic: *hepatotoxicity,* jaundice.
Respiratory: dyspnea, *respiratory failure.*

INTERACTIONS
Herb-drug. *Antacids, H_2-blockers (such as famotidine and ranitidine), proton pump inhibitors (including lansoprazole and omeprazole), other alkalinizing drugs:* Inactivates the acid components of the herb due to the alkaline pH. Instruct patient to separate administration times by at least 2 hours.
Drugs that increase liver enzyme levels, such as 3-hydroxy-3-methyl-glutaryl-coenzyme A (HMG-CoA) reductase inhibitors (atorvastatin, simvastatin): Increases risk of hepatocellular damage. Advise patient to avoid using the herb and drug together.
Herb-food. *Fats and oils, including castor oil:* Increases absorption

---

*Liquid contains alcohol.

and risk of toxicity. Advise patient to avoid using the two together.
Herb-lifestyle. *Alcohol use:* Increases absorption and risk of toxicity. Advise patient to avoid using the herb and alcohol together.

EFFECTS ON LAB TEST RESULTS
• May alter liver enzyme levels, including increasing the bilirubin level.
• May cause albuminuria.

CAUTIONS
Pregnant women shouldn't use this herb because it may stimulate uterine muscle. Breast-feeding patients, infants and children younger than age 4, geriatric patients, and debilitated patients should also avoid use, as should patients who are sensitive to herb or its components or who have anemia, GI ulceration, CV disease, diabetes, or hepatic or renal failure.

NURSING CONSIDERATIONS
ALERT: Male fern is toxic. Ingestion isn't recommended. Poisoning or overdose may cause optic neuritis, blindness, seizures, psychosis, paralysis, respiratory or cardiac failure, coma, or death—and thus requires emergency medical care. Poisoning should be treated with activated charcoal; fatty and oily cathartics should be avoided. Patient may need a benzodiazepine to control seizures along with respiratory and cardiac support. Vision should be tested during and after exposure.
• Explore patient's knowledge of this herb.

• The draught form is considered a more effective anthelmintic than the capsule form.
• Monitor patient's liver enzyme levels and renal function.
• If patient develops vomiting and diarrhea, monitor his fluid intake and electrolyte loss.

PATIENT TEACHING
• Inform patient that toxic effects can occur with normal doses.
• Advise patient that conventional anthelmintics are safer than male fern.
• If patient suspects he has a tapeworm, advise him not to treat the condition with male fern before seeking medical evaluation.
• If patient has persistent abdominal pain or yellowing of the skin and eyes, advise him to seek medical evaluation right away.
• If patient is pregnant or breast-feeding or has anemia, a GI condition, or a heart, liver, or kidney problem, advise her not to use this herb.
• Warn patient to keep all herbal products away from children and pets.

mallow

Malva sylvestris, blue mallow, cheeseflower, high mallow, mallow flower (*Malvae flos*), mallow leaf (*Malvae folium*), mauls

Common trade names
Malvedrin, Malveol

AVAILABLE FORMS
Available as an extract and as dried herb.

Bold italic type indicates that reaction may be life-threatening.

ACTIONS & COMPONENTS

Mallow contains glycosides, flavonoids, mucilage, anthocyanin, and tannins. The mucilage component, made up largely of glucuronic acid, galacturonic acid, rhamnose, and galactose, is responsible for emollient and demulcent action. Mallow may also act as an astringent and expectorant.

USES

Used as demulcent to treat oral and pharyngeal mucosal irritation, cough, hoarseness, bronchitis, laryngitis, and tonsillitis. Used topically as an emollient for skin irritation and swelling. Also used as a laxative, as a pain reliever for children who are teething and, when combined with yarrow, as a vaginal douche.

DOSAGE & ADMINISTRATION

Dried herb: 5 g daily.
Infusion: For mallow flower, 1.5 to 2 g of dried flower added to cold water, boiled, then strained after 10 minutes. For mallow leaf, 5 ounces of boiling water poured over 3 to 5 g and steeped for 2 to 3 hours; stirred occasionally.

ADVERSE REACTIONS

Musculoskeletal: muscle tremors.

INTERACTIONS

None reported.

EFFECTS ON LAB TEST RESULTS

None reported.

CAUTIONS

Pregnant and breast-feeding patients shouldn't use this herb, nor should those who are sensitive to it.

NURSING CONSIDERATIONS

• Explore patient's knowledge of this herb.
⚠ **ALERT:** Don't confuse mallow with the herb marshmallow.
• Little data exist to support this herb's use or establish its safety.

PATIENT TEACHING

• Advise patient to consult a health care provider before using an herbal preparation because another treatment may be available.
• Tell patient that when filling a new prescription he should inform pharmacist of any herbal or dietary supplement he's taking.
• Advise patient to consult his health care provider if he develops a persistent cough or throat or mouth pain or irritation.
• Warn patient that little data exist to support this herb's use or establish its safety.
• Advise patient to notify her health care provider before continuing to use the herb if she suspects or knows that she's pregnant or if she plans to become pregnant.
• Warn patient to keep all herbal products away from children and pets.

---

*Liquid contains alcohol.

marigold

Calendula officinalis, garden marigold, goldbloom, golds, holligold, marybud, marygold, mary gowles, pot marigold, ruddes

Common trade names
Calendula Gel, Calendula Ointment, California Calendula Gel, Kneipp's Calendula Ointment

AVAILABLE FORMS
Available as ointment, cream, gel, shampoo, tincture*, tea, and mouthwash; obtained from powdered flowers, shoots, and leaves of *C. officinalis.*

ACTIONS & COMPONENTS
Contains lutein, volatile oils, flavonoids, carotenoid pigments, and sterols. Topical use of extract promotes wound healing. The herb has antibacterial, antifungal, antiviral, antimitotic, antimutagenic, antioxidant, cancerostatic, and immunostimulating properties. The extracts also have a systemic anti-inflammatory effect.

USES
Ointments are used for wounds, burns, chapped lips, dry nipples from breast-feeding, skin inflammation, furunculosis, eczema, acne, and varicose veins; tinctures or teas, for peptic ulcers, dysmenorrhea, and sore throat; and extracts, for cancer therapy and for immunostimulation in patients with viral or bacterial infection. Other reported uses include diuresis and treatment of fever, toothache, and eye inflammation.

Volatile oil is used in perfumes; plant pigments, in cosmetics.

DOSAGE & ADMINISTRATION
Ointment: 2 to 5 g powdered herb in 100 g ointment for external use.
Tea: 1 to 2 g per cup of water daily, ingested or used as a gargle.
Tincture: 1:9 with 20% alcohol-water mixture for external use.

ADVERSE REACTIONS
Other: allergic reaction.

INTERACTIONS
Herb-drug. *Disulfiram, metronidazole:* May cause a disulfiram-like reaction if herbal preparation contains alcohol. Advise patient to avoid using the herb and drug together.

EFFECTS ON LAB TEST RESULTS
None reported.

CAUTIONS
Patients who are pregnant or breast-feeding shouldn't use the herb, nor should patients who have a history of environmental allergies or are sensitive to the herb.

NURSING CONSIDERATIONS
• Explore patient's knowledge of this herb.
☑**ALERT:** Don't confuse marigold *(C. officinalis)* with African Inca, or French marigold *(Tagetes),* which is commonly used in gardens to repel insects.
• Tinctures and extracts typically contain between 15% to 60% alcohol and may be unsuitable for children, patients with a history of alcoholism or liver disease, or patients taking certain drugs.

Bold italic type indicates that reaction may be life-threatening.

PATIENT TEACHING
- Advise patient to consult a health care provider before using an herbal preparation because another treatment may be available.
- Tell patient that when filling a new prescription he should inform pharmacist of any herbal or dietary supplement he's taking.
- If patient has a history of alcoholism or liver disease, inform him that some herbal products contain alcohol.
- Warn patient about the risk of allergic reaction.
- If patient has a chronic illness, advise him not to put off seeking appropriate medical evaluation, because doing so can delay diagnosis of a potentially serious medical condition.
- Advise patient to notify her health care provider before continuing to use the herb if she suspects or knows that she's pregnant or if she plans to become pregnant.
- Warn patient to keep all herbal products away from children and pets.

marjoram

Origanum marjorana, common marjoram, knotted marjoram, sweet marjoram, wild marjoram

Common trade names
Marjoram, Marjoram Essential Oil, Sweet Marjoram

AVAILABLE FORMS
Available as tea from dried leaves and flowers of *O. marjorana,* and as essential oil of marjoram (extracted by distillation).

ACTIONS & COMPONENTS
Marjoram contains thymol, carvacrol, tannins, flavonoids, hydroquinone, and phenolic glycosides. Extracts decrease response to acetylcholine, histamine, serotonin, and nicotine. Antiviral, bactericidal, antiseptic, and antifungal effects are attributed to thymol, carvacrol, and the essential oil.

USES
Used to treat headaches, depression, dizziness, insomnia, motion sickness, conjunctivitis, and GI complaints, such as gastritis, flatulence, and colic. Also used for symptomatic treatment of rhinitis and colds. Essential oil is used externally for musculoskeletal pain and aromatherapy.

DOSAGE & ADMINISTRATION
Essential oil: Apply externally, p.r.n.
Tea: 1 to 2 teaspoons of dried leaves in 1 cup water, daily to t.i.d.

ADVERSE REACTIONS
GI: nausea, vomiting, diarrhea.

INTERACTIONS
None reported.

EFFECTS ON LAB TEST RESULTS
None reported.

CAUTIONS
Patients who have had an allergic reaction to oregano or thyme shouldn't use this herb. Women who are pregnant or breast-feeding shouldn't use this herb in amounts larger than those used in cooking. The essential oil shouldn't be used for children.

*Liquid contains alcohol.

NURSING CONSIDERATIONS
• Explore patient's knowledge of this herb.
• There are no reported cases of toxicity. However, marjoram essential oils contain thymol, arbutin, and hydroquinone in low concentrations, which may be toxic during extended use.
• Safety in children hasn't been established for amounts greater than those used for cooking.
• Patient should avoid using the essential oil internally.

PATIENT TEACHING
• Advise patient to consult a health care provider before using an herbal preparation because another treatment may be available.
• Tell patient that when filling a new prescription he should inform pharmacist of any herbal or dietary supplement he's taking.
• Warn patient not to take herb for headaches, insomnia, or depression before seeking medical attention because doing so may delay diagnosis of a potentially serious medical condition.
• Advise patient to stop taking herb if he develops nausea, vomiting, or diarrhea. Tell him to notify his health care provider if these signs or symptoms last more than 2 to 3 days because they may indicate toxicity.
• Advise patient to avoid use of volatile oils. If he uses them anyway, tell him to keep them away from eyes.
• Counsel patient not to use more of the herb than is normally used for cooking.
• Discourage patient from using the herb for a prolonged period.

marshmallow

Athaea officinalis, althea, cheeses, mallards, Moorish mallow, mortification root, Schloss tea, sweet weed, white maoow, wymote

Common trade names
Marshmallow Root

AVAILABLE FORMS
Available as whole dried root, dried leaves or flowers, capsules, extracts, syrup, and tea.

ACTIONS & COMPONENTS
Contains mucilage, pectin, and starch. Herb has emollient, demulcent, anti-inflammatory, anticomplement, and urinary analgesic activity. Inhibits mucociliary activity and stimulates phagocytosis and immune activity.

USES
Used as a cough suppressant to alleviate irritation of oral and pharyngeal tissue. Also used to treat inflammation and burns and to relieve mild gastric inflammation, irritable bowel syndrome, diarrhea, and constipation.

DOSAGE & ADMINISTRATION
Leaf: 5 g P.O. daily.
Root: 6 g P.O. daily.
Syrup: 10 g in a single dose.
Tea: 10 to 15 g in 5 ounces of cold water, freshly prepared several times daily.

ADVERSE REACTIONS
Metabolic: *hypoglycemia.*

Bold italic type indicates that reaction may be life-threatening.

INTERACTIONS
Herb-drug. *Insulin, sulfonylureas:*
May enhance hypoglycemic activity. Advise patient to avoid using the herb and drug together, and monitor glucose level closely.
Other drugs: May delay absorption of other drugs. Advise patient to separate administration times by at least 2 hours.

EFFECTS ON LAB TEST RESULTS
• May decrease glucose level.

CAUTIONS
Patients who are pregnant or breast-feeding shouldn't use this herb, nor should those who are sensitive to it or its components.

NURSING CONSIDERATIONS
• Explore patient's knowledge of this herb.
• Diabetic patients should use herb cautiously and be monitored closely for hypoglycemia.

PATIENT TEACHING
• Advise patient to consult a health care provider before using an herbal preparation because another treatment may be available.
• Tell patient that when filling a new prescription he should inform pharmacist of any herbal or dietary supplement he's taking.
• Although no chemical interactions have been reported in clinical studies, advise patient that herb may interfere with therapeutic effects of conventional drugs.
• Advise pregnant and breast-feeding patients and women of childbearing age to avoid using this herb because information about its safety is lacking.

• Warn patient that little data exist to support this herb's use or establish its safety.
• If patient has diabetes, advise him to avoid using marshmallow. If he chooses to use it anyway, tell him to frequently monitor his glucose level.
• Advise patient to store herb away from light.
• Warn patient to keep all herbal products away from children and pets.

mayapple

Podophyllum peltatum, devil's apple, duck's foot, ground lemon, hog apple, Indian apple, mandrake, raccoon berry, umbrella plant, vegetable mercury, wild lemon

Common trade names
Condylox, Podocon-25, Podofilm, Podofin, Warix, Wartex

AVAILABLE FORMS
Available as dried roots and rhizomes, powder, tincture*, and resin extract*.
Concentrated tincture: 5% to 25% in alcohol or benzoin available by prescription for topical use
Resinous extract: 0.5% in alcohol available by prescription for topical use

ACTIONS & COMPONENTS
Contains podophyllic acid, picropodophyllin, alpha- and beta-peltatin, and podophyllotoxin. These components demonstrate antimitotic effects, thereby inhibiting tumor growth. Some components decrease mitochondrial cy-

*Liquid contains alcohol.

tochrome activity as well. Various anticarcinogenics contain a synthetic component of the plant (podophyllin). Dried root irritates colonic mucosa, acting as a purgative cathartic.

USES
Mayapple extracts are included in prescription keratolytics used to treat condyloma acuminatum, external and perianal warts, keratoses, laryngeal papilloma, and plantar warts. Some plant components are included in anticarcinogenics used to treat testicular, ovarian, and small-cell lung cancer.

Mayapple is used as a stimulant laxative, cathartic, purgative, counterirritant, and anthelmintic. It's also used to treat tinea capitis, rheumatoid arthritis, and amenorrhea. Topical tincture and extract are FDA approved for treating warts. Podophyllum is recommended by the Centers for Disease Control and Prevention as an alternative to cryotherapy for external warts.

DOSAGE & ADMINISTRATION
Dried root: 1.5 to 3 g P.O. daily.
Tincture (25% in benzoin): Applied to dry skin with dropper or applicator. A health care provider should apply the solution. To avoid toxicity, the treated area shouldn't exceed 4 square inches (25 cm²). Dried resin is removed with soap and water after 1 to 4 hours.
Topical solution (0.5%): Applied b.i.d. with cotton-tipped applicator to wart surface for 3 days and then discontinued for 4 days. Cycle may be repeated up to four times.

ADVERSE REACTIONS
CNS: mental status changes, *seizures,* stupor, dizziness, hallucinations, decreased reflexes, fever, peripheral neuropathy, *coma.*
CV: hypotension, tachycardia.
EENT: conjunctivitis, keratitis.
GI: nausea, vomiting, diarrhea, abdominal pain, paralytic ileus.
GU: *nephrotoxicity,* urine retention.
Hematologic: anemia, *leukopenia, thrombocytopenia, myelosuppression.*
Hepatic: *hepatotoxicity.*
Metabolic: hypokalemia.
Respiratory: shortness of breath, tachypnea.
Skin: hair loss, ulcerative skin lesion.

INTERACTIONS
Herb-drug. *Disulfiram, metronidazole:* May cause a disulfiram-like reaction if herbal preparation contains alcohol. Advise patient to avoid using the herb and drug together.

EFFECTS ON LAB TEST RESULTS
• May increase liver enzyme, BUN, and creatinine levels. May decrease potassium level.
• May decrease CBC.

CAUTIONS
Patients who are pregnant or breast-feeding shouldn't take this herb, nor should patients with diabetes mellitus, circulatory problems, inflamed surrounding tissue, open warts, or sensitivity to the herb.

Bold italic type indicates that reaction may be life-threatening.

NURSING CONSIDERATIONS
⚠️**ALERT:** This entire herb is considered toxic and should be used only under the supervision of a qualified health care provider. Only the ripe fruits are edible.
- Explore patient's knowledge of this herb.
- Tinctures and extracts typically contain between 15% and 60% alcohol and may be unsuitable for children, patients with a history of alcoholism or liver disease, or patients taking certain drugs.
- Patients shouldn't use the herb topically for areas larger than 4 square inches (25 cm^2) because of the risk of resorptive poisoning.
- Resin extracts are for external use only.
- Topical solutions should be washed off genital and perianal warts in 1 to 4 hours; meatal warts, in 1 to 2 hours.
- Patients should apply occlusive dressing or urea around treated area to avoid contact with healthy skin.

PATIENT TEACHING
- Advise patient to consult a health care provider before using an herbal preparation because another treatment may be available.
- Tell patient that when filling a new prescription he should inform pharmacist of any herbal or dietary supplement he's taking.
- If patient has a history of alcoholism or liver disease, inform him that some herbal products contain alcohol.
- Advise patient to report any irritation or increase in bleeding or bruising to his health care provider.

- Warn patient not to use mayapple near the eyes.
- Caution patient about ingesting large amounts of the dried root to avoid excess laxative effects or poisoning.
- Warn patient to keep all herbal products away from children and pets.

meadowsweet

Filipendula ulmaria, Spireaea ulmaria, bridewort, dolloff, dropwort, lady of the meadow, meadow queen, meadow-wort, meadsweet, meadwort, queen of the meadow

Common trade names
Arkocaps, Artival, Neutracalm, Rheuma-Tee, Rheumex

AVAILABLE FORMS
Available as dried flowers, stems, leaves, and roots; tablets, infusion, powder, liquid extract, and tincture*.
Tablets: 300 mg

ACTIONS & COMPONENTS
Meadowsweet contains flavonoids, salicylates, coumarins, tannins, methyl salicylate, mucilage, ascorbic acid, and carbohydrates. It displays analgesic, antipyretic, antiemetic, antiulcerative, antirheumatic, antiflatulent, laxative, sedative, diuretic, and antiinflammatory actions. A heparin complex found in the plant demonstrates in vitro fibrinolytic and anticoagulant properties. Extracts from the flower exhibit in vitro bactericidal activity against *Staphylococcus aureus, S. epider-*

*Liquid contains alcohol.

midis, Escherichia coli, Pseudo-monas aeruginosa, and *Proteus vulgaris.* Astringent properties have been attributed to the tannins in the plant. Extracts demonstrate antitumorigenic, sedative, and urinary antiseptic properties as well.

USES
Used as an analgesic and anti-inflammatory for conditions such as toothache, rheumatoid arthritis, headache, tendinitis, and sprains. Used for GI complaints such as gastritis, diarrhea, peptic ulcer, heartburn, and irritable bowel syndrome. Also used as a diuretic or astringent and to relieve cough, colds, and bronchitis.

DOSAGE & ADMINISTRATION
Dried flowers: 2.5 to 3.5 g P.O. daily.
Dried herb: 4 to 5 g P.O. daily.
Infusion: 3 to 6 g prepared with 100 ml boiling water, strained after 10 minutes, taken P.O. t.i.d., p.r.n.
Liquid extract (1:1 in 25% alcohol): 1.5 to 6 ml P.O. t.i.d.
Powder: ½ teaspoon in a small amount of water P.O. t.i.d.
Tincture (1:5 in 25% alcohol): 2 to 4 ml P.O. t.i.d.

ADVERSE REACTIONS
GI: nausea.
Respiratory: *bronchospasm.*

INTERACTIONS
Herb-drug. *Disulfiram, metronidazole:* May cause a disulfiram-like reaction if herbal preparation contains alcohol. Advise patient to avoid using the herb and drug together.

Salicylate, salicylate derivatives: May cause additive effects of salicylates. Advise patient to avoid using the herb and drug together.
Warfarin: May cause an additive effect. Advise patient to avoid using the herb and drug together.

EFFECTS ON LAB TEST RESULTS
None reported.

CAUTIONS
Patients who have a history of salicylate or sulfite sensitivity or who are undergoing warfarin or aspirin therapy (for example, for a cardiac condition) shouldn't use the herb, nor should patients who are pregnant or breast-feeding. The herb also shouldn't be used for children.

NURSING CONSIDERATIONS
● Explore patient's knowledge of this herb.
● Tinctures and extracts typically contain between 15% and 60% alcohol and may be unsuitable for children, patients with a history of alcoholism or liver disease, or patients taking certain drugs.
● If patient has asthma, advise him to use this herb cautiously.
▨ALERT: This product contains methyl salicylate, which is fatal in high doses.

PATIENT TEACHING
● Advise patient to consult a health care provider before using an herbal preparation because another treatment may be available.
● Tell patient that when filling a new prescription he should inform pharmacist of any herbal or dietary supplement he's taking.

Bold italic type indicates that reaction may be life-threatening.

- If patient has a history of alcoholism or liver disease, inform him that some herbal products contain alcohol.
- Although no chemical interactions have been reported in clinical studies, advise patient that herb may interfere with therapeutic effects of conventional drugs.
- If patient has a history of asthma or sensitivity to aspirin, advise him to avoid using the herb.

☑**ALERT:** Tell patient to stop using salicylates if using meadowsweet. The herb can cause salicylate poisoning.

- If patient has a chronic illness, advise him not to put off seeking medical evaluation, because doing so can delay diagnosis of a potentially serious medical condition.
- Advise patient to notify her health care provider before continuing to use the herb if she suspects or knows that she's pregnant or if she plans to become pregnant.

milk thistle

Silybum marianum, cardui mariae fructus, holy thistle, lady's thistle, Marian thistle, Mary thistle, silymarin, St. Mary thistle

Common trade names
Liver Formula with Milk Thistle, Milk Thistle Extract, Milk Thistle Phytosome, Milk Thistle Plus, Milk Thistle Power, Milk Thistle Super Complex, Silybin Phytosome, Silymarin Milk Thistle, Simply Milk Thistle, Thisilyn

AVAILABLE FORMS
Obtained from seeds of *S. marianum.* Available as capsules, soft gels, liquid, extract*, tincture*, and I.V. silbinin (I.V. form unavailable in the United States).
Capsules: 70 mg, 120 mg, 175 mg, 280 mg, 350 mg, 525 mg, 1,050 mg
Liquid caps: 75 mg, 150 mg
Liquid extract: 1:1, 1:2 (70% silymarin extract)
Softgels: 100 mg, 150 mg
Tablets: 50 mg, 500 mg
Tincture: 80 mg, 140 mg

ACTIONS & COMPONENTS
Contains silymarin, which consists of hepatoprotective flavonolignans, including silibinin (silybin), isosilibinin, silidyanin, and silychristin. Silymarin stabilizes liver cell membranes and acts as an antioxidant by scavenging free radicals. It also stimulates protein synthesis in the liver, promoting liver cell generation. Silymarin's antiinflammatory and immunomodulatory activity may add to its protective actions on the liver. Silibinin blocks toxin binding on liver cell membranes, reducing severe liver damage. It also reduces intracellular forms of prostate-specific antigen and inhibits cell growth via G_1 arrest in the cell cycle in hormone-refractory prostate cancer.

Milk thistle components reduce histamine release from basophils through membrane stabilization, inhibit T-lymphocyte activation, increase neutrophil motility, and alter polymorphonuclear leukocyte function. Silibinin administration decreases biliary cholesterol levels.

---

*Liquid contains alcohol.

Milk thistle reduces insulin resistance in patients with alcoholic cirrhosis.

USES
Used for dyspepsia, liver damage from chemicals, *Amanita* mushroom poisoning, supportive therapy for inflammatory liver disease and cirrhosis, loss of appetite, prostate disorders, and gallbladder and spleen disorders. It's also used as a liver protectant.

DOSAGE & ADMINISTRATION
Dried fruit or seed: 12 to 15 g P.O. daily.
Injection (not available in the United States) for Amanita phalloides *mushroom poisoning:* 20 to 50 mg/kg I.V. over 24 hours, divided into four doses infused over 2 hours each.
Oral: Doses of milk thistle extract vary from 70 to 1,050 mg of silibinin (70% silymarin extract) P.O. daily in divided doses.

ADVERSE REACTIONS
GI: nausea, vomiting, diarrhea.

INTERACTIONS
Herb-drug. *Aspirin:* May improve aspirin metabolism in patients with liver cirrhosis. Advise patient to consult his health care provider before using the herb.
Cisplatin: May prevent kidney damage by cisplatin. Advise patient to consult his health care provider before using the herb.
Disulfiram, metronidazole: May cause a disulfiram-like reaction if herbal preparation contains alcohol. Advise patient to avoid using the herb and drug together.

Hepatotoxic drugs: May prevent liver damage from butyrophenones, phenothiazines, phenytoin, acetaminophen, or halothane. Advise patient to consult his health care provider before using the herb.
Tacrine: Reduces adverse cholinergic effects from the herb. Advise patient to consult his health care provider before using the herb.

EFFECTS ON LAB TEST RESULTS
• May decrease liver enzyme and glucose levels.
• May increase clotting times.

CAUTIONS
Patients who are pregnant or breast-feeding and those who are sensitive to the herb shouldn't use it. Those with decompensated liver disease also should avoid use.

NURSING CONSIDERATIONS
• Explore patient's knowledge of this herb.
• Mild allergic reactions may occur, especially in those who are allergic to members of the Asteraceae family, including ragweed, chrysanthemums, marigolds, and daisies.
⚠ **ALERT:** Don't confuse milk thistle seeds or fruit with other parts of the plant or with blessed thistle *(Cnictus benedictus).*
• Silymarin has poor water solubility; therefore, efficacy when prepared as a tea is questionable.

PATIENT TEACHING
• Advise patient to consult a health care provider before using an

---

Bold italic type indicates that reaction may be life-threatening.

herbal preparation because another treatment may be available.

• Tell patient that when filling a new prescription he should inform pharmacist of any herbal or dietary supplement he's taking.

• Although no chemical interactions have been reported in clinical studies, advise patient that herb may interfere with therapeutic effects of conventional drugs.

• If patient is pregnant or breast-feeding, advise her to avoid using this herb.

• Tell patient to stay alert for possible allergic reactions, especially if he's allergic to ragweed, chrysanthemums, marigolds, or daisies.

• Tell patient to report signs or symptoms of low glucose levels.

• Warn patient to stop taking the herb and notify his health care provider if he notices easy bruising or bleeding from gums, which may be signs of overdose.

• Warn patient not to take herb for liver inflammation or cirrhosis before seeking medical evaluation, because doing so may delay diagnosis of a potentially serious medical condition.

• Tell patient to keep the herb at room temperature, away from heat and moisture.

• Warn patient to keep all herbal products away from children and pets.

mistletoe

Phoradendron serotinum, Viscum album, all-heal, American mistletoe, birdlime, devil's fuge, European mistletoe, mistelkraut, mystyldene, visci

Common trade names
Helixor, Iscador, Plenosol

AVAILABLE FORMS
Available as dried leaves, stems, flowers, and fruit; extract* and injectable form (I.V. form unavailable in the United States) are obtained from American mistletoe (*Phoradendron* sp.) and European mistletoe (*Viscum* sp.).

ACTIONS & COMPONENTS
Phoratoxins and viscotoxins are toxic proteins isolated from American and European mistletoe, respectively. Phoratoxins from American mistletoe can cause hypertension, hypotension, bradycardia, and increased uterine and intestinal motility. Phoratoxins may also cause depolarization of skeletal muscle, smooth-muscle contraction, vasoconstriction, and cardiac arrest. Lectins and viscotoxins from European mistletoe may have anticarcinogenic and immunostimulation activity. Other effects include hypotension, bradycardia, and sedation. As an immunomodulator, *V. album* may stimulate DNA repair through lymphokines and cytokines in cancer patients. A lectin from mistletoe extract increases secretion of tumor necrosis factor (TNF), interleukin-1, interleukin-6, and TNF-alpha.

*Liquid contains alcohol.

USES

American mistletoe is used as a smooth-muscle stimulant for increasing blood pressure and uterine and intestinal contractions. European mistletoe is used to treat hypertension, cancer, internal bleeding, major blood loss, arteriosclerosis, epilepsy, gout, and hysteria; it's also used to purify the blood.

DOSAGE & ADMINISTRATION

Not well documented.

ADVERSE REACTIONS

CNS: delirium, hallucinations.
CV: *bradycardia,* hypertension, vasoconstriction, *cardiac arrest.*
EENT: double vision.
GI: nausea, vomiting, diarrhea, acute gastroenteritis.
Hepatic: *hepatitis.*
Skin: infiltration after S.C. injection.

INTERACTIONS

Herb-drug. *Anticoagulants, coagulants:* May alter drug efficacy from European mistletoe. Advise patient to avoid using the herb and drug together.
Antidepressants: May interfere with drug therapy from European mistletoe. Advise patient to avoid using the herb and drug together.
Antihypertensives: May decrease blood pressure from European mistletoe. Monitor blood pressure frequently.
Immunosuppressants: May interfere with drug therapy. Advise patient to avoid using the herb and drug together.

EFFECTS ON LAB TEST RESULTS

- May increase liver enzyme levels. May alter electrolyte levels.
- May increase clotting times.

CAUTIONS

All components of mistletoe, including berries, are considered toxic. Because mistletoe contains tyramine, which stimulates the uterus, neither pregnant nor breastfeeding patients should use it.

NURSING CONSIDERATIONS

- Explore patient's knowledge of this herb.
- ☑ALERT: Signs and symptoms of toxicity include nausea, bradycardia, gastroenteritis, hypertension, delirium, and hallucinations. Diarrhea and vomiting can lead to serious dehydration, hypovolemic shock, and CV collapse. Monitor blood pressure and heart rate closely. If patient ingested any berries, perform gastric lavage. Adverse effects seem to be dose related.
- Teach patient to monitor his blood pressure, pulse, and respirations daily, and instruct him to report trends to his health care provider.
- The pharmacologic effects of mistletoe vary depending on the type. Ask the patient whether he's taking American mistletoe or European mistletoe.

PATIENT TEACHING

☑ALERT: Inform patient that the FDA has forbidden marketing this herb as a food additive until proven safe, and has seized or barred the sale of commercial products

---

Bold italic type indicates that reaction may be life-threatening.

known to contain it. Tell him that mistletoe is a highly toxic herb.
• If patient has chosen to take the herb, tell him to notify his health care provider if he experiences any adverse reactions, especially chest pain or tightness, nausea, vomiting, diarrhea, hallucinations, double vision, or slowed heart rate.
• Warn patient to keep all herbal products away from children and pets.

monascus

red rice yeast, red yeast, xuezhikang, zhitai

Common trade names
Cholester-Reg, CholesteSure, Cholestin, Ruby Monascus

AVAILABLE FORMS
Obtained from a yeast, *Monascus purpureus,* grown on cooked, nonglutinous rice. Available as capsules and extract.
Capsules: 500 mg, 600 mg (0.4% or 2.4 mg of 3-hydroxy-3-methyl-glutaryl-coenzyme A [HMG-CoA] reductase inhibitors)
Ethanol extract: 1.1% HMG-CoA reductase inhibitors

ACTIONS & COMPONENTS
Yeast contains HMG-CoA reductase inhibitors, primarily lovastatin (or monacolin K). Lovastatin is available as a prescription cholesterol-lowering drug. Monacolin K is converted in the body to mevinolinic acid, which competitively binds to HMG-CoA reductase in place of the endogenous substance, HMG-CoA, thus inhibiting cholesterol formation.

USES
Used to reduce total cholesterol, low-density-lipoprotein cholesterol, and triglyceride levels; to increase high-density-lipoprotein levels in patients with hypercholesterolemia; and to sustain desirable cholesterol levels in healthy people. Also used to treat indigestion and diarrhea, to improve blood circulation, and to promote stomach and spleen health.

DOSAGE & ADMINISTRATION
Hypercholesterolemia: 1,200 mg (7.2 mg of lovastatin, 9.6 mg of HMG Co-A reductase inhibitors) P.O. b.i.d. with food. One manufacturer recommends 600 mg daily and another recommends 1,000 mg daily.

ADVERSE REACTIONS
GI: gastritis, abdominal discomfort.
GU: *nephrotoxicity.*
Musculoskeletal: *rhabdomyolysis,* muscle pain, tenderness, weakness.

INTERACTIONS
Herb-drug. *Cholesterol-lowering drugs, including gemfibrozil and niacin:* May increase risk of adverse reactions. To determine whether combination therapy is more effective, monitor patient closely.
Cytochrome P-450-3A inhibitors, such as fluconazole, itraconazole, ketoconazole, and theophylline: May increase blood levels and adverse reactions from the herb. Monitor patient for adverse reactions and efficacy.
HMG-CoA reductase inhibitors: May increase risk of adverse reac-

*Liquid contains alcohol.

tions without added benefit. Advise patient to avoid using the herb and drug together.

Levothyroxine: Rarely, may alter thyroid function. Monitor thyroid function test results.

Herb-food. *Grapefruit juice:* Increases bioavailability of lovastatin, increasing the risk of adverse reactions. Monitor patient closely for adverse reactions.

Herb-lifestyle. *Alcohol use:* May increase risk of liver toxicity. Advise patient to avoid using the herb and alcohol together.

EFFECTS ON LAB TEST RESULTS
• May increase liver enzyme, BUN, creatinine, and CK levels. May decrease cholesterol and triglyceride levels. May alter electrolyte levels.
• May alter thyroid function test results.

CAUTIONS
Patients at risk for liver disease, with active liver disease, or with a history of liver disease shouldn't take monascus. Pregnant patients should avoid use because cholesterol is important for fetal development; patients who are breast-feeding also should avoid use.

The makers of the Cholestin brand warn patients not to take the product if they consume more than two alcoholic drinks per day; have a serious infection, serious disease, or physical disorder; or have undergone an organ transplant or a recent major surgery.

Patients younger than age 18 should use the herb cautiously because safety hasn't been established.

NURSING CONSIDERATIONS
• Explore patient's knowledge of this herb.
• Monitor lipid panel for treatment efficacy and liver function test results for liver toxicity at regular intervals.
• If patient develops muscle pain or weakness, check creatine kinase levels to test for rhabdomyolysis.
• Review patient's current drug regimen. Many drugs, especially cytochrome P-450-3A inhibitors, can interact with the herb.

PATIENT TEACHING
• Advise patient to consult a health care provider before using an herbal preparation because another treatment may be available.
• Tell patient that when filling a new prescription he should inform pharmacist of any herbal or dietary supplement he's taking.
• Advise patient that the herb should be taken with food.
• If patient has liver disease, warn him not to use the herb.
• Recommend that patient abstain from alcohol or limit its use.
• Advise pregnant and breast-feeding patients to avoid using this herb.
• Urge patient to seek medical attention if he experiences brown urine, muscle pain, or weakness.
• Teach patient the importance of having regular laboratory tests to monitor for efficacy and toxicity.
• Warn patient to keep all herbal products away from children and pets.

Bold italic type indicates that reaction may be life-threatening.

morinda

Morinda citrifolia, ba ji tian, hog apple, Indian mulberry, mengkudu, mora de la India, noni, pain killer, ruibarbo caribe, wild pine

Common trade names
Morinda, Morinda Citrifolia Capsules, Noni, Noni Nectar, Noni Juice, Tahitian Noni Juice

AVAILABLE FORMS
Obtained from the root of *M. citrifolia;* leaves, fruit, and juice also are used. Available in many forms, including fruit leather, capsules, tincture*, oil, fiber, and combination foods, such as protein wafers, juices, and nutritional supplements.

ACTIONS & COMPONENTS
Aboveground portions contain essential oils with hexoic and octoic acids, paraffin and esters of methyl, and ethyl alcohols. Root contains anthraquinones, alizarin, morindone, xeronine, and damnacanthal. Xeronine, a digestive enzyme, may be responsible for herb's ability to repair damaged cells in digestive, respiratory, and skeletal systems, possibly by affecting shape of protein molecules and by enhancing immune function.

Damnacanthal exerts antitumorigenic activity by inhibiting the reticular activating system oncogene, a protein partially responsible for cell proliferation. Alcoholic extracts have anthelmintic and central analgesic activity. Tannins contained in morinda may have hypoglycemic properties.

USES
Used to treat diabetes, high blood pressure, GI and liver conditions, chronic fatigue syndrome, premenstrual syndrome, and ankylosing spondylitis. Used topically for soothing headaches and arthritic joints by wrapping leaves around affected areas. Also used for its sedative, immunostimulant, anticarcinogenic, and anthelmintic effects.

DOSAGE & ADMINISTRATION
Dosage can range from 3 to 6 g daily in two divided doses P.O. on an empty stomach.
Compress: Dried leaves steeped in hot water and applied on chest and stomach for fever and stomachache.
Tea: Prepared by adding 5 to 9 g herb to 3 to 4 cups of water, boiling until volume is reduced by half, and cooling. Taken in two divided doses on empty stomach.
Tincture: 30 to 60 g steeped in 1 L of ethanol for 2 to 3 months. 30 ml taken P.O. b.i.d. on empty stomach in afternoon and h.s.

ADVERSE REACTIONS
CNS: sedation.
GU: discoloration of urine.
Metabolic: *hyperkalemia in patients with chronic renal failure.*

INTERACTIONS
Herb-drug. *ACE inhibitors, angiotensin II receptor antagonists, beta blockers, potassium-sparing diuretics, trimethoprim-sulfamethoxazole:* Causes additive effect of hyperkalemia. Monitor patient closely for increased potassium level.

* Liquid contains alcohol.

Disulfiram, metronidazole: May cause a disulfiram-like reaction if herbal preparation contains alcohol. Advise patient to avoid using the herb and drug together.
Immunosuppressants: May counteract drug effect. Advise patient to avoid using the herb and drug together.

EFFECTS ON LAB TEST RESULTS
• May increase potassium level. May decrease glucose level.

CAUTIONS
Patients who are pregnant or breast-feeding shouldn't use the herb, nor should patients with end-stage renal disease (noni juice form contains potassium) or those sensitive to the herb. Organ transplant recipients also should avoid use because of the increased risk of rejection, resulting from the herb's immune system–enhancing properties.

NURSING CONSIDERATIONS
• Explore patient's knowledge of this herb.
• Morinda shouldn't replace conventional therapies that are known to be effective in treating different cancers and CV and endocrine disorders.
• Tinctures and extracts typically contain between 15% and 60% alcohol and may be unsuitable for children, patients with a history of alcoholism or liver disease, or patients taking certain drugs.
• Carefully monitor patient for adverse reactions.

PATIENT TEACHING
• Advise patient to consult a health care provider before using an herbal preparation because another treatment may be available.
• Tell patient that when filling a new prescription he should inform pharmacist of any herbal or dietary supplement he's taking.
• If patient has a history of alcoholism or liver disease, inform him that some herbal products contain alcohol.
• Although no chemical interactions have been reported in clinical studies, advise patient that herb may interfere with therapeutic effects of conventional drugs.
• If patient has a chronic illness, advise him not to put off seeking medical evaluation, because doing so can delay diagnosis of a potentially serious medical condition.
• Inform patient that the anthraquinone component of the herb may turn urine a pink or rust color.
• Instruct patient to take herb on an empty stomach so intestines can activate the enzyme.
• Advise patient to use caution when performing activities that require mental alertness until he knows how the herb affects his CNS.
• If patient has kidney failure, caution him that noni juice is a source of potassium and that he shouldn't use it.
• Warn pregnant or breast-feeding patients to avoid using this herb.
• Warn patient to keep all herbal products away from children and pets.

Bold italic type indicates that reaction may be life-threatening.

motherwort

Leonurus cardiaca, heart heal, heartwort, lion's ear, lion's tail, mother herb, Roman motherwort, throw-wort

Common trade names
Motherwort Flowering Tops, Motherwort Flowers, Motherwort Herb—Organic Alcohol

AVAILABLE FORMS
Obtained from aboveground parts of *L. cardiaca*. Available as powdered herb, leaf and flowering tops, fluidextract*, solid extract, and alcohol extract*.

ACTIONS & COMPONENTS
Contains leocardin, ajugoside (leonuride), ajugol, galiridoside, reptoside and other components, including flavonoids, leonurin, betaine, caffeic acid derivative, tannins, and traces of volatile oil. Alkaloids responsible for major herb activity include stachydrine, betonicine, turicin, leonurine, leonuridin, and leonurinine. Herb has mild negative chronotropic properties, and hypotonic, cardiac-inhibitory, antispasmodic, and sedative actions. Leonurine may stimulate uterine tone and blood flow, and stachydrine may stimulate oxytocin release. Ursolic acid may have antiviral, antitumorigenic, and cytotoxic activity. "K substance," an extract of motherwort, may decrease blood viscosity by inhibiting platelet aggregation and cardiac function.

USES
Used to manage mild to moderate cardiac insufficiency (New York Heart Association classes I and II) and to improve reproductive health. Used to treat hyperthyroidism, arrhythmias such as tachycardia and other nervous cardiac conditions, flatulence, amenorrhea, itching, and shingles. Used topically to improve eyesight and as a generalized tonic and antiplatelet agent. Combined with other herbs to treat signs and symptoms of BPH. Also used as a uterine stimulant.

DOSAGE & ADMINISTRATION
Acute conditions: 5 gtt, 1 tablet, or 10 pellets P.O. every 30 to 60 minutes.
Dietary supplement: Fluidextract 1:1 (g/ml) 1 to 2 ml P.O. t.i.d. (extract contains 12% to 15% organic alcohol).
Dried above-ground parts: 2 g P.O. t.i.d.
Infusion for internal use: Average total daily dose, 4.5 g herb.
Long-term use: 5 gtt, 1 tablet, or 10 pellets P.O. daily to t.i.d.
Tea: Prepared by steeping 2 g dried aboveground part in 5 ounces boiling water for 5 to 10 minutes, then straining. 1 cup taken t.i.d.
Tincture: 1:5 (g/ml) 22.5 ml (tincture contains 56% to 62% grain alcohol).

ADVERSE REACTIONS
CNS: sedation.
GI: diarrhea, stomach irritation.
GU: uterine bleeding.
Skin: contact dermatitis, photosensitivity reaction.
Other: allergic reactions.

*Liquid contains alcohol.

INTERACTIONS

Herb-drug. *Antihistamines, CNS depressants:* May increase sedation. Monitor patient.

Cardiac glycosides: May cause additive effect and possible drug toxicity. Advise patient to use the herb only under the supervision of a health care provider.

Disulfiram, metronidazole: May cause a disulfiram-like reaction if herbal preparation contains alcohol. Advise patient to avoid using the herb and drug together.

Herb-herb. *Herbs containing cardiac glycosides, such as black hellebore, Canadian hemp roots, digitalis leaf, figwort, hedge mustard, lily-of-the-valley roots, oleander leaf, pheasant's-eye plant, pleurisy root, squill bulb leaf scales, strophanthus seeds, and uzara:* May cause additive effect and possible cardiac glycoside toxicity. Advise patient to use the herb only under the supervision of a health care provider.

Herb-lifestyle. *Alcohol use:* May potentiate sedative effect. Advise patient not to use the herb and alcohol together.

Sun exposure: May cause photosensitivity reaction. Advise patient to wear protective clothing and sunscreen and to limit exposure to direct sunlight.

EFFECTS ON LAB TEST RESULTS
- May alter cardiac enzyme levels.
- May increase clotting times. May alter thyroid function test results.

CAUTIONS
Pregnant patients shouldn't use the herb because of its uterine stimulant activity. Breast-feeding patients should avoid use because clinical and safety data are lacking.

Patients receiving treatment for cardiac dysfunction or arrhythmias should use herb only under the supervision of a health care provider.

NURSING CONSIDERATIONS
- Explore patient's knowledge of this herb.
- Because herb has sedative effects, monitor geriatric patients for excessive drowsiness, confusion, or falls.
- Monitor vital signs.
- Tinctures and extracts typically contain between 15% and 60% alcohol and may be unsuitable for children, patients with a history of alcoholism or liver disease, or patients taking certain drugs.

PATIENT TEACHING
- Advise patient to consult a health care provider before using an herbal preparation because another treatment may be available.
- Tell patient that when filling a new prescription he should inform pharmacist of any herbal or dietary supplement he's taking.
- Advise patient that motherwort has an unpleasant odor.
- Advise patient to notify her health care provider before continuing to use the herb if she suspects or knows that she's pregnant or if she plans to become pregnant. Also advise her not to take the herb if she breast-feeds.
- Tell patient that higher-than-recommended doses may cause diarrhea, stomach irritation, uterine bleeding, low blood pressure, or low pulse rate.

Bold italic type indicates that reaction may be life-threatening.

- Advise patient to avoid performing activities that require mental alertness until he knows how the drug affects his CNS.
- Warn patient to keep all herbal products away from children and pets.

mugwort

Artemisiae vulgaris radix,
Artemisia vulgaris, carline thistle, felon herb, hierba de San Juan, sailor's tobacco, St. John's plant

Common trade names
Mugwort

AVAILABLE FORMS
Obtained from leaves and roots of *A. vulgaris.* Available as leaves, tablets, fluidextract, and powder. Also used in food products such as pasta.
Mugwort tincture*: (1:5, 50% alcohol)

ACTIONS & COMPONENTS
Contains volatile oils (including 1,8-cineol, camphor, linalool, and thujone), sesquiterpene lactones, lipophilic flavonoids, polyenes, umbelliferone, aesculetin, and hydroxycoumarins. Aqueous extract and essential oil have antimicrobial activity. Thujone may be responsible for uterine stimulant and abortifacient activity.

USES
Used to treat many GI complaints, such as colic, diarrhea, constipation, cramps, weak digestion, and persistent vomiting. Also used as a laxative for obesity, as a therapeutic hand soak, and as a tonic for asthenia. Also used to treat worm infestations, epilepsy, poor circulation, sedation, and menstrual problems and to stimulate gastric juice and bile secretion. Used with other herbs to treat psychoneuroses, neurasthenia, depression, hypochondria, autonomic neuroses, general irritability, restlessness, insomnia, and anxiety states.

DOSAGE & ADMINISTRATION
Hand soak: 2 handfuls of dried mugwort steeped in 10 ounces of raw apple cider vinegar. Then, 1 to 2 tablespoons of this infusion added to warm water; hands are soaked for 10 minutes.
Tea: 0.5 to 2 g of the dried herb steeped in 8 ounces of boiling water and strained. 2 to 3 cups of tea are taken daily before meals.
Tincture: Dosages vary depending on formulation and reason for treatment.

ADVERSE REACTIONS
Skin: rarely sensitization through skin contact.
Other: *hypersensitivity reactions.*

INTERACTIONS
Herb-drug. *CNS depressants:* May increased sedative effect. Monitor patient.
Disulfiram, metronidazole: May cause a disulfiram-like reaction if herbal preparation contains alcohol. Advise patient to avoid using the herb and drug together.
Herb-lifestyle. *Alcohol use:* May potentiate sedative effect. Advise patient to avoid using the herb and alcohol together.

---

*Liquid contains alcohol.

EFFECTS ON LAB TEST RESULTS
None reported.

CAUTIONS
Patients who are pregnant or breast-feeding shouldn't use this herb because of its uterine stimulant properties.

Patients who are sensitive to members of the Asteraceae family (such as ragweed, chrysanthemums, marigolds, daisies, sage, and wormwood) or who are allergic to tobacco, honey, or royal jelly may have an allergic reaction to mugwort and, thus, should use the herb cautiously.

NURSING CONSIDERATIONS
• Explore patient's knowledge of this herb.
• Allergic immunoglobulin E–mediated reactions via histamine release may occur in patients with allergies to plants of the same family.
• Tinctures and extracts typically contain between 15% and 60% alcohol and may be unsuitable for children, patients with a history of alcoholism or liver disease, or patients taking certain drugs.

PATIENT TEACHING
• Advise patient to consult a health care provider before using an herbal preparation because another treatment may be available.
• Tell patient that when filling a new prescription he should inform pharmacist of any herbal or dietary supplement he's taking.
• Advise patient that mugwort root has a pleasant, tangy taste and that the belowground parts (root) are sweet and pungent.

• Caution patient that skin contact with the herb may lead to sensitization.
• If patient is allergic to herbs of the Asteraceae family, tobacco, honey, or royal jelly, warn of a possible hypersensitivity reaction to mugwort.
• Advise patient to notify her health care provider before continuing to use the herb if she suspects or knows that she's pregnant or if she plans to become pregnant. Also advise her not to take the herb if she breast-feeds.
• Warn patient to keep all herbal products away from children and pets.

mullein

Verbascum densiflorum, Aaron's rod, Adam's flannel, ag-leaf, ag-paper, American mullein, beggar's blanket, blanket herb, blanketleaf, bouillon blanc, candleflower, candlewick plant, clot-bur, clown's lungwort, cuddy's lungs, duffle, European mullein, feltwort, flannelflower, fluffweed, golden rod, hag's taper, hare's beard, hedgetaper, Jacob's staff, Jupiter's staff, longwort, orange mullein, Our Lady's flannel, rag paper, shepherd's club, shepherd's staff, torches, torch weed, velvet plant, verbasci flos, wild ice leaf, woollen

Common trade names
Alcohol-Free Mullein Leaves, Mullein Extract, Mullein Leaf, Mullein Tea

---

Bold italic type indicates that reaction may be life-threatening.

AVAILABLE FORMS

Obtained from dried flowers and leaves. Available as extracts*, dried herb, capsules, teas, and oil. Available in many tea preparations and in combination with other herbs.

Capsules: 330 mg dried leaf

Extracts in grain alcohol (70%): 250 mg dry leaves = 1 ml liquid extract

Oil: Fresh flowers in pure virgin oil

ACTIONS & COMPONENTS

Contains mucilage, triterpene saponins (including songarosaponin D, E, and F) iridoide monoterpenes, tannins, caffeic acid derivatives, flavonoids, and invert sugar. Tannins, saponins, and mucilage are responsible for herb's effects. Saponins have expectorant actions, mucin has antibiotic actions, and the combination alleviates irritation from colds. Demulcent properties may be useful for treating sore throats. Mullein extract may have activity against influenza types A and B and against herpes simplex virus type I.

USES

Used to treat respiratory tract inflammation, cough, sore throat, bronchitis, croup, asthma, and tuberculosis. Also used internally as a diuretic, antibiotic, sedative, narcotic, and antirheumatic. Used topically to treat hemorrhoids, burns, bruises, frostbite, and erysipelas. Oil is used to soothe earaches, and leaves are used to soften and protect the skin. Mullein is also used as a flavoring agent in alcoholic beverages.

DOSAGE & ADMINISTRATION

Capsules (330 mg): 2 or 3 capsules P.O. b.i.d. with meals.

Decoction: 1.5 to 2 g of herb placed in 5 to 8 ounces cold water and boiled for 10 minutes. Taken b.i.d.

Fluidextract: 1:1 (g/ml) 1.5 to 2 ml P.O. b.i.d. (contains 45% to 55% grain alcohol).

Mullein extract: 3 to 4 ml P.O. t.i.d. Use half this dose in children.

Mullein flower oil: 5 to 10 gtt of extract in a little water P.O. b.i.d. to t.i.d.

Mullein leaves liquid: 4 to 8 gtt in a little water P.O. b.i.d.; liquid is alcohol-free.

Tea: Prepared by pouring boiling water over 1.5 to 2 g (1 teaspoon = 0.5 g drug) finely cut petals, steeping for 10 to 15 minutes, then straining. 1 cup taken daily.

Tincture: 1:5 (g/ml) 7.5 to 10 ml P.O. b.i.d. May dilute in warm water.

ADVERSE REACTIONS

None reported.

INTERACTIONS

Herb-drug. *CNS depressants:* May potentiate sedative effect. Monitor patient.

Disulfiram, metronidazole: May cause a disulfiram-like reaction if herbal preparation contains alcohol. Advise patient to avoid using the herb and drug together.

Herb-lifestyle. *Alcohol use:* May potentiate sedative effect. Advise patient to avoid using the herb and alcohol together.

EFFECTS ON LAB TEST RESULTS

None reported.

*Liquid contains alcohol.

CAUTIONS
Patients who are pregnant or breast-feeding shouldn't use the herb, nor should those who are sensitive to it.

NURSING CONSIDERATIONS
• Explore patient's knowledge of this herb.
• Tinctures and extracts typically contain between 15% and 60% alcohol and may be unsuitable for children, patients with a history of alcoholism or liver disease, or patients taking certain drugs.

⚡ALERT: Don't confuse mullein with goldenrod (*Solidago* sp.), which is also known as Aaron's rod.

PATIENT TEACHING
• Advise patient to consult a health care provider before using an herbal preparation because another treatment may be available.
• Tell patient that when filling a new prescription he should inform pharmacist of any herbal or dietary supplement he's taking.
• Although no chemical interactions have been reported in clinical studies, advise patient that herb may interfere with therapeutic effects of conventional drugs.
• Tell patient to store herb in a cool, dry place protected from light. If herb comes into contact with light or moisture, it discolors to brown or dark brown.
• Advise patient to refrigerate mullein extract after opening it.
• Advise patient to notify her health care provider before continuing to use the herb if she suspects or knows that she's pregnant or if she plans to become pregnant.

Also advise her not to take the herb if she breast-feeds.
• Warn patient to keep all herbal products away from children and pets.

mustard

Synapis alba, black mustard, brown mustard, Chinese mustard, Indian mustard, mustard oil, white mustard, yellow mustard

Common trade names
Dr. Singha's Mustard Bath, Dr. Singha's Mustard Rub, Mustard, Essence of Mustard

AVAILABLE FORMS
Mustard preparations are extracted from the dried ripe seeds of *S. alba* or *Brassica alba* (white mustard) or *Brassica nigra* (black mustard) powder. Also available as essential oil of mustard and essence of mustard* (27% alcohol).

ACTIONS & COMPONENTS
The therapeutic action of mustard is achieved when the enzyme myrosin hydrolyzes the glucosinolates, and the active components are released, which occurs upon chewing or grinding the seeds and mixing them with warm water. Sinalbin is the glucosinolate found in white mustard; sinigrin, in black or brown mustard. Sinalbin is hydrolyzed to p-hydroxybenzyl isothiocyanate or *p*-hydroxybenzylamine, whereas sinigrin is hydrolyzed to allyl isothiocyanate. These substances, which are the active components responsible for the characteristic pungent odor, are po-

tent skin irritants and bacteriostatics, and may possess anticarcinogenic properties. Mustard also contains fatty oil, proteins, and phenylpropane derivatives. Mustard acts as a counterirritant when diluted to a 1:50 ratio. Mustard oil is absorbed through the skin and eliminated through the lungs.

USES

Mustard has been used for upper respiratory tract conditions including the common cold, cough, bronchitis, sinusitis, fevers and colds, and inflammation of the mouth and pharynx. It's also used in a poultice for catarrhs of the respiratory tract, hyperemization of the skin, and chronic degenerative disorders.

Black mustard oil or mustard seed is used topically for pulmonary congestion, rheumatism, and arthritis; as a counterirritant; and in baths for soothing aching feet and paralytic conditions. Black mustard oil is used as a flavoring agent in foods and drinks, a lubricant and illuminant in soaps, and in cat and dog repellents. Mustard seed, a culinary spice, is also a flavoring agent in many foods, including condiments and beverages.

White mustard is used to clear the voice and for those with a tendency for infection.

DOSAGE & ADMINISTRATION

Average daily doses of mustard range from 60 to 240 g.
For external use: 50 to 70 g (4 tablespoons) of powdered seeds are mixed with warm water, wrapped in gauze, and applied to affected area for 10 to 15 minutes for adults and 5 to 10 minutes for children older than age 6.
For tired, aching feet: 20 to 30 g of mustard flour is mixed with 1 quart (1 L) of water for a footbath.
Mustard plaster: For adults, 100 g of black mustard flour (ground mustard) is mixed with warm water to form a paste. The paste is packed in linen, applied to the affected area, and left in place for 10 to 15 minutes.
To clear the voice: Mustard flour is mixed with honey, and then formed into balls. 1 or 2 balls are taken P.O. on an empty stomach daily.
To soothe paralytic signs and symptoms: 150 g of mustard flour is placed in a pouch and dropped into bath water.

ADVERSE REACTIONS

CNS: nerve damage, *coma,* somnolence.
CV: *heart failure.*
GI: vomiting, diarrhea, stomach pain.
Respiratory: coughing or sneezing (with mustard flour), breathing difficulties.
Skin: blistering, urticaria, ulceration, necrosis.
Other: goiter, allergic reaction, *anaphylactoid reactions, angioedema.*

INTERACTIONS

Herb-drug. *Antacids, H_2 antagonists, sucralfate, and proton pump inhibitors:* May decrease drug effect because of increased stomach acid production. Monitor patient for increased abdominal signs and symptoms.

---

*Liquid contains alcohol.

EFFECTS ON LAB TEST RESULTS
• May increase stomach acid levels. May decrease BUN and creatinine levels. May alter cardiac enzyme levels.

CAUTIONS
Patients allergic to mustard shouldn't use herbal mustard preparations. Patients with gastric or duodenal ulcers or reflux conditions shouldn't use mustard because of the irritant GI effects. Patients with inflammatory kidney disease should avoid use because of the potential for irritant poisoning. Pregnant patients shouldn't use mustard because of possible abortifacient actions; breast-feeding patients also should avoid use. Mustard shouldn't be used in children younger than age 6.

Patients with allergies to coriander and curry should use mustard cautiously.

NURSING CONSIDERATIONS
• Explore patient's knowledge of this herb.
• Small amounts of mustard can cause allergic reaction, ranging from contact dermatitis to anaphylaxis.
• Monitor electrolyte and cardiac enzymes levels.
• If patient has eczema, he may experience an exacerbation of his condition if he uses mustard externally.
ALERT: Don't confuse this mustard with hedge mustard.
ALERT: Irritant poisoning may occur if mustard oil is used in its undiluted form or ingested in large quantity.

PATIENT TEACHING
• Advise patient to consult a health care provider before using an herbal preparation because another treatment may be available.
• Tell patient that when filling a new prescription he should inform pharmacist of any herbal or dietary supplement he's taking.
• Explain to the patient that to release the active component he must rub the powder on with *warm* water; hot water will destroy the active enzymes.
• Warn patient to wash his hands after preparing the herb and not to touch his eyes, mouth, or nose until his hands are washed.
• Inform patient that mustard oil is highly irritating and shouldn't be tasted or inhaled undiluted.
• Tell patient not to use mustard on open wounds or cuts.
• Tell patient that herb may cause pain and increased inflammation of the skin when applied topically.
• Tell patient not to use herb topically for more than 2 weeks and not to leave it on the skin at any time for more than 30 minutes, less if the patient has sensitive skin.
• Warn patient that he may experience coughing or sneezing when handling mustard flour.
• Tell patient that the results of a soak or bath may be improved if followed by a brief, cold shower.
• Advise patient to store the herb in a cool, dry place and protect it from light.
• Warn patient to keep all herbal products away from children and pets.

Bold italic type indicates that reaction may be life-threatening.

myrrh

Commiphora molmol, C. myrrha (nees), African myrrh, Arabian myrrh, Balsamodendron myrrha, bola, comniphora, didin, didthin, guggal gum, guggal resin, heerabol, Somali myrrh, Yemen myrrh

Common trade names
Myrrh Gum Commiphora, Myrrh Extract Liquid, Myrrh Gum Capsules, Myrrh Gum Extract, Myrrh Gum Resin, Myrrh Tincture, Medicinol

AVAILABLE FORMS
The active constituent of myrrh is obtained from the oleo-gum resin, which is exuded from the stems of *C. molmol*. This resin is air dried and then crushed into a powder or dissolved in liquid. Myrrh can also originate from other *Commiphora* species if the chemical composition is comparable to the official drug. Available as oil, tincture, mouth rinse, liquid extract, gum capsules (1 g), dental powder (10%), and home antifungal lotion.

ACTIONS & COMPONENTS
The active constituents of myrrh are obtained from the resin, gum, and volatile oils. Myrrh is reported to have mild astringent properties on mucous membranes. The phenol component of the volatile oils may account for the antimicrobial activity in vitro. Myrrh was found to be an active component in a multiplant extract that exhibited antidiabetic activity. The mode of action is thought to involve a de-crease in gluconeogenesis and an increase in peripheral glucose use.

USES
Myrrh is used to treat mouth and throat ulcers, pharyngitis, laryngitis, respiratory and sinus congestion, the common cold, sore throats, canker sores, herpes, athlete's foot, and gingivitis. It's used as an antiflatulent. It's also used topically to treat pressure ulcers, muscle pain, wounds, and abrasions.

DOSAGE & ADMINISTRATION
Athlete's foot: Applied topically to affected area b.i.d. to q.i.d.
Capsules: 657 mg to 1 g P.O. t.i.d.
Dental powder (10%): Applied topically to affected area b.i.d. to q.i.d.
Undiluted tincture as a rinse or gargle: 5 to 10 gtt in a glass of water.

ADVERSE REACTIONS
CNS: apprehension, restlessness.
GI: diarrhea.
Respiratory: hiccups.
Skin: dermatitis.

INTERACTIONS
Herb-drug. *Antidiabetics:* May increase drug action. Advise patient to avoid using the herb and drug together.

EFFECTS ON LAB TEST RESULTS
• May decrease glucose level. May alter electrolyte levels (because of prolonged diarrhea).

CAUTIONS
Patients with diabetes shouldn't use the herb, nor should patients

---

*Liquid contains alcohol.

who are pregnant or breast-feeding. Large doses may stimulate the uterus, increase pulse rate, and cause gastric burning.

NURSING CONSIDERATIONS
● Explore patient's knowledge of this herb.
● Myrrh is an active ingredient in many herbal combination products. Patient may not realize he's using a product that contains myrrh.
● Monitor glucose level.
● At excessive doses, the herb may produce hiccups, diarrhea, restlessness, and apprehension.

PATIENT TEACHING
● Advise patient to consult a health care provider before using an herbal preparation because another treatment may be available.
● Tell patient that when filling a new prescription he should inform pharmacist of any herbal or dietary supplement he's taking.
● Teach patient signs and symptoms of low blood glucose level, and instruct him to notify his health care provider if he experiences them.
● Tell patient that if he experiences prolonged diarrhea he should report it immediately to his health care provider.
● Tell patient to protect herb from light and moisture and to store it in a sealed container away from exposure to water.
● Warn patient that myrrh resin is sticky.
● Warn patient to keep all herbal products away from children and pets.

myrtle

Myrtus communis, Myrti folium, Myrti aetheroleum, myrtle oil

Common trade names
Myrtle Essential Oil

AVAILABLE FORMS
The medicinal parts of myrtle are obtained from the leaves and the branches. *M. folium* are the dried leaves of *M. communis; M. aetheroleum,* the essential oil of *M. communis.* The essential oil is extracted from the leaves and branches by steam distillation; the percentage extracted ranges from 0.1% to 0.5%. Other preparations are available; however, information is limited.

ACTIONS & COMPONENTS
The chief components of myrtle are volatile oils, tannins, and acetylphloroglucinols. Myrtol is the active component. It's absorbed in the intestine, stimulates the mucous membranes of the stomach, and deodorizes the breath. This component also has fungicidal, disinfectant, antibacterial, and antimicrobial effects.

USES
Internally, myrtle is used to treat acute and chronic infections of the respiratory tract, such as bronchitis, whooping cough, and tuberculosis. Other uses include bladder conditions, diarrhea, worm infestation, muscle spasms, and hemorrhoids. Externally, myrtle is used to treat acne and varicose veins.

Bold italic type indicates that reaction may be life-threatening.

DOSAGE & ADMINISTRATION

Dosage varies according to manufacturer and indication. Dosage may be as high as 200 mg P.O. q.i.d. for internal use.

Infusion: 15 to 30 g steeped in 1 quart (1 L) of water for 15 minutes.

ADVERSE REACTIONS

GI: *glottal spasm,* nausea, vomiting, diarrhea.
Respiratory: *bronchial spasm.*

INTERACTIONS

None reported.

EFFECTS ON LAB TEST RESULTS

None reported.

CAUTIONS

Patients with GI, biliary, or liver disease shouldn't use myrtle, nor should patients who are pregnant or breast-feeding. Topical use in children may stimulate an asthma-like response.

NURSING CONSIDERATIONS

• Explore patient's knowledge of this herb.

⚠ **ALERT:** Overdose of myrtle oil (more than 10 g) can lead to a rapid fall in blood pressure, and circulatory and respiratory collapse. Vomiting shouldn't be induced because of the danger of aspiration. Following administration of activated charcoal, give diazepam and atropine to treat signs and symptoms. Intubation and oxygen may be needed.

PATIENT TEACHING

• Advise patient to consult a health care provider before using an herbal preparation because another treatment may be available.

• Tell patient that when filling a new prescription he should inform pharmacist of any herbal or dietary supplement he's taking.

• If patient has a chronic illness, advise him not to put off seeking medical evaluation, because doing so can delay diagnosis of a potentially serious medical condition.

• Warn patient not to use the herb topically on the faces of children because this may cause glottal and bronchial spasm.

• Advise patient that this product should be stored away from light.

• Warn patient to keep all herbal products away from children and pets.

---

* Liquid contains alcohol.

N

nettle

Urtica dioica, U. urens, Urticae herba, Urticae radix, annual nettle, brennesselkraut, nettle herb, nettle root, nettle weed, small nettle, stinging nettle

Common trade names
Freeze-Dried Nettle Capsules, Fresh Nettle Leaf, Nettle Blend, Nettle Leaf, Nettle Leaf Tea, Nettle Organic Tea, Nettle Root, Nettle Seed

AVAILABLE FORMS
Available as tea, tablets, capsules, tincture*, and liquid extract*.
Capsules: 50 mg, 100 mg

ACTIONS & COMPONENTS
Obtained from fresh or dried roots and aboveground parts of *U. dioica, U. urens,* and hybrids of these species. Contains acids, amines, histamine, flavonoids, choline acetyltransferase, and lectins. Aqueous extract yields five immunologically active polysaccharides and some lectins, which may also have anti-inflammatory and immunostimulant properties. The lectin agglutinin has antifungal activity. Two of the five polysaccharides have antihemolytic effects. Nettle leaves have diuretic, analgesic, and immunomodulating pharmacologic actions in vivo.

USES
Used to treat allergic rhinitis, osteoarthritis, rheumatoid arthritis, kidney stones, asthma, BPH, eczema, hives, bursitis, tendinitis, laryngitis, sciatica, and premenstrual syndrome. Also used as a diuretic, an expectorant, a general health tonic, a blood builder and purifier, a pain reliever and anti-inflammatory, and a lung tonic for ex-smokers. Nettle is being investigated for treatment of hay fever and irrigation of the urinary tract.

DOSAGE & ADMINISTRATION
Allergic rhinitis: 600 mg freeze-dried leaf P.O. at onset of signs and symptoms.
BPH: 4 g root extract P.O. daily, or 600 to 1,200 mg P.O. encapsulated extract daily.
Fresh juice: 5 to 10 ml P.O. t.i.d.
Infusion: 1.5 g powdered nettle in cold water; heated to boiling for 1 minute, then steeped covered for 10 minutes and strained (1 teaspoon = 1.3 g herb). Dose is 1 to 4 g.
Liquid extract (1:1 in 25% alcohol): 2 to 8 ml P.O. t.i.d.
Osteoarthritis: 1 leaf applied to affected area daily.
Rheumatoid arthritis: 8 to 12 g leaf extract P.O. daily.
Tea: 1 tablespoon fresh young plant steeped in 1 cup boiled water for 15 minutes. 3 or more cups taken daily.
Tincture (1:5 in 45% alcohol): 2 to 6 ml P.O. t.i.d.

ADVERSE REACTIONS
CV: edema.
GI: gastric irritation, gingivostomatitis.
GU: decreased urine formation; oliguria; increased diuresis in pa-

---

Bold italic type indicates that reaction may be life-threatening.

tients with arthritic conditions and those with myocardial or chronic venous insufficiency.
Skin: topical irritation, burning sensation, urticaria.

INTERACTIONS

Herb-drug. *Diclofenac:* Increases anti-inflammatory effect of diclofenac. Monitor patient for effect.

Disulfiram, metronidazole: May cause a disulfiram-like reaction if herbal preparation contains alcohol. Advise patient to avoid using the herb and drug together.

Herb-lifestyle. *Alcohol use:* May cause additive effect from liquid extract and tincture. Advise patient not to use the herb and alcohol together.

EFFECTS ON LAB TEST RESULTS
• May decrease BUN and creatinine levels. May alter electrolyte levels.

CAUTIONS
Patients with fluid retention caused by reduced cardiac or renal activity, patients sensitive to herb, and patients who are pregnant or breast-feeding shouldn't use the herb.

NURSING CONSIDERATIONS
• Explore patient's knowledge of this herb.
• Tinctures and extracts typically contain between 15% and 60% alcohol and may be unsuitable for children, patients with a history of alcoholism or liver disease, or patients taking certain drugs.
• Nettle is reported to be an abortifacient and may affect the menstrual cycle.

• Allergic reactions from internal use are rare.

PATIENT TEACHING
• Advise patient to consult a health care provider before using an herbal preparation because another treatment may be available.
• Tell patient that when filling a new prescription he should inform pharmacist of any herbal or dietary supplement he's taking.
• If patient has a history of alcoholism or liver disease, inform him that some herbal products contain alcohol.
• Warn patient that skin contact may cause external adverse reactions, such as burning and stinging, which could last for 12 hours or more.
• Advise patient to monitor fluid balance by checking his weight regularly.
• Advise patient to notify her health care provider before continuing to use the herb if she suspects or knows that she's pregnant or if she plans to become pregnant. Also advise her not to take the herb if she breast-feeds.
• Inform patient that capsules and extracts should be stored at room temperature, away from heat and direct light.
• Warn patient to keep all herbal products away from children and pets.

*Liquid contains alcohol.

night-blooming cereus

Cactus grandiflorus,
Selenicereus grandiflorus, large-flowered cactus, sweet-scented cactus, vanilla cactus

Common trade names
Liquid Extract of Cereus, Tincture of Cereus

AVAILABLE FORMS
Available as liquid extract* and tincture*.

ACTIONS & COMPONENTS
Obtained from fresh or dried flowers and fresh young stems or shoots of *S. grandiflorus,* a cactus cultivated in greenhouses. Contains flavonoids, amines (mainly tyramine, which produces a digitalis effect), and betacyans. May induce a positive inotropic effect, causing cardiac stimulation and coronary and peripheral vessel dilation. May also stimulate motor neurons of the spinal cord. Herb contains hordenine, which may increase blood pressure by liberating norepinephrine or inhibiting its uptake.

USES
Used for nervous cardiac disorders, angina pectoris, stenocardia, urinary ailments, hemoptysis, menorrhagia, dysmenorrhea, and hemorrhage. Juice of whole plant is used for cystitis, shortness of breath, and edema. Used externally as astringent for rheumatism.

DOSAGE & ADMINISTRATION
Liquid extract: 0.06 ml to 6 ml P.O. 1 to 10 times daily.
Tincture of cereus: 0.12 to 2 ml P.O. b.i.d. to t.i.d.
Tincture in sweetened water (1:10): 10 gtt P.O. three to five times daily.

ADVERSE REACTIONS
CV: decreased heart rate.
GI: nausea, vomiting, diarrhea.
Skin: burning sensation, irritation.

INTERACTIONS
Herb-drug. *Digoxin:* May increase effect. Monitor digoxin levels.
MAO inhibitors, OTC cold and flu drugs: May cause additive effect and potentiation of cardiac effects. Advise patient to use caution if using the herb and drug together.

EFFECTS ON LAB TEST RESULTS
• May alter ECG results.

CAUTIONS
Patients who are sensitive to the herb shouldn't use it, nor should patients who are pregnant or breast-feeding. Patients who take a MAO inhibitor or have a cardiac disorder shouldn't take this herb.

NURSING CONSIDERATIONS
• Explore patient's knowledge of this herb.
• An overdose of the herb can cause severe nausea, vomiting, and diarrhea.
• Herb may decrease heart rate. Monitor cardiac function.

PATIENT TEACHING
• Advise patient to consult a health care provider before using an herbal preparation because another treatment may be available.
• Tell patient that when filling a new prescription he should inform

---

Bold italic type indicates that reaction may be life-threatening.

pharmacist of any herbal or dietary supplement he's taking.

• Although no chemical interactions have been reported in clinical studies, advise patient that herb may interfere with therapeutic effects of conventional drugs.

• Advise patient that if he experiences prolonged nausea, vomiting, or diarrhea, he should immediately notify his health care provider.

• Advise patient to notify her health care provider before continuing to use the herb if she suspects or knows that she's pregnant or if she plans to become pregnant.

• Warn patient to keep all herbal products away from children and pets.

nutmeg

Myristica fragrans, mace, moschata, Myristicea nux

Common trade names
Nutmeg Essential Oil, Nutmeg Tincture, Oil of Nutmeg, Powdered Nutmeg, Spirits of Nutmeg

AVAILABLE FORMS
Available as essential oil, extracts, dried seeds, powder, pressed seed cake, and syrups.

ACTIONS & COMPONENTS
Obtained from nuts and seeds of an evergreen tree *(M. fragrans).* Nutmeg oil, also known as myristica oil, is distilled from the nuts. The dried aril of the nutmeg seed produces another herbal product, known as mace. Nuts contain 20% to 40% of a fixed oil called nutmeg butter. Oil contains myristic acid, starch, protein, saponin, alcohols, phenlypropane derivatives, fatty oils, saponins, volatile oils, sterols, catechins, and glycerides of laureic, tridecanoic, stearic, and palmitic acids. The nut also contains 8% to 15% of an aromatic oil believed to be partially responsible for nutmeg intoxication. This aromatic oil contains *d*-camphene (60% to 80%), dipentene (8%), and myristicin (4% to 8%).

Nutmeg is known for its psychoactive and hallucinogenic properties resulting from CNS effects. Ingestion can produce amphetamine derivatives from conversion of phenylpropanes. Nutmeg may play a role in inhibiting prostaglandin synthesis and platelet aggregation.

USES
Used internally to treat diarrhea, indigestion, loss of appetite, colic, flatulence, and insomnia. It's also used as a larvicidal and as a hallucinogen. Used externally for rheumatoid arthritis. Nutmeg butter is used in soaps and perfumes.

DOSAGE & ADMINISTRATION
Dried seed powder: 300 mg to 1,000 mg P.O. daily.
Fluidextract: 10 to 30 gtt P.O. up to q.i.d.
Powder: 5 to 20 grains applied topically to affected area up to t.i.d.
Syrup: 10 to 40 ml daily.
Oil: 1 to 3 gtt b.i.d. to t.i.d.

ADVERSE REACTIONS
CNS: hypothermia, hallucinations, giddiness, fear of impending death, disorientation, loss of feeling in limbs, depolarization.

*Liquid contains alcohol.

CV: tachycardia, decreased pulse, feeling of pressure in chest.
GI: dry mouth.
Skin: flushing, allergic contact dermatitis.

INTERACTIONS
Herb-drug. *MAO inhibitors, psychoactive drugs:* May potentiate effect of these drugs via the herb's mild MAO-inhibiting action. Advise patient to avoid using the herb and drug together.

EFFECTS ON LAB TEST RESULTS
● May alter electrolyte levels.

CAUTIONS
Patients who are pregnant or breast-feeding, who have a cardiac or neurologic disorder, or who are sensitive to the herb shouldn't use this herb.

NURSING CONSIDERATIONS
● Explore patient's knowledge of this herb.
● Misuse and abuse of nutmeg are a growing problem.
🔳**ALERT:** Ingestion of several tablespoons of nutmeg can lead to a stuporous intoxication that may be severe. Signs and symptoms of overdose (nausea and violent vomiting) occur 3 to 8 hours after ingestion of the herb. Episodes are characterized by weak pulse, intense thirst, reddening and swelling of the face, hypothermia, disorientation, giddiness, and a feeling of pressure in the chest or lower abdomen. For up to 24 hours, an extended period of alternating delirium and stupor persists, ending in heavy sleep. The patient may have a sensation of loss of limbs and a

terrifying fear of death. Gastric lavage and supportive therapy, such as haloperidol, may be necessary. Recovery usually occurs within 24 hours but may take several days. Monitor renal function and electrolyte levels.

PATIENT TEACHING
● Advise patient to consult a health care provider before using an herbal preparation because another treatment may be available.
● Tell patient that when filling a new prescription he should inform pharmacist of any herbal or dietary supplement he's taking.
🔳**ALERT:** Caution patient to use nutmeg in moderation because intoxication and death can occur after ingesting large doses.
● Advise patient to notify her health care provider before continuing to use the herb if she suspects or knows that she's pregnant or if she plans to become pregnant. Also advise her not to take the herb if she breast-feeds.
● Warn patient not to take herb for diarrhea, indigestion, or chronic GI distress before seeking medical evaluation, because doing so may delay diagnosis of a potentially serious medical condition.
● Warn patient to keep all herbal products away from children and pets.

Bold italic type indicates that reaction may be life-threatening.

O

oak bark

Quercus alba, English oak, common oak, oak, stave oak, stone oak, tanner's oak, white oak

Common trade names
Combination products: *Alvita White Bark Tea, Conchae Compound, Kernosan Elixir, Menodoron, Nature's Way White Oak Bark Capsules and Powders, Peerless Composition Essence*

AVAILABLE FORMS
Available as chopped or powdered bark, capsules, liquid extracts, teas, compress, decoction, extract, gargles, lotions, mouthwash, and poultices.

ACTIONS & COMPONENTS
White oak bark contains the tannin, quercitannic acid, which is thought to have astringent, antiviral, antiseptic, anthelmintic, and anti-inflammatory properties.

USES
Used to treat inflammatory skin diseases, mild oropharyngeal and GI inflammation, inflammation of genital and anal areas, and acute diarrhea. Also used as a stomach tonic.
External uses include treatment of hemorrhoid bleeding, varicose veins, vaginal discharge, rashes, chronic itching, eczema, and eye inflammation.

DOSAGE & ADMINISTRATION
Baths: 5 g of herb or 1 to 3 teaspoons of bark extract to every quart (1 L) of water.
For diarrhea: 3 g P.O. daily of powdered oak bark, or 1 cup of tea t.i.d. Tea is prepared by adding 1 g of powdered bark or 1 to 2 teaspoons of chopped bark to 17 ounces (500 ml) of water, boiling for 15 minutes, straining, then cooling. Taken undiluted. Herb shouldn't be used for more than 3 days.
Rinses, compresses, and gargles: 20 g of bark boiled in 1 quart (1 L) of water for 10 to 15 minutes; the liquid is taken strained and undiluted.
Tea: 3 g herb/1 cup t.i.d.

ADVERSE REACTIONS
GI: constipation, nausea or vomiting, stomach upset, abdominal pain.
GU: renal damage.
Hepatic: liver damage.
Respiratory: *respiratory failure.*

INTERACTIONS
Herb-drug. *Atropine, digoxin, heavy metal salts (such as iron or gold), morphine, nicotine, quinine:* May decrease drug absorption. Advise patient to avoid using the herb and drug together.

EFFECTS ON LAB TEST RESULTS
• May increase liver enzyme, BUN, and creatinine levels.

---

*Liquid contains alcohol.

CAUTIONS

Patients allergic to oak bark pollen shouldn't use any products containing oak. Those with skin damage over large areas shouldn't use topical oak products. Those with weeping eczema, febrile or infectious disease, asthma, COPD, renal or hepatic insufficiency, or New York Heart Association class III or IV heart failure shouldn't take full baths containing oak.

NURSING CONSIDERATIONS

● Explore patient's knowledge of this herb.
● Oak and other tannin-containing herbs shouldn't be used for prolonged periods because the cancer risks are poorly understood.
● Short-term external use of oak preparations may be effective for skin conditions; however, safety and efficacy of internal use haven't been studied.
● Geriatric and pediatric patients may be more sensitive to the herb's adverse effects.

PATIENT TEACHING

● Advise patient to consult a health care provider before using an herbal preparation because another treatment may be available.
● Tell patient that when filling a new prescription he should inform pharmacist of any herbal or dietary supplement he's taking.
● Warn patient not to apply topical oak bark preparations on large areas of damaged skin.
● Advise patient to stop taking herb and contact a health care provider if diarrhea lasts for more than 3 days.

● Tell patient to keep oak preparation out of eyes. If contact occurs, advise flushing eyes with water for at least 15 minutes.
● Warn patient to keep all herbal products away from children and pets.

oats

Avena sativa, Avenae fructus, oat herb, wild oat herb

Common trade names
Aveeno Cleansing Bar, Aveeno Colloidal, Aveeno Dry, Aveeno Lotion, Aveeno Oilated Bath, Aveeno Regular Bath, Oat Bran, Oats and Honey, Oatstraw, Oat Straw Tea, Quaker Oat Bran, Wild Oats

AVAILABLE FORMS

Available as tablets, whole grains, cereals, wafers, teas, soaps, gels, powders, lotions, creams, colloidal oatmeal, and bath preparations.
Tablets: 850 mg, 1,000 mg

ACTIONS & COMPONENTS

Contains fresh or dried above-ground parts or flowers of *A. sativa.* Foods are made from the grains (seeds) of the plant, and oat bran is made from the inner husks of the seeds. Oats contain gluten, which forms a sticky mass that holds moisture in skin when mixed with liquid. Oat bran also contains beta-glucan, which may have blood lipid-reducing properties.

USES

Used to treat dry, itchy skin; chickenpox; diarrhea; and constipation. Dietary oat bran may lower choles-

---

terol levels. Also used to treat opium and cigarette addiction, but mechanism of action is unknown. May also be used to stabilize the glucose level. Oral intake of oats may be effective in preventing colon cancer, but that has yet to be proven.

DOSAGE & ADMINISTRATION
Baths: Follow package labeling.
Cholesterol level reduction: 3 to 5 g soluble oat fiber P.O. daily.

ADVERSE REACTIONS
GI: increased stool bulk, frequent bowel movements, flatulence, abdominal bloating.

INTERACTIONS
Herb-drug. *Morphine:* May alter analgesic effect (with green seed extracts). Advise patient to avoid using the herb and drug together. *Oral drugs:* May interfere with drug absorption (with large amounts of oats or oatmeal). Tell patient to take oral drugs 1 hour before or 2 hours after eating oats or oatmeal.

EFFECTS ON LAB TEST RESULTS
• May alter glucose and cholesterol levels.

CAUTIONS
Patients allergic to the *A. sativa* plant should avoid using oat products. Patients with celiac disease also should avoid them because gluten damages digestive and absorptive cells in the intestines in these patients.
    Patients with dermatitis herpetiformis should avoid diets high in gluten because they may cause intestinal abnormalities.

NURSING CONSIDERATIONS
• Explore patient's knowledge of this herb.
• Patients with intestinal problems should use oat products cautiously.
• As with all fiber products, oats should be taken with plenty of fluids to ensure adequate hydration and dispersion of fiber in the GI tract.
• Patients may experience frequent bowel movements, resulting in anogenital irritation.

PATIENT TEACHING
• Advise patient to consult a health care provider before using an herbal preparation because another treatment may be available.
• Tell patient that when filling a new prescription he should inform pharmacist of any herbal or dietary supplement he's taking.
• Tell patient to drink plenty of water to help regulate bowel movements.
• Caution patient that skin care products containing oats shouldn't be used near eyes or on inflamed skin.
• Warn patient to keep all herbal products away from children and pets.

---

*Liquid contains alcohol.

oleander

Nerium oleander, adelfa, laurier rose, rosa fancesca, rose laurel, rosebay

Common trade names
None known

AVAILABLE FORMS
Available as leaf extract and tincture.

ACTIONS & COMPONENTS
Obtained from a flowering ornamental shrub *(N. oleander)* grown widely throughout the southern and southwestern United States and Hawaii. Oleander is a natural cardiac glycoside that has positive inotropic and negative chronotropic effects on cardiac muscle. Its actions mimic digoxin.

USES
Reported uses include treating heart and skin diseases, but oleander's effectiveness hasn't been proven. Traditionally, it has been used to treat leprosy, malaria, ringworm, venereal disease, and indigestion; it has also been used as an abortifacient.

DOSAGE & ADMINISTRATION
Oleander isn't recommended for use. Dosages aren't well documented.

ADVERSE REACTIONS
CNS: enlarged pupils, *seizures.*
CV: irregular pulse, *heart failure.*
GI: abdominal pain, appetite loss, nausea, vomiting, bloody diarrhea.
Respiratory: *respiratory paralysis.*

INTERACTIONS
Herb-drug. *Beta blockers, calcium channel blockers, digoxin:* May cause additive effect. Advise patient to avoid using the herb and drug together.

EFFECTS ON LAB TEST RESULTS
None reported.

CAUTIONS
Oleander shouldn't be used in any form.

NURSING CONSIDERATIONS
● Explore patient's knowledge of this herb.
🗹**ALERT:** All plant parts are toxic and shouldn't be used. Adults and children have died after ingesting flowers, nectar, and leaves— even after using oleander branches to roast foods. Ingesting water that the plant has soaked in and inhaling smoke from burning oleander wood also can be toxic.
● Patients who ingest oleander will need immediate medical attention. Accidental poisonings may require gastric lavage, activated charcoal, and ipecac syrup. Digoxin-specific FAB fragments (Digibind) used in digoxin overdoses have been used with some success in oleander poisonings. Patients should have continuous ECG monitoring, and respiratory resuscitation equipment should be close at hand.
🗹**ALERT:** Don't confuse oleander *(N. oleander)* with yellow oleander *(Thevetia peruviana),* which may also be toxic.

PATIENT TEACHING
● Advise patient that if he swallows any part of the oleander plant

---

Bold italic type indicates that reaction may be life-threatening.

he should contact a poison control center or seek immediate medical attention.

● Advise patient not to burn oleander branches and leaves in poorly ventilated areas because the smoke is toxic.

● Warn patient to keep all herbal products away from children and pets. Plants should be clearly labeled.

olive (oil and leaf)

Olea europaea

Common trade names
Bertolli Olive Oil, Colavita Olive Oil, East Park D-Lenolate Olive Leaf Extract Capsules, Italica Olive Oil, Natrol Olive Leaf Extract, Nature's Herb Olive Leaf Powder, Olive Leaf PE 10%, Pompeian Olive Oil, Solgar Olive Leaf Extract Capsules, Villa Blanca Olive Oil, Virtanen, Wellness Olive Leaf

AVAILABLE FORMS
Available as oil, capsules, and powder.
Olive leaf extract capsules: 60 mg to 500 mg

ACTIONS & COMPONENTS
Obtained from leaves and fruits of *O. europaea.* Contains phenolic compound oleuropein, which has anti-inflammatory and antioxidant properties. Oleuropein may exert its anti-inflammatory activity by damping the expression of intercellular adhesion molecule-1, involved in adhesion of leukocytes to endothelial cells. The antioxidant properties of oleuropein may prevent the oxidative modification of low-density-lipoprotein cholesterol. Olive oil also inhibits platelet aggregation. All of these mechanisms indicate that olive-derived products may help prevent atherosclerosis.

Oleuropein may also have vasodilatory, hypoglycemic, and antimicrobial properties. Although the exact mechanism of vasodilation is unknown, the hypoglycemic activity may result from either a potentiation of insulin release or increased peripheral uptake of glucose. Olive polyphenols have antimicrobial activity against certain gram-positive and gram-negative bacteria.

USES
Used as an emollient and topical lubricant. Used to treat skin irritations (such as burns and psoriasis), to soften earwax, to relieve constipation, to moisturize dry hair and itchy scalp, and to prevent stretch marks caused by pregnancy. Recent evidence suggests that olive oil, when part of a diet high in monounsaturated fats, may lower cholesterol levels. It has also been used to prevent CV disease, breast cancer, and rheumatoid arthritis.

Olive leaf preparations have been used to lower blood pressure, reduce glucose levels in diabetic patients, and treat various bacterial, viral, and fungal infections.

DOSAGE & ADMINISTRATION
Cholesterol level reduction: Used in moderation as part of a diet low in saturated fat.
Hair and skin problems: Rub undiluted oil into affected area, p.r.n.

---

*Liquid contains alcohol.

Infections: 60 to 500 mg of olive leaf preparation P.O. every 6 hours.
Laxative: 1 to 2 ounces of oil P.O. p.r.n.

ADVERSE REACTIONS
CV: hypotension.
GI: stomach irritation.
Metabolic: *hypoglycemia.*

INTERACTIONS
Herb-drug. *Antidiabetics:* May cause additive effect. Monitor glucose level closely.
Antihypertensives: May cause additive effect. Monitor blood pressure closely.

EFFECTS ON LAB TEST RESULTS
• May decrease glucose level.

CAUTIONS
Patients allergic to any part of the olive plant shouldn't use these products. Olive oil may cause biliary colic in patients with gallstones.

NURSING CONSIDERATIONS
• Explore patient's knowledge of this herb.
• Patients who are immunocompromised shouldn't use olive leaf products because clinical and safety data are lacking.
• Diabetic patients who choose to use olive leaf preparations should check their glucose level more frequently because of the risk of hypoglycemia.
• Olive oil should be part of a diet that is low in saturated fat and cholesterol.
• Monitor blood pressure closely for hypotension.

PATIENT TEACHING
• Advise patient to consult a health care provider before using an herbal preparation because another treatment may be available.
• Tell patient that when filling a new prescription he should inform pharmacist of any herbal or dietary supplement he's taking.
• Tell patient that olive leaf preparations should be taken with food to avoid stomach upset.
⚡**ALERT:** If patient has HIV or another condition that weakens the immune system, diabetes, or blood pressure abnormalities, advise him to consult a health care provider before using olive for medicinal purposes.
• If patient thinks he has diabetes, encourage him to consult a health care provider for proper management.
• If patient has a history of gallstones, advise him to limit his intake of olive oil.
• Review the signs and symptoms of low blood glucose level, including a fast heart rate, sweating, nausea, and hunger.
• Warn patient to keep all herbal products away from children and pets.

onion

Allii cepae bulbus, allium cepa

Common trade names
None known

AVAILABLE FORMS
Available as leaves and bulbs.

Bold italic type indicates that reaction may be life-threatening.

ACTIONS & COMPONENTS
Contains essential oils, organosulfur compounds, cysteine sulfoxide, quercetin glycosides, thiosulfinates, and diphenylamine. The organosulfur compound may have antimicrobial and anticancer effects. Cysteine sulfoxide is responsible for flavor and lacrimation effects. Quercetin glycosides impart antioxidant properties. Thiosulfinates inhibit mediators of bronchoconstriction, such as leukotriene and thromboxane; extracts containing the compound have reduced bronchial constriction in patients with asthma. The herb inhibits platelet aggregation, lowers cholesterol levels, decreases blood pressure, enhances fibrinolysis, and has hypoglycemic and antifungal effects.

USES
Used as raw herb for anemia, exhaustion, appetite loss, stomach gas, furuncles, warts, bruises, bronchitis, asthma, atherosclerosis, diabetes, dyspepsia, fever, colds, hypertension, hypercholesterolemia, infection, inflammation, angina, dehydration, and menstrual problems. Also used as a mucolytic agent, an anthelmintic, a diuretic, and a gallbladder stimulant. Onion water is used as tea to relieve sore throat and cough.

Used topically as a poultice for sores, bites, and burns. Fishermen have used onion to treat stingray and fish-spine wounds. Onion is also used as a food flavoring.

DOSAGE & ADMINISTRATION
Externally: Onion slices or poultices containing onion juice are placed on the skin and covered with a cloth.
Internally: Typically, 50 g fresh onion or juice from 50 g of fresh onion P.O. daily; 20 g of dried onion daily can also be used. Maximum recommended dose of diphenylamine is 35 mg daily if use is intended over several months.

ADVERSE REACTIONS
EENT: excessive tearing.
GI: nausea.
Skin: eczema.

INTERACTIONS
Herb-drug. *Antilipemics:* May alter serum cholesterol levels. Monitor cholesterol levels.
Antiplatelet drugs: May increase risk of bleeding. Observe and monitor patient for evidence of bleeding. Advise patient at risk for bleeding to use herb cautiously.
Hypoglycemics: May affect blood glucose level. Monitor glucose level.
Herb-herb. *Other herbs with antiplatelet and anticoagulant properties:* Increases risk of bleeding. Advise caution.
Other herbs with hypoglycemic effects: Increases risk of hypoglycemia. Advise caution. Monitor blood glucose level in diabetic patients.

EFFECTS ON LAB TEST RESULTS
• May decrease glucose, cholesterol, and lipid levels.
• May affect PT, INR, and platelet count.

---

*Liquid contains alcohol.

CAUTIONS
Patients sensitive to onions should avoid these products.

NURSING CONSIDERATIONS
- Find out why patient is using the herb.
- Herb should be used cautiously by patients with diabetes, bleeding disorders, and eczema.
- Monitor blood glucose level carefully in diabetic patients.
- Observe patient for evidence of bleeding.

PATIENT TEACHING
- Advise patient to consult a health care provider before using an herbal preparation because a standard treatment that has been proven effective may be available.
- Tell patient that when filling a new prescription he should remind pharmacist of any herbal and dietary supplements he's taking.
- Tell patient that information on the use of onion during pregnancy and breast-feeding is lacking, and that amounts greater than those used in foods should be avoided.
- Urge diabetic patient to monitor blood glucose level carefully and to stay alert for signs of hypoglycemia, such as sweating, a racing heart, hunger, and nausea.
- Warn patient of potential for flare of eczema.
- Instruct patient to wash hands after handling onion.
- If patient takes an antiplatelet drug or anticoagulant, warn him about the increased risk of bleeding caused by onion.

oregano

*Origani vulgaris herba,
Origanum vulgare,* dostenkraut,
mountain mint, orgianum,
origano, wild marjoram, winter
marjoram, wintersweet

Common trade names
*Oil of Oregano, Oregamax,
Oregano, Oregano Powder*

AVAILABLE FORMS
Available as oil and dried herb.
Oil: 0.15% to 1%

ACTIONS & COMPONENTS
Obtained from leaves of *O. vulgare.* Chief components of oil are carvacrol 40% to 70%, gamma-terpinene 8% to 10%, *p*-cymene 5% to 10%, alpha-pinene, myrcene, and thymol. Other species may contain linalool, caryophyllene, or germacren D. Carvacrol has antifungal and antibacterial action against gram-positive and gram-negative bacteria and against yeast. Oregano also has anthelmintic, antispasmodic, irritant, diuretic, bile stimulant, and expectorant properties. It also has antioxidant effects and may act at progesterone receptors in intact human breast cancer cells.

USES
Used for urinary tract disorders, respiratory tract ailments, cough, painful menstruation, arthritis, diuresis, scrofulosis, GI disorders, dyspepsia, and bloating. Also used as an expectorant, a sedative, a diaphoretic, and a stimulant of appetite, digestion, and bile excretion.

Bold italic type indicates that reaction may be life-threatening.

DOSAGE & ADMINISTRATION

Bath: 1 quart (1 L) of water poured over 100 g of oregano; strained after 10 minutes and added to a full bath.

Tea: 8 ounces of boiling water poured over 1 heaping teaspoon and strained after 10 minutes; tea may be sweetened with honey. Unsweetened tea may be used as a gargle and a mouthwash.

ADVERSE REACTIONS

GI: upset stomach.
Other: allergic reaction.

INTERACTIONS

Herb-drug. *Iron:* May decrease iron absorption. Advise patient to separate administration of oregano and iron supplements by at least 2 hours.

EFFECTS ON LAB TEST RESULTS

None reported.

CAUTIONS

Patients sensitive to oregano or other members of the mint family should avoid using this herb. Pregnant women should also avoid use because of its possible abortifacient and menstruation-stimulant effects.

NURSING CONSIDERATIONS

• Find out why patient is using the herb.
• Stay alert for evidence of an allergic reaction.
• Patients should take oregano and iron supplements at least 2 hours apart.
• Patients allergic to other plants in the same plant family may show cross-sensitivity. Other herbs that belong to the mint family include thyme, hyssop, basil, marjoram, mint, sage, and lavender.

PATIENT TEACHING

• Advise patient to consult a health care provider before using an herbal preparation because a standard treatment that has been proven effective may be available.
• Tell patient that when filling a new prescription he should remind pharmacist of any herbal and dietary supplements he's taking.
⚠ALERT: Symptoms of allergic reaction include difficulty breathing, speaking, or swallowing. Other symptoms may include facial swelling and itching.
• Tell patient to notify his health care provider if he takes an iron supplement.
• Counsel pregnant women to avoid excessive use of tea and not to use herb in the bath.

Oregon grape

Mahonia aquifolium, barberry, blue barberry, creeping barberry, holly barberry, holly-leaved berberis, holly mahonia, mahonia aquifolium, mountain grape, Oregon barberry, Oregon grapeholly, trailing mahonia, water-holly

Common trade names
Oregon Grape Root, Prime Relief

AVAILABLE FORMS

Available as capsules, powder, tincture, ointment, and creams.
Capsules: 400 mg

*Liquid contains alcohol.

ACTIONS & COMPONENTS
Obtained from rhizome and root of Oregon grape. Physiologic activity stems from alkaloids berberine, berbamine, and oxyacanthine. Berberine and oxyacanthine have antibacterial properties. Berberine also has activity against amoebas and trypanosomes, as well as anticonvulsant, sedative, and uterine-stimulant properties. Berbamine and berberine may have anticancer activity. Berbamine has a hypotensive effect. Berbamine and oxyacanthine are potent lipoxygenase inhibitors. Herb may also have anti-inflammatory and antifungal activity.

USES
Used topically for psoriasis. Also used in small doses for ulcers, heartburn, and stomach problems. Larger doses have a cathartic effect. Used for dry rashes, for general debility, and to improve appetite.

DOSAGE & ADMINISTRATION
Powder: 0.5 to 1 g P.O. t.i.d.
Tincture: 2 to 4 ml P.O. t.i.d.
Topical: Apply bark extract (10%) ointment to affected areas b.i.d. or t.i.d. for psoriasis. Massage root extract (10%) cream into affected areas t.i.d. or as directed by a health care provider.

ADVERSE REACTIONS
CNS: lethargy.
CV: hypotension, *cardiac damage.*
EENT: epistaxis, eye irritation.
GI: upset stomach.
GU: kidney irritation, *hemorrhagic nephritis.*

Respiratory: dyspnea, *respiratory spasm and arrest.*
Skin: itching, burning, irritation.
Other: allergic reaction.

INTERACTIONS
Herb-drug. *Antihypertensives:* May cause additive effect. Advise patient to avoid using together.
Herb-herb. *Other herbs containing berberine, including amur cork tree, bloodroot, celandine, Chinese corktree, Chinese goldthread, European barberry, goldenseal, and goldthread:* May increase risk of toxicity. Advise patient to avoid using together.

EFFECTS ON LAB TEST RESULTS
● May increase creatinine levels. May alter cardiac enzyme levels.
● May decrease creatinine clearance.

CAUTIONS
Pregnant and breast-feeding women shouldn't use Oregon grape. Berberine may cause or worsen kidney irritation and induce nephritis. Patients hypersensitive to Oregon grape or to related plants shouldn't use it.

NURSING CONSIDERATIONS
● Find out why patient is using the herb.
● This herb should be used cautiously by patients with kidney problems.
⚡**ALERT:** Don't confuse Oregon grape with "European barberry" *(Berberis vulgaris).*

PATIENT TEACHING
● Advise patient to consult a health care provider before using an

---

Bold italic type indicates that reaction may be life-threatening.

herbal preparation because a standard treatment that has been proven effective may be available.
• Tell patient that when filling a new prescription he should remind pharmacist of any herbal and dietary supplements he's taking.
• Tell patient not to use Oregon grape if she's pregnant or breast-feeding.

✍ALERT: Advise patient that poisoning and death have resulted from excessive doses of berberine.

pansy

Viola tricolor, Violae tricoloris herba, European wild pansy, heartsease, heart's ease herb, Johnny-jump-up, wild pansy

Common trade names
None known

AVAILABLE FORMS
Available as extract, tea, and poultice.

ACTIONS & COMPONENTS
Obtained from dried and fresh leaves, stems, and flowers of *V. tricolor.* Contains flavonoids (0.2%), mucilage (10%), tannins (2% to 5%), and hydroxycoumarins. Pansy has antioxidant and anti-inflammatory properties.

USES
Used orally to promote metabolism, treat respiratory disorders, and provide mild laxative effect. Used topically for mild seborrheic skin and scalp disorders, warts, skin inflammation, acne, exanthema, eczema, impetigo, and pruritus vulvae.

DOSAGE & ADMINISTRATION
Poultice: Applied t.i.d.
Tea: 1 cup t.i.d. Prepared by steeping 1.5 g of herb in 5 ounces (148 ml) of boiling water for 5 to 10 minutes and then straining.

ADVERSE REACTIONS
Hepatic: *hepatotoxicity (with excessive ingestion).*

INTERACTIONS
Herb-drug. *Anticoagulants, antiplatelet drugs:* May increase risk of bleeding. Advise patient to use caution if using the herb and drug together.

EFFECTS ON LAB TEST RESULTS
• May increase liver enzyme levels.
• May increase PT and INR.

CAUTIONS
Patients who are pregnant or breast-feeding shouldn't use this herb. Patients with liver disease should use caution when using the herb.

NURSING CONSIDERATIONS
• Explore patient's knowledge of this herb.
• Pansy may be effective for mild seborrheic disorders, but information on its use for other conditions is lacking.
• Although no chemical interactions have been reported in clinical studies, advise patient that herb may interfere with therapeutic effects of conventional drugs.

PATIENT TEACHING
• Advise patient to consult a health care provider before using an herbal preparation because another treatment may be available.
• Tell patient that when filling a new prescription he should inform pharmacist of any herbal or dietary supplement he's taking.
• If patient is taking an anticoagulant or an antiplatelet drug, warn

---

Bold italic type indicates that reaction may be life-threatening.

him to consult his health care provider before taking this herb.
• Advise patient to store herb in well-sealed container to limit exposure to moisture and light.
• Tell patient to seek medical help if excessive bleeding or bruising occurs.
• Warn patient to keep all herbal products away from children and pets.

papaya

Carica papaya, Caricae papayae folium, mamaerie, melon tree, papaw

Common trade names
Papaya Digestive Enzyme, Papaya Digestive Enzyme–Double Strength, Papaya Enzyme, Papaya Enzyme with Chlorophyll, Papaya Leaf, Papaya with Papain, Super Papaya Enzyme, Super Papaya–Plex

AVAILABLE FORMS
Available as tablets, tea, and as combination products.
Chewable tablets: 25 mg
Tablets: 5 mg

ACTIONS & COMPONENTS
Obtained from leaves and fruits of *C. papaya.* Leaf contains 2% papain and carpain. Papain is a mixture of proteolytic enzymes found in the fruit latex and the leaf with a fairly broad spectrum of activity. It hydrolyzes proteins, peptides, amides, and some esters. Carpain may have amoebicidal properties. Other components of the enzyme blend hydrolyze fats and carbohydrates. Papaya has bacteriostatic and antioxidant activity and may also have antisickling properties.

USES
Used to promote digestion, to expel intestinal parasites, and to treat inflammation, gastroduodenal ulcers, pancreatic excretion insufficiency, chronic infected ulcers, and keloid scars. Also used as a sedative and a diuretic. Used in preparations to control edema and inflammation from surgical, accidental, or sports trauma. Chymopapain, obtained from papain, is used to treat intervertebral disc hernia in a procedure called chemonucleolysis. Papain is also used as a meat tenderizer.

DOSAGE & ADMINISTRATION
For enhancing digestion: 10 to 50 mg of papain tablets P.O. Or chewable tablets containing 250 mg of papaya powder, 150 mg of pineapple juice powder, and 10 mg of papain P.O. t.i.d. after meals.

ADVERSE REACTIONS
CNS: *paralysis,* sedation.
CV: *bradycardia.*
GI: gastritis, esophageal perforation (with ingestion of large amounts of papain).
Respiratory: *asthma attack.*
Other: allergic reaction.

INTERACTIONS
Herb-drug. *Anisindione, dicumarol, warfarin:* May increase INR. Advise patient to avoid using the herb and drug together.
CNS depressants: May cause additive effect. Tell patient to avoid using the herb and drug together.

*Liquid contains alcohol.

Digoxin, diltiazem, verapamil:
May increase potential for brady-cardia. Tell patient to use cautious-ly if using the herb and drug to-gether.
Herb-herb. *Papain:* May potenti-ate effect. Advise patient to avoid using the two together.

EFFECTS ON LAB TEST RESULTS
• May increase PT and INR.

CAUTIONS
Patients who are pregnant or breast-feeding shouldn't use this herb because it may be harmful to the developing fetus and may in-duce menstruation. Patients aller-gic to papaya and those with a his-tory of Crohn's disease or chronic gastritis should avoid the herb as well.

NURSING CONSIDERATIONS
• Explore patient's knowledge of this herb.
• Monitor patient for allergic reac-tions to papaya.
• Although no chemical interac-tions have been reported in clinical studies, advise patient that herb may interfere with therapeutic ef-fects of conventional drugs.

PATIENT TEACHING
• Advise patient to consult a health care provider before using an herbal preparation because another treatment may be available.
• Tell patient that when filling a new prescription he should inform pharmacist of any herbal or di-etary supplement he's taking.
• If patient takes warfarin, digoxin, diltiazem, or verapamil, tell him to

consult his health care provider before taking papaya.

pareira

Chondrodendron tomentosum, ice vine, pareira brava, velvet leaf

Common trade names
None known

AVAILABLE FORMS
Available as powder, granules, and in various combination products. Not commercially available in the United States.

ACTIONS & COMPONENTS
Obtained from fresh or dried bark, roots, and stems of *C. tomentosum.* Effects of pareira depend on the toxic derivatives that enter the bloodstream and cause systemic effects. Pareira contains dibenzoyl isoquinoline alkaloids, such as *D*-tubocurarine, chondrocurarine, curine, chondrofoline, chondro-curine, and isochondrodendrine. These alkaloids have emmenagog-ic, diuretic, and muscle-relaxing effects. Tubocurarine chloride is used medicinally as a muscle re-laxant during anesthesia. It works as a nondepolarizing (competitive) neuromuscular blocker by compet-ing with acetylcholine for cholin-ergic receptors, thus decreasing the response to acetylcholine and in-hibiting skeletal muscle contrac-tion. Unless large quantities are in-gested or cuts or ulcerations are present in the mouth or GI tract, oral absorption is poor. However, it may be enough to cause muscle paralysis.

Bold italic type indicates that reaction may be life-threatening.

USES
Used as a laxative, tonic, and diuretic. Also used to relieve kidney inflammation and induce menstruation. Brazilians use pareira for snakebites by drinking an infusion of the plant and applying bruised leaves to the bite. The herb is also used to make curare, a paralyzing arrow poison used during hunting.

DOSAGE & ADMINISTRATION
Not commercially available in the United States. Dosages not well documented.

ADVERSE REACTIONS
CNS: sedation.
CV: flushing, hypotension, tachycardia.
EENT: blurred vision.
GI: decreased GI motility, nausea.
Musculoskeletal: skeletal muscle relaxation, jaw weakness.
Respiratory: *bronchospasm, apnea.*

INTERACTIONS
Herb-drug. *Anticonvulsants, such as phenytoin; calcium channel blockers, such as diltiazem and verapamil; ketamine; procainamide; quinidine; skeletal muscle relaxants, including vecuronium; other drugs containing tubocurarine:* May potentiate neuromuscular blocking action of pareira. Advise patient to avoid using the herb and drug together.

EFFECTS ON LAB TEST RESULTS
None reported.

CAUTIONS
The plant is considered poisonous and shouldn't be consumed.

NURSING CONSIDERATIONS
• Explore patient's knowledge of this herb.
• The FDA doesn't recommend using this herb.
• Nausea and heavy urine flow have been observed in patients poisoned with tubocurare.

PATIENT TEACHING
✒ **ALERT:** Advise patients not to use this poisonous herb.

parsley

Petroselinum crispum, garden parsley, Hamburg parsley, persely, petersylinge, rock parsley

Common trade names
Parsley Herb, Parsley Leaf

AVAILABLE FORMS
Available as dried herb, seeds, liquid extract, capsules, tincture*, and tea. Also available in combination with other herbs such as garlic.
Leaf and root: 430-mg capsules
Leaf extract: In vegetable glycerin and grain neutral spirit (12% to 14%)
Leaves: 450-mg, 455-mg capsules

ACTIONS & COMPONENTS
Obtained from leaves, roots, and seeds of *P. crispum.* Contains carotene and vitamins B, C, E, and K; iron and calcium; flavonoids with anti-inflammatory and antioxidant activity; coumarins with anticoagulant properties; psoralens; and two volatile oils, apiole and myristicin. The volatile oils are the most active components. Leaves

*Liquid contains alcohol.

contain 0.3% to 0.5% and seeds contain 2% to 7% oils.

Myristicin and apiole act as diuretics and strong uterine stimulants. They may act as MAO inhibitors, causing decreased intracellular metabolism of norepinephrine, serotonin, and other biogenic amines. Sympathetic activity of myristicin and renal irritation of apiole contribute to diuretic effects. Myristicin may be metabolized to compounds with stimulating effects in the body, explaining the CNS effects seen with higher doses.

USES
Used for indigestion, flatulence, dyspepsia, colic, kidney ailments, diuresis, cystitis, liver and spleen disorders, functional amenorrhea, uterine contraction, and dysmenorrhea. Used to increase milk production, freshen breath, promote hair growth, and provide antiseptic effects. Also used as an antirheumatic, analgesic, antispasmodic, expectorant, and decongestant.

DOSAGE & ADMINISTRATION
Breath freshener: Sprigs are dipped into vinegar and chewed slowly before swallowing.
Decoction: 1 to 2 teaspoons of dried leaves or root or 1 teaspoon of bruised seeds dissolved in a cup of water.
Diuresis: 6 g daily of root or leaves P.O. 1 teaspoon of chopped herb = 2 g.
Dried root: 2 to 4 g P.O. or by oral infusion t.i.d.
Hair-growth promoter: Crushed parsley leaves are rubbed over scalp.

Leaf: 2 to 4 g P.O. t.i.d.
Leaf capsules: 2 capsules (450 mg each) P.O., b.i.d. or t.i.d.; 3 capsules (455 mg each) P.O. t.i.d.
Leaf extract in vegetable glycerin and grain neutral spirit (12% to 14%): 10 to 15 gtt with water P.O. b.i.d. or t.i.d.
Liquid extract (1:1 in 25% alcohol): 2 to 4 ml P.O. t.i.d.
Seeds: 1 to 2 g P.O. t.i.d.
Uterine contractions: Parsley juice (85%).

ADVERSE REACTIONS
CNS: sedation, headache, loss of balance, *seizures,* giddiness, hallucinations.
CV: hypotension, *bradycardia,* flushing, tachycardia, hypotension, *ventricular arrhythmias, shock.*
EENT: hearing loss.
GI: nausea, vomiting, GI irritation.
GU: menstruation, miscarriages, irritation of the kidneys, nephrosis.
Hematologic: *hemolytic anemia, thrombocytopenic purpura.*
Hepatic: fatty degeneration of the liver, hepatic dysfunction.
Musculoskeletal: *paralysis,* neuropathy.
Skin: pruritus, pigmentation, photosensitivity reactions.

INTERACTIONS
Herb-drug. *Antidepressants, hormonal drugs:* May cause phototoxicity. Advise patient to avoid using the herb and drug together.
Antihypertensives, diuretics: May enhance sodium absorption and alter blood pressure with large amounts of parsley. Tell patient to avoid using the herb and drug together.

Bold italic type indicates that reaction may be life-threatening.

Disulfiram, metronidazole: May cause a disulfiram-like reaction if herbal preparation contains alcohol. Advise patient to avoid using the herb and drug together.

MAO inhibitors, such as isocarboxazid, moclobemide, phenelzine, selegiline, tranylcypromine: May potentiate drug effect. Advise patient to avoid using the herb and drug together.

Warfarin: May decrease drug effect. Monitor patient closely, and advise him to avoid using the herb and drug together.

Herb-lifestyle. *Sun exposure:* May cause additive photosensitivity risk because of the psoralens component. Advise patient to wear protective clothing and sunscreen and to limit exposure to direct sunlight.

EFFECTS ON LAB TEST RESULTS
● May alter PT and INR.

CAUTIONS
Patients who are pregnant or breast-feeding shouldn't use this herb. Patients should avoid consuming high doses of seed products because of the high volatile oil content. High doses may also potentiate MAO inhibitor therapy. Patients with kidney and liver disease shouldn't use this herb because some forms may contain alcohol. Patients with hypertension shouldn't use large amounts of parsley because it may interfere with their drug therapy.

NURSING CONSIDERATIONS
● Explore patient's knowledge of this herb.
● Tinctures and extracts typically contain between 15% and 60% alcohol and may be unsuitable for children, patients with a history of alcoholism or liver disease, or patients taking certain drugs.
● Consuming high doses of parsley can cause serious adverse reactions.
● Because parsley seeds contain higher amounts of volatile oils, they may increase the risk of adverse reactions.

PATIENT TEACHING
● Advise patient to consult a health care provider before using an herbal preparation because another treatment may be available.
● Tell patient that when filling a new prescription he should inform pharmacist of any herbal or dietary supplement he's taking.
● If patient has a chronic illness, advise him not to put off seeking medical evaluation, because doing so can delay diagnosis of a potentially serious medical condition.
● Inform patient that parsley seeds contain the highest amount of volatile oils, so he should use them cautiously.
● Tell patient to avoid high doses or prolonged use of parsley because of the risk of adverse reactions.
● If patient is pregnant, caution her that parsley components may cause uterine stimulation and may complicate pregnancy or cause miscarriage.
● If patient has a history of alcoholism or liver disease, inform him that some herbal products contain alcohol.
● Warn patient to keep all herbal products away from children and pets.

*Liquid contains alcohol.

parsley piert

Aphanes arvensis, field lady's mantle, parsley breakstone, parsley piercestone

Common trade names
None known

AVAILABLE FORMS
Available as dried herb, liquid extract*, tincture*, and infusion.
Liquid extract: 1:1 in 25% alcohol
Tincture: 1:5 in 45% alcohol

ACTIONS & COMPONENTS
Obtained from *A. arvensis.* Contains tannin (a styptic and an astringent) similar to a related species, *Alchemilla vulgaris* (lady's mantle). May have diuretic and demulcent properties.

USES
Used as a diuretic and demulcent. Also used to dissolve kidney or bladder calculi, to reduce fever, and to treat dysuria, edema of renal or hepatic origin, bladder inflammation, and recurrent UTI.

DOSAGE & ADMINISTRATION
Dried herb: 2 to 4 g P.O. t.i.d.
Infusion: 1 cup t.i.d. or q.i.d. Prepared by boiling 1 ounce dried herb in 1 pint of water, simmering for 1 minute, cooling, and straining.
Liquid extract (1:1 in 25% alcohol): 2 to 4 ml P.O. t.i.d.
Tincture (1:5 in 45% alcohol): 2 to 10 ml P.O. t.i.d.
  Parsley piert is also combined with other products, such as mullein flowers, sweet flag root, marshmallow root, comfrey root, slippery elm, gravel root, and pellitory.

ADVERSE REACTIONS
CNS: headache.
CV: flushing, tachycardia, hypotension, *ventricular arrhythmias.*
GI: nausea, vomiting.
Other: *shock.*

INTERACTIONS
Herb-drug. *Disulfiram, metronidazole:* May cause a disulfiram-like reaction if herbal preparation contains alcohol. Advise patient to avoid using the herb and drug together.

EFFECTS ON LAB TEST RESULTS
None reported.

CAUTIONS
Patients who are pregnant or breast-feeding shouldn't use this herb because information about its safety and efficacy is lacking. Patients with a history of alcoholism or liver disease shouldn't use it because liquid extract and tincture both contain alcohol.

NURSING CONSIDERATIONS
• Explore patient's knowledge of this herb.
• Tinctures and extracts typically contain between 15% and 60% alcohol and may be unsuitable for children, patients with a history of alcoholism or liver disease, or patients taking certain drugs.
• Parsley piert shouldn't be confused with the true parsley used in cooking.

Bold italic type indicates that reaction may be life-threatening.

PATIENT TEACHING
• Advise patient to consult a health care provider before using an herbal preparation because another treatment may be available.
• Tell patient that when filling a new prescription he should inform pharmacist of any herbal or dietary supplement he's taking.
• If patient has a history of alcoholism or liver disease, inform him that some herbal products contain alcohol.
• Warn patient not to use parsley piert tincture or liquid extracts together with disulfiram, metronidazole, or any other drugs that interact with alcohol.
• Advise patient not to exceed recommended doses.
• Warn patient to keep all herbal products away from children and pets.

passion flower

Passiflora incarnata, grenadille, maypop, passiflora, passion vine, purple passion flower, wild passionflower

Common trade names
Passion Flower, Alcohol Free Passion Flower Liquid

AVAILABLE FORMS
Available as fruits, flowers, extracts*, capsules, tincture*, and tea.
Capsules: 400 mg
Liquid: 1:1 (in 25% alcohol)

ACTIONS & COMPONENTS
Obtained from leaves, fruits, and flowers of *P. incarnata.* Contains indole alkaloids, including harman and harmine, flavonoids, and maltol. Indole alkaloids are the basis of many biologically active substances, such as serotonin and tryptophan. Exact effect of these alkaloids is unknown; however, they can cause CNS stimulation via MAO inhibition, thereby decreasing intracellular metabolism of norepinephrine, serotonin, and other biogenic amines. Flavonoids can reduce capillary permeability and fragility. Maltol can cause sedative effects and potentiate hexobarbital and anticonvulsive activity.

USES
Used as a sedative, a hypnotic, an analgesic, and an antispasmodic for treating muscle spasms caused by indigestion, menstrual cramping, pain, or migraines. Also used for neuralgia, generalized seizures, hysteria, nervous agitation, and insomnia. Crushed leaves and flowers are used topically for cuts and bruises.

DOSAGE & ADMINISTRATION
Dried herb: 250 mg to 1 g P.O., two to three 100-mg capsules P.O. b.i.d., or one 400-mg capsule P.O. daily.
For cuts and bruises: Crushed leaves and flowers are applied topically, p.r.n.
For anxiety: 100 mg P.O. b.i.d. to t.i.d.
For hemorrhoids: Prepared by soaking 20 g dried herb in 200 ml of simmering water, straining, then cooling before use. Applied topically, as indicated.
For insomnia: 200 mg P.O. h.s.

---

*Liquid contains alcohol.

Infusion: 5 ounces (150 ml) of hot water poured over 0.25 to 2 g of herb. Strained after standing for 10 minutes. Taken b.i.d. or t.i.d., with a final dose about 30 minutes before h.s.
Liquid extract (1:1 in 25% alcohol): 0.5 to 1 ml P.O. t.i.d.
Solid extract: Taken in doses of 150 to 300 mg/day P.O.
Tincture (1:8 in 45% alcohol): 0.5 to 2 ml P.O. t.i.d. or ½ to 1 teaspoon P.O. t.i.d.

ADVERSE REACTIONS
CNS: drowsiness, headache, flushing, agitation, confusion, psychosis.
CV: tachycardia, hypotension, *ventricular arrhythmias.*
GI: nausea, vomiting.
Respiratory: asthma.
Other: allergic reaction, *shock.*

INTERACTIONS
Herb-drug. *Anticoagulants, antiplatelet drugs:* May increase risk of bleeding. Advise patient to avoid using the herb and drug together.
CNS depressants: May cause additive effect. Advise patient to avoid using the herb and drug together.
Disulfiram, metronidazole: May cause a disulfiram-like reaction if herbal preparation contains alcohol. Advise patient to avoid using the herb and drug together.
Hexobarbital, phenobarbital: May increase sleeping time or potentiation of other barbiturate effects. Monitor patient's level of consciousness carefully.
Isocarboxazid, moclobemide, phenelzine, selegiline, tranylcypromine: May potentiate drug action. Advise patient to avoid using the herb and drug together.

EFFECTS ON LAB TEST RESULTS
● May alter PT and INR.

CAUTIONS
Excessive doses may cause sedation and may potentiate MAO inhibitor therapy. Pregnant patients shouldn't take this herb.

NURSING CONSIDERATIONS
● Explore patient's knowledge of this herb.
● No adverse reactions have been observed with recommended doses.
● Monitor patient for adverse CNS reactions.
● Tinctures and extracts typically contain between 15% and 60% alcohol and may be unsuitable for children, patients with a history of alcoholism or liver disease, or patients taking certain drugs.
🖅 **ALERT:** A disulfiram-like reaction may produce nausea, vomiting, flushing, headache, hypotension, tachycardia, ventricular arrhythmias, and shock leading to death.

PATIENT TEACHING
● Advise patient to consult a health care provider before using an herbal preparation because another treatment may be available.
● Tell patient that when filling a new prescription he should inform pharmacist of any herbal or dietary supplement he's taking.
● Advise patient to use caution when performing activities that require mental alertness until he knows how the herb affects his

---

Bold italic type indicates that reaction may be life-threatening.

CNS. Also advise him to avoid taking the herb with alcohol or other CNS depressants.

● If patient has a chronic illness, advise him not to put off seeking medical evaluation because doing so can delay diagnosis of a potentially serious medical condition.

● Advise patient to notify her health care provider before continuing to use the herb if she suspects or knows that she's pregnant or if she plans to become pregnant.

● Warn patient to keep all herbal products away from children and pets.

pau d'arco

Tabebuia avellanedae, T. impetiginosa, ipe roxo, lapacho, tabebuia ipe, taheebo, tahuari, tajy, queshua

Common trade names
Amazon Support, Antifungal Formula, BP-X, Caprylimune, Pau d'Arco Power Pack, Red Clover Blend Defense Maintenance

AVAILABLE FORMS
Available as capsules, extracts*, tincture*, and tea.
Capsules: 300 mg

ACTIONS & COMPONENTS
Obtained from bark and heartwood of *T. avellanedae.* Contains anthraquinones, naphthoquinones (such as lapachol), flavonoids, alkaloids, and traces of saponins. Lapachol compounds may be effective against psoriasis. Compounds of the lapachol fraction block electron transport in the mitochondria and have shown activity against colon, breast, and lung cancer cells. Lapachol may also interact directly with nucleic acids, thereby blocking DNA replication. The beta-lapachone component of the extract stimulates lipid peroxidation, producing toxic derivatives that further weaken cell proliferation.

Herb is active against *Bacillus subtilis, Mycobacterium pyogenes aureus, Trypanosoma cruzi,* and certain viruses, such as herpesvirus, avian myeloblastosis, Rous sarcoma, and murine leukemia virus. Lapachol acts as a mild sedative; it has hypotensive action and may be blended with other decongestants.

USES
Used to treat ulcers, diarrhea, rheumatism, cancers, vaginal infections with *Candida albicans* or *Trichomonas vaginalis,* inflammation, and other infections, such as colds, flu, and bladder infections. Also used to kill vaginal parasites and to reduce fever and arthritis pain.

DOSAGE & ADMINISTRATION
Alcoholic tincture: 1.2 to 1.5 ml diluted in 4 ounces (118 ml) of warm water P.O. t.i.d.
Bark decoction: ½ to 1 cup taken once to t.i.d. Prepared by adding bark to 8 ounces (237 ml) of water, bringing to a boil, and simmering for 5 minutes.
Capsules: Average dose is 250 mg to 1 g P.O. Typically, 5 capsules = 2 cups of tea.
Colds and flu: 1 to 2 cups of tea daily as a preventive measure.

*Liquid contains alcohol.

Tea: Should be freshly prepared and taken at least b.i.d.

Vaginal infections: Gauze tampons soaked in the extract inserted vaginally and changed every 12 hours to heal swollen mucous membranes and kill parasites.

ADVERSE REACTIONS
GI: nausea, diarrhea.
Hematologic: anemia, anticoagulation.

INTERACTIONS
Herb-drug. *Disulfiram, metronidazole:* May cause a disulfiram-like reaction if herbal preparation contains alcohol. Advise patient to avoid using the herb and drug together.
Warfarin, other anticoagulants: May cause additive effect. Advise patient to avoid using the herb and drug together.
Herb-herb. *Yerba maté:* May potentiate pau d'arco products. Advise patient to avoid using the herbs together.

EFFECTS ON LAB TEST RESULTS
• May increase PT and INR.

CAUTIONS
Patients who are pregnant or breast-feeding or who have a thyroid or hematologic disorder shouldn't use this herb.

NURSING CONSIDERATIONS
• Explore patient's knowledge of this herb.
• Tinctures and extracts typically contain between 15% and 60% alcohol and may be unsuitable for children, patients with a history of alcoholism or liver disease, or patients taking certain drugs.
• Overdose may alter blood values. Advise patients with anemia and those whose WBC count changes during herb treatment to stop taking the herb.
• Monitor patient's thyroid function because the lapachol component can interfere with the body's use of iodine.
• Adverse reactions usually occur at higher-than-recommended doses.
• Herb may act against vitamin K, causing signs and symptoms of anemia.

PATIENT TEACHING
• Advise patient to consult a health care provider before using an herbal preparation because another treatment may be available.
• Tell patient that when filling a new prescription he should inform pharmacist of any herbal or dietary supplement he's taking.
• Tinctures and extracts typically contain between 15% and 60% alcohol and may be unsuitable for children, patients with a history of alcoholism or liver disease, or patients taking certain drugs.
• Duration of treatment may exceed 3 weeks but is usually shorter than 6 months. One manufacturer warns that product shouldn't be used more than 7 days.
• Advise patient with a thyroid problem to consult his health care provider before taking the herb. The lapachol component may interfere with absorption of iodine. If patient chooses to use the herb, advise him to have his thyroid function checked regularly.

Bold italic type indicates that reaction may be life-threatening.

• Warn patient to keep all herbal products away from children and pets.

peach

Prunus persica, amygdalin, laetrile, vitamin B_{17}

Common trade names
Laetrile, Vitamin B_{17}

AVAILABLE FORMS
Available as persic oil, peach kernel oil, seeds, dried bark, leaves, and flowers.

ACTIONS & COMPONENTS
Obtained from *P. persica.* Mechanism of action is unknown. Contains cyanogenic glycosides (amygdalin), volatile oils that are carminatives and GI irritants, and phloretin. A 1-g peach seed also contains about 2.6 mg of hydrocyanic acid. Phloretin may have antibacterial activity against gram-positive and gram-negative organisms.

USES
Used for constipation, cough, bad breath, blisters, boils, bronchitis, bruises, burns, dysentery, earache, eczema, edema, headache, hemorrhage, hypertension, tetanus, menstrual pain, minor wounds, nervousness, pain, pinworm, tapeworm, pneumonia, scurvy, shingles, skin irritation and inflammation, sore throat, stomach upset, warts, and kidney or liver problems. In the past, peach seed was thought to be a cancer remedy, but National Cancer Institute studies failed to show clinical effectiveness.
⚡**ALERT:** Laetrile (also known as amygdalin, or vitamin B_{17}) was touted as an anticarcinogenic but is banned by the FDA because of its high cyanide content and potential for overdosing or poisoning.

DOSAGE & ADMINISTRATION
Indigestion and bladder inflammation: Tea is prepared from ½ ounce dried bark or 1 ounce dried leaves in 16 ounces (473 ml) boiling water, steeped for 15 minutes, then taken t.i.d.
Sores and wounds: Peach leaves are applied as a poultice, p.r.n.

ADVERSE REACTIONS
CNS: peripheral neuropathy.
EENT: hearing loss.
Musculoskeletal: muscle spasms.
Other: *cyanide poisoning.*

INTERACTIONS
None reported.

EFFECTS ON LAB TEST RESULTS
None reported.

CAUTIONS
Patients who are pregnant or who are sensitive to the herb shouldn't use it. Anyone who uses the herb should do so with caution because the seeds contain cyanogenic glycosides.

NURSING CONSIDERATIONS
• Explore patient's knowledge of this herb.
⚡**ALERT:** Monitor patient for signs and symptoms of cyanide poisoning, such as vomiting, se-

---

*Liquid contains alcohol.

vere stomach pain, fainting, drowsiness, seizures, or coma.
• If cyanide toxicity is suspected, give sodium thiosulfate immediately, and obtain laboratory confirmation of cyanide levels.

PATIENT TEACHING
• Warn patient that laetrile is banned by the FDA and that high doses or long-term use of the seeds could cause cyanide poisoning.
• Review with patient signs and symptoms of cyanide poisoning, such as vomiting, severe stomach pain, fainting, drowsiness, seizures, and coma.
• Warn patient to keep all herbal products away from children and pets.

pennyroyal

Mentha pulegium, American pennyroyal, European pennyroyal, lurk-in-the-ditch, mosquito plant, piliolerial, pudding grass, pulegium, run-by-the-ground, squaw balm, squawmint tickweed

Common trade names
Pennyroyal, Pennyroyal Extract, Pennyroyal Tea

AVAILABLE FORMS
Available as tea, tincture*, loose dried herb, and capsules.

ACTIONS & COMPONENTS
Leaves and flowering tops contain pennyroyal oil. The oil contains *D*-pulegione (60% to 90%), methone, isomethone, tannins, and flavonoids. Pulegione depletes glutathione in the liver.

USES
Used for digestive disorders, liver and gallbladder disorders, bowel disorders, pneumonia, gout, and colds. Used topically for skin diseases. Also used as an abortifacient (in high doses), insect repellent, antiseptic, flavoring agent, and fragrance in detergents, soaps, and perfumes.

DOSAGE & ADMINISTRATION
Dried herb: 1 to 4 g P.O. t.i.d.
Insect repellent: Oil is applied sparingly to skin, p.r.n.
Tea: 1 cup P.O. daily.

ADVERSE REACTIONS
CNS: lethargy, delirium, unconsciousness, *seizures,* hallucinations.
CV: hypertension, tachycardia.
GI: abdominal pain, nausea, vomiting.
GU: irreversible renal damage.
Hematologic: *DIC.*
Hepatic: *hepatotoxicity, liver damage.*
Skin: dermatitis.
Other: *shock.*

INTERACTIONS
Herb-drug. *Disulfiram, metronidazole:* May cause a disulfiram-like reaction if herbal preparation contains alcohol. Advise patient to avoid using the herb and drug together.

EFFECTS ON LAB TEST RESULTS
• May increase liver enzyme, BUN, and creatinine levels. May alter electrolyte levels.

Bold italic type indicates that reaction may be life-threatening.

• May alter CBC and coagulation studies.

CAUTIONS
Patients who are pregnant or breast-feeding or who have liver or kidney disease shouldn't use this herb.

NURSING CONSIDERATIONS
• Explore patient's knowledge of this herb.

🔲 **ALERT:** Drinking 5 g of oil to induce abortion or drinking the alcoholic extract repeatedly over 2 weeks has resulted in severe poisoning. Overdose may cause vomiting, hypertension, anesthetic-like paralysis, and respiratory failure.

• Tinctures and extracts typically contain between 15% and 60% alcohol and may be unsuitable for children, patients with a history of alcoholism or liver disease, or patients taking certain drugs.

PATIENT TEACHING
• Advise patient to consult a health care provider before using an herbal preparation because another treatment may be available.

• Tell patient that when filling a new prescription he should inform pharmacist of any herbal or dietary supplement he's taking.

• Caution patient against consuming herb because of its toxic effects on the liver. If he takes herb internally, tell him to do so only under the close supervision of a health care provider.

• Warn patient to use the oil as a flavoring only in small amounts.

• If patient is pregnant, advise her not to use the herb because it may induce abortion.

• Although no chemical interactions have been reported in clinical studies, advise patient that herb may interfere with therapeutic effects of conventional drugs.

• Warn patient to keep all herbal products away from children and pets.

pepper, black

Piper nigrum, pepper bark, pimenta, piper

Common trade names
None known

AVAILABLE FORMS
Available as dried berries, powder, and ointment for external use.

ACTIONS & COMPONENTS
Obtained from berries of *P. nigrum.* The shell is removed, and the green fruit is sun-dried or roasted. This yields volatile oils (1.2% to 2.6%), limonene (15% to 20%), sabinene (15% to 25%), caryophyllene (10% to 15%), betaphinene (10% to 12%), alpha-pinene (8% to 12%), acid amides (pungent substances), and fatty oils. Pepper stimulates thermal receptors and increases secretion of saliva and gastric mucus. May have abortifacient, analgesic, diaphoretic, diuretic, sedative, emetic, hypnotic, mydriatic, narcotic, sudorific, insecticidal, and antimicrobial effects.

USES
Used for constipation, gonorrhea, dyspepsia, colic, headache, cholera, diarrhea, scarlatina, paralytic disorders, asthma, bronchitis,

---

*Liquid contains alcohol.

delirium, dysmenorrhea, insomnia, pertussis, tuberculosis, flatulence, nausea, vertigo, and arthritic conditions. Also used to ease signs and symptoms of nicotine withdrawal during smoking cessation. Used externally for neuralgia and scabies. Used extensively as a domestic spice and flavoring ingredient.

DOSAGE & ADMINISTRATION
Scabies: Ointment applied externally, p.r.n.
To improve digestive function: 1.5 g P.O. daily; divided doses 0.3 to 0.6 g P.O. per dose.

ADVERSE REACTIONS
CNS: tremors, numbness.
EENT: eye irritation, mucous membrane irritation, salivation.
GI: nausea, gastric pain.
Skin: irritation, sweating.

INTERACTIONS
Herb-drug. *Drugs metabolized by cytochrome P-450 system, such as acetaminophen, erythromycin, ibuprofen, ketoconazole, naproxen:* May reduce drug effect. Monitor patient, and advise him to avoid using the herb and drug together.
Phenobarbital, phenytoin, propranolol, rifampin, theophylline: May increase absorption. Monitor patient closely for adverse reactions and signs and symptoms of toxicity. Advise patient to avoid using the herb and drug together.
Warfarin: May alter drug metabolism. Monitor INR closely to maintain therapeutic value. Advise patient to avoid using the herb and drug together.

EFFECTS ON LAB TEST RESULTS
• May increase phenytoin, propranolol, and theophylline levels.
• May alter INR.

CAUTIONS
Patients who are pregnant or sensitive to black pepper shouldn't use it.

NURSING CONSIDERATIONS
• Explore patient's knowledge of this herb.
• Black pepper is an irritant when inhaled or allowed into the eyes. If black pepper gets into the eyes, they should be flushed with water to lessen the irritation.
• Exceeding recommended internal dose may cause GI irritation.
• No health hazards or adverse effects have been reported with proper use of standard amounts.

PATIENT TEACHING
• Advise patient to consult a health care provider before using an herbal preparation because another treatment may be available.
• Tell patient that when filling a new prescription he should inform pharmacist of any herbal or dietary supplement he's taking.
• Advise patient to be careful of nasal or eye irritation if using powder.
• Tell patient not to exceed recommended amounts without consulting his health care provider. Explain that higher-than-recommended amounts can cause GI irritation.

Bold italic type indicates that reaction may be life-threatening.

peppermint

Mentha x piperita, Menthae piperitae folium (leaves), *Menthae piperitae aetheroleum* (oil), brandy mint, lamb mint

Common trade names
Peppermint Capsules, Peppermint Plus Menthoril, Peppermint Tea

AVAILABLE FORMS
Available as essential oil, ointment, liniment, extract, tincture*, leaves, dried herb, and capsules.
Aqueous alcohol preparation: 5% to 10% essential oil
Enteric-coated capsules: 0.2/ 0.02 ml
Ointment: 1% to 5% essential oil
Semisolid and oily preparations: 5% to 20% essential oil
Tincture: 1:10

ACTIONS & COMPONENTS
Obtained from dried leaves and flowering branch tips of *Mentha x piperita*. The oil contains more than 100 components, including menthol (29% to 48%), methyl acetate (3% to 10%), menthone (20% to 31%), caffeic acid, azulene, and flavonoids. Actions include antibacterial, antiviral, and spasmolytic effects on smooth muscles. When taken as enteric-coated capsules, peppermint oil may have antispasmodic effects on smooth muscle of the intestines; antispasmodic activity results from calcium antagonist effect of menthol. Flavonoids may cause bile-stimulating effect. Azulene may have anti-inflammatory and antiulcerative action.

USES
Used for irritable bowel syndrome, colitis, ileitis, Crohn's disease, and other spasmodic conditions of the bowel. Also used for liver and gallbladder complaints, cramps of the upper GI tract and bile ducts, menstrual cramps, colds and flu, inflammation of the oral and pharyngeal mucosa, loss of appetite, dyspepsia, flatulence, and gastritis. Used externally for myalgia, neuralgia, itching, and skin irritation. Oil is applied to forehead to relieve tension and migraine headaches.

DOSAGE & ADMINISTRATION
Dry normalized extract: 0.44 to 0.57 g P.O. b.i.d. or t.i.d.
Enteric-coated capsules: 0.6 ml of essential oil in enteric-coated capsules P.O. daily for irritable bowel syndrome.
Essential oil: 0.2 ml P.O. daily.
Fluidextract: 2 ml P.O. b.i.d. or t.i.d.
Infusion: 2 g dried leaf in 5 ounces (150 ml) of water P.O. b.i.d. or t.i.d.; 3 to 6 g daily of cut leaf for infusions and extracts.
Liniment: 5% to 20% essential oil in vegetable oil, applied with friction to area of joint or bone pain.
Nasal ointment: 1% to 5% essential oil, applied topically, p.r.n.
Ointment: 5% to 20% essential oil in petroleum or lanolin used topically, p.r.n.
Tincture: 2 to 3 ml P.O. t.i.d. For topical use, aqueous-alcoholic preparation of 5% to 10% essential oil.

ADVERSE REACTIONS
CNS: headache.
CV: flushing.

*Liquid contains alcohol.

EENT: spasm of tongue, eye irritation, *glottal spasm.*
GI: gastroesophageal reflux.
Respiratory: *bronchospasm, respiratory arrest.*
Skin: contact dermatitis or inflammation (with the oil), irritation.
Other: allergic reaction.

INTERACTIONS
Herb-drug. *Antacids, H_2 antagonists:* Increases gastric pH and possible premature dissolution of enteric-coated capsules. Tell patient to take enteric-coated capsules on an empty stomach.
Calcium channel blockers, such as amlodipine, bepridil, diltiazem, felodipine, isradipine, nicardipine, nifedipine, nimodipine, nitrendipine, verapamil: Decreases drug effects. Monitor patient closely.

EFFECTS ON LAB TEST RESULTS
None reported.

CAUTIONS
Patients with gallstones, obstructed bile ducts, gallbladder inflammation, or severe liver damage shouldn't take this herb. Peppermint oil shouldn't be applied to the face or nasal passages of infants or children because of the risks of tongue spasms and respiratory arrest.

NURSING CONSIDERATIONS
• Explore patient's knowledge of this herb.
• If patient has a hiatal hernia, monitor him closely because peppermint weakens the esophageal sphincters.

• When the herb is being used to treat irritable bowel syndrome or another intestinal disorder, the enteric-coated capsule must be used; otherwise, the peppermint oil will not reach the intestines in its active form.

PATIENT TEACHING
• Advise patient to consult a health care provider before using an herbal preparation because another treatment may be available.
• Tell patient that when filling a new prescription he should inform pharmacist of any herbal or dietary supplement he's taking.
• Advise parents not to use peppermint oil on an infant's or child's face, especially around nose openings, because it may cause glottal or bronchial spasm.
• If patient has a hiatal hernia, advise him to contact his health care provider before using peppermint internally.
• If patient is taking peppermint for irritable bowel syndrome or another bowel disorder, make sure he's using the enteric-coated capsules.
• Stress that patient should consult his health care provider if symptoms don't improve in a reasonable length of time.
• Warn patient that using peppermint oil on the skin may cause inflammation.
• Warn patient to keep all herbal products away from children and pets.

Bold italic type indicates that reaction may be life-threatening.

peyote

Lophophora williamsii, devil's root, dumpling cactus, mescal buttons, mescaline, pellote, sacred mushroom

Common trade names
None known

AVAILABLE FORMS
Available as buttons, extracts, and tinctures.

ACTIONS & COMPONENTS
Root and hair tufts of the cactus *L. williamsii* are removed and the mescaline-rich center is sliced and dried, making mescaline buttons. A button contains up to 7% mescaline (trimethoxyphenethylamine), the main active ingredient. It has an emetic and hallucinogenic effect. Mescaline may cause visual, auditory, gustatory, kinesthetic, and synesthetic hallucinations.

USES
Peyote isn't currently used as a medicinal herb. It's illegally used for its psychogenic and hallucinogenic effects.

DOSAGE & ADMINISTRATION
No dosages are available for internal ingestion.

ADVERSE REACTIONS
CNS: visual, aural, kinesthetic, and synesthetic hallucinations.
CV: hypotension, *bradycardia,* vasodilation.
GI: nausea, vomiting.
Respiratory: *bronchospasm, respiratory depression.*

INTERACTIONS
Herb-drug. *Drugs with sedative properties:* Increases sedation. Advise patient not to take the herb.

EFFECTS ON LAB TEST RESULTS
None reported.

CAUTIONS
Peyote is categorized as controlled substance schedule I and has no proven medicinal use.

NURSING CONSIDERATIONS
• Explore patient's knowledge of this herb.
🗹 **ALERT:** Mescaline doses above 20 mg may cause hypotension, bradycardia, vasodilation, and respiratory depression. Nausea and vomiting may occur 30 to 60 minutes after ingestion.
• Peyote has no medicinal value. It's ingested illegally for its hallucinogenic effects.

PATIENT TEACHING
• Warn patient that the herb shouldn't be taken for any reason.
• If the patient chooses to take the herb, advise him not to perform activities that require mental alertness.
• Warn patient to keep all herbal products away from children and pets.

*Liquid contains alcohol.

pill-bearing spurge

Euphorbia pilulifera, asthma weed, Euphorbia, garden spurge, milkweed, snakeweed

Common trade names
None known

AVAILABLE FORMS
Available as dried herb, extract*, and tincture*.
Liquid extract: 1:1 in 45% alcohol
Tincture: 1:5 in 50% alcohol

ACTIONS & COMPONENTS
Contains 0.4% of a glycosidal substance, tannin, fatty acids, phorbic acid, sterols, euphosterol, jambulol, melissic acid, and sugars.

USES
Used for upper respiratory catarrh, bronchial asthma, bronchitis, laryngeal spasm, and intestinal amebiasis.

DOSAGE & ADMINISTRATION
Dried herb: 120 to 300 mg infusion P.O.
Liquid extract: 0.12 to 0.3 ml P.O.
Tincture: 0.6 to 2 ml P.O.

ADVERSE REACTIONS
GI: nausea, vomiting.
Respiratory: *respiratory failure.*
Skin: contact dermatitis.

INTERACTIONS
Herb-drug. *ACE inhibitors, such as clonidine, enalapril, and quinapril:* Potentiates hypotension. Monitor patient's blood pressure closely. Advise patient to avoid using the herb and drug together.

Anticholinergics, such as atropine, ipratropium, and scopolamine: Decreases drug effect. Advise patient to avoid using the herb and drug together.
Anticholinesterases, such as donepezil and edrophonium: Causes additive effect. Monitor patient for adverse reactions. Advise patient to avoid using the herb and drug together.
Arecoline, methacholine, muscarine, and muscarinic agonists: Causes additive effect. Monitor patient for adverse reactions. Advise patient to avoid using the herb and drug together.
Disulfiram, metronidazole: May cause a disulfiram-like reaction if herbal preparation contains alcohol. Advise patient to avoid using the herb and drug together.
Drugs metabolized by the CYP3A enzyme system, such as cyclosporine and erythromycin: Decreases absorption. Advise patient to avoid using the herb and drug together.
Barbiturates, such as phenobarbital: Increases central hypnotic effects. Advise patient to avoid using the herb and drug together.
Warfarin: Potentiates effect. Monitor patient's INR. Advise patient to avoid using the herb and drug together.

EFFECTS ON LAB TEST RESULTS
None reported.

CAUTIONS
Patients who are pregnant or breast-feeding shouldn't use this herb. Pill-bearing spurge may decrease platelet aggregation, so al-

---

Bold italic type indicates that reaction may be life-threatening.

coholic patients, patients who take an anticoagulant, and patients with bleeding a disorder or liver disease should use it cautiously.

NURSING CONSIDERATIONS
- Explore patient's knowledge of this herb.
- The FDA doesn't recognize this herb as a safe and effective treatment for asthma.
- The tincture and extract contain more than 40% alcohol and so may be unsuitable for children, patients with a history of alcoholism or liver disease, or patients taking certain drugs.

PATIENT TEACHING
- Advise patient to consult a health care provider before using an herbal preparation because another treatment may be available.
- Tell patient that when filling a new prescription he should inform pharmacist of any herbal or dietary supplement he's taking.
- If patient has a history of alcoholism or liver disease, inform him that some herbal products contain alcohol.
- If patient has a bleeding disorder and takes an anticoagulant, tell him not to take herb without consulting his health care provider.
- Warn patient to keep all herbal products away from children and pets.

pineapple

Ananas comosus, bromelainum, pineapple enzyme

Common trade names
Ananas, Bromelain, Mega Bromelain

AVAILABLE FORMS
Available as capsules, syrup, extracts, juices, candy, and whole fruit.

ACTIONS & COMPONENTS
Contains bromelain, a proteolytic enzyme used commercially as a meat tenderizer and medically for its soft tissue anti-inflammatory effect. Bromelain prolongs PT and bleeding time because it enhances fibrinolytic activity. It also lowers serum bradykinin and kininogen levels. It may influence prostaglandin synthesis, thus explaining its effect in burn debridement and wound healing. It's also active against nematodes and may reduce the risk of cancer.

USES
Used for acute postoperative and posttraumatic swelling, especially in nasal and paranasal sinuses. When combined with trypsin, amylase, and lipase enzymes, it's used for dyspepsia and exocrine hepatic insufficiency. Also used for constipation, jaundice, edema, inflammation, and wound debridement.

DOSAGE & ADMINISTRATION
Capsules: For acute postoperative or posttraumatic swelling, 80 to

*Liquid contains alcohol.

320 mg P.O. b.i.d. to t.i.d. for 8 to 10 days unless instructed otherwise.

ADVERSE REACTIONS
GI: nausea, vomiting, diarrhea, stomatitis.
GU: menorrhagia, uterine contractions.
Skin: rash, loss of fingerprints after prolonged contact.
Other: allergic reaction.

INTERACTIONS
Herb-drug. *ACE inhibitors, such as clonidine, enalapril, and quinapril:* May alter bradykinin levels. Monitor patient. Advise patient to avoid using the herb and drug together.
Tetracycline: Increases plasma and urine drug levels. Advise patient to avoid using the herb and drug together.
Warfarin and other anticoagulants, antiplatelets: Potentiates effect. Advise patient to avoid using the herb and drug together.

EFFECTS ON LAB TEST RESULTS
None reported.

CAUTIONS
Patients who are pregnant or intend to become pregnant, who take an anticoagulant, or who are sensitive to pineapple shouldn't use this herb.

NURSING CONSIDERATIONS
• Explore patient's knowledge of this herb.
• Fruit packers who cut pineapple have reported a loss of their fingerprints because of bromelain's keratolytic effects.

PATIENT TEACHING
• Advise patient to consult a health care provider before using an herbal preparation because another treatment may be available.
• Tell patient that when filling a new prescription he should inform pharmacist of any herbal or dietary supplement he's taking.
• If patient is taking an anticoagulant, advise him not to take this herb because it thins the blood.
• Caution patient not to combine pineapple and aspirin.
• Advise patients taking tetracycline not to use pineapple unless advised by his health care provider.
• Warn patient not to take pineapple for constipation, inflammation, or swelling before seeking medical attention, because doing so may delay diagnosis of a potentially serious medical condition.
• Warn patient to keep all herbal products away from children and pets.

pipsissewa

Chimaphila umbellata, bitter wintergreen, butter winter, ground holly, King's cure, love in winter, Prince's pine, rheumatism weed, wintergreen

Common trade names
Pipsissewa

AVAILABLE FORMS
Available as decoction, tincture, extract, and syrup.

ACTIONS & COMPONENTS
Obtained from aboveground parts of *C. umbellata.* Active components include ericolin, chimaphilin, ursolic acid, tannin, gallic acid, and arbutin, a hydroquinone glycoside. Arbutin and chimaphilin are reported to function as urinary antiseptics. May also have hypoglycemic activity.

USES
Used to treat tuberculosis of the lymph nodes, cardiac and kidney disease, chronic gonorrhea, catarrh of the bladder, gallstones, kidney stones, and ascites. Combined with other treatments, herb is used for dropsy. Used topically to redden the skin. Also used as a diuretic and astringent, and as a flavoring agent in beverages.

DOSAGE & ADMINISTRATION
Syrup: 1 to 2 tablespoons, as directed, P.O.
Tincture: 1 to 5 grains per dose, P.O.
Tubercular sores: Decoction applied topically to external sores, p.r.n.

ADVERSE REACTIONS
Hepatic: *hepatotoxicity.*
Skin: redness, vesication, irritation.

INTERACTIONS
None reported.

EFFECTS ON LAB TEST RESULTS
• May increase liver enzyme levels.

CAUTIONS
Patients who are pregnant or breast-feeding shouldn't use this herb. Pipsissewa contains the hydroquinone glycoside arbutin; therefore, it isn't recommended for long-term use because of risk of hepatotoxicity.

NURSING CONSIDERATIONS
• Explore patient's knowledge of this herb.
• Although no chemical interactions have been reported in clinical studies, advise patient that herb may interfere with therapeutic effects of conventional drugs.
• Topical application may cause skin irritation, redness, and vesication.

PATIENT TEACHING
• Advise patient to consult a health care provider before using an herbal preparation because another treatment may be available.
• Tell patient that when filling a new prescription he should inform pharmacist of any herbal or dietary supplement he's taking.
• Advise patient not to take this herb internally for prolonged periods because of potential liver damage.
• Tell patient that applying herb on the skin may cause irritation.
• Warn patient to keep all herbal products away from children and pets.

plantain

Plantago lanceolata, P. ovata, P. psyllium, black psyllium, blond plantago, broad leaf plantain, common plantain, flea seed, French psyllium, greater plantain, Indian plantago, lance leaf plantain, narrow leaf plantain, psyllium seed, ribwort plantain, Spanish psyllium

Common trade names
Effer-Syllium, Ground Psyllium, Hydrocil, Konsyl, Metamucil, Perdiem, Psyllium, Psyllium Seed

AVAILABLE FORMS
Available as powder, seeds, extract, infusion, pressed juice, and poultice.
Extract: 1 g:1 ml

ACTIONS & COMPONENTS
Obtained from seed of *P. ovata, P. psyllium,* and other species. When seeds are mixed with water, a mucilaginous mass is formed. Seeds provide bulk to aid in treating constipation while the mucilage—2% to 6% of glucomannans, arabinogalactane, and rhamnogalacturontane—acts as a mild laxative. Taken in dry form, it decreases intestinal motility and is useful in treating diarrhea and irritable bowel syndrome. Plantain also contains aglycone and aucubigenin, which give psyllium an antimicrobial action. Cholesterol-lowering action is caused by a polyphenolic compound contained in the herb.

USES
Used as a bulk-forming laxative for constipation. For irritable bow-el syndrome or diarrhea, plantain is taken with a small amount of water to decrease intestinal motility. Regular use may slightly reduce cholesterol levels. Also used internally to treat respiratory tract catarrh and oropharyngeal inflammation, and topically to treat skin inflammation.

DOSAGE & ADMINISTRATION
Compress: Applied to affected area, p.r.n. Prepared by soaking 1.4 g cut herb in 5 ounces (148 ml) of cold water for 1 to 2 hours, stirring often.
Infusion: 1 cup P.O. t.i.d. to q.i.d. Prepared by steeping 1.4 g of herb in 5 ounces (148 ml) of boiled water for 10 to 15 minutes.
Powder: 3 to 6 g P.O. daily.
Rinse or gargle: Swished t.i.d. to q.i.d.; not swallowed. Prepared by soaking 1.4 g cut herb in 5 ounces (148 ml) cold water for 1 to 2 hours, stirring often.
Tincture (1 g:5 ml): 7 ml P.O. t.i.d. to q.i.d.

ADVERSE REACTIONS
EENT: watery eyes.
GI: diarrhea, flatulence, constipation, *GI obstruction (if consumed without water).*
Respiratory: sneezing, chest congestion.
Other: allergic reaction, *anaphylaxis.*

INTERACTIONS
Herb-drug. *Calcium, feosol, iron supplements, vitamin B$_{12}$, zinc:* Decreases absorption of these vitamin and mineral supplements. Advise patient to take the supple-

---

Bold italic type indicates that reaction may be life-threatening.

ments either 1 hour before or 4 hours after plantain.

Carbamazepine, digoxin, lithium, warfarin: Decreases absorption. Advise patient to avoid using the herb and drug together.

Oral drugs: May decrease absorption. Advise patient to take all oral drugs 1 hour before or 4 hours after plantain.

EFFECTS ON LAB TEST RESULTS
• May decrease postprandial glucose, total cholesterol, and LDL cholesterol levels.

CAUTIONS
Patients who are sensitive to plantain products shouldn't use this herb.

NURSING CONSIDERATIONS
• Explore patient's knowledge of this herb.
• Plantain should be taken with plenty of fluids to avoid constipation because the herb removes liquid from the GI tract.

ALERT: Don't confuse the herb plantain with the edible plantain or banana, *Musa paradisiacal.*

PATIENT TEACHING
• Advise patient to consult a health care provider before using an herbal preparation because another treatment may be available.
• Tell patient that when filling a new prescription he should inform pharmacist of any herbal or dietary supplement he's taking.
• Advise patient to not use this product if he has trouble swallowing.
• If patient is taking lithium, carbamazepine, digoxin, or warfarin, ad-

vise him to consult his health care provider before taking plantain.
• If patient is using the herb as a bulk laxative, warn him to drink plenty of fluids with each dose to prevent his constipation from worsening.
• Inform patient that if allergic signs and symptoms occur, including sneezing, itching, and swollen eyes, he should stop using product and consult his health care provider.

pokeweed

Phytolacca americana, American nightshade, American spinach, bear's grape, branching phytolacca, cancerroot, cankerroot, coakumchongras, crowberry, garget, inkberry, jalap, pigeon berry, poke, poke berry, red-ink plant, scoke, Virginian poke

Common trade names
Pokeweed

AVAILABLE FORMS
Available as powder, liquid, extract*, and tincture.

ACTIONS & COMPONENTS
Contains triterpene, saponins, esculinic acid, and pokeweed mitogen. Mechanisms of action aren't known. Pokeweed mitogen has been linked to blood cell abnormalities. Extracts containing pokeweed mitogens may alter T and B lymphocytes. May also have antiinflammatory, antirheumatic, and digestive activity.

*Liquid contains alcohol.

USES
Used as an emetic because of its saponin content. Under investigation for its antiviral effects in flu, herpes simplex virus type I, and polio. Also used to treat rheumatism, cough, tonsillitis, itching, laryngitis, and swollen glands. Berries are used as a food coloring. Young spring plant shoots are used as an edible vegetable, but only after careful boiling.

DOSAGE & ADMINISTRATION
Emetic: 60 to 300 mg of dried root P.O.
Extract (1:1 in 45% alcohol): 0.1 to 0.5 ml P.O.

ADVERSE REACTIONS
CNS: dizziness, somnolence, ***seizures.***
CV: hypotension, tachycardia.
GI: nausea, vomiting, severe stomach cramping, diarrhea.
Respiratory: ***bronchospasm, apnea.***

INTERACTIONS
Herb-drug. *Disulfiram, metronidazole:* May cause a disulfiram-like reaction if herbal preparation contains alcohol. Advise patient to avoid using the herb and drug together.

EFFECTS ON LAB TEST RESULTS
None reported.

CAUTIONS
Roots, berries, and purple bark of stems are poisonous. Because of its high toxicity, this herb shouldn't be used for any medical conditions. The FDA has classified pokeweed as an herb of undefined safety with demonstrated narcotic effects.

NURSING CONSIDERATIONS
• Explore patient's knowledge of this herb.
⚡**ALERT:** Even properly prepared, pokeweed has caused toxicity. Signs and symptoms of poisoning or overdose include dizziness, nausea, vomiting, diarrhea, and stomach cramps. Mild overdose usually subsides within 24 hours, but severe poisoning may last up to 48 hours. Gastric decontamination and symptomatic and supportive treatment have been suggested. Death has been reported.
• Because pokeweed mitogens can alter blood cells, gloves should be worn when handling this herb.
• Tinctures and extracts typically contain between 15% and 60% alcohol and may be unsuitable for children, patients with a history of alcoholism or liver disease, or patients taking certain drugs.

PATIENT TEACHING
• Caution patient not to consume any part of this herb because it's highly toxic.
• Warn patient to keep all herbal products away from children and pets.

Bold italic type indicates that reaction may be life-threatening.

pomegranate

Punica granatum, grenadier

Common trade names
Pomegranate

AVAILABLE FORMS
Available as juice, powder, and bark extract.

ACTIONS & COMPONENTS
Obtained from flowers, stems, bark, rind, and rhizomes of *P. granatum.* Contains tannins (20% to 25%) and piperidine alkaloids (0.4%). Piperidine alkaloids are the basis for use in treating tapeworm. Tannins may be beneficial in treating hemorrhoids when applied externally.

USES
Used to treat tapeworm and other worm infestations. Also used as a gargle rinse for sore throat and topically for hemorrhoids. Herb may have abortifacient properties.

DOSAGE & ADMINISTRATION
Hemorrhoids: Juice or extract applied topically, p.r.n.
Tapeworm: 20 g of bark juice extract P.O. as a single dose. Or, prepared by adding 60 parts herb and 400 parts water, then macerating for 12 hours to half initial volume. 65 ml of extract instilled via duodenal probe every 30 minutes for three doses, followed by a laxative 1 hour after the third dose.

ADVERSE REACTIONS
CNS: dizziness, chills.
CV: *circulatory collapse with overdose.*

EENT: vision disorders.
GI: gastric irritation, vomiting.
Respiratory: *apnea with overdose.*

INTERACTIONS
None reported.

EFFECTS ON LAB TEST RESULTS
None reported.

CAUTIONS
Patients who are pregnant or breast-feeding shouldn't use this herb.

NURSING CONSIDERATIONS
• Explore patient's knowledge of this herb.
• Although no chemical interactions have been reported in clinical studies, advise patient that herb may interfere with therapeutic effects of conventional drugs.
• Patients who use pomegranate to treat tapeworm need medical supervision and proper follow-up.
☑ ALERT: Overdoses of rind, stem, or root may lead to vomiting (possibly bloody), dizziness, chills, visual disturbances (including blindness), circulatory collapse, and death. Treatment includes gastric emptying by inducing vomiting (if patient is conscious) or performing gastric lavage and instilling activated charcoal. Provide supportive treatment for shock. Patient may need intubation and mechanical ventilation. Monitor renal function closely.

PATIENT TEACHING
• Advise patient to consult a health care provider before using an

---

*Liquid contains alcohol.

herbal preparation because another treatment may be available.

• Tell patient that when filling a new prescription he should inform pharmacist of any herbal or dietary supplement he's taking.

• Caution patient that consuming higher doses of pomegranate may cause respiratory, visual, and GI problems. Advise patient to seek medical attention from a health care provider immediately if any such signs or symptoms develop.

• Warn patient to keep all herbal products away from children and pets.

poplar

Populus alba, P. gileadensis, P. nigra, P. tremuloides, black poplar, Canadian poplar, European aspen, poplar bud (balm of Gilead buds), Populi cortex et folium, Populi gemma, quaking aspen, trembling poplar, white poplar

Common trade names
None known

AVAILABLE FORMS
Available as buds, ointment, extract*, powder, and dried bark (in combination products).

ACTIONS & COMPONENTS
Obtained from bark and leaves of *Populus* species. Contains essential oil, flavonoids, phenol glycosides, and salicylate glycosides. Volatile oil has expectorant properties. Leaves of *P. alba* may contain up to 6% of glycosides and esters that yield salicylic acid. Populus bark contains about 2% salicylate compounds such as salicortin and salicin. Salicylate compounds contribute to herb's analgesic, anti-inflammatory, and antispasmodic properties. Caffeic acid, found in poplar buds, provides antibacterial properties. Zinc lignins contained in poplar may have a beneficial effect on micturition in prostatic hyperplasia.

USES
Used to treat pain, rheumatism, respiratory tract infections, and micturition complaints in prostatic hyperplasia and to stimulate wound healing. Used topically for superficial skin injuries, external hemorrhoids, frostbite, and sunburn. Also used as an antiseptic and as a gargle for laryngitis.

DOSAGE & ADMINISTRATION
Dried bark: 1 to 4 g, or as a tea P.O. t.i.d.
Ground drug and galenic preparations of Populi cortex et folium: As directed. Maximum, 10 g daily.
Liquid bark extract (1:1 in 25% alcohol): 1 to 4 ml (20 to 80 gtt) P.O. t.i.d.
Topical, semisolid, or ointment preparations: Applied as directed.

ADVERSE REACTIONS
Hematologic: depression of clotting factors.
Skin: rash.

INTERACTIONS
Herb-drug. *Antarthritics, aspirin, warfarin:* May increase bleeding time. Monitor patient for signs and symptoms of bleeding. Advise patient to avoid using the herb and drug together.

Bold italic type indicates that reaction may be life-threatening.

Disulfiram, metronidazole: May cause a disulfiram-like reaction if herbal preparation contains alcohol. Advise patient to avoid using the herb and drug together.
Feosol and other iron supplements: May increase iron absorption. Advise patient to avoid using the herb and supplement together.

EFFECTS ON LAB TEST RESULTS
None reported.

CAUTIONS
Patients sensitive to poplar products, salicylates, or Peruvian balsam shouldn't take this herb. Patients with heart disease or a history of bleeding disorders should use this herb cautiously.

NURSING CONSIDERATIONS
● Explore patient's knowledge of this herb.
● If patient takes aspirin, an antarthritic, or an anticoagulant, closely monitor his PT and INR.
● Tinctures and extracts typically contain between 15% and 60% alcohol and may be unsuitable for children, patients with a history of alcoholism or liver disease, or patients taking certain drugs.

PATIENT TEACHING
● Advise patient to consult a health care provider before using an herbal preparation because another treatment may be available.
● Tell patient that when filling a new prescription he should inform pharmacist of any herbal or dietary supplement he's taking.
● If patient has a history of alcoholism or liver disease, inform

him that some herbal products contain alcohol.
● Tell patient to stop using topical preparation if it causes a rash or skin irritation.
● Inform patient that poplar contains aspirin-like compounds that can increase the risk of bleeding when taken orally with other drugs.
● Advise patient not to take iron supplements with poplar tea.

prickly ash

Zanthoxylum clava-herculis, Z. americanum, northern prickly ash, suterberry, toothache tree, yellow wood

Common trade names
Prickly Ash Autumn-Harvested

AVAILABLE FORMS
Available as extract*, tablets, dried bark, tincture*, and in various combination products.
Extract: 65% to 70% grain alcohol

ACTIONS & COMPONENTS
Obtained from bark and berries of the *Z. clava-herculis* tree. Contains pyranocoumarins, such as xanthoxyletin; isoquinoline alkaloids, including berberine and *N*-methylisocorydin; volatile oil; and resins. Prickly ash has anti-inflammatory, antirheumatic, diaphoretic, and circulatory stimulant properties.

USES
Used for cramps, hypotension, rheumatism, soreness, toothache, intermittent claudication, Reye's syndrome, fever, and inflammation. Also used topically for treat-

*Liquid contains alcohol.

ing indolent ulcers and wound healing.

DOSAGE & ADMINISTRATION
Dried bark: 1 to 2 g as a tea, P.O. t.i.d.
For toothache: Dried bark or berries, chewed p.r.n.
Liquid extract (1:1 in 45% alcohol): 1 to 3 ml (20 to 60 gtt) of extract in a little water P.O. t.i.d.
Tincture (1:5 in 45% alcohol): 2 to 5 ml (40 to 100 gtt) P.O. t.i.d.

ADVERSE REACTIONS
None reported.

INTERACTIONS
Herb-drug. *Antihypertensives:* May potentiate effect. Monitor blood pressure, and advise patient to avoid using the herb and drug together.
Disulfiram, metronidazole: May cause a disulfiram-like reaction if herbal preparation contains alcohol. Advise patient to avoid using the herb and drug together.
Iron supplements, such as ferrous sulfate: Decreases iron absorption. Advise patient to avoid using the herb and supplement together.
Scopolamine and other muscle relaxants: May potentiate effect. Advise patient to avoid using the herb and drug together.

EFFECTS ON LAB TEST RESULTS
None reported.

CAUTIONS
Patients who are pregnant or breast-feeding shouldn't use this herb. Patients with cardiac disease, especially those who take antihy-pertensives, should use the herb cautiously.

NURSING CONSIDERATIONS
● Explore patient's knowledge of this herb.
● If patient has cardiac disease or takes an antihypertensive, monitor vital signs, particularly blood pressure, during and after use of prickly ash.
● Some prickly ash extracts contain 65% to 70% grain alcohol and may be unsuitable for children, patients with a history of alcoholism or liver disease, or patients taking certain drugs.
🗲 **ALERT:** Don't confuse the true species of prickly ash trees *(Z. americanum, Z. clava-herculis, Z. fagara)* with Devil's walkingstick *(Aralia spinosa),* a shrub also commonly known as prickly ash.

PATIENT TEACHING
● Advise patient to consult a health care provider before using an herbal preparation because another treatment may be available.
● Tell patient that when filling a new prescription he should inform pharmacist of any herbal or dietary supplement he's taking.
● If patient has cardiac disease or takes blood pressure medication, tell him to monitor his blood pressure during and after use of prickly ash.
● If patient has a history of alcoholism or liver disease, warn him to avoid extracts because they may contain 65% to 70% grain alcohol.
● Tell patient to seek medical attention if his signs and symptoms worsen or last longer than 7 days.

Bold italic type indicates that reaction may be life-threatening.

- Warn patient to keep all herbal products away from children and pets.

pulsatilla

Anemone pulsatilla, Pulsatilla pratensis, P. vulgaris, Easter flower, meadow anemone, passe flower, pasque flower, pulsatillae herba, wild flower

Common trade names
Boiron Pulsatilla 9c, Pulsatilla 200ck, Pulsatilla Nig. 30c. Also available in combination products.

AVAILABLE FORMS
Available as dried herb, pellets, extracts*, tincture*, and tablets.

ACTIONS & COMPONENTS
Obtained from dried aboveground parts of *A. pulsatilla (P. vulgaris)* and *P. pratensis*. Contains protoanemonin, ranunculin, and degradation products of ranunculin, including anemonin, anemoninic acid, and anemonic acid. Protoanemonin may cause stimulation and paralysis of the CNS; its alkylating action may inhibit cell regeneration, leading to kidney irritation. Protoanemonin also has anti-infective activity. Abortion and birth defects have been reported among grazing animals who consumed large amounts of protoanemonin-containing plants.

USES
Used for inflammatory and infectious diseases of the skin and mucosa, diseases and functional disorders of the GI tract, and functional urogenital disorders. Also used for neuralgia, migraine, and general restlessness.

DOSAGE & ADMINISTRATION
Dried herb: 100 to 300 mg as a tea P.O. t.i.d.
Liquid extract (1:1 in 25% alcohol): 0.1 to 0.3 ml (2 to 6 gtt) P.O. t.i.d.
Oral tablets and pellets: P.O., as directed.
Tincture (1:10 in 40% alcohol): 0.5 to 3 ml (10 to 60 gtt) P.O. t.i.d.

ADVERSE REACTIONS
GI: irritation of mucous membranes, nausea, vomiting, abdominal pain, colic, diarrhea.
GU: irritation of kidneys and urinary tract.
Skin: rash.

INTERACTIONS
Drug-herb. *Disulfiram, metronidazole:* May cause a disulfiram-like reaction if herbal preparation contains alcohol. Advise patient to avoid using the herb and drug together.

EFFECTS ON LAB TEST RESULTS
- May alter urinalysis results.

CAUTIONS
Patients who are pregnant or breast-feeding shouldn't use this herb. Alcoholic patients and those with liver disease shouldn't use forms that contain alcohol.

NURSING CONSIDERATIONS
- Explore patient's knowledge of this herb.
- ⚠ALERT: Fresh pulsatilla plant parts can cause severe skin and mucosal irritation in susceptible

*Liquid contains alcohol.

patients. Irrigate affected area with dilute potassium permanganate solution, and then apply mucilage preparation. Overdose may cause renal and urinary tract irritation and severe stomach irritation with colic and diarrhea. Urge patient to go to the emergency department, where he may undergo gastric lavage with activated charcoal.
- Tinctures and extracts typically contain between 15% and 60% alcohol and may be unsuitable for children, patients with a history of alcoholism or liver disease, or patients taking certain drugs.

PATIENT TEACHING
- Advise patient to consult a health care provider before using an herbal preparation because a standard treatment that has been proven effective may be available.
- Tell patient that when filling a new prescription he should remind pharmacist of any herbal and dietary supplements he's taking.
- Tell patient that fresh pulsatilla is considered poisonous and shouldn't be ingested or placed on the skin. If patient uses pulsatilla, it should be dried.
- Warn patient that kidney and urinary tract irritation can occur at higher-than-recommended doses.
- Caution patients who are pregnant or planning pregnancy not to use this herb.
- Tell patients with liver disease or alcoholism to avoid forms that contain alcohol.
- Tell patient to consult his health care provider if signs or symptoms last longer than 7 days or if they worsen.

- Warn patient to keep all herbal products away from children and pets.

pumpkin

Cucurbita pepo, field pumpkin, pompion, semina cucurbitae, yellow pumpkin

Common trade names
None known

AVAILABLE FORMS
Available as extract and seeds.
Extract: Water, coconut glycerin, 12% to 15% certified organic alcohol

ACTIONS & COMPONENTS
Contains cucurbitacin, tocopherol, and selenium. Seeds contain fatty acids (50%). Curcubitacin may provide anthelmintic activity. Tocopherol and selenium may inhibit oxidative degradation of lipids, vitamins, hormones, and enzymes. Pumpkin also has anti-inflammatory, diuretic, antioxidative, and antiandrogenic actions. Delta-7 sterols in the fatty oils of the seeds may block dihydrotestosterone from androgen receptors and prevent hyperproliferation of prostate cells in an enlarged prostate.

USES
Used to treat irritable bladder, micturition problems associated with BPH stages I and II, childhood nocturnal enuresis, and intestinal worms. Also used as a diuretic.

Bold italic type indicates that reaction may be life-threatening.

DOSAGE & ADMINISTRATION

As a dietary supplement: 2 to 4 ml of liquid extract (56 to 112 gtt) P.O. t.i.d.

As a diuretic: 200 to 400 g of un-peeled seeds pounded or ground into a pulp. Mixed with milk and honey to form a porridge. Ingested on an empty stomach in 2 doses in the morning, followed by castor oil 2 to 3 hours later.

Whole and coarse-ground seeds: Average dose is 10 g of ground seeds P.O., half in the morning and half in the evening with 1 to 2 tea-spoons of fluid. Outer covering from hard seeds is removed before eating.

ADVERSE REACTIONS
None known.

INTERACTIONS
None known.

EFFECTS ON LAB TEST RESULTS
None reported.

CAUTIONS
Patients sensitive to pumpkin or its components shouldn't take this herb.

NURSING CONSIDERATIONS
• Explore patient's knowledge of this herb.
• Although no adverse reactions are known, diuretics may cause fluid and electrolyte imbalances. Monitor patient as appropriate.
• Monitor patient's renal status. Ir-ritable bladder signs and symp-toms may signal a more serious problem.

PATIENT TEACHING
• Advise patient to consult a health care provider before using an herbal preparation because another treatment may be available.
• Tell patient that when filling a new prescription he should inform pharmacist of any herbal or di-etary supplement he's taking.
• Inform patient that although pumpkin may relieve irritable bladder and urination problems caused by benign prostatic hyper-plasia stages I and II, the herb doesn't reduce prostate enlarge-ment, so he should use it only un-der the supervision of his health care provider.
• Advise patient to store pumpkin preparations away from light and moisture.
• Tell patient to contact his health care provider if signs or symptoms worsen or last longer than 7 days.
• Warn patient to keep all herbal products away from children and pets.

*Liquid contains alcohol.

Q

Queen Anne's lace

Daucus carota, bees' nest, bird's nest, carrot, wild carrot

Common trade names
None known

AVAILABLE FORMS
Available as tea, seeds, dried herb, infusion, oil, and liquid extract*.

ACTIONS & COMPONENTS
Obtained from all plant parts of *D. carota.* Contains a volatile oil that may have diuretic and hypotensive properties.

USES
Used for kidney stones, bladder infections, gout, and swollen joints. Seeds are used for flatulence, windy colic, hiccups, dysentery, renal calculi, bowel obstruction, edema, and chronic coughs. Poultices of roots are used for pain of cancerous ulcers.

DOSAGE & ADMINISTRATION
Dried herb: 2 to 4 g as a tea P.O. t.i.d.
Flatulence, windy colic, hiccups, dysentery, and chronic cough: ⅓ teaspoon of bruised seeds P.O., p.r.n.
Gout: Tea brewed from the whole root and taken P.O. b.i.d., in morning and evening.
Infusion: 1 ounce of herb in 1 pint of water. 1 wineglassful taken b.i.d., in morning and evening.

Liquid extract (1:1 in 25% alcohol): 2 to 4 ml (40 to 80 gtt) P.O. t.i.d.
Seeds: ⅓ to 1 teaspoon P.O. p.r.n.

ADVERSE REACTIONS
GU: renal irritation.
Skin: rash and photosensitivity reactions (with essential oil).

INTERACTIONS
Herb-drug. *Antihypertensives, cardiac drugs:* May cause additive effects. Monitor patient's blood pressure closely. Advise patient to avoid using the herb and drug together.
Disulfiram, metronidazole: May cause a disulfiram-like reaction if herbal preparation contains alcohol. Advise patient to avoid using the herb and drug together.
Herb-lifestyle. *Sun exposure:* May cause additive photosensitivity risk. Advise patient to wear protective clothing and sunscreen and to limit exposure to direct sunlight.

EFFECTS ON LAB TEST RESULTS
None reported.

CAUTIONS
Patients who are pregnant or breast-feeding shouldn't use this herb.

NURSING CONSIDERATIONS
• Explore patient's knowledge of this herb.
• Tinctures and extracts typically contain between 15% and 60% alcohol and may be unsuitable for children, patients with a history of

alcoholism or liver disease, or patients taking certain drugs.

PATIENT TEACHING
• Advise patient to consult a health care provider before using an herbal preparation because another treatment may be available.
• Tell patient that when filling a new prescription he should inform pharmacist of any herbal or dietary supplement he's taking.
• If patient has a history of alcoholism or liver disease, inform him that some herbal products contain alcohol.
• Advise patient to avoid using excessive amounts of the herb if she suspects or knows that she's pregnant or if she plans to become pregnant.
• Encourage patient to monitor his blood pressure during and after consuming Queen Anne's lace.
• Teach patient the symptoms of low blood pressure, including fatigue, light-headedness, and rapid heart rate.
• Inform patient that the essential oil may cause a rash and increase the risk of sunburn. Advise him to take precautions.
• Warn patient to keep all herbal products away from children and pets.

quince

Cydonia oblongata

Common trade names
None known

AVAILABLE FORMS
Available as powder, lotion, extract, fruit syrup, and *Decoctum*

Cydoniae, B.P. (decoction from seeds).

ACTIONS & COMPONENTS
Obtained from fruits and seeds of *C. oblongata.* Fresh fruits and syrup have astringent properties. Seeds contain mucilage and a small amount of amygdalin, a cyanogenic glycoside. When soaked in water, the seeds swell to form a mucilaginous mass or gum that has demulcent properties.

USES
Used as a demulcent in digestive disorders and diarrhea. Raw fruits are used for diarrhea. Decoction of seeds is used internally for dysentery, diarrhea, gonorrhea, thrush, and mucous membrane irritation. Decoction is also used as an adjunct to boric acid eye lotions and as a compress or poultice for skin wounds and injuries or inflammation of the joints and nipples.

DOSAGE & ADMINISTRATION
Decoctum Cydoniae: Prepared by boiling 2 drams of seed in 1 pint of water in a tightly covered container for 10 minutes and then straining. Amount of liquid to be ingested varies and should be consumed only under the supervision of a knowledgeable practitioner.
For external use: Poultice is prepared from ground macerated seeds.

ADVERSE REACTIONS
None reported.

INTERACTIONS
None reported.

*Liquid contains alcohol.

EFFECTS ON LAB TEST RESULTS
None reported.

CAUTIONS
Patients who are pregnant or breast-feeding shouldn't use this herb. Geriatric patients and those with a history of immune disorders or peptic ulcers should use the herb cautiously.

NURSING CONSIDERATIONS
• Explore patient's knowledge of this herb.
🗲 **ALERT:** Seeds may be toxic because they contain cyanogenic glycoside.

PATIENT TEACHING
• Advise patient to consult a health care provider before using an herbal preparation because another treatment may be available.
• Tell patient that when filling a new prescription he should inform pharmacist of any herbal or dietary supplement he's taking.
• Warn patient not to eat the seeds because of the possible toxic effects.
• Warn patient not to take herb for a digestive disorder before seeking medical evaluation, because doing so can delay diagnosis of a potentially serious medical condition.
• If patient is breast-feeding, caution her not to use this herb.
• Advise patient to store herb away from heat and direct sunlight.
• Warn patient to keep all herbal products away from children and pets.

Bold italic type indicates that reaction may be life-threatening.

R

ragwort

Senecio jacoboea, cankerwort, dog standard, ragweed, staggerwort, stammerwort, stinking nanny, St. James wort, tansy ragwort

Common trade names
None known

AVAILABLE FORMS
Available as fresh and dried herb, and lotion*.

ACTIONS & COMPONENTS
Contains pyrrolizidine alkaloids (0.1% to 0.9%) and a volatile oil. The juice has cooling and astringent properties.

USES
Used as a wash in burns, eye inflammation, sores, bee stings, and cancerous ulcers. Also used for rheumatism, painful menstruation, chronic cough, urinary tract inflammation, anemia, anemic headaches, sciatica, and gout. Leaves made into a poultice are applied to painful joints to reduce inflammation and swelling. Ragwort is gargled, but not swallowed, for ulcers of the throat and mouth. A decoction of the root has been used for inward bruises and wounds.

DOSAGE & ADMINISTRATION
Rheumatoid arthritis: Lotion is made from 1 part herb and 5 parts 10% alcohol. Applied topically, p.r.n.

ADVERSE REACTIONS
Hepatic: *hepatotoxicity.*
Other: allergic reaction.

INTERACTIONS
None reported.

EFFECTS ON LAB TEST RESULTS
• May increase liver enzyme levels.

CAUTIONS
Patients who are pregnant or breast-feeding shouldn't use this herb.

NURSING CONSIDERATIONS
• Explore patient's knowledge of this herb.
⚡**ALERT:** Ragwort may have hepatotoxic and carcinogenic properties as a result of its pyrrolizidine alkaloid content.
• Although no chemical interactions have been reported in clinical studies, advise patient that herb may interfere with therapeutic effects of conventional drugs.
• Herb shouldn't be taken internally.

PATIENT TEACHING
• Advise patient to consult a health care provider before using an herbal preparation because another treatment may be available.
• Tell patient that when filling a new prescription he should inform pharmacist of any herbal or dietary supplement he's taking.
• Tell patient the herb is for external use only. Caution patient about the risk of liver failure and cancer if herb is taken internally.

*Liquid contains alcohol.

• Advise patient not to use the herb on broken skin.
• Warn patient to keep all herbal products away from children and pets.

raspberry

Rubus idaeus, bramble of Mount Ida, hindberry, raspbis

Common trade names
Alcohol-Free Red Raspberry Leaf, Certified Organic Red Raspberry, Red Raspberry, Red Raspberry Leaves, Red Raspberry Leaves Glycerine, Wild Countryside Red Raspberry Leaves

AVAILABLE FORMS
Available as tea, extract*, dried leaf, and infusion.

ACTIONS & COMPONENTS
Obtained from leaves and fruits of *R. idaeus.* Contains tannins, flavonoids, vitamin C, crystallizable fruit sugar, fragrant volatile oil, pectin, manganese, citric acid, malic acid, and mineral salts. Tannins have astringent activity.

USES
Leaves are used as a gargle for sore mouths and canker sores and as a wash for wounds and ulcers. Infusion of leaves, taken cold, is used to treat diarrhea. Herb is also used to normalize glucose level and to treat various disorders of the GI, CV, and respiratory systems. Leaf tea is taken regularly during pregnancy to prevent complications and tone the uterus in preparation for childbirth. Raspberry is reputed to relieve heavy menstrual bleeding and increase milk production in breast-feeding mothers.

DOSAGE & ADMINISTRATION
Dried leaf: 4 to 8 g P.O. t.i.d.
Liquid extract (1:1 in 25% alcohol): 4 to 8 ml (80 to 160 gtt) P.O. t.i.d.
Tea: Prepared by scalding 1.5 g finely cut herb (1 teaspoon = 0.8 g herb), steeping for 5 minutes, then straining. Taken t.i.d.

ADVERSE REACTIONS
None reported.

INTERACTIONS
Herb-drug. *Antidepressants, hypnotics, sedatives, tranquilizers:* Decreases absorption of drug. Advise patient to avoid using the herb and drug together.
Calcium and magnesium supplements; iron supplements, such as ferrous sulfate: Decreases absorption of supplement. Advise patient to avoid using the herb and supplement together.
Disulfiram, metronidazole: May cause a disulfiram-like reaction if herbal preparation contains alcohol. Advise patient to avoid using the herb and drug together.

EFFECTS ON LAB TEST RESULTS
None reported.

CAUTIONS
Patients who are pregnant or breast-feeding or sensitive to raspberry products shouldn't use this herb.

NURSING CONSIDERATIONS
• Explore patient's knowledge of this herb.

Bold italic type indicates that reaction may be life-threatening.

• Safety in pregnant or breast-feeding women, young children, and patients with severe liver or kidney disease hasn't been established.

• If patient has trouble breathing or develops a rash, he may be allergic to raspberry. He should immediately stop taking the herb and seek medical attention.

PATIENT TEACHING
• Advise patient to consult a health care provider before using an herbal preparation because another treatment may be available.

• Tell patient that when filling a new prescription he should inform pharmacist of any herbal or dietary supplement he's taking.

• If patient is taking red raspberry for GI symptoms, discuss with him other proven medical treatments for his condition.

• Inform patient that little evidence exists to support the use of herbal raspberry during pregnancy, childbirth, or menstruation.

• Advise patient to store herb away from heat and direct sunlight.

• Warn patient to keep all herbal products away from children and pets.

rauwolfia

Rauwolfia serpentina, Indian snakeroot, snakeroot

Common trade names
None known

AVAILABLE FORMS
Available as dried root, powder, and extracts.

ACTIONS & COMPONENTS
Contains reserpine, ajmalicine, and numerous other alkaloids. The herb exerts hypotensive and antiarrhythmic effects. It depletes catecholamine and serotonin stores. The whole extract is more easily tolerated with reserpine than the isolated substance, indicating the importance of the accompanying substances, or coeffectors.

USES
Used internally to treat nervousness, insomnia, anxiety, tension states, and other mental health disorders. Also used to treat flatulence, vomiting, liver disease, hypertension, and eclampsia, and to assist with contractions during childbirth. Used topically to treat wounds, snakebite, dysuria, and colic.

DOSAGE & ADMINISTRATION
Daily dose: 600 mg of powdered whole root (equivalent to 6 mg total alkaloids) P.O. daily

ADVERSE REACTIONS
CNS: depression, fatigue, drowsiness, nightmares, decreased libido.
CV: tachycardia and hypertension progressing to ***bradycardia*** and hypotension.
EENT: nasal congestion.
GI: nausea, vomiting.
GU: erectile dysfunction.

INTERACTIONS
Herb-drug. *Antihypertensives:* Increases hypotension. Monitor patient's blood pressure. Advise patient to avoid using the herb and drug together.

*Liquid contains alcohol.

Barbiturates, neuroleptic drugs:
Causes synergistic effect. Monitor
patient's laboratory values, and advise patient to avoid using the herb
and drug together.
Cardiac glycosides: Causes severe
bradycardia. Advise patient to
avoid using the herb and drug together.
Levodopa: Decreases effect. Advise patient to avoid using the herb
and drug together.
*OTC cold medicines, flu remedies,
and appetite suppressants:* Increases blood pressure. Advise patient to avoid using the herb and
drug together.
Sympathomimetics: Causes initially significant increase in blood
pressure. Advise patient to avoid
using the herb and drug together.
Herb-lifestyle. *Alcohol use:* Increases impairment of motor reactions. Advise patient not to consume foods or beverages that
contain alcohol.

EFFECTS ON LAB TEST RESULTS
• May decrease 17-hydroxycorti-
costeroid and T_4 levels.
• May interfere with urinary catecholamine tests.

CAUTIONS
Patients sensitive to rauwolfia
products should avoid this herb, as
should pregnant patients, breast-
feeding patients, and patients with
depression, GI ulceration, gallbladder disease, or pheochromocytoma. Patients receiving electro-
convulsive therapy also shouldn't
use this herb.

NURSING CONSIDERATIONS
• Explore patient's knowledge of
this herb.
• Monitor patient's blood pressure
closely.

PATIENT TEACHING
• Advise patient to consult a health
care provider before using an
herbal preparation because another
treatment may be available.
• Tell patient that when filling a
new prescription he should inform
pharmacist of any herbal or dietary supplement he's taking.
• Warn patient not to take herb for
insomnia before seeking medical
attention, because doing so may
delay diagnosis of a potentially serious medical condition.
• If patient is to receive electrocon-
vulsive therapy, advise him to stop
taking the herb 1 week before the
therapy.
• Tell patient to store herb away
from heat and direct sunlight.
• Warn patient to keep all herbal
products away from children and
pets.

red clover

Trifolium pratense, purple
clover, trefoil, wild clover

Common trade names
*EuroQuality Red Clover Blossoms,
NuVeg Red Clover Concentrate,
Promensil, Red Clover Blossom,
Red Clover Herb, Red Clover
Liquid*

AVAILABLE FORMS
Available as liquid extract*, tincture*, and tea.

Bold italic type indicates that reaction may be life-threatening.

ACTIONS & COMPONENTS

Obtained from dried and fresh flower heads of *T. pratense*. Contains volatile oil, isoflavones, coumarin derivatives, and cyanogenic glycosides. It has antispasmodic and expectorant effects and promotes skin healing. It also has hormonal effects similar to estrogen caused by isoflavones.

USES

Used internally to treat dry coughs and similar respiratory problems. It's also used to relieve menopausal signs and symptoms, prevent osteoporosis, and treat BPH and some cancers. Used externally to treat chronic skin diseases such as eczema and psoriasis.

DOSAGE & ADMINISTRATION

Dried flower heads: 4 g P.O., or as a tea, up to t.i.d.
Liquid extract (1:1 in 25% alcohol): 1.5 to 3 ml (30 to 60 gtt) P.O. t.i.d.
Tincture (1:10 in 45% alcohol): 1 to 2 ml (20 to 40 gtt) P.O. t.i.d.

ADVERSE REACTIONS

Metabolic: weight gain.
Respiratory: dyspnea.
Other: breast tenderness or enlargement; allergic reaction including hives, swelling, and itching.

INTERACTIONS

Herb-drug. *Drugs metabolized by the liver:* May decrease drug metabolism and increase drug levels. Advise patient against using the herb and drug together.
Heparin, warfarin, and other anticoagulants or antiplatelet drugs: May increase INR. Monitor laboratory values and patient closely for bleeding. Advise patient to avoid using the herb and drug together.
Hormonal contraceptives, hormone replacement therapy: May enhance or antagonize estrogen effect. Advise patient to avoid using the herb and drug together.
Disulfiram, metronidazole: May cause a disulfiram-like reaction if herbal preparation contains alcohol. Advise patient to avoid using the herb and drug together.

EFFECTS ON LAB TEST RESULTS

● May increase levels of drugs metabolized by the liver.
● May increase PT, INR, and PTT.

CAUTIONS

Patients who are pregnant or breast-feeding shouldn't use this herb, nor should patients who are sensitive to red clover products. Patients with breast or uterine cancer shouldn't use the herb because it could cause hormonal effects, which may increase the metabolism of cancer cells.

Safety in young children or patients with severe liver or kidney disease hasn't been established.

NURSING CONSIDERATIONS

● Explore patient's knowledge of this herb.
● Monitor patient for evidence of bleeding, especially if he takes warfarin or aspirin.
● Tinctures and extracts typically contain between 15% and 60% alcohol and may be unsuitable for children, patients with a history of alcoholism or liver disease, or patients taking certain drugs.

*Liquid contains alcohol.

PATIENT TEACHING

• Advise patient to consult a health care provider before using an herbal preparation because another treatment may be available.

• Tell patient that when filling a new prescription he should inform pharmacist of any herbal or dietary supplement he's taking.

• If patient has a history of alcoholism or liver disease, inform him that some herbal products contain alcohol.

• Caution patient to watch for signs and symptoms of bleeding, including easy bruising, bleeding gums, black tarry stools, and tea-colored urine, especially when taking large amounts of herb with warfarin.

• If patient is a woman, advise her to watch for estrogen-like effects, such as breast tenderness, breast enlargement, and weight gain.

• Tell patient to store herb away from heat and direct sunlight.

• Warn patient to keep all herbal products away from children and pets.

red poppy

Papaver rhoeas, copperose, corn poppy, corn rose, cup-puppy, headache poppy, headwark, rhoeados flos

Common trade names
None known

AVAILABLE FORMS

Available as dried flower petals, powder, and teas.

ACTIONS & COMPONENTS

Obtained from flowers of *P. rhoeas.* Contains small amounts of isoquinoline alkaloids (0.1%) and anthocyanin glycosides. Mechanism of action isn't well defined.

USES

Used for respiratory tract diseases and discomforts, for disturbed sleep, for sedation, and for pain relief. Also used in children's cough syrup, as a tea for insomnia, and as a colorant.

DOSAGE & ADMINISTRATION

Bronchial irritation: Prepared by steeping 2 teaspoons dried petals in 1 cup boiling water for 5 to 10 minutes and then straining. 1 cup taken b.i.d. to t.i.d. May be sweetened with honey. 1 teaspoon = about 8 g of herb.

ADVERSE REACTIONS

GI: vomiting, stomach pain.

INTERACTIONS

None reported.

EFFECTS ON LAB TEST RESULTS

None reported.

CAUTIONS

Patients who are pregnant or breast-feeding shouldn't use this herb. The herb also shouldn't be used in children.

NURSING CONSIDERATIONS

• Explore patient's knowledge of this herb.

⚠ALERT: Poisoning has occurred in children who consumed fresh leaves and blossoms, with signs and symptoms including

---

Bold italic type indicates that reaction may be life-threatening.

vomiting and stomach pain. The powdered herb has a low alkaloid content and is considered nontoxic.

PATIENT TEACHING
● Advise patient to consult a health care provider before using an herbal preparation because another treatment may be available.
● Tell patient that when filling a new prescription he should inform pharmacist of any herbal or dietary supplement he's taking.
● Warn patient to keep all herbal products away from children and pets.

rhatany

Krameria triandra, krameria root, mapato, Peruvian rhatany, ratanhiae radix, ratanhiawurzel, red rhatany, rhatania

Common trade names
None known

AVAILABLE FORMS
Available as powder, tincture*, and tea.

ACTIONS & COMPONENTS
Obtained from dried root of *K. triandra.* Contains high levels of proanthocyanidin tannins, which give the herb astringent properties.

USES
Used internally as an antidiarrheal for enteritis. Used externally for mild inflammation of the oral and pharyngeal mucosa and gums. Also used for fissures of the tongue, stomatitis, pharyngitis, noninfectious canker sores, chilblains, hemorrhoids, and leg ulcers.

DOSAGE & ADMINISTRATION
Decoction: 1 g of powdered root in 1 cup of water.
For external sores and ulcers: Undiluted tincture painted on affected area, b.i.d. to t.i.d.
Mouthwash and gargle: Prepared by simmering 1 to 1.5 g powdered root in 5 ounces boiling water for 10 to 15 minutes, then straining. Swished, not swallowed, b.i.d. to t.i.d.
Tea: Prepared by scalding 1.5 to 2 g coarsely powdered rhatany in 1 cup boiling water for 10 to 15 minutes, then straining. 1 teaspoon = about 3 g of powdered rhatany.
Tincture: 5 to 10 gtt in 1 glass of water. Swished, not swallowed, b.i.d. to t.i.d.

ADVERSE REACTIONS
GI: digestive complaints.
Other: allergic mucous membrane reactions.

INTERACTIONS
Herb-drug. *Disulfiram, metronidazole:* May cause a disulfiram-like reaction if herbal preparation contains alcohol. Advise patient to avoid using the herb and drug together.
Iron supplements such as ferrous sulfate, and calcium and magnesium: Decreases absorption if taken with rhatany tea. Advise patient to avoid using the herb and drug together.
Tretinoin: May cause skin irritation if used with topical rhatany. Advise patient to avoid using the herb and drug together.
Herb-herb. *Echinacea:* May potentiate echinacea's antibiotic activity. Monitor patient closely.

*Liquid contains alcohol.

Advise patient to avoid using the herbs together.

Herb-food. *Milk or cream:* May inactivate the tannins in rhatany tea. Advise patient to avoid using the two together.

EFFECTS ON LAB TEST RESULTS
None reported.

CAUTIONS
Patients who are pregnant or breast-feeding shouldn't use this herb. The herb also shouldn't be used for more than 2 weeks if taken without medical advice.

NURSING CONSIDERATIONS
• Explore patient's knowledge of this herb.
• Rhatany is difficult to find, and adulteration with other *Krameria* species is common.

PATIENT TEACHING
• Advise patient to consult a health care provider before using an herbal preparation because another treatment may be available.
• Tell patient that when filling a new prescription he should inform pharmacist of any herbal or dietary supplement he's taking.
• Advise patient not to use rhatany for more than 2 weeks without a health care provider's advice.
• Warn patient to keep all herbal products away from children and pets.

rose hip

Rosa canina, R. centifolia, brier hip, brier rose, dog rose, heps, hip, hipberry, hip fruit, hip sweet, hop fruit, rose hip and seed, rosehips, sweet brier, wild boar fruit, witches' brier

Common trade names
Ascorbate C, Chewable Honey C, Ester-C 1000, Hi-Potent-C, Mega-Stress Complex, Vitamin C 500 mg (special)

AVAILABLE FORMS
Available as capsules, tablets, powder, and tea, and in combination products.

ACTIONS & COMPONENTS
Obtained from fruits (hips) and seeds of various species of *Rosa.* Contains pectins and fruit acids, such as malic and citric acids, which are responsible for diuretic and laxative effects, as well as tannins, vitamin C, carotenoids, and flavonoids. Fresh rose hip contains 0.5% to 1.7% vitamin C but, because it deteriorates in processing, many natural vitamin supplements have some vitamin C added to them. Rose hip also contains vitamins A, B_1, B_2, B_3, and K.

USES
Used to treat diarrhea, respiratory disorders such as colds and flu, vitamin C deficiency (scurvy), gastric spasms and inflammation, intestinal diseases, edema, arthritis, sciatica, diabetes, metabolic disorders of uric acid metabolism (including gout), lower urinary tract and gallbladder ailments, gall-

---

Bold italic type indicates that reaction may be life-threatening.

stones, kidney stones, and inadequate peripheral circulation. Also used as a diuretic, a laxative, an astringent, and a booster of immune function during exhaustion. Has recently been used to treat osteogenesis imperfecta in children.

DOSAGE & ADMINISTRATION
Osteogenesis imperfecta: 250 to 600 mg/day P.O.
Tea: Prepared by steeping 1 to 2.5 g of crushed rose hip in 5 ounces boiling water for 10 to 15 minutes and then straining; 1 teaspoon = 3.5 g of herb. Taken as a diuretic, p.r.n.

ADVERSE REACTIONS
CNS: insomnia, headache, fatigue.
CV: flushing.
GI: nausea, vomiting, abdominal cramps, esophagitis, gastroesophageal reflux, diarrhea.
GU: kidney stones.
Respiratory: severe respiratory allergies (after exposure to herb dust).
Skin: itching, prickly sensations.
Other: *anaphylaxis.*

INTERACTIONS
Herb-drug. *Antacids that contain aluminum:* May increase aluminum absorption. Advise patient to avoid using the herb and drug together.
Aspirin, salicylates: May increase excretion of ascorbic acid and decrease excretion of salicylates. Monitor patient for salicylate toxicity. Advise patient to avoid using the herb and drug together.
Barbiturates, estrogens, hormonal contraceptives, tetracyclines: May increase vitamin C requirements. Advise patient to avoid using the herb and drug together.
Iron: May increase iron absorption. Advise patient to avoid using the herb and drug together.
Tretinoin: May cause additive effect. Advise patient to avoid using the herb and drug together.
Warfarin: May decrease effect. Monitor patient's INR. Advise patient to avoid using the herb and drug together.
Herb-herb. *Echinacea:* May potentiate antibiotic activity of echinacea. Monitor patient closely. Advise patient to avoid using the herbs together.
Herb-food. *Milk or cream:* May inactivate rose hip tea. Advise patient to avoid using the two together.

EFFECTS ON LAB TEST RESULTS
• May increase AST levels measured by color reactions (redox reactions) and Technicon SMA 12/60, bilirubin level measured by colorimetric methods or Technicon SMA 12/60, carbamazepine level measured by Ames ARIS method, urine glucose level measured by Clinitest, and serum or urine creatinine level. May decrease LDH level measured by Technicon SMA 12/60 and Abbott 100 methods, theophylline level measured by ARIS system or Ames Seralyzer photometer, and blood glucose level measured by Clinistix.
• May cause false-negative results for occult blood tests.

CAUTIONS
Patients who are pregnant or breast-feeding shouldn't use more of this herb than is found in foods; patients with asthma shouldn't use this herb at all.

NURSING CONSIDERATIONS
• Explore patient's knowledge of this herb.
• Rose hip is nontoxic in recommended amounts; most people don't have adverse reactions from ingesting small quantities.
• Rose hip interactions depend on the amount of vitamin C present.
• German Commission E has listed no known risks of using rose hip, but there have been reports of severe respiratory allergies with mild to moderate anaphylaxis in production workers exposed to rose hip dust during the manufacturing process. Plant fibers may also cause itching and a prickly sensation, resulting from mechanical irritation rather than allergic reaction.
• Herb may cause precipitation of urate, oxalate, or cysteine stones or drugs in the urinary tract, causing kidney stones.

PATIENT TEACHING
• Advise patient to consult a health care provider before using an herbal preparation because another treatment may be available.
• Tell patient that when filling a new prescription he should inform pharmacist of any herbal or dietary supplement he's taking.
• If patient has asthma and chooses to use rose hip, advise him to do so cautiously and to stop herb immediately and consult a health care provider if he experiences wheezing or shortness of breath.
• Inform patient that many rose hip–derived natural vitamin C supplements are fortified with synthetic vitamin C.
• Warn patient to keep all herbal products away from children and pets.

rosemary

Rosmarinus officinalis, compass plant, compass-weed, old man, polar plant, romero

Common trade names
Barlean's Flax Oil, Breast Health Formula, Bright-Eyes, Complete Cleanse, Easy Now, Female Sage, Respi-Oil, RoseOx

AVAILABLE FORMS
Available as dried leaves, essential oil, lotion, extracts*, and tea.
Capsules: 250 mg, 300 mg
Extracts: 1:1 in 45% alcohol

ACTIONS & COMPONENTS
Obtained from leaves of *R. officinalis*. Contains 1% to 2.5% of a volatile oil, made up of monoterpene hydrocarbons, camphor, borneol, and cineol. Leaves also contain rosmaricine; the flavonoid pigments diosmin, diosmentin, genkwanin, and related compounds; and various volatile and aromatic components. Diosmin decreases capillary permeability and fragility. Herb exerts some antibacterial activity as well as spasmolytic effects on smooth muscle. It also may have a positive inotropic effect, increasing coronary blood flow. Rosemary may also have

---

Bold italic type indicates that reaction may be life-threatening.

antifungal, antioxidant, anticarcinogenic, and abortifacient properties as well as stimulant effects on uterine muscle and menstrual flow. When applied topically, rosemary is an irritant and may increase circulation.

USES
Used for flatulence, gout, toothache, cough, eczema, and as a poultice for poor wound healing. Also used to aid digestion, ease dyspepsia, promote menstrual flow, induce abortion, increase appetite, and relieve headaches, liver and gallbladder complaints, and blood pressure problems. Used topically to repel insects and to treat baldness, circulatory disturbances, joint or musculoskeletal pain, myalgia, sciatica, and neuralgia. Rosemary is also popularly used in cooking, cosmetics, and various teas.

DOSAGE & ADMINISTRATION
Bath: 50 g of leaves added to 1 quart (1 L) of hot water and added to bath water.
Liquid extract (1:1 in 45% alcohol): 2 to 4 ml P.O. t.i.d.
Oral: 4 to 6 g of leaves P.O. daily.
Tea: Prepared by steeping 1 to 2 g of leaves in 5 ounces (148 ml) boiling water for 15 minutes, then straining; typically 1 cup is taken t.i.d.
Topical: 6% to 10% essential oil in semisolid or liquid preparations.

ADVERSE REACTIONS
CNS: *seizures.*
Respiratory: asthma (from repeated occupational exposure).

Skin: contact dermatitis, photosensitivity.

INTERACTIONS
Herb-drug. *Disulfiram, metronidazole:* May cause a disulfiram-like reaction if herbal preparation contains alcohol. Advise patient to avoid using the herb and drug together.
Herb-lifestyle. *Sun exposure:* May cause photosensitivity with use of topical forms. Advise patient to wear protective clothing and sunscreen and to limit exposure to direct sunlight.

EFFECTS ON LAB TEST RESULTS
None reported.

CAUTIONS
Patients who are pregnant or breast-feeding shouldn't use this herb, nor should patients with seizure disorders or sensitivity to rosemary products. The herb shouldn't be used medicinally for children.

NURSING CONSIDERATIONS
• Explore patient's knowledge of this herb.
⚠ **ALERT:** Undiluted oil shouldn't be ingested. Overdose may cause spasms, vomiting, gastroenteritis, uterine bleeding, kidney irritation, deep coma, and possibly death.
• Seizures can occur with high doses.
• Rosemary is unlikely to produce adverse reactions when the leaves and oil are used in amounts typically found in foods—that is, a maximum level 0.41% of leaves in baked goods and 0.003% in oil.

*Liquid contains alcohol.

The FDA generally recognizes the herb as safe.
• Repeated occupational exposure to rosemary may lead to asthma.

PATIENT TEACHING
• Advise patient to consult a health care provider before using an herbal preparation because another treatment may be available.
• Tell patient that when filling a new prescription he should inform pharmacist of any herbal or dietary supplement he's taking.
• Warn patient not to ingest undiluted rosemary oil.
• Advise pregnant patients, patients trying to get pregnant, and breast-feeding patients not to use rosemary in amounts greater than those found in food.
• If patient has a seizure disorder, advise him not to consume large amounts of rosemary.
• Inform patient that repeated occupational exposure to rosemary may lead to asthma.
• Advise parents not to give children amounts of rosemary greater than those found in food.
• Warn patient to keep all herbal products away from children and pets.

royal jelly

Common trade names
Bee Complete, Bee Pollen Complex, Energy Elixir, Pure Energy, Royal Bee Power, Super Energy Up, Ultra Virile-Actin

AVAILABLE FORMS
Available as capsules, creams, lotions, milk baths, and honey.

Capsules: 62.5 mg, 100 mg, 125 mg, 250 mg, 500 mg

ACTIONS & COMPONENTS
Obtained from milky white secretion produced by worker bees of the species *Apis mellifera* for exclusive growth and development of the queen bee. Contains a complex mixture of proteins, sugar, fats, and variable amounts of minerals, vitamins, and pheromones. It's rich in B vitamins, especially pantothenic acid. About 15% of royal jelly is 10-hydroxy-trans-(2)-decanoic acid, which has weak antimicrobial activity. Royal jelly may also have antitumorigenic activity.

USES
Used orally as a health tonic and for reducing cholesterol levels, promoting rejuvenation, enhancing sexual performance, improving the immune system, and treating bronchial asthma, liver disease, kidney disease, pancreatitis, insomnia, stomach ulcers, bone fractures, skin disorders, and hyperlipidemia. Applied topically to tone the skin and to stimulate hair growth.

DOSAGE & ADMINISTRATION
Hyperlipidemia: 50 to 100 mg P.O. daily.

ADVERSE REACTIONS
Respiratory: asthma.
Skin: rash, dermatitis, irritation.
Other: *anaphylaxis.*

INTERACTIONS
None reported.

Bold italic type indicates that reaction may be life-threatening.

EFFECTS ON LAB TEST RESULTS
• May decrease cholesterol levels.

CAUTIONS
Patients who are pregnant or breast-feeding shouldn't use this herb, nor should patients who are sensitive to related products or have seasonal allergies or dermatitis.

Patients with asthma should use the herb cautiously.

NURSING CONSIDERATIONS
• Explore patient's knowledge of this herb.

☑ALERT: Patients with asthma should use extreme caution because allergic reactions to this herb have led to anaphylaxis and death.
• One case of severe adverse GI reactions has been reported; reactions included abdominal pain, hemorrhagic colitis, diarrhea, GI hemorrhage, and mucosal edema of the sigmoid colon.
• Topical application may worsen existing dermatitis.

☑ALERT: Don't confuse royal jelly with bee pollen or honey bee venom.

PATIENT TEACHING
• Advise patient to consult a health care provider before using an herbal preparation because a standard treatment that has been proven effective may be available.
• Tell patient that when filling a new prescription he should remind pharmacist of any herbal and dietary supplements he's taking.
• If patient has asthma, tell patient that royal jelly may worsen his condition and lead to anaphylaxis. Warn patient to seek medical at-

tention if he develops shortness of breath after taking the herb.
• Advise patient that topical use of royal jelly may worsen existing skin inflammation.
• Warn patient to keep all herbal products away from children and pets.

rue

Ruta graveolens, herb of grace, herbygrass

Common trade names
Rue

AVAILABLE FORMS
Available as dried leaves, compresses, capsules, tincture*, oil, and tea. Because of the risk of toxicity, rue is available only from specialty herb suppliers.

ACTIONS & COMPONENTS
Obtained from aboveground plant parts of *R. graveolens.* Contains such essential oils as limonene, pinene, anisic acid, and phenol. Flavonoids such as rutin and quercitin may have a strengthening effect on capillaries; alkaloids arborinine, gamma-fagarine, and graveoline may have antispasmodic and abortifacient activity. Furanocoumarins such as bergapten, psoralen, and xanthotoxin have a photosensitizing effect with topical use. Chalepensin inhibits fertility, and coumarin derivatives and alkaloids have a spasmolytic effect. Rue also contains hypericin, tannin, pectin, choline, and iron.

*Liquid contains alcohol.

USES

Used internally for amenorrhea, Bell's palsy, colic, cough, epilepsy, hypertension, hysteria, multiple sclerosis, skin inflammation, oral and pharyngeal cavities, cramps, hepatitis, dyspepsia, diarrhea, intestinal parasites, and worm infections. Also used as a uterine stimulant for abortions. Used externally for backache, ear infection, eye soreness, gout, headache, muscle spasms, varicose veins, sprains, bruising, rheumatism, sore throat, and wounds. Applied topically as an insect repellent.

DOSAGE & ADMINISTRATION

Daily internal dosage: 0.5 to 1 g P.O. daily.
Tea: 1 heaping teaspoon (about 3 g) to ¼ L of water P.O.

ADVERSE REACTIONS

CNS: dizziness, vertigo, tremors, depression, sleep disorders, delirium, melancholic mood, fatigue.
CV: *bradycardia.*
EENT: swelling of the tongue.
GI: vomiting, epigastric pain, abdominal pain.
GU: *severe kidney damage.*
Hepatic: *hepatotoxicity.*
Skin: contact dermatitis (with topical use), photosensitivity reactions (with large doses), clammy skin, phototoxicity.

INTERACTIONS

Drug-herb. *Disulfiram, metronidazole:* May cause a disulfiram-like reaction if herbal preparation contains alcohol. Advise patient to avoid using the herb and drug together.

EFFECTS ON LAB TEST RESULTS

• May increase liver enzyme, BUN, and creatinine levels.

CAUTIONS

Patients who are pregnant or breast-feeding shouldn't use this herb; large doses of rue used as an abortifacient can be toxic or fatal to the mother. Patients with kidney or liver disease or GI inflammatory disorders also shouldn't use the herb.

NURSING CONSIDERATIONS

• Explore patient's knowledge of this herb.
• Discourage use of rue for any reason because of its toxic effects.
• Tinctures and extracts typically contain between 15% and 60% alcohol and may be unsuitable for children, patients with a history of alcoholism or liver disease, or patients taking certain drugs.
• If patient chooses to use rue, he should do so only under the strict supervision of a health care provider with extensive herbal experience.
⚠ALERT: Women have died after using rue to induce miscarriage.
• Using the prepared oil or rubbing fresh leaves on the skin can lead to phototoxic reactions causing dermatoses.

PATIENT TEACHING

• Advise patient to consult a health care provider before using an herbal preparation because another treatment may be available.
• Tell patient that when filling a new prescription he should inform

---

Bold italic type indicates that reaction may be life-threatening.

pharmacist of any herbal or dietary supplement he's taking.
• If patient has a history of alcoholism or liver disease, inform him that some herbal products contain alcohol.
• Caution patient not to use rue because of its potential toxicity and the availability of safer treatments.
• Warn patient to keep all herbal products away from children and pets.

*Liquid contains alcohol.

S

safflower

Carthamus tinctorius, American saffron, bastard saffron, dyer's saffron, fake saffron, false saffron, hoang-chi, koosumbha, parrot plant, zaffer

Common trade names
Safflower, Safflower Oil

AVAILABLE FORMS
Available as oil and powdered flowers.

ACTIONS & COMPONENTS
Obtained from flowers of *C. tinctorius.* Oil contains unsaturated fatty acids, including linoleic (76% to 79%), oleic (13%), palmitic (6%), and stearic (3%) acids. It also contains lignans, polysaccharides, carthamone, and carthamin. Linoleic acid is an omega-6 fatty acid that may help lower cholesterol.

USES
Oil is commonly used in cooking as a source of polyunsaturated fats to help lower dietary cholesterol levels. Also used to treat wounds, amenorrhea, stomach tumors, scabies, arthritis, and chest pain. Also used to help stimulate movement of stagnant blood and to help alleviate pain when used topically and systemically.

DOSAGE & ADMINISTRATION
Decoction: Average daily dose is 1 g P.O. t.i.d.

ADVERSE REACTIONS
Other: *allergic reactions* (in patients sensitive to plants in the ragweed family).

INTERACTIONS
Herb-drug. *Warfarin, heparin, other anticoagulants and antiplatelet drugs:* May increase the risk of bleeding. Monitor patient for bleeding tendencies; monitor PT and INR.

EFFECTS ON LAB TEST RESULTS
• May increase PT and INR.

CAUTIONS
Pregnant or breast-feeding women shouldn't use flowers and seeds. Purified oil is probably safe to use during pregnancy in amounts normally found in food. Patients with bleeding disorders should avoid herb.

NURSING CONSIDERATIONS
• Find out why patient is using the herb.
• Excessive intake of omega-6 oils (such as safflower) without appropriate amounts of omega-3 fatty acids can negatively affect patient's health.
• Monitor patient's cholesterol levels, as needed.

PATIENT TEACHING
• Tell patient to consult his health care provider before using an herbal preparation because a standard treatment that has been proven effective may be available.

Bold italic type indicates that reaction may be life-threatening.

• Tell patient that when filling a new prescription he should remind pharmacist of any herbal and dietary supplements he's taking.

• Advise patients with bleeding disorders and those taking anticoagulants and antiplatelet drugs to avoid taking safflower.

• Tell patient to avoid excessive use of omega-6 oils, such as safflower, without appropriate intake of omega-3 fatty acids.

• Advise patient to seek medical evaluation before taking any herbal or dietary supplement.

• Tell patient to notify a health care provider immediately about new or worsened symptoms.

• Advise women to notify a health care provider about planned, suspected, or known pregnancy.

• Warn patient to keep all herbal products away from children and pets.

saffron

Crocus sativus, nagakeshara, saffron crocus, Spanish saffron, zang hong hua

Common trade names
Saffron

AVAILABLE FORMS
Available as dried powder and dried stigmas; often adulterated with American saffron.

ACTIONS & COMPONENTS
Obtained from flower stigmas and styles of *C. sativus,* grown mainly in Spain and France. Contains crocetin, a xanthophyll carotenoid, which increases oxygen diffusion in blood plasma and, in turn, may help prevent or treat atherosclerosis. The low incidence of CV disease in parts of Spain may result from daily consumption of saffron. Saffron also contains essential oils such as cineole, safranal, and terpenes; crocin, a bitter glycoside; and vitamins B_1 and B_2.

Purified crocetin products in development are more likely than the crude herb to help increase plasma oxygen levels.

USES
Used to stimulate digestion and to treat amenorrhea, atherosclerosis, bronchitis, sore throat, headache, vomiting, and fever. Also used as an abortifacient and a sedative.

DOSAGE & ADMINISTRATION
Dosages aren't well documented. Some sources suggest an infusion of 6 to 10 stigmas in ½ cup of water to be taken as ½ cup to 1 cup P.O. daily. Other sources suggest a decoction of 12 to 15 stigmas in 1 cup of boiling water, which is then strained and taken as 1 cup P.O. daily.

ADVERSE REACTIONS
None reported.

INTERACTIONS
None reported.

EFFECTS ON LAB TEST RESULTS
None reported.

CAUTIONS
Pregnant or breast-feeding women shouldn't use this herb except in amounts normally found in food; 10 g can induce abortion.

*Liquid contains alcohol.

NURSING CONSIDERATIONS
• Find out why patient is using the herb.

�€ALERT: Saffron may be lethal at doses above 12 g. Overdose may cause central paralysis, dizziness, stupor, vomiting, intestinal colic, bloody diarrhea, and hemorrhaging of skin on the nose, lips, and eyelids. Treatment involves emptying the stomach by gastric lavage and giving activated charcoal, if needed. Symptomatic treatment includes diazepam to control seizures and sodium bicarbonate to correct acidosis. In severe cases, patient may need mechanical ventilation.

• Saffron is generally safe for use as a spice.

PATIENT TEACHING
• Advise patient to consult his health care provider before using an herbal preparation because a standard treatment that has been proven effective may be available.
• Tell patient that when filling a new prescription he should remind pharmacist of any herbal and dietary supplements he's taking.
• Instruct patient to promptly notify a health care provider about new or worsened symptoms.
• Warn patient not to take herb before seeking medical attention because doing so may delay diagnosis of a potentially serious medical condition.
• Warn patient to keep all herbal products away from children and pets.

sage

Salvia officinalis, Dalmatian sage, garden sage, meadow sage, red sage, scarlet sage, tree sage

Common trade names
Alcohol-Free Sage, Sage

AVAILABLE FORMS
Available as dried leaves, extract*, tincture*, and essential oil. Also used in shampoos and conditioners.

ACTIONS & COMPONENTS
Contains volatile oils (including thujone, cineole, and camphor), tannins, diterpene bitter principles, triterpenes, steroids, flavones, and flavonoid glycosides. Herb has antibacterial, fungistatic, virustatic, astringent, antioxidative, antispasmodic, secretion-promoting, and perspiration-inhibiting properties.

USES
Used topically to treat itching from insect bites, herpes lesions, shingles, and psoriasis. Also used to prevent hair loss and preserve hair color. Used internally for loss of appetite, excessive perspiration, laryngitis, tonsillitis, pharyngitis, halitosis, canker sores, gum disease, fatigue, and Alzheimer's disease. Also used as a vaginal douche to treat vaginal yeast infection.

DOSAGE & ADMINISTRATION
Dry herb (leaves): 4 to 6 g P.O. daily.

Bold italic type indicates that reaction may be life-threatening.

Essential oil: 0.1 to 0.3 g P.O. daily.

For halitosis: A few leaves chewed, as necessary.

For inflamed mucous membranes: Undiluted alcohol extract, applied p.r.n.

For inflammation of bronchial mucous membranes: 50 g of powdered herb mixed with 80 g honey and used as an expectorant.

Gargle or mouth rinse: 2.5 g dry herb or 2 or 3 gtt essential oil in 100 ml of water, or 9 ml of alcoholic extract in 1 glass of water.

Liquid extract or tincture (1:2 and 1:5 alcohol): 6 to 12 ml P.O. in divided doses, t.i.d.

ADVERSE REACTIONS
CNS: *seizures,* vertigo.
CV: tachycardia.

INTERACTIONS
Herb-drug. *Disulfiram, metronidazole:* Herbal products that contain alcohol may cause a disulfiram-like reaction. Advise patient to avoid using together.

EFFECTS ON LAB TEST RESULTS
None reported.

CAUTIONS
Pregnant or breast-feeding women shouldn't use this herb. It should be used cautiously by patients with a history of epilepsy or other seizure disorders.

NURSING CONSIDERATIONS
• Find out why patient is using the herb.
• Although no chemical interactions have been reported, consider the pharmacologic properties of the herbal product and the risk that it will interfere with therapeutic effects of conventional drugs.
• Chemical content of the dry herbal product is likely to vary widely, depending on where the herb is grown, time of harvest, storage time, and drying method used.

PATIENT TEACHING
• Advise patient to consult a health care provider before using an herbal preparation because a standard treatment that has been proven effective may be available.
• Tell patient that when filling a new prescription he should remind pharmacist of any herbal and dietary supplements he's taking.
🖉 **ALERT:** Advise patient to avoid using large amounts of sage, especially tincture or essential oil, because large amounts of thujone may be toxic.
• Warn patient not to take herb before seeking medical attention because doing so may delay diagnosis of a potentially serious medical condition.
• Tell patient to promptly notify health care provider about new symptoms or adverse effects.
• Warn patient to keep all herbal products away from children and pets.

---

*Liquid contains alcohol.

St. John's wort

Hypericum perforatum, amber, goatweed, hardhay, herb John, hexenkraut, Johanniskraut, John's wort, klamath weed, millepertuis, Saint John's word, tipton weed

Common trade names
Alterra, Hypercalm, Kira, Quanterra Emotional Balance, St. John's Wort Extracts, Tension Tamer

AVAILABLE FORMS
Available as tablets, pellets, capsules of standardized extract, powdered or dried herb, liquid extract*, tincture, and transdermal forms. Also available in various combination products.
Capsules (extended-release, standardized at 0.3% hypericin): 450 mg, 900 mg, 1,000 mg
Capsules (standardized at 0.3% hypericin): 125 mg, 150 mg, 250 mg, 300 mg, 350 mg, 370 mg, 375 mg, 400 mg, 424 mg, 434 mg, 450 mg, 500 mg, 510 mg
Extract: 1:1
Injection: 1%
Liquid: 250 mg/ml, 300 mg/5 ml
Liquid dilutions: 3x, 6x, 30x, 12c, 30c
Pellets: 3x, 6x, 12x, 12c, 30c
Tablets (standardized at 0.3% hypericin): 100 mg, 150 mg, 300 mg, 450 mg
Tincture: 1:10
Transdermal: 900 mg/24 hr

ACTIONS & COMPONENTS
Obtained from *H. perforatum.* Contains naphthodianthrones, including hypericin and pseudohypericin; hyperoside; quercitrin; rutin; isoquercitrin; bioflavonoids, including amentoflavone; 1,3,6,7-tetrahydroxy-xanthone; hyperforin; adhyperforin; aliphatic hydrocarbons, including 2-methyloctane and undecane; dodecanol; mono- and sesquiterpenes, including alphapinene and caryophyllene; 2-methyl-3-but-3-en-2-ol, oligomeric procyanidins; catechin tannins; and caffeic acid derivatives, including chlorogenic acid. St. John's wort may have a slight inhibitory effect on MAO with more inhibition of the reuptake of serotonin, dopamine, and norepinephrine. Hypericin inhibits catecholmethyltransferase and receptors for adenosine, benzodiazepines, GABA-A, GABA-B, and inositol triphosphate. Hypericin has antiviral activity and other constituents have shown antibacterial activity; can also stimulate or inhibit the cyclic P-450 enzyme system.

USES
Used orally for mild to moderate depression, anxiety, restlessness, sciatica, and viral infections, including herpes simplex virus types 1 and 2, hepatitis C, influenza virus, murine cytomegalovirus, poliovirus, and Epstein-Barr. Has also been used to treat bronchitis, asthma, gallbladder disease, nocturnal enuresis, gout, and rheumatism, although it hasn't proven effective in these cases. Used topically for contusions, inflammation, myalgia, burns, hemorrhoids, vitiligo, herpetic lesions, and shingles. In traditional Chinese medicine, St. John's wort has been used as a gargle for tonsillitis and as a lotion for dermatoses.

Bold italic type indicates that reaction may be life-threatening.

DOSAGE & ADMINISTRATION

Capsules or tablets for mild to moderate depression: Initially, 300 mg P.O. t.i.d.; maintenance, 300 to 600 mg P.O. daily.
For depression: 2 to 4 g dried herb P.O. daily, or 0.2 to 1 mg hypericin.
For wounds, bruising, and swelling: Applied topically to affected area.
Liquid extract: 2 to 4 ml P.O. daily.
Tea: 2 or 3 g of dried herb in boiling water.
Tincture: 2 to 4 ml P.O. daily.

ADVERSE REACTIONS

CNS: fatigue, neuropathy, restlessness, headache.
GI: digestive complaints, fullness sensation, constipation, diarrhea, nausea, abdominal pain, dry mouth.
Skin: photosensitivity reaction, pruritus.
Other: delayed hypersensitivity.

INTERACTIONS

Herb-drug. *Amitriptyline; chemotherapy drugs; cyclosporine; digoxin; drugs metabolized by the cytochrome P-450 enzyme system; hormonal contraceptives; protease inhibitors, including amprenavir, indinavir, nelfinavir, ritonavir, saquinavir; theophylline; warfarin:* Decreases effectiveness, requiring possible dosage adjustment. There have been reports of failed drug therapy when these drugs are used with St. John's wort. Advise patient to avoid using together. If patient stops taking the herb during drug therapy, check his blood drug levels because these levels may rise.

Anesthetics: May have synergistic or unpredictable effects. Discourage use together.
MAO inhibitors, including phenelzine and tranylcypromine: May increase effects and cause possible toxicity and hypertensive crisis. Advise patient to avoid using together.
Nonnucleoside reverse transcriptase inhibitors, such as delavirdine, efavirenz, nevirapine: May enhance metabolism of these drugs, causing treatment failure. Advise patient to avoid using together.
Reserpine: Antagonizes effects of reserpine. Advise patient to avoid using together.
Selective serotonin reuptake inhibitors, such as citalopram, fluoxetine, paroxetine, sertraline: Increases risk of serotonin syndrome, causing confusion, agitation, tachycardia, hypertension, nausea, hyperreflexia, muscle rigidity, restlessness, diaphoresis and, rarely, death. Advise patient to avoid using together.
Herb-herb. *Herbs with sedative effects, such as calamus, calendula, California poppy, capsicum, catnip, celery, couch grass, elecampane, German chamomile, goldenseal, gotu kola, Jamaican dogwood, kava, lemon balm, sage, sassafras, skullcap, shepherd's purse, Siberian ginseng, stinging nettle, valerian, wild carrot, wild lettuce:* May enhance effects of either herb. Monitor patient closely, and advise him to avoid using together.
Herb-food. *Tyramine-containing foods such as beer, cheese, dried meats, fava beans, liver, yeast, and*

---

*Liquid contains alcohol.

wine: May cause hypertensive crisis when used together. Advise patient to separate administration times.

Herb-lifestyle. *Alcohol use:* May increase sedative effects. Advise patient to avoid using together. *Sun exposure:* May increase risk of photosensitivity reactions. Urge patient to avoid unprotected sun exposure.

EFFECTS ON LAB TEST RESULTS
None reported.

CAUTIONS
Pregnant patients and men and women planning pregnancy shouldn't take St. John's wort because of the mutagenic risk to developing cells and fetus. Transplant patients maintained on cyclosporine therapy should avoid this herb because of the risk of organ rejection.

NURSING CONSIDERATIONS
• Find out why patient is using the herb.
• Herb should be used with caution, if at all, in patients at high risk for, or who have had, skin cancer related to photosensitivity.
• St. John's wort is effective in treating mild to moderate depression. Recommended duration of trial for depression is 4 to 6 weeks. Monitor patient for response to herbal therapy, as evidenced by improved mood and lessened depression. If no improvement occurs, a different therapy should be considered.
• By using standardized extracts, patient can better control the dosage. Formulations of standard-ized 0.3% hypericin as well as hyperforin-stabilized version of the extract have been used.
• St. John's wort interacts with many prescription or OTC products. Patient must consider the possibility of interactions before taking herb with other products.
• Because St. John's wort decreases the effect of certain prescription drugs, watch for signs of drug toxicity if patient stops using the herb. Drug dosage may need to be reduced.
• Serotonin syndrome may cause dizziness, nausea, vomiting, headache, epigastric pain, anxiety, confusion, restlessness, and irritability.
• Because St. John's wort has mutagenic effects on sperm cells and oocytes and adversely affects reproductive cells, it shouldn't be used by pregnant patients or those planning pregnancy (including men).
• Topically, the volatile plant oil is an irritant. Monitor affected site for adverse effects and improvement.
• Monitor patient for sedative effects and GI complaints.

PATIENT TEACHING
• Advise patient to consult a health care provider before using an herbal preparation because a standard treatment that has been proven effective may be available.
• Tell patient that when filling a new prescription he should remind pharmacist of any herbal and dietary supplements he's taking.
• Advise patient to discontinue herb several weeks before elective surgery.

Bold italic type indicates that reaction may be life-threatening.

• Encourage patient to discuss depression and to seek professional psychiatric help, as indicated.
• If patient takes St. John's wort for mild to moderate depression, explain that several weeks may pass before beneficial effects occur. Tell patient that a new therapy may be needed if no improvement occurs after 4 to 6 weeks.
• Inform patient that St. John's wort interacts with many prescription and OTC products and may reduce their effectiveness.
• Tell patient that St. John's wort may cause increased sensitivity to direct sunlight. Recommend protective clothing, sunscreen, and limited sun exposure.
• Inform patient that he needs to wait a certain amount of time (determined by a health care provider) between stopping an antidepressant and starting St. John's wort .
• Tell patient to report adverse effects to a health care provider.
• Warn patient to keep all herbal products away from children and pets.

santonica

Artemisia cina, levant, sea wormwood, wormseed

Common trade names
None known

AVAILABLE FORMS
Available as powder, lozenges, and in combination products.

ACTIONS & COMPONENTS
Obtained from *A. cina.* Contains sesquiterpene lactones, including alpha-santonin, artemisin, and beta-santonin, which gives herb its action against intestinal worms, particularly ascarids. Alpha-santonin paralyzes the muscles of worms. It also may reduce fever.

USES
Used to treat intestinal parasites such as *Ascaris* and *Oxyuris.*

DOSAGE & ADMINISTRATION
For intestinal worms: For adults, 25 mg powder P.O. For children, dose is based on child's weight.

ADVERSE REACTIONS
CNS: headache, muscle twitching, stupor.
EENT: visual disorders (xanthopsia).
GI: gastroenteritis, nausea, vomiting.
GU: kidney irritation.
Other: *allergic reactions.*

INTERACTIONS
None known.

EFFECTS ON LAB TEST RESULTS
• May increase BUN and creatinine levels.

CAUTIONS
Patients allergic to members of the Compositae family, which includes ragweed, chrysanthemums, marigolds, and daisies, should avoid this herb. In general, this herb should be avoided because of the high potential for poisoning.

NURSING CONSIDERATIONS
• Find out why patient is using the herb.

---

*Liquid contains alcohol.

⚡**ALERT:** Fatal poisonings have occurred with doses of less than 10 g of this herb. Poisoning can occur with therapeutic dosages.

• To treat intestinal worms, herb must be taken with a laxative to ensure expulsion.

• Monitor patient's response to the herb.

• Although no chemical interactions have been reported, consider the pharmacologic properties of the herb and its potential to interfere with therapeutic effects of conventional drugs.

PATIENT TEACHING

• Advise patient to consult a health care provider before using an herbal preparation because a standard treatment that has been proven effective may be available.

• Tell patient that when filling a new prescription he should remind pharmacist of any herbal and dietary supplements he's taking.

• Advise patient to avoid using this herb if he is allergic to members of the Compositae family, which includes ragweed, chrysanthemums, marigolds, daisies, and other herbs.

• Warn patient not to take herb before seeking medical attention because doing so may delay diagnosis of a potentially serious medical condition.

• Instruct patient to promptly notify health care provider about new symptoms or adverse effects.

sarsaparilla

Smilax officinalis, anantamul, anantamula, gopakanya, Indian sarsaparilla, khao yen, nagajihva, sariva, sarsa, smilax

Common trade names
EveCare, Renalka, Sarsaparilla Root, Styplon

AVAILABLE FORMS
Available as dried root, capsules, and tablets.

ACTIONS & COMPONENTS
Obtained from dried root of *S. officinalis.* Contains saponins, phytosterols, resin, shikimic acid, terpene alcohols, glycosides, tannins, and essential oils. Detoxifying effect of herb is based on its ability to bind endotoxins. Antimicrobial and antipsoriatic activity may be caused by saponins. Herb also may act against *Treponema pallidum,* the organism that causes syphilis. It also has diuretic, antiinflammatory, and hepatoprotective effects.

USES
Used to treat psoriasis, rheumatisms (including arthritis, arthralgia, bursitis, and gout), kidney problems (including kidney stones), other urinary problems, syphilis, and venereal disease. Used as a tonic to improve appetite, digestion, vitality, and virility; it's popular among body-builders. Used to improve ailments and excrete waste from the blood. Sarsaparilla can be used with other herbs, such as burdock root, sassafras, red clover, gotu cola, and

yellow dock, to enhance desired effect. Also used as a flavoring agent in medicines.

DOSAGE & ADMINISTRATION
Capsules or tablets: 9 g of dried root P.O. t.i.d. in divided doses. Or 6 to 10 g of dried root P.O. daily in divided doses. Or, one to six 500-mg capsules P.O. daily in divided doses.
Cold water extract: 500 ml P.O. in a.m. and p.m.
Decoction: 3 cups P.O. daily. Prepared by placing 1 or 2 teaspoons root in 1 cup of water and simmering for 10 to 15 minutes. Or 1 to 5 g P.O. t.i.d.
Liquid extract: 8 to 15 ml P.O. daily.
Powder: 0.3 to 1.5 g daily.
Tincture: 1 or 2 ml in 1 cup of warm water P.O. t.i.d.

ADVERSE REACTIONS
GI: GI irritation, nausea.
GU: kidney irritation.
Respiratory: asthma from root dust.

INTERACTIONS
Herb-drug. *Oral drugs:* May affect absorption of oral drugs. Advise patient to separate administration times by 2 hours.

EFFECTS ON LAB TEST RESULTS
• May increase BUN and creatinine levels.

CAUTIONS
Patients with recurrent kidney stones should avoid this herb. No one should take large doses for long periods.

NURSING CONSIDERATIONS
• Find out why patient is using the herb.
• Monitor patient's response to herbal therapy.

PATIENT TEACHING
• Advise patient to consult a health care provider before using an herbal preparation because a standard treatment that has been proven effective may be available.
• Tell patient that when filling a new prescription he should remind pharmacist of any herbal and dietary supplements he's taking.
• Tell patient not to combine sarsaparilla with drugs that contains digitalis or bismuth.
• Advise patient to avoid heavy meals and animal-based foods.
• Tell patient to drink enough fluids to help flush out urinary system.
• Urge patient to promptly notify a health care provider about new symptoms or adverse effects.

sassafras

Sassafras albidum, S. officinale, S. radix, S. variifolia, ague tree, cinnamon wood, kuntze saloop, laurus sassafras, saloop, sassafrax, saxifras

Common trade names
None known

AVAILABLE FORMS
Available as dried root.

ACTIONS & COMPONENTS
Obtained from root of *S. albidum.* Volatile oil contains safrole (up to 90%); other constituents include

---

*Liquid contains alcohol.

anethole, asarone, camphor, eugenol, myristicin, and pinene apiole. Herb elicits a mild antidiuretic response. Safrole and its major metabolite, 1-hydroxysafrole, are carcinogenic and neurotoxic.

USES
Used orally to treat eye or mucous membrane inflammation, catarrh, bronchitis, high blood pressure, kidney disorders, arthritis, cancers, and syphilis; as a tonic and blood purifier; as a diuretic; and as a flavoring agent. Used topically as an antiseptic and to treat skin eruptions, insect bites and stings, rheumatism, gout, sprains, and swelling.

DOSAGE & ADMINISTRATION
Infusion: 50 g added to 1 L of water.
Tea: 1 teaspoon added to boiling water and strained after 10 minutes.

ADVERSE REACTIONS
CNS: ataxia, CNS depression, hallucinations, hot flashes, paralysis, shakes, stupor, exhaustion, spasm.
CV: hypertension, tachycardia, *CV collapse.*
EENT: dilated pupils, ptosis.
GI: vomiting.
GU: miscarriage, *renal toxicity.*
Hepatic: *liver cancer.*
Skin: contact dermatitis, diaphoresis.
Other: *carcinogenesis, hypersensitivity,* hypothermia.

INTERACTIONS
Herb-drug. *Barbiturates, sedatives:* May cause additive effects.

Advise patient to avoid using together.
Drugs metabolized by cytochrome P-450 and P-488, phenytoin: Increases metabolism and decreases blood levels of drugs metabolized by these pathways. Advise patient to avoid using together.
Herb-herb. *Herbs with sedative effects, including calamus, calendula, California poppy, capsicum, catnip, celery, couch grass, elecampane, German chamomile, goldenseal, gotu kola, hops, Jamaican dogwood, kava, lemon balm, sage, shepherd's purse, Siberian ginseng, skullcap, stinging nettle, St. John's wort, valerian, wild carrot, wild lettuce:* May enhance therapeutic and adverse effects. Advise patient to avoid using together.
Safrole-containing herbs, including basil, camphor, cinnamon, nutmeg: May have additive toxicity. Advise patient to avoid using together.
Herb-lifestyle. *Alcohol use:* May enhance CNS depressant effects. Advise patient to avoid using together.

EFFECTS ON LAB TEST RESULTS
• May increase BUN, creatinine, and liver enzyme levels. May alter phenytoin levels.

CAUTIONS
Because of its carcinogenic potential, safrole shouldn't be used in any form.

NURSING CONSIDERATIONS
• Find out why patient is using the herb.
⚡ALERT: Safrole has been banned by the FDA as a drug or

Bold italic type indicates that reaction may be life-threatening.

food product; it may be carcinogenic and has caused death.

PATIENT TEACHING
• Warn patient not to take herb before seeking medical attention because doing so may delay diagnosis of a potentially serious medical condition.
• Advise patient that safrole has been banned by the FDA as a potential carcinogen with numerous adverse effects.

saw palmetto

Serenoa repens, American dwarf palm tree, cabbage palm, sabal, shrub palmetto

Common trade names
Centrum Saw Palmetto, Herbal Sure Saw Palmetto, Permixon, PlusStrogen, Premium Blend Saw Palmetto, Proactive Saw Palmetto, Propalmex, Quanterra Prostate, Saw Palmetto Power, Standardized Saw Palmetto ExtractCap, Super Saw Palmetto

AVAILABLE FORMS
Available as tablets, capsules, fresh and dried berries, and as extracts*.
Extracts: 60% to 70% grain alcohol

ACTIONS & COMPONENTS
Obtained from berries of *S. repens.* Contains fatty acids, fatty acid esters, sitosterols, and phytosterols. Exact mechanism of action isn't known, but sitosterols may inhibit conversion of testosterone to dihydrotestosterone (DHT), reducing prostate enlargement. May also inhibit androgenic activity by competing with DHT for androgen receptors, affecting testosterone metabolism and may have antiestrogenic effect, which may also contribute to its use with BPH. The antispasmodic activity is related to the inhibition of calcium influx and activation of the sodium/calcium exchanger. Herb also has antiinflammatory and astringent properties and inhibits prolactin and growth factor-induced cell proliferation. Said to improve urine flow rate and postvoid residual urine and relieve nocturia by up to 73% in BPH.

USES
Used to treat symptoms of BPH (stages I and II) and coughs and congestion from colds, bronchitis, or asthma. Also used as a mild diuretic, urinary antiseptic (for UTIs and interstitial cystitis), and astringent.

DOSAGE & ADMINISTRATION
Average daily dose: 160 mg P.O. b.i.d. or 320 mg P.O. daily (1 or 2 g fresh berries or 320 mg of lipophilic extract).
Decoction of berries: 1 or 2 g of fresh berries in 1 cup of water, boiled, then simmered for 5 minutes. Taken t.i.d., possibly for longer than 3 months but less than 6 months.

ADVERSE REACTIONS
CNS: headache.
CV: hypertension.
GI: nausea, abdominal pain, diarrhea.
GU: urine retention.
Musculoskeletal: back pain.

*Liquid contains alcohol.

INTERACTIONS

Herb-drug. *Adrenergics, hormones, hormone-like drugs:* May block alpha receptors, estrogen, and androgen. Drug dosages may need adjustment if patient takes this herb. Monitor patient closely.

EFFECTS ON LAB TEST RESULTS

None reported.

CAUTIONS

Pregnant or breast-feeding women and women of childbearing age shouldn't use this herb. Adults and children with hormone-dependent illnesses other than BPH or breast cancer should avoid this herb.

NURSING CONSIDERATIONS

• Find out why patient is using the herb.
• Herb should be used cautiously for conditions other than BPH because data about its effectiveness in other conditions are lacking.
• Obtain a baseline prostate-specific antigen (PSA) test before patient starts taking herb because it may cause a false-negative PSA result. PSA laboratory values didn't change significantly in clinical trials using dosages of 160 to 320 mg daily.
• Saw palmetto may not alter prostate size. Some sources report that herb does reduce prostate swelling and further progression.

PATIENT TEACHING

• Advise patient to consult a health care provider before using an herbal preparation because a standard treatment that has been proven effective may be available.

• Tell patient that when filling a new prescription he should remind pharmacist of any herbal and dietary supplements he's taking.
• Warn patient not to take herb for bladder or prostate problems before seeking medical attention because doing so could delay diagnosis of a potentially serious medical condition.
• Tell patient to take herb with food to minimize GI effects.
• Caution patient to promptly notify health care provider about new or worsened adverse effects.
• Warn women to avoid herb if pregnant or planning pregnancy or if breast-feeding.

scented geranium

Pelargonium

Common trade names
None known

AVAILABLE FORMS

Available as whole plant and essential oil.

ACTIONS & COMPONENTS

Obtained from leaves of certain *Pelargonium* species. Contains *l*-citronellol, alcohols, esters, aldehydes, and ketones. Mechanism of antibacterial and antifungal effects is unknown.

USES

Used for citronellol effects as mosquito repellant and for antibacterial and antifungal effects. Also used as an analgesic, antidepressant, expectorant, astringent, diuretic, sedative, flavoring agent, and fragrance.

Bold italic type indicates that reaction may be life-threatening.

DOSAGE & ADMINISTRATION
Dosages aren't well documented.

ADVERSE REACTIONS
CV: edema.
Skin: dermatitis, erythema, vesiculation, cheilitis.

INTERACTIONS
None known.

EFFECTS ON LAB TEST RESULTS
None reported.

CAUTIONS
Patients sensitive to members of the geranium family should avoid this herb.

NURSING CONSIDERATIONS
• Find out why patient is using the herb.
• *Pelargonium* includes common annuals and houseplants of many different species and varieties. They shouldn't be confused with plants of the genus *Geranium*.

PATIENT TEACHING
• Advise patient to consult a health care provider before using an herbal preparation because a standard treatment that has been proven efficacy may be available.
• Tell patient that when filling a new prescription he should remind pharmacist of any herbal and dietary supplements he's taking.
• Inform patient that few data are available regarding medicinal use of geraniums. Tell him that scented geranium has questionable effectiveness as a topical mosquito repellant and may cause skin irritation.

• Instruct patient to promptly notify a health care provider about new or worsened adverse effects.
• Warn patient to keep all herbal products away from children and pets.

schisandra

Schisandra chinensis, gomishi, hoku-gomishi, kita-gomishi, omicha, schizandra, wu-wei-zu

Common trade names
Bilberry/Schizandra Plus, Clarity, Immunity, Milk Thistle/Schizandra Plus, NutraPack, ParaCleanse, Schizandra Plus

AVAILABLE FORMS
Available as dried berries, seeds, and liquid extract*.
Capsules: 500 mg, 560 mg, 600 mg
Extract: 1:1 in 12% to 15% grain alcohol or glycerin base

ACTIONS & COMPONENTS
Obtained from *S. chinensis.* Contains 10% organic acids, including carboxylic, malic, citric, tartaric, and nigranoic acids, as well as vitamins A, C, and E. More than 30 lignins have been identified in seeds and fruit (about 2% of fruit by weight), including schizandrin and related compounds and many gomisin compounds. Lignins may have pronounced liver-protecting effects. Schizandrol A may have neuroleptic, anticonvulsant, and sedative effects. Herb may have astringent and nervous system stimulant effects.

---

*Liquid contains alcohol.

USES
Used to treat dry cough, asthma, night sweats, chronic fatigue, nocturnal seminal emissions, chronic diarrhea, and various lung, liver, and kidney disorders. Also used to improve mental alertness and memory and reflex responses, relieve eye fatigue, increase visual acuity, and ease depression caused by adrenergic exhaustion.

DOSAGE & ADMINISTRATION
Capsules: Up to six 500-mg capsules P.O. daily.
Decoction: 1 cup taken every 8 hours. Prepared by adding 5 g crushed berries to 100 ml water, boiling, and then simmering.
Liquid extract (1:1 alcohol or glycerin base): 1.25 to 3 ml P.O. t.i.d.
Tea: 2 or 3 cups P.O. daily. Prepared by adding 2 to 4 tablespoons dried berries to 2 cups of water, boiling, and then simmering until liquid is reduced to 1 cup.

ADVERSE REACTIONS
CNS: restlessness, insomnia, **CNS depression.**
GI: heartburn.
Respiratory: dyspnea.

INTERACTIONS
Herb-drug. *Amphetamines, other CNS stimulants:* May increase CNS adverse effects. Advise patient to avoid using together.
Barbital, pentobarbital: May potentiate action of the drug. Advise patient to report herbal use and to avoid using herb.
Body-strengthening drugs: May potentiate drug effects and raise blood pressure. Advise patient to avoid using together.
Herb-food. *Caffeine:* May increase CNS adverse effects. Advise patient to avoid using together.

EFFECTS ON LAB TEST RESULTS
● May alter ALT levels.

CAUTIONS
Pregnant or breast-feeding patients should avoid this herb, as should patients with epilepsy, peptic ulcers, fever, or high blood pressure.

NURSING CONSIDERATIONS
● Find out why patient is using the herb.
● Patients with peptic ulcer may develop increased acidity.
● Monitor liver function test results.
● Advise patient to avoid taking schisandra before having liver function tests because herb may alter ALT test results.
● Some Chinese call this herb *wuwei-zu* (five-taste fruit) because berries are sweet, sour, bitter, pungent (hot), and salty. Plant is considered balanced because of this wide range of flavors.

PATIENT TEACHING
● Advise patient to consult a health care provider before using an herbal preparation because a standard treatment that has been proven effective may be available.
● Tell patient that when filling a new prescription he should remind pharmacist of any herbal and dietary supplements he's taking.
● Tell patient to take herb with meals to minimize GI upset.

Bold italic type indicates that reaction may be life-threatening.

• Advise women to avoid using this herb when pregnant or breast-feeding.
• Warn patient to keep all herbal products away from children and pets.

sea holly

Eryngium campestre, eryngio herba, eryngo, sea holme, sea hulver

Common trade names
None known

AVAILABLE FORMS
Available as leaves, powdered root, and extract*.

ACTIONS & COMPONENTS
Obtained from *E. campestre.* Above-ground parts contain triterpene saponins, caffeic acid esters such as chlorogenic acid and rosmaric acid, and flavonoids. Roots also contain procoumarins, pyranocoumarins, and oligosaccharides. Above-ground plant parts have a mild diuretic effect. Roots have antispasmodic and mild expectorant effects.

USES
Above-ground parts are used to treat UTIs, prostatitis, and inflamed bronchial mucous membranes. Roots are used to treat kidney and bladder stones, renal colic, kidney and urinary tract inflammation, urine retention, edema, cough, bronchitis, and skin and respiratory disorders.

DOSAGE & ADMINISTRATION
Decoction: 2 or 3 cups daily. Prepared by boiling 4 teaspoons ground root in 1 L water for 10 minutes, steeping 15 minutes, and then straining.
Tea: 3 or 4 cups daily. Prepared by steeping 1 teaspoon ground root in 150 ml boiling water until cold, and then straining.
Tincture: 50 to 60 gtt P.O. daily, divided into three or four doses. Prepared by soaking 20 g powdered root in 80 g of 60% alcohol for 10 days.

ADVERSE REACTIONS
None known.

INTERACTIONS
Herb-drug. *Disulfiram:* Herbal products that contain alcohol may cause a disulfiram-like reaction. Advise patient to avoid using together.

EFFECTS ON LAB TEST RESULTS
None reported.

CAUTIONS
Pregnant or breast-feeding women shouldn't use this herb.

NURSING CONSIDERATIONS
• Find out why patient is using the herb.
• Monitor patient's response to herbal therapy.

PATIENT TEACHING
• Advise patient to consult a health care provider before using an herbal preparation because a standard treatment that has been proven effective may be available.

*Liquid contains alcohol.

• Tell patient that when filling a new prescription he should remind pharmacist of any herbal and dietary supplements he's taking.
• Advise patient to promptly notify health care provider about adverse effects or changes in symptoms.

self-heal

Prunella vulgaris, all-heal, blue curls, brownwort, brunella, carpenter's herb, carpenter's weed, heal-all, heart of the earth, Hercules woundwort, hock-heal, hook-heal, sicklewort, siclewort, slough-heal, woundwort

Common trade names
Prunella, Self-Heal

AVAILABLE FORMS
Available as dried herb, capsules, tea, and tincture*.

ACTIONS & COMPONENTS
Obtained from *P. vulgaris*. Contains oleanolic acid, urosolic acid, rutin, hyperoside, caffeic acid, vitamins, carotenoids, tannins, essential oils, and alkaloids. Urosolic acid is cytotoxic against lymphocytic leukemia cells and human lung cancer cells. Also contains rosmarinic acid, an antioxidant, and prunellin, which may have anti-HIV activity. Some marginal cytotoxicity against human colon and mammary tumor cells has also been reported.

USES
Used to treat wounds, stop bleeding, control diarrhea, support the liver, and aid circulation. Also used as a gargle for mouth and throat infections, as a cooling tea, and as a treatment for tuberculosis, jaundice, infectious hepatitis, bacillary dysentery, pleuritis with effusion, and cancer. Also used as an antibiotic, antihypertensive, antimutagenic, and antioxidant, especially in patients with HIV and cancer.

DOSAGE & ADMINISTRATION
Infusion: 6 to 15 g of dried herb steeped for 10 minutes in 8 ounces of water, P.O. t.i.d.
Tincture: 1 or 2 ml P.O. t.i.d.
Topical: Juice or poultice applied to affected area.

ADVERSE REACTIONS
None known.

INTERACTIONS
Herb-drug. *Disulfiram:* Herbal products that contain alcohol may cause a disulfiram-like reaction. Advise patient to avoid using together.

EFFECTS ON LAB TEST RESULTS
None reported.

CAUTIONS
Patients sensitive to any part of self-heal shouldn't take the herb. Pregnant or breast-feeding women shouldn't use this herb. Safety in children isn't known.

NURSING CONSIDERATIONS
• Find out why patient is using the herb.
• Because entire plant is used, sensitivity reactions are possible.
• Patients may combine topical and liquid forms of self-heal with

---

Bold italic type indicates that reaction may be life-threatening.

other herbal products. Read product ingredients carefully.

• Although no chemical interactions have been reported, consider the pharmacologic properties of the herb and its potential to interfere with therapeutic effects of conventional drugs.

PATIENT TEACHING
• Advise patient to consult a health care provider before using an herbal preparation because a standard treatment that has been proven effective may be available.
• Tell patient that when filling a new prescription he should remind pharmacist of any herbal and dietary supplements he's taking.
• Advise patients with such allergies as hay fever and ragweed to use this herb cautiously.
• Urge patient to consult a health care provider before taking self-heal.
• Tell patient to promptly notify a health care provider about adverse effects or changes in symptoms.

senega

Polygala senega, milkwort, mountain flax, northern senega, plantula marilandica, poligala raiz, polygala virginiana, polygalae radix, polygale de virginie, rattlesnake root, senega snakeroot, senegawurzel, snake root, snakeroot yuan zhi

Common trade names
Seneca, Senega
Combination products: *Antibron, Asthma 6-N, Bronchial, Bronchiplant, Bronchiplant Light, Bronchozone, Broncofluid,*

Broncovial, Calmarum, Chest Mixture, Cocillana-Etyfin, Combitorax, Desbly, Dinacode, Dinacode avae Codeine, Expectoran Codeine, Fluidin Antiasmatico, Fluidin Infantil, Hederix, Makatussin, Makatussin forte, Neo-Codion, Nyl Bronchitis, Pastillas Pectoral Kely, Patussol, Pectocalamine, Pectoral N, Phol-Tux, Polery, Pulmofasa, Pulmofasa Antihist, Quintopan, Senega and Ammonia, Sirop Pectoral Adulte, Sirop Santitussif Wyss a Base de Codeine, Sirop Wyss Contre La Toux, Stodol, Tussimont, Wampole Bronchial Cough Syrup

AVAILABLE FORMS
Available as dried root, liquid extract*, infusion, syrup, lozenges, tea, and tincture*.

ACTIONS & COMPONENTS
Obtained from *P. senega.* Contains triterpenoid saponins (senegenin, polygalin, and polygalic acid), which exert expectorant action on the lining of the upper GI tract and stomach. Irritation of the gastric mucosa may lead to reflex stimulation of bronchial mucous gland secretion.

USES
Used with other expectorants for chronic bronchitis and for treating pneumonia or the second stage of acute bronchial catarrh. Used mainly as an expectorant by patients with bronchitis. Also used as an antidote for some poisons, as a poultice for external wounds, and as an abortifacient. Also used for general ailments.

---

*Liquid contains alcohol.

DOSAGE & ADMINISTRATION

Fluidextract (1:1 in 60% alcohol): 0.3 to 1 ml (6 to 20 gtt) P.O. t.i.d. or 1.5 to 3 g P.O. daily.

Infusion: 0.5 to 1 g of herb in 1 cup of water P.O. b.i.d. or t.i.d. In severe cases, q 2 hours as long as patient is being monitored for adverse effects.

Root: 1.5 to 3 g P.O. daily.

Tincture (1:4 in 60% alcohol): 2.5 to 5 ml (50 to 100 gtt) P.O. t.i.d. or 2.5 to 7.5 g P.O. daily.

ADVERSE REACTIONS

GI: nausea, vomiting, GI irritation, diarrhea.
Respiratory: increased bronchial secretion.
Skin: diaphoresis.

INTERACTIONS

Herb-drug. *Disulfiram:* Herbal products that contain alcohol may cause a disulfiram-like reaction. Advise patient to avoid using together.

EFFECTS ON LAB TEST RESULTS

None reported.

CAUTIONS

Patients sensitive to senega shouldn't use this herb. Patients with GI disorders (such as peptic ulcer disease and inflammatory bowel disease) and women who are pregnant or breast-feeding also shouldn't use this herb. Pediatric effects are unknown and use in children isn't recommended.

NURSING CONSIDERATIONS

● Find out why patient is using the herb.

● Prolonged use has been linked to GI irritation.

☑**ALERT:** Monitor patient for nausea, diaphoresis, vomiting, GI complaints, and diarrhea. These problems may indicate an overdose, an adverse reaction, or sensitivity to senega. Emetic properties of the herb at high doses make further toxicity self-limiting.

● Monitor patients, especially those with diagnosed respiratory conditions, for shortness of breath or other respiratory difficulties from increased bronchial secretions.

PATIENT TEACHING

● Advise patient to consult a health care provider before using an herbal preparation because a standard treatment that has been proven effective may be available.

● Tell patient that when filling a new prescription he should remind pharmacist of any herbal and dietary supplements he's taking.

● Tell patient to read product labels carefully because senega is usually taken with other herbs or substances.

● Caution patient against prolonged use.

● Recommend that patient stop taking senega if he develops nausea, GI discomfort, vomiting, diarrhea, or increased breathing problems.

● Tell patient that liquid forms may contain alcohol, which can interact with other drugs.

Bold italic type indicates that reaction may be life-threatening.

senna

Cassia acutifolia, Alexandria senna, Alexandrian senna, Cassia senna, India senna, Khartoum senna, sennae folium, tinnevelly senna

Common trade names
Black Draught, Dr. Caldwell Senna Laxative, Fletcher's Castoria, Gentlax, Senexon Senna-Gen, Senokot, SenokotXTRA, Senolax, X-Prep Bowel Evacuant

AVAILABLE FORMS
Available as granules, liquid extract, suppository, syrup, and tablets.
Granules: 326 mg/teaspoon, 1.65 g/half teaspoon
Suppositories: 652 mg
Syrup: 218 mg/5 ml
Tablets: 187 mg, 217 mg, 600 mg

ACTIONS & COMPONENTS
Obtained from dried leaves and pods of *C. acutifolia* or *C. angustifolia.* Contains 1.2% to 6% dianthrone glycosides—primarily sennosides A, A_1, and B with lesser amounts of C, D, E, F, and G—with other anthraquinone derivatives that contribute to the laxative effect. Senna increases peristalsis, probably by direct effect on intestinal smooth muscle. It probably either irritates the muscles or stimulates the colonic intramural plexus. Senna is activated in the colon to rheinanthrone. Because activation takes 6 to 12 hours, a bedtime dose typically produces a morning bowel movement. It also promotes fluid accumulation in the colon and small intestine.

USES
Used as a laxative to treat constipation or ease bowel evacuation after rectal-anal surgery or if patient has anal fissures or hemorrhoids. Also used for colon evacuation before rectal and bowel examinations or surgery. It's commonly used to treat constipation caused by narcotics. Senna has been investigated as a treatment for fecal soiling, herpes simplex, and infections with *Escherichia coli* or *Candida albicans.*

DOSAGE & ADMINISTRATION
The following are general ranges; dosage should be individualized to the smallest dose needed to produce a soft stool. Elderly, debilitated, antepartum, and postpartum patients start with smallest doses. If comfortable elimination doesn't occur by the second day, dosage can be adjusted until evacuation occurs.
For adults, to evacuate colon for rectal and bowel examinations: Single 75-ml dose of a standardized senna preparation (1 ml standardized to 26 mg sennoside B).
For adults with constipation: 0.5 to 3 g crude herb or 15 to 40 mg sennosides (standardized preparations) P.O., ideally h.s.
For children: Several OTC products are available for children older than age 6 or who weigh more than 27 kg (60 lb). See product labels.
Infusion: Prepared either by adding 0.5 to 2 g of powdered herb to 150 ml hot (not boiling) water for 10 to 15 minutes and then straining or by steeping macerated herb in cold water for 10 to 12 hours and then straining.

*Liquid contains alcohol.

ADVERSE REACTIONS

CNS: tetany.
CV: *arrhythmias (prolonged use),* disorders of heart function.
EENT: rhinoconjunctivitis.
GI: cramping, diarrhea, nausea, perianal irritation, aggravated constipation.
GU: yellowish brown or red urine, nephritis, nephropathies, albuminuria, hematuria, damage to renal tubules.
Metabolic: hyperaldosteronism.
Musculoskeletal: accelerated bone deterioration, muscle weakness.
Respiratory: asthma.
Other: reversible finger clubbing, immunoglobulin E–mediated allergy, colon cancer (prolonged use).

INTERACTIONS

Herb-drug. *Antiarrhythmics, cardiac glycosides, including digoxin, lanoxin:* Overuse or abuse of senna may interfere with drug action via loss of potassium, leading to an increase in arrhythmias. For extended use, monitor patient's potassium levels and heart rate. Advise patient to avoid using together.
Corticosteroids: May increase risk of hypokalemia and potentiation of cardioactive steroids, and may rarely cause arrhythmias. For extended use, monitor patient's potassium levels, vital signs, and ECG.
Estrogen: Decreases estrogen levels. Advise patient to avoid using together.
NSAIDs: May decrease effect of senna. Advise patient to avoid using together.
Oral drugs: May decrease absorption of some drugs by rapid transit time in the colon. Monitor patient for loss of therapeutic response, especially patient previously well controlled.
Thiazide diuretics, including furosemide: May increase risk of hypokalemia. For extended use, monitor patient's potassium levels and ECG.
Herb-herb. *Potassium-depleting herbs such as gossypol, horsetail plant, licorice:* Increases risk of hypokalemia. For extended use together, monitor patient's potassium levels.
Stimulant laxative herbs such as aloe dried leaf sap, black root, blue flag rhizome, butternut bark, cascara bark, castor oil, colocynth fruit pulp, gamboge bark exudate, jalap root, manna bark exudate, podophyllum, rhubarb root, senna leaves and pods, wild cumber fruit, yellow dock root: Increases risk of hypokalemia. For extended use, monitor patient's potassium levels.

EFFECTS ON LAB TEST RESULTS

• May increase BUN, creatinine, and aldosterone levels. May decrease electrolyte levels, especially potassium.
• Albumin and blood may appear in urine.

CAUTIONS

Senna should be avoided by patients with intestinal obstruction, diarrhea, abdominal pain of unknown origin, fluid or electrolyte imbalance, and acute inflammatory intestinal diseases, such as appendicitis, colitis, Crohn's disease, and irritable bowel syndrome. Those with renal disease should use the herb cautiously.

Bold italic type indicates that reaction may be life-threatening.

There is no consensus in international labeling regarding use of senna by pregnant or breast-feeding women. In Britain and Germany, senna is contraindicated for these conditions. In the United States, no label restrictions appear on standardized OTC products. It hasn't been shown that standardized senna products stimulate uterine contractions in pregnant women.

The German Commission E doesn't recommend senna for children younger than age 12; however, several OTC products available in the United States provide dose recommendations for children older than age 6 or who weigh more than 60 pounds.

NURSING CONSIDERATIONS
• Find out why patient is using the herb.
• Although senna may be taken as a tea, dosages are difficult to determine or adjust using this unstandardized form. Many OTC products with standardized ingredients and doses are available. Adult dosages for senna can range from 20 to 60 mg of hydroxyanthracene derivatives.
• Infusions made in cold water may contain less of the compounds suspected to cause abdominal pain.
• Geriatric patients are usually advised to start with half the typical adult dose.
• Herb takes effect 6 to 8 hours after administration and isn't suitable for rapid emptying of the bowels.
• Long-term use is undesirable; however, if patient has chronic constipation, long-term use may

be warranted with proper care, including potassium replacement.
• Long-term use may reduce spontaneous bowel function and lead to "cathartic colon" and laxative-dependency syndrome.
• Typical symptoms of laxative abuse include abdominal pain, weakness, fatigue, thirst, vomiting, edema, bone pain caused by osteomalacia, fluid and electrolyte imbalance, hypoalbuminemia caused by protein-losing gastroenteropathy, and syndromes that mimic colitis.
• Evidence of overdose includes vomiting, severe GI spasms, and thin, watery stools. Large overdoses may also cause nephritis.
• Melanosis coli develops in about 5% of people who use anthranoids long-term (4 to 13 months). It resolves after discontinuation. There's no definite link between anthracene drugs and colon cancer.
• Other anthranoids, such as cassic acid, appear in breast milk in small amounts and may give milk a brownish tint. No data exist to determine whether the anthranoid level causes diarrhea in breast-fed infants.
• Senna preparations may contain alcohol or sugar.
• Monitor patient's serum potassium level when senna and cardiac glycosides, thiazide diuretics, corticosteroids, antiarrhythmics, licorice, potassium-depleting herbs, or other stimulant laxative herbs are used together.

PATIENT TEACHING
• Advise patient to consult a health care provider before using an herbal preparation because a stan-

*Liquid contains alcohol.

dard treatment that has been proven effective may be available.

• Tell patient that when filling a new prescription he should remind pharmacist of any herbal and dietary supplements he's taking.

• Encourage patient to first try lifestyle changes, such as increasing dietary fiber, fluid intake, and exercise, to restore normal bowel function. Patient can also use a bulk laxative.

• Tell patient that senna may turn urine yellowish brown or red.

• Recommend that pregnant or breast-feeding patients consult a health care provider before using senna.

• Inform patient that senna preparations may contain alcohol or sugar; advise patient to check product label if he has alcohol or sugar restrictions.

• Instruct patient not to take stimulant laxatives for longer than 2 weeks without seeking medical advice.

• Warn patient not to exceed maximum recommended dose.

• Advise patient that overuse of laxatives can lead to severe electrolyte imbalances, intestinal sluggishness, and a dependency on laxatives.

• Advise patient that rectal bleeding or failure to have a bowel movement after using a laxative may indicate a serious condition.

• Instruct patient to stop using senna if he has or develops nausea, vomiting, abdominal pain, loose stools, or diarrhea.

• Tell patient to contact a health care provider if his bowel habits change suddenly after 2 or more weeks.

• Warn patient to keep all herbal products away from children and pets.

shepherd's purse

Capsella bursa-pastoris, bursae pastoris herba, blindweed, capsella, case-weed, cocowort, lady's purse, mother's heart, pepper-and-salt, pick-pocket, poor man's parmacettie, rattle pouches, sanguinary, shepherd's heart, shepherd's purse herb, shepherd's scrip, shepherd's sprout, shovelweed, St. James' weed, toywort, witches' pouches

Common trade names
None known

AVAILABLE FORMS
Available as dried herb and liquid extract*.

ACTIONS & COMPONENTS
Obtained from *C. bursa-pastoris.* Contains the amino acid proline, cardioactive steroids, and a peptide with hemostatic oxytocin-like activity. Also contains saponins, flavonoids, large amounts of potassium salts, oxalates, vitamin C, and sinigrin. Sinigrin can be degraded to allyl isothiocyanate, which is linked to goiter and abnormal thyroid function. Shepherd's purse increases uterine contractions by stimulating smooth muscle. Cardioactive steroids in the seeds cause positive and negative inotropic and chronotropic effects. Muscarine-like, dose-dependent hypertensive and antihypertensive effects have also been reported.

Bold italic type indicates that reaction may be life-threatening.

USES
Used internally to treat dysmenorrhea, mild menorrhagia, and metrorrhagia. Also used for headache, mild cardiac insufficiency, arrhythmia, hypotension, nervous heart complaints, premenstrual complaints, hematemesis, hematuria, diarrhea, and acute catarrhal cystitis. Topically, it's used as a styptic for nosebleeds and other superficial bleeding injuries.

DOSAGE & ADMINISTRATION
Dried above-ground parts: 10 to 15 g P.O. daily. May be taken as 1 to 4 g of dried herb t.i.d.
Fluidextract (1:1 in 25% alcohol): 5 to 8 g or 1 to 4 ml P.O. t.i.d.
Tea: 1 to 4 g dried herb steeped in 150 ml of boiling water for 15 minutes and then strained.
Topical form: 3 to 5 g of herb steeped in 180 ml of boiling water for 10 to 15 minutes and then strained. Fluid is applied to affected area.

ADVERSE REACTIONS
CNS: sedation.
CV: palpitations, hypertension, hypotension.
GU: increased uterine contractions, abnormal menstruation.
Metabolic: abnormal thyroid function.

INTERACTIONS
Herb-drug. *Antihypertensives, antihypotensives:* May reduce or enhance effect as related to blood pressure; herb has positive inotropic and chronotropic effects. Monitor blood pressure closely.

CV drugs: May reduce effect. Monitor vital signs, and assess patient for palpitations.
Disulfiram: Herbal products that contain alcohol may cause a disulfiram-like reaction. Advise patient to avoid using together.
Sedatives: Has additive effects. Monitor patient for sedation.
Thyroid drugs: Allyl isothiocyanate may interfere with thyroid therapy. Monitor thyroid function in patients previously well controlled.
Herb-herb. *Herbs with sedative effects, including calamus, calendula, California poppy, capsicum, catnip, celery, cough grass, elecampane, German chamomile, goldenseal, gotu kola, hops, Jamaican dogwood, kava, lemon balm, sage, St. John's wort, sassafras, Siberian ginseng, skullcap, stinging nettle, valerian, wild carrot, wild lettuce, yerba maté:* May have additive effects. Monitor patient for sedation.

EFFECTS ON LAB TEST RESULTS
• May cause abnormal thyroid function test results.

CAUTIONS
Shepherd's purse is a uterine stimulant and may induce miscarriage; it shouldn't be used by women planning pregnancy or those who are pregnant or breast-feeding. Patients with a history of kidney stones should use shepherd's purse cautiously because of its oxalate content. Shepherd's purse commonly harbors endophytic fungi such as *Albugo candida* and *Peronospora parasitica.* Because it may contain mycotoxins, patients with compro-

*Liquid contains alcohol.

mised immune systems should use the herb cautiously.

NURSING CONSIDERATIONS

● Find out why patient is using the herb.

● The use of shepherd's purse instead of ergot for uterine bleeding is inappropriate because of inadequate activity.

● Monitor blood pressure, which may increase or decrease, and thyroid function in patients taking thyroid medication who were previously well controlled.

● Monitor patient for palpitations, especially if susceptible to arrhythmias.

● Monitor patient for changes in menstruation.

PATIENT TEACHING

● Advise patient to consult a health care provider before using an herbal preparation because a standard treatment that has been proven effective may be available.

● Tell patient that when filling a new prescription he should remind pharmacist of any herbal and dietary supplements he's taking.

● Warn patient not to use alcohol-containing forms if he takes disulfiram, metronidazole, or other drugs that interact with alcohol.

● Inform women that shepherd's purse may cause abnormal menstruation.

● Tell patient that this herb may aggravate kidney stones, cerebrovascular therapy, thyroid therapy, and treatment for low or high blood pressure. Affected patients should use shepherd's purse cautiously and only under direct supervision

by a knowledgeable health care provider.

● Advise patient that herb may cause or increase sedation and the adverse effects of other herbs or drugs that cause sedation.

● Caution patient to avoid hazardous tasks until full sedative effects of herb are known.

● Urge patient to promptly notify health care provider about new symptoms or adverse effects.

● Tell patient to store herb away from light and moisture, and to keep it away from children and pets.

shiitake

Lentinula edodes, Lentinan edodes, Lentinus edodes, Tricholomopsis edodes, forest mushroom, Hua Gu, Lentinula, pasania fungus, shitake, snake butter

Common trade names
None known

AVAILABLE FORMS

Available as tea bags and fresh mushrooms.
Capsules: 325 mg

ACTIONS & COMPONENTS

Shiitake contains very low concentrations of lentinan (0.02%), which has antitumor effects. Shiitake may reduce plasma levels of free cholesterol, triglycerides, and phospholipids.

USES

In general, shiitake is used for boosting the immune system and

---

Bold italic type indicates that reaction may be life-threatening.

reducing cholesterol levels, and as an anti-aging agent.

DOSAGE & ADMINISTRATION
Capsules: 325 P.O. twice daily.
Decoctions: Prepared by boiling either whole or powdered mushroom in water, concentrating the extract and then drinking it.

ADVERSE REACTIONS
GI: abdominal discomfort, *intestinal obstruction.*
Hematology: *eosinophilia.*
Respiratory: hypersensitivity pneumonitis due to spore inhalation.
Skin: contact dermatitis, photosensitivity.

INTERACTIONS
None reported.

EFFECTS ON LAB TEST RESULTS
• May decrease eosinophil count.

CAUTIONS
Women who are pregnant or breast-feeding should avoid ingesting amounts greater than normally consumed in food. One case study has reported the development of eosinophilia after daily ingestion of 4 g shiitake powder for 10 weeks.

NURSING CONSIDERATIONS
• Find out why patient is taking shiitake.
• Adverse reactions to shiitake are rare.
• Shiitake is commonly used in Japanese cooking.

PATIENT TEACHING
• Advise patient to consult a health care provider before using an herbal preparation because a standard treatment that has been proven effective may be available.
• Tell patient that when filling a new prescription he should remind pharmacist of any herbal or dietary supplement he's taking.
• Warn patient not to take herb before seeking medical attention because doing so may delay diagnosis of a potentially serious medical condition.
• Instruct patient to promptly notify health care provider about any new symptoms or adverse effects.
• Warn patient to keep all herbal products away from children and pets.

skullcap

Scutellaria lateriflora, blue pimpernel, helmet flower, hoodwort, mad-dog weed, madweed, Quaker bonnet, scullcap, Virginian skullcap

Common trade names
Skullcap, Wild American Skullcap, Wild Countryside Skullcap

AVAILABLE FORMS
Available as dried herb, extracts, and capsules.
Capsules: 425 mg, 430 mg

ACTIONS & COMPONENTS
Obtained from roots and leaves of *S. lateriflora* and *S. baicalensis.* Contains such flavonoids as apigenin, baicalein, baicalin, hispidulin, scutellarein, and scutellarin. Also contains sesquiterpenes such as cadinene, caryophyllene, catapol, limonene, and terpineol. Other compounds include wogonin

*Liquid contains alcohol.

and its glucuronide, which can inhibit sialidase, an enzyme linked to some cancers. Lignin and various tannins are also present. Extracts from *S. baicalensis* may modulate hematopoiesis, scavenge free radicals, and increase nitric oxide production. Extracts may have some bacteriostatic, bactericidal, anti-inflammatory, and antiviral activity.

USES
Used as an anticonvulsant, antispasmodic, anti-inflammatory, and sedative. Also used as an adjunct to chemotherapy to enhance immune response.

DOSAGE & ADMINISTRATION
Dried herb: 1 or 2 g as a tea P.O. t.i.d.
Liquid extract (1:1 in 25% alcohol): 2 to 4 ml P.O. t.i.d.

ADVERSE REACTIONS
CNS: confusion, headache, *seizures.*
CV: *arrhythmias.*
Hepatic: *hepatotoxicity.*

INTERACTIONS
Herb-drug. *Disulfiram:* Herbal products that contain alcohol may cause a disulfiram-like reaction. Advise patient to avoid using together.

EFFECTS ON LAB TEST RESULTS
• May increase liver enzyme levels.

CAUTIONS
Pregnant or breast-feeding women shouldn't use this herb.

NURSING CONSIDERATIONS
• Find out why patient is using the herb.
• Skullcap preparations may be contaminated with other substances.
• Monitor patient for adverse effects and response to herbal treatment.

PATIENT TEACHING
• Advise patient to consult a health care provider before using an herbal preparation because a standard treatment that has been proven effective may be available.
• Tell patient that when filling a new prescription he should remind pharmacist of any herbal and dietary supplements he's taking
• Warn patient not to take herb before seeking medical attention because doing so may delay diagnosis of a potentially serious medical condition.
• Instruct patient to promptly notify health care provider about any new symptoms or adverse effects.
• Warn patient to keep all herbal products away from children and pets.

skunk cabbage

Symplocarpus foetidus,
dracontium, meadow cabbage, polecat cabbage, polecatweed, skunkweed

Common trade names
None known

AVAILABLE FORMS
Available as powdered root, extract*, and tincture.

Bold italic type indicates that reaction may be life-threatening.

ACTIONS & COMPONENTS

Obtained from seeds, rhizomes, and roots of *S. foetidus.* Contains starch, gum sugar, fixed and volatile oils, iron, various alkaloids, phenolic compounds, glycosides, and tannins. The leaves are also said to contain *n*-hydroxytryptamine. The root contains calcium oxalate.

USES

Used for treating chest tightness (as in asthma and bronchitis) and as an antispasmodic, diaphoretic, emetic, expectorant, and sedative.

DOSAGE & ADMINISTRATION

Liquid extract (1:1 in 25% alcohol): 0.5 to 1 ml P.O. t.i.d.

ADVERSE REACTIONS

CNS: headache, vertigo.
EENT: burning of mucous membranes or a hot sensation when taken orally; vision impairment.
GI: nausea, vomiting.
GU: renal damage.
Skin: irritation.

INTERACTIONS

Herb-drug. *Disulfiram:* Herbal products that contain alcohol may cause a disulfiram-like reaction. Advise patient to avoid using together.

EFFECTS ON LAB TEST RESULTS

• May increase BUN and creatinine levels.

CAUTIONS

Pregnant or breast-feeding women shouldn't use this herb.

NURSING CONSIDERATIONS

• Find out why patient is using the herb.
• Monitor patient's response to herbal therapy.

PATIENT TEACHING

• Advise patient to consult a health care provider before using an herbal preparation because a standard treatment that has been proven effective may be available.
• Tell patient that when filling a new prescription he should remind pharmacist of any herbal and dietary supplements he's taking
• Warn patient not to take herb for asthma or bronchitis before seeking medical attention because doing so may delay diagnosis of a potentially serious medical condition.
• Instruct patient to seek appropriate medical attention if he is short of breath or has a persistent cough.
• Warn patient to keep all herbal products away from children and pets.

slippery elm

Ulmus rubra, American elm, Indian elm, moose elm, red elm, sweet elm

Common trade names
None known

AVAILABLE FORMS

Available as powdered bark, liquid extract*, lozenges, capsules, tablets, and tincture.
Capsules, tablets: 370 mg, 400 mg, 500 mg
Liquid extract: 1:1 in 60% alcohol

---

*Liquid contains alcohol.

ACTIONS & COMPONENTS
Obtained from inner bark of *U. rubra*. Contains mucilage composed of hexoses, methylpentoses, pentoses, and polyuronides. Other constituents include phytosterols, sesquiterpenes, calcium oxalate, cholesterol, and tannins that may have astringent activity.

USES
Used externally as a demulcent to soothe and soften skin and as an emollient that coats and protects irritated tissues. Also used to treat wounds, burns, and various skin conditions. Used internally to treat diverticulitis, gastritis, gastric and duodenal ulcers, herpes, and syphilis. Also used as an abortifacient, a lubricant to ease labor, and a nutritional source in baby food.

DOSAGE & ADMINISTRATION
Capsules: Up to 12 400-mg capsules P.O. daily. Or two or more 400- to 500-mg capsules P.O. t.i.d. or q.i.d.
Decoction (1:8 with alcohol): 4 to 16 ml P.O. daily.
Tea: 1 teaspoon powdered bark steeped in 8 ounces cool water for 1 hour, taken b.i.d. to t.i.d. Or ½ to 2 g of bark in 200 ml boiling water for 10 to 15 minutes, then cooled. 3 to 4 cups P.O. daily.
Tincture: 5 ml P.O. t.i.d.
For GI discomfort: 5 ml liquid extract P.O. t.i.d.
Topical use: Poultice is prepared from powdered bark in boiling water. Applied to affected area.

ADVERSE REACTIONS
Skin: contact dermatitis.
Other: *allergic reaction.*

INTERACTIONS
Herb-drug. *Disulfiram:* Herbal products that contain alcohol may cause a disulfiram-like reaction. Advise patient to avoid using together.
Oral drugs: Herb is mucilaginous. Advise patient to separate oral drugs from herbal consumption by at least 2 hours.

EFFECTS ON LAB TEST RESULTS
None reported.

CAUTIONS
Pregnant or breast-feeding women shouldn't use this herb.

NURSING CONSIDERATIONS
• Find out why patient is using the herb.
• Although no chemical interactions have been reported, consider the pharmacologic properties of the herb and its potential to interfere with therapeutic effects of conventional drugs.
• Monitor patient's response to herbal therapy.

PATIENT TEACHING
• Advise patient to consult a health care provider before using an herbal preparation because a standard treatment that has been proven effective may be available.
• Tell patient that when filling a new prescription he should remind pharmacist of any herbal and dietary supplements he's taking
• Warn patient not to use herb for burns or wounds before seeking

medical attention because doing so may delay diagnosis of a potentially serious medical condition.
● Instruct patient to promptly notify health care provider about new symptoms and adverse effects.
● Warn patient to keep all herbal products away from children and pets.

soapwort

Saponaria officinalis, bouncing bet, bruisewort, crow soap, dog cloves, Fuller's herb, latherwort, old maid's pink, soap root, soapwood, sweet Betty, wild sweet William

Common trade names
None known

AVAILABLE FORMS
Available as dried leaves, root, and liquid extract.

ACTIONS & COMPONENTS
Obtained from leaves, roots, and rhizomes of *S. officinalis.* Contains saponin, sapotoxin, saponarine, and other saporins. Other components include flavonoids, resin, and gum. Saponins are cytotoxic compounds that may be active against various cancers, including lymphoma, leukemia, melanoma, and breast cancer. The seeds of *S. officinalis* have ribosome-inactivating activity.

USES
Used as an expectorant for cough and other respiratory tract disorders, a gargle for tonsillitis, a diaphoretic, and a diuretic. Also used for GI complaints, liver and kidney disorders, rheumatic gout, and such skin conditions as acne, eczema, psoriasis, and poison ivy. Also used to alter metabolism. Externally, its lathering action has led to use in shampoo and bath preparations.

DOSAGE & ADMINISTRATION
soapwort herb
For constipation: Decoction of leaves, 2 glasses P.O. daily.
Daily dose: Aqueous extract, 1 or 2 g daily.
soapwort root
Decoction: 10 to 180 g root added to 1 g sodium carbonate and simple syrup to make 200 g.
Expectorant: 9 ml (about 2 teaspoons) of the decoction P.O. q 2 hours.
Tea: 0.4 g of medium fine cut root; 1 teaspoon contains about 2.6 g of herb.

ADVERSE REACTIONS
CNS: neurotoxicity.
GI: GI irritation, nausea, vomiting, diarrhea.
GU: *nephrotoxicity.*
Hepatic: *hepatotoxicity.*
Skin: localized irritation, mucous membrane irritations.

INTERACTIONS
None reported.

EFFECTS ON LAB TEST RESULTS
● May increase BUN and creatinine levels.
● May increase liver function test values.

CAUTIONS
Internal use isn't recommended because herb is purgative and mildly

---

*Liquid contains alcohol.

poisonous. Women who are pregnant or breast-feeding shouldn't use this herb. Patients with GI disorders should avoid using this herb because it irritates the gastric mucosa.

NURSING CONSIDERATIONS
• Find out why patient is using the herb.
• Although no chemical interactions have been reported, consider the pharmacologic properties of the herb and its potential to interfere with therapeutic effects of conventional drugs.
• Patients who take soapwort should have liver and renal function monitored periodically.
• If patient takes herb internally, watch for adverse effects, such as vomiting and diarrhea.
• Observe patient for localized skin reactions.

PATIENT TEACHING
• Advise patient to consult a health care provider before using an herbal preparation because a standard treatment that has been proven effective may be available.
• Tell patient that when filling a new prescription he should remind pharmacist of any herbal and dietary supplements he's taking.
• Warn patient not to take herb for extended periods before seeking medical attention because a persistent cough may indicate a potentially serious medical condition.
• Instruct patient to notify a health care provider about adverse effects, such as localized skin reactions or nausea.

• Tell patient to store herb in a tightly sealed container that protects it from light and moisture.
• Warn patient to keep all herbal products away from children and pets.

sorrel

Rumex acetosa, cuckoo's meate, cuckoo sorrow, dock, garden sorrel, green sauce, green sorrel, sour dock, sourgrass, sour sauce, soursuds

Common trade names
None known

AVAILABLE FORMS
Available as a tea, liquid extract*, and coated tablets.

ACTIONS & COMPONENTS
Obtained from leaves, berries, and roots of *R. acetosa*. Contains oxalates (such as oxalic acid and calcium oxalate) and anthracene derivatives, such as physcion, chryosphanol, emodin, and rhein. Other components include ascorbic acid, tartaric acid, and tannins.

USES
Used for acute and chronic inflammation of nasal passages and respiratory tract. Also used as an adjunct to antibacterial therapy and as an antiseptic, an astringent, and a diuretic.

DOSAGE & ADMINISTRATION
Liquid extract (19% alcohol):
50 gtt P.O. t.i.d.
Tablets: For adults, 2 coated tablets t.i.d.

Bold italic type indicates that reaction may be life-threatening.

ADVERSE REACTIONS
CNS: headache.
GI: nausea, flatulence.
GU: renal damage.
Hepatic: liver damage.

INTERACTIONS
Herb-drug. *Disulfiram:* Herbal products that contain alcohol may cause a disulfiram-like reaction. Advise patient to avoid using together.

EFFECTS ON LAB TEST RESULTS
• May increase BUN and creatinine levels.
• May increase liver function test values.

CAUTIONS
Pregnant or breast-feeding women shouldn't use this herb.

NURSING CONSIDERATIONS
• Find out why patient is using the herb.
◪ **ALERT:** High oxalate salt content may lead to significant toxicity and even death if enough herb is ingested. Such oxalate poisoning can occur with consumption of large quantities of leaves as a salad.
• Closely monitor patient's response to herbal therapy.

PATIENT TEACHING
• Advise patient to consult a health care provider before using an herbal preparation because a standard treatment that has been proven effective may be available.
• Tell patient that when filling a new prescription he should remind pharmacist of any herbal and dietary supplements he's taking.

• Warn patient not to take herb for inflammatory or respiratory symptoms before seeking medical attention because doing so may delay diagnosis of a potentially serious medical condition.
• Instruct patient to promptly notify his health care provider about adverse effects or a change in symptoms.
• Warn patient to keep all herbal products away from children and pets.

southernwood

Artemisia abrotanum, appleringie, boy's love, garde robe, lad's love, old man, southern wormwood

Common trade names
None known

AVAILABLE FORMS
Available as dried herb and fluid extract.

ACTIONS & COMPONENTS
Obtained from *A. abrotanum.* Contains a volatile essential oil, mostly absinthol, as well as artemisitin, hydroxycoumarins such as umbelliferone and isofraxidin, and tannins. Four flavonols possessing spasmolytic activity have recently been isolated. Herb has tonic, antiseptic, antimicrobial, anthelmintic, and stimulant effects.

USES
Used internally to treat fever, infections, irregular menstruation, and worm infestations, especially roundworm and pinworm in children, and as a bitter to improve di-

---

*Liquid contains alcohol.

gestion. Applied externally to treat baldness and dandruff, poorly healing or gangrenous wounds, ulcers, and insect bites. Also used to repel moths, fleas, flies, and mosquitoes.

DOSAGE & ADMINISTRATION

Liquid extract: ½ to 1 dram.
To stimulate menstruation: 1 ounce of herb added to 1 pint boiling water P.O. t.i.d.
To treat worm infestations: 1 teaspoon powdered herb P.O. a.m. and h.s.

ADVERSE REACTIONS

Hepatic: liver damage.

INTERACTIONS

Herb-drug. *Alkaloids, glycosides, heavy metal ions such as aluminum and zinc:* Tannic acid may form insoluble complexes. Advise patient to avoid using together.
Antiplatelet drugs such as aspirin, heparin, low-molecular-weight heparin, warfarin: Alters coagulation. Monitor PT and INR closely.

EFFECTS ON LAB TEST RESULTS

• May increase liver function test values.
• May alter PT and INR.

CAUTIONS

Pregnant or breast-feeding women should avoid this herb, as should patients with a history of liver disease. Using herb to treat burns has caused toxicity.

NURSING CONSIDERATIONS

• Find out why patient is using the herb.

• Southernwood shouldn't be consumed in large amounts.
• Significant amounts of tannic acid present in the plant may lead to liver damage.
• Monitor patient for signs of bleeding, especially if he takes an anticoagulant.
• Monitor patient's response to herbal therapy.
⚠ALERT: Don't confuse southernwood with a related species, field southernwood *(A. campestris).*

PATIENT TEACHING

• Advise patient to consult a health care provider before using an herbal preparation because a standard treatment that has been proven effective may be available.
• Tell patient that when filling a new prescription he should remind pharmacist of any herbal and dietary supplements he's taking.
• Instruct patient to have a medical evaluation before taking this herb and not to consume large quantities of it.
• Tell patient to consult a health care provider if he takes the herb for any medical condition that doesn't improve in 2 weeks.
• Tell patient to store herb in a sealed container protected from light.
• Warn patient to keep all herbal products away from children and pets.

Bold italic type indicates that reaction may be life-threatening.

soy

Glycine max, G. soja, soya, soyabean, soybean

Common trade names
None known

AVAILABLE FORMS
Available as soy protein or isoflavone supplements in powder, capsules, or tablets. Also available as beans, flour, and many food items such as sprouts, tofu, tempeh, soy milk, textured and hydrolyzed vegetable protein, meat substitutes, miso, and soy sauce.

ACTIONS & COMPONENTS
Obtained from beans (seeds) of *G. max.* Contains soy protein; isoflavones; saponins; phenolic acids; lecithin; phytoestrols; vitamins A, E, K, and some B; minerals such as calcium, potassium, iron, and phosphorus; and amino acids.

Isoflavones are molecularly similar to natural body estrogens. The isoflavones in soy, particularly genistein and daidzen, have antioxidant and phytoestrogenic properties. Saponins enhance immune function and bind to cholesterol to limit its absorption in the intestines. Phenolic acids have antioxidant properties. Phytoestrols and other components, including lecithin, may lower cholesterol levels.

Isoflavones may reduce the risk of hormone-dependent cancers, such as breast and prostate cancer, as well as other forms of cancer. Increased consumption of soy in Asian populations helps account for decreased rates of CV disease.

Soy-based diets lead to significant decreases in total cholesterol, high-density lipoprotein, and low-density lipoprotein levels. The FDA officially supports the claim that soy protein may decrease cholesterol levels.

The mild estrogenic activity of soy isoflavones may help to alleviate menopausal symptoms in some women. However, no data exist concerning the effect of soy on other symptoms of menopause, such as night sweats, insomnia, vaginal dryness, or changes in sexual desire. Soy consumption may also help regulate hormone levels in premenopausal women. Soy may also have a beneficial effect on GI function.

USES
Used to treat cancers, CV disease, menopausal symptoms, and osteoporosis. Also used as a detoxicant, a circulatory stimulant, and a popular dietary protein supplement.

DOSAGE & ADMINISTRATION
No consensus exists. The FDA currently recommends 25 g soy protein P.O. daily. Other sources suggest beneficial CV effects with doses of 25 to 50 g P.O. daily (to lower cholesterol).
For menopausal symptoms: 25 to 60 g P.O. daily.

ADVERSE REACTIONS
GI: stomach pain, flatulence, loose stools, diarrhea.
Respiratory: *asthma.*
Other: *allergic reaction.*

---

*Liquid contains alcohol.

INTERACTIONS

Herb-drug. *Calcium, iron, zinc:* Decreases absorption. Advise patient to avoid using together.
Estrogen, raloxifene, tamoxifen: May reduce effects. Advise patient to avoid using together.

EFFECTS ON LAB TEST RESULTS

None reported.

CAUTIONS

Patients sensitive to soy or soy-containing products shouldn't use this herb. High doses of soy protein may have harmful effects in women with breast cancer. Soy isoflavones shouldn't be used by those with thyroid problems; these agents may inhibit thyroid hormone synthesis. Infants shouldn't be fed soy-based formulas because of high isoflavone content. Inhalation of soy dust led to an asthma outbreak in 26 workers exposed to soy powder when unloading the product.

NURSING CONSIDERATIONS

• Find out why patient is using the herb.
• Certain constituents of soy may interfere with thyroid function, but the clinical importance of this problem is unclear.
• Long-term safety of unfermented soy and soy isoflavones may be potentially harmful because of trypsin inhibitors, hemaglutinin, and phytic acid content.
• Soybeans and soybean products are an excellent source of protein, vitamins, and minerals.
• Monitor patient's response to herbal therapy.

PATIENT TEACHING

• Advise patient to consult a health care provider before using an herbal preparation because a standard treatment that has been proven effective may be available.
• Tell patient that when filling a new prescription he should remind pharmacist of any herbal and dietary supplements he's taking
• Tell patient who takes estrogen, tamoxifen, or raloxifene to inform a health care provider if she also takes soy, which may interfere with therapeutic effects of these drugs.
• To avoid disturbed absorption, instruct patient to consume zinc, iron, or calcium supplements several hours apart from any soy products.
• Warn patient to keep all herbal products away from children and pets.

spirulina

Spirulina maxima, S. platensis, blue green algae, blue-green micro-algae, dihe, tecuitlatl

Common trade names
Chinese Spirulina, Green Earth Food, Spirulina

AVAILABLE FORMS

Available as a powder, flakes, capsules, and tablets.
Capsules: 380 mg
Tablets: 500 mg

ACTIONS & COMPONENTS

Obtained from the blue-green algae *S. maxima* and *S. platensis*. Contains about 65% protein and all essential amino acids. Spirulina is a concentrated source of other nutrients, including chlorophyll, beta-carotene, other carotenoids, high levels of B-complex vitamins, minerals, essential fatty acids, including gamma linolenic acid and omega-3 fatty acid, and iron. Spirulina may enhance disease resistance, inhibit allergic reactions, and exert hepatoprotective and hypocholesteremic effects.

The protein content of spirulina is comparable to other sources, such as meat and milk. The vitamin B_{12} in spirulina has no activity in humans and may even block assimilation of regular vitamin B_{12}.

USES
Used as a nutritional supplement and energy booster and to treat obesity, diabetes mellitus, and oral cancers.

DOSAGE & ADMINISTRATION
Average daily dose: 2 to 3 g P.O. daily in divided doses.

ADVERSE REACTIONS
Metabolic: inhibited vitamin B_{12} absorption.
Other: *allergic reaction.*

INTERACTIONS
None reported.

EFFECTS ON LAB TEST RESULTS
None reported.

CAUTIONS
Spirulina grown in contaminated water may concentrate such toxic metals as lead, mercury, and cadmium.

NURSING CONSIDERATIONS
• Find out why patient is using the herb.
• Assess patient's knowledge of herb use.
• Monitor patient's response to herbal therapy.

PATIENT TEACHING
• Advise patient to consult a health care provider before using an herbal preparation because a standard treatment that has been proven effective may be available.
• Tell patient that when filling a new prescription he should remind pharmacist of any herbal and dietary supplements he's taking.
• Advise patient to store product in a cool, dry place, not to freeze it, and to keep it away from children and pets.

squaw vine

Mitchella repens, checkerberry, deerberry, deer berry, one berry, partridgeberry, partridge berry, squawberry, squawvine, winter clover

Common trade names
None known

AVAILABLE FORMS
Available as dried herb, extract, and tincture.

ACTIONS & COMPONENTS
Obtained from above-ground parts of *M. repens.* Contains resin, dextrin, mucilage, saponin, wax, alkaloids, glycosides, and tannins. Herb has tonic, antispasmodic, diuretic, and astringent effects.

---

*Liquid contains alcohol.

USES
Used to treat dysmenorrhea or amenorrhea and to aid labor and childbirth. After delivery, herb is used to treat sore nipples. Also used to stimulate lactation and to treat insomnia, colitis, dysuria, diarrhea, heart failure, liver failure, and seizures.

DOSAGE & ADMINISTRATION
For sore nipples: 2 ounces fresh herb added to 1 pint boiling water, strained, and added to an equal amount of cream. Mixture is boiled to a soft consistency, allowed to cool, then applied to nipples after each breast-feeding session.
Infusion: 1 teaspoon of herb added to 1 cup boiling water, steeped for 10 to 15 minutes and taken t.i.d.
Strong decoction: 2 to 4 ounces fresh herb added to 1 pint boiling water; then strained and cooled; 2 to 4 ounces taken P.O. b.i.d. or t.i.d.
Tincture: 1 or 2 ml P.O. t.i.d.

ADVERSE REACTIONS
Hepatic: liver damage.

INTERACTIONS
Herb-drug. *Cardiac glycosides:* May have increased effects. Advise patient to avoid using together.

EFFECTS ON LAB TEST RESULTS
• May increase liver enzyme levels.
• May increase liver function test values.

CAUTIONS
Pregnant or breast-feeding women should use herb cautiously.

NURSING CONSIDERATIONS
• Find out why patient is using the herb.
• Toxicity is rare and is only likely to occur after ingestion of large amounts of tannic acid.
• Monitor patient's response to herbal therapy.

PATIENT TEACHING
• Advise patient to consult a health care provider before using an herbal preparation because a standard treatment that has been proven effective may be available.
• Tell patient that when filling a new prescription he should remind pharmacist of any herbal and dietary supplements he's taking.
• Advise patient to consult a health care provider if taking the herb for any condition that doesn't improve within 2 weeks. Chronic symptoms may indicate a more serious problem.
• Instruct patient to promptly notify a health care provider about new symptoms or adverse effects.
• Tell patient not to exceed recommended dosage.
• Advise patient to store herb in a cool, dry place, not to freeze it, and to keep it away from children and pets.

squill

Urginea indica, U. maritima, European squill, Indian squill, Mediterranean squill, red squill, sea onion, sea squill, white squill

Common trade names
None known

Bold italic type indicates that reaction may be life-threatening.

AVAILABLE FORMS
Available as powder and syrup.

ACTIONS & COMPONENTS
Obtained from bulbs of *U. maritima* and *U. indica*. Contains several cardioactive steroid glycosides, including scillaren A, glucoscillaren A, scillaridin A, and scilliroside and proscillaridin A that exert digitalis-like activity. Squill components also have diuretic, natriuretic (increases urinary sodium excretion), stimulant, expectorant, and emetic action. One component, silliglaucosidin, has shown anticancer activity.

USES
Used to treat cancer, arthritis, gout, dysmenorrhea, and warts. Also used to treat mild (New York Heart Association Class I and II) cardiac insufficiency, arrhythmias, and reduced kidney capacity. However, squill extracts have been superseded by widespread use of cardiac glycosides. Squill is a component of some cough preparations because of its weak expectorant effect.

Red squill has been used externally in hair tonics for dandruff and seborrhea; however, it's mainly used as a rodenticide.

DOSAGE & ADMINISTRATION
Cardiotonic: 0.1 to 0.5 g standardized squill powder P.O.
Expectorant (syrup): Dosage varies depending on liquid formulation used.

ADVERSE REACTIONS
CNS: fatigue, dizziness, *seizures, coma,* headache, psychosis, hallucinations.
CV: *arrhythmias, ventricular tachycardia, bradycardia, AV block,* hypotension.
GI: vomiting, nausea, diarrhea, loss of appetite.

INTERACTIONS
Herb-drug. *Calcium, digoxin, diuretics, extended glucocorticoid therapy, laxatives, quinidine:* Increases risk of digitalis-like toxicity. Advise patient to avoid using together.
Methylxanthines, such as theophylline; phosphodiesterase inhibitors, including cilostazol, inamrinone, and milrinone; quinidine; sympathomimetics, including epinephrine and phenylephrine: Increases risk of cardiac arrhythmias. Advise patient to avoid using together. Monitor ECG closely if these drugs are taken together.

EFFECTS ON LAB TEST RESULTS
• May decrease potassium level. May alter electrolyte levels.

CAUTIONS
Squill should be avoided by patients with second- or third-degree AV block, hypercalcemia, hypokalemia, hypertrophic cardiomyopathy, carotid sinus syndrome, ventricular tachycardia, thoracic aortic aneurysm, or Wolff-Parkinson-White syndrome.

NURSING CONSIDERATIONS
• Find out why patient is using the herb.

*Liquid contains alcohol.

☑ALERT: All squill species can cause digitalis-like toxicity, which may cause nausea, vomiting, diarrhea, fatigue, dizziness, arrhythmias, bradycardia, hypotension, seizures, and coma.

● Treatment of overdose includes gastric lavage and instillation of activated charcoal. Treat adverse effects symptomatically, such as potassium replacement for potassium loss; phenytoin for ventricular ectopic formation; lidocaine for ventricular extrasystole; atropine or orciprenaline for bradycardia. A pacemaker may be necessary. Hemoperfusion may be used to eliminate glycosides; cholestyramine may be used to interrupt enterohepatic circulation.

● In patients with GI symptoms and bradyarrhythmias from presumed herbal poisoning, suspect cardiac glycoside poisoning as the cause.

● Because of the narrow therapeutic index of squill glycosides, adverse effects could occur rapidly in some patients even at therapeutic doses.

● Monitor vital signs and ECG.

PATIENT TEACHING

● Advise patient to consult a health care provider before using an herbal preparation because a standard treatment that has been proven effective may be available.

● Tell patient that when filling a new prescription he should remind pharmacist of any herbal and dietary supplements he's taking.

● Instruct patient to consult a health care provider if taking the herb for any condition that doesn't improve within 2 weeks. Chronic symptoms may indicate a more serious medical condition.

● Warn patient to contact a health care provider if he has an irregular heartbeat, fainting, difficulty breathing, nausea, appetite loss, vomiting, diarrhea, or unusual weakness, tiredness, or drowsiness.

● Instruct patient to store herb in a cool, dry place, not to freeze it, and to keep it away from children and pets.

stone root

Collinsonia canadensis, citronella, hardback, hardhack, heal-all, horseweed, knob grass, knob root, knobweed, richleaf, richweed

Common trade names
Stoneroot Extract

AVAILABLE FORMS

Available as dried root or rhizome, tea, liquid extract*, and tincture*.

ACTIONS & COMPONENTS

Obtained from *C. canadensis.* Contains volatile oils, tannins, saponins, resin, mucilage, and caffeic acid derivatives.

USES

Used for bladder inflammation, kidney stones, water retention, hyperuricuria, edema, GI disorders, headaches, and indigestion. In homeopathic medicine, stone root is used for hemorrhoids and constipation.

Bold italic type indicates that reaction may be life-threatening.

DOSAGE & ADMINISTRATION
Dried root: 1 to 4 g in 150 ml boiling water, steeped 5 to 10 minutes, and then strained. Consumed t.i.d.
Liquid extract (1:1 in 25% alcohol): 1 to 4 ml P.O. t.i.d.
Tincture (1:5 in 40% alcohol): 2 to 8 ml P.O. t.i.d.

ADVERSE REACTIONS
CNS: dizziness, numbness with ingestion of large quantities.
GI: irritation, abdominal pain, nausea.
GU: painful urination.

INTERACTIONS
Herb-drug. *Diuretics, including acetazolamide, furosemide, hydrochlorothiazide:* May have additive effects. Advise patient to use cautiously with other diuretics.
Herb-herb. *Herbs with diuretic action, such as gum acacia, Chinese cucumber, ginkgo, sassafras:* May have additive effects. Advise patient to use cautiously with other herbs with diuretic action.

EFFECTS ON LAB TEST RESULTS
• May alter electrolyte levels.

CAUTIONS
Pregnant or breast-feeding women should avoid this herb.

NURSING CONSIDERATIONS
• Find out why patient is using the herb.
• Stone root citronella is not the same as true citronella oil *(Cymbopogon),* which is used as an insect repellent.
• Because stone root may have diuretic effects, caution should be used when patient takes it with other herbs or drugs that have diuretic effects.
• Although no chemical interactions have been reported, consider the pharmacologic properties of the herb and its potential to interfere with therapeutic effects of conventional drugs.
• Monitor intake and output, as indicated.
• Monitor patient's response to herbal therapy.

PATIENT TEACHING
• Advise patient to consult a health care provider before using an herbal preparation because a standard treatment that has been proven effective may be available.
• Tell patient that when filling a new prescription he should remind pharmacist of any herbal and dietary supplements he's taking.
• Inform patient that stone root normally has a strong, unpleasant odor.
• Advise pregnant and breast-feeding patients not to take stone root.
• Tell patients taking a diuretic herb or drug to consult a health care provider before using stone root.
• Warn patient not to take herb for urinary or abdominal complaints before seeking medical attention because doing so may delay diagnosis of a potentially serious medical condition.
• Instruct patient to promptly notify health care provider about adverse effects or new symptoms.
• Warn patient to keep all herbal products away from children and pets.

*Liquid contains alcohol.

sundew

Drosera ramentacea, D. rotundifolia, dew plant, drosera, lustwort, red rot, ros solis, round-leafed sundew, sonnenthau, youthwort

Common trade names
B&T Natural Relief-Cough

AVAILABLE FORMS
Available as dried herb, tea, liquid extract*, and tincture*.

ACTIONS & COMPONENTS
Obtained from *D. ramentacea, D. rotundifolia, D. intermedia,* and *D. anglica.* Contains naphthoquinone, and is thought to have antitussive, antimicrobial, secretolytic, and bronchospasmolytic effects. May also have immunostimulant effects.

USES
Used orally for bronchitis, asthma, pertussis, coughing fits, and dry cough. May be used topically for warts.

DOSAGE & ADMINISTRATION
Average daily dose: 3 g dried plant P.O.
Liquid extract (1:1 in 25% alcohol): 0.5 to 2 ml P.O. t.i.d.
Tea: 1 or 2 g in 150 ml boiling water, steeped for 5 to 10 minutes, strained, and taken t.i.d.
Tincture (1:5 in 60% alcohol): 0.5 to 1 ml P.O. t.i.d.

ADVERSE REACTIONS
None known.

INTERACTIONS
Herb-drug. *Disulfiram:* Herbal products that contain alcohol may cause a disulfiram-like reaction. Advise patient to avoid using together.

EFFECTS ON LAB TEST RESULTS
None reported.

CAUTIONS
Pregnant or breast-feeding women shouldn't use this herb.

NURSING CONSIDERATIONS
• Find out why patient is using the herb.
• Although few chemical interactions have been reported, consider the pharmacologic properties of the herb and its potential to interfere with therapeutic effects of conventional drugs.
• Monitor patient's response to herbal therapy.

PATIENT TEACHING
• Advise patient to consult a health care provider before using an herbal preparation because a standard treatment that has been proven effective may be available.
• Tell patient that when filling a new prescription he should remind pharmacist of any herbal and dietary supplements he's taking.
• Warn patient not to take herb before seeking medical attention because doing so may delay diagnosis of a potentially serious medical condition.
• Advise women not to use this herb while pregnant or breast-feeding.
• Warn patient that herb has a bitter, sour, hot taste.

Bold italic type indicates that reaction may be life-threatening.

• Warn patient not to take herb for persistent cough or difficulty breathing before seeking medical attention because doing so may delay diagnosis of a potentially serious medical condition.

• Instruct patient to promptly notify a health care provider about adverse effects or changes in symptoms.

• Warn patient to keep all herbal products away from children and pets.

sweet cicely

Myrrhis odorata, British myrrh, cow chervil, the Roman plant, shepherd's needle, smooth cicely, sweet bracken, sweet chervil, sweet-cus, sweet-fern, sweet-humlock, sweets

Common trade names
None known

AVAILABLE FORMS
Available as ground root, tonic, infusion, and salve.

ACTIONS & COMPONENTS
Obtained from *M. odorata.* Volatile oils and flavonoids may act as a digestive aid, an expectorant, and a carminative.

USES
Used orally for asthma, breathing difficulties, intestinal gas and colic, and for urinary tract, chest, and throat complaints. Also used as an expectorant, a blood purifier, and a digestive aid. Used topically to treat gout pain and acute wounds and sores.

DOSAGE & ADMINISTRATION
For wounds, sores, pain of gout:
Fresh herb salve applied topically, p.r.n.

ADVERSE REACTIONS
None known.

INTERACTIONS
None reported.

EFFECTS ON LAB TEST RESULTS
None reported.

CAUTIONS
Pregnant and breast-feeding women shouldn't use this herb.

NURSING CONSIDERATIONS
• Find out why patient is using the herb.

• Herb is generally thought to be harmless in typical quantities.

• Although no chemical interactions have been reported, consider the pharmacologic properties of the herb and its potential to interfere with therapeutic effects of conventional drugs.

• Monitor patient's response to herbal therapy.

PATIENT TEACHING
• Advise patient to consult a health care provider before using an herbal preparation because a standard treatment that has been proven effective may be available.

• Tell patient that when filling a new prescription he should remind pharmacist of any herbal and dietary supplements he's taking.

• Warn patient not to take herb for breathing problems before seeking medical attention because doing so

---

* Liquid contains alcohol.

may delay diagnosis of a potentially serious medical condition.

• Discuss alternative, proven therapies with patient.

• Tell patient to promptly notify his health care provider about adverse effects or changes in symptoms.

• Warn patient to keep all herbal products away from children and pets.

sweet flag

Acorus calamus, beewort, calamus, cinnamon sedge, gladdon, myrtle-flag, myrtle-grass, myrtle sedge, rat root, sweet cane, sweet grass, sweet myrtle, sweet root, sweet rush, sweet sedge

Common trade names
None known

AVAILABLE FORMS
Available as oil, extract*, tincture*, and dried and powdered rhizome.

ACTIONS & COMPONENTS
Obtained from *A. calamus* or *A. gramineus.* There are four types of sweet flag, based on their content of asarone, a carcinogen. The North American type (*A. calamus* var. *americanus*) contains none of this component, but varieties from India do. Sweet flag also contains acorin, choline, resin, starch, calcium oxalate, tannins, mucilage, and asarone. Asarone is chemically related to reserpine.

USES
Used orally for childhood colic, digestive complaints, fever, and sore throat. Also used as a sweat inducer. Used topically to treat rheumatism, angina, and gingivitis. Use of sweet flag as a flavoring agent in dental products, drinks, and medicines has been banned in the United States.

DOSAGE & ADMINISTRATION
Average daily dose: 1 to 3 g P.O. t.i.d.
Liquid extract (1:1 in 60% alcohol): 1 to 3 ml P.O. t.i.d.
Tea: 1 cup P.O. t.i.d. Made from 1 to 3 g rhizome in 150 ml boiling water, steeped for 5 to 10 minutes, and strained.
Tincture (1:5 in 60% alcohol): 2 to 4 ml P.O. t.i.d.
Wash: 250 to 500 g added to bath water.

ADVERSE REACTIONS
CNS: sedation, tremors, *seizures.*
CV: *arrhythmias,* chest pain, syncope.

INTERACTIONS
Herb-drug. *CNS depressants, MAO inhibitors:* May have additive adverse reactions. Monitor patient closely if used together.
H_2-receptor antagonists, proton pump inhibitors: Decreases effect caused by acidifying effect of herb. Monitor patient closely if used together.
Reserpine: Increases adverse effects if herb contains asarone (usually not found in North American varieties). Advise patient to avoid use together.
Herb-herb. *Herbs that cause sedation, including calendula, California poppy, capsicum, catnip, celery, couch grass, elecampane,*

German chamomile, goldenseal, gotu kola, hops, Jamaican dogwood, kava, lemon balm, sage, St. John's wort, sassafras, shepherd's purse, Siberian ginseng, skullcap, stinging nettle, valerian, wild carrot, wild lettuce, withania root, yerba maté: Has additive effects. Advise patient to use together cautiously.
Herb-lifestyle. *Alcohol use:* May have additive sedative effects. Advise patient to avoid using together.

EFFECTS ON LAB TEST RESULTS
• May increase BUN and creatinine levels.

CAUTIONS
Pregnant or breast-feeding women shouldn't use this herb.

NURSING CONSIDERATIONS
• Find out why patient is using the herb.
⚠ALERT: Because of its potential cancer-causing properties, sweet flag is banned by the FDA for use in foods, medicine, and beverages in the United States. The cancer-causing component of sweet flag, asarone, usually isn't found in the North American variety; however, sweet flag from India (Indian calmus oils) contains large amounts of this chemical.
• Chemical content of the supplement—and its safety—can't be assured.
• If a patient is taking sweet flag, he should avoid other sedative herbs or drugs because of possible additive effects.

PATIENT TEACHING
• Advise patient to avoid this herb in any form because of its cancer-causing potential.
• Inform patient taking sweet flag that other herbs or drugs that cause drowsiness should be avoided because of possible additive effects.
• Caution patient to avoid hazardous tasks until full sedative effects of herb are known.
• Tell patient to avoid alcohol while taking sweet flag because of possible additive sedative effects.
• Instruct patient to promptly notify his health care provider about adverse effects or change in symptoms.
• Warn patient to keep all herbal products away from children and pets.

sweet violet

Viola odorata, garden violet, sweet violet herb, violet

Common trade names
Acnetonic, Herbal Pumpkin, Sweet Violet Lotion

AVAILABLE FORMS
Available as dried or fresh root, dried flowers, and leaves.

ACTIONS & COMPONENTS
Obtained from *V. odorata.* Contains saponins that, in high doses, can irritate mucous membranes. In low doses, they act as expectorants. Also contains salicylic acid, methyl esters, and alkaloids. Herb has antimicrobial and bronchosecretolytic effects caused by saponin content.

*Liquid contains alcohol.

USES

Used as an expectorant in acute and chronic bronchitis, bronchial asthma, cough and cold symptoms, and late flu symptoms. Also used as a sedative or relaxant, for urinary incontinence, and for GI complaints, such as heartburn, flatulence, and digestion problems.

DOSAGE & ADMINISTRATION

Average daily dose of root: 1 g.
Decoction: 1 tablespoon in boiling water in proportion to make a 5% water to volume preparation, steeped for 10 to 15 minutes, and then strained. 1 tablespoon taken P.O. five to six times daily.
Tea: 2 teaspoons herb in 250 ml boiling water, steeped for 10 to 15 minutes, then strained. Taken P.O. b.i.d. to t.i.d.

ADVERSE REACTIONS

None known.

INTERACTIONS

None reported.

EFFECTS ON LAB TEST RESULTS

None reported.

CAUTIONS

Because full effects of sweet violet haven't been studied, pregnant and breast-feeding women shouldn't use this herb.

NURSING CONSIDERATIONS

● Find out why patient is using the herb.
● Sweet violet is often used in combination preparations for oral and topical use.
● Although no chemical interactions have been reported, consider the pharmacologic properties of the herb and its potential to interfere with therapeutic effects of conventional drugs.
● Monitor patient's response to herbal therapy.

PATIENT TEACHING

● Advise patient to consult a health care provider before using an herbal preparation because a standard treatment that has been proven effective may be available.
● Tell patient that when filling a new prescription he should remind pharmacist of any herbal and dietary supplements he's taking
● If patient takes sweet violet for respiratory problems, tell him to seek medical attention if it fails to relieve symptoms.
● Instruct patient not to use more than recommended amounts because higher amounts can irritate the lining of the mouth, stomach, intestines, and lungs.
● Urge pregnant and breast-feeding women to consult a health care provider before using sweet violet.
● Warn patient to keep all herbal products away from children and pets.

Bold italic type indicates that reaction may be life-threatening.

T

tansy

Chrysanthemum vulgare,
Tanacetum vulgare, bitter
buttons, buttons, daisy,
hindheal, parsley fern, tansy
flower, tansy herb

Common trade names
None known

AVAILABLE FORMS
Available as oil, extract, and combination products.

ACTIONS & COMPONENTS
Obtained from leaves and flowers of *T. vulgare.* Contains volatile oil with thujone, a neurotoxin. Other components include sesquiterpenes and flavones. Caffeic acid may have bile-inducing effects. Thujone is probably responsible for liver toxicity. Tansy toxicity varies greatly among subtypes.

USES
Used orally to stimulate menstrual flow, induce abortion, improve digestion, and treat migraines and GI worm infestations in children. Used topically for scabies, sunburn, toothache, sores, sprains, and insect repellent. Also used in perfumes and as a green dye source, but the toxic potential of the herb precludes its use in herbal medicine.

DOSAGE & ADMINISTRATION
Tansy use is strongly discouraged. Deaths have been reported after ingestion of oil, powdered form, or tea. Lethal dosage is 15 to 30 g of essential oil.
Average daily dose: 0.1 g P.O.

ADVERSE REACTIONS
CNS: *seizures,* tremors, vertigo, restlessness, loss of consciousness, tonic-clonic spasms.
CV: tachycardia, irregular heart rate.
EENT: dilated pupils.
GI: vomiting, gastroenteritis, abdominal pain.
GU: *kidney damage,* uterine bleeding.
Hepatic: *liver toxicity.*
Skin: local mucous membrane irritation, contact dermatitis, severe facial flushing.
Other: *allergic reaction.*

INTERACTIONS
Herb-drug. *Hypoglycemics:* Alters control of glucose level and increases effect of hypoglycemics. Monitor glucose level closely. Advise patient to avoid use.
Herb-herb. *Herbs that may contain thujone, including cedar leaf oil, oak moss, oriental arborvitae, sage, tree moss, and wormwood:* Increases toxicity. Warn patient to avoid use.
Herb-lifestyle. *Alcohol use:* Because of the thujone component, tansy may increase and change the effects of alcohol. Advise patient to avoid use.

EFFECTS ON LAB TEST RESULTS
• May increase BUN, creatinine, and liver enzyme levels.

---

*Liquid contains alcohol.

CAUTIONS

Pregnant or breast-feeding women shouldn't use this herb. Tansy products shouldn't be used by patients allergic to ragweed, chrysanthemums, arnica, sunflowers, yarrow, marigolds, daisies, or similar plants.

Administration of therapeutic doses of agent with high thujone content can lead to poisoning.

NURSING CONSIDERATIONS

- Find out why patient is using the herb.
- **ALERT:** People have died from taking as little as 10 gtt of oil. Take a careful history if a patient uses tansy. Make sure to note if patient has also taken other herbs containing thujone, a potent toxin.
- **ALERT:** Tansy poisoning may cause vomiting, abdominal pain, gastroenteritis, severe reddening of the face, mydriasis, fixed pupils, cardiac arrhythmias, violent spasms, seizures, uterine bleeding, and kidney and liver damage. Death can occur in 1 to 3½ hours.
- Gastric lavage and emesis have been used to treat symptomatic toxicity.
- **ALERT:** Don't confuse tansy (*T. vulgare*) with tansy ragwort (*Senecio jacoboea*).

PATIENT TEACHING

- **ALERT:** Warn patient that tansy is toxic at very low doses and is unsafe for any medicinal use.
- **ALERT:** If patient takes tansy, caution him to watch for signs of toxicity, such as a rapid and weak pulse, severe abdominal pain, and seizures. Urge patient to seek emergency care immediately if adverse effects or toxic reactions develop.
- Advise patient that tansy may cause severe skin irritation.
- Tell patients with a history of allergy to any member of the Compositae family, such as arnica, yarrow, or sunflower, not to take tansy because a cross-reaction may occur.
- Warn patient to keep all herbal products away from children and pets.

tea tree

Melaleuca alternifolia,
paperbark tree

Common trade names
Tea Tree Oil, Tea Tree Oil Lotion, Tea Tree Soap

AVAILABLE FORMS
Available as essential oil, creams, lotions, suppositories, and soaps.

ACTIONS & COMPONENTS
Obtained from leaves of *M. alternifolia.* Contains 2% of a pale yellow volatile oil. Oil contains cineole and terpinen-4-ol. The latter supplies most antifungal and antibacterial activity of tea tree oil. Tea tree oils with high cineole content are lower quality and more likely to cause skin irritation. Therapeutic concentrations range from 0.25% to 0.5%, but may contain up to 10% essential oil.

USES
Used as a topical antiseptic that is more effective than phenol for superficial skin infections (bacterial, viral, or fungal), minor burns, cuts,

---

Bold italic type indicates that reaction may be life-threatening.

sore throats, ingrown or infected toenails, sunburn, tinea (athlete's foot), *Candida* species (including *C. albicans*), impetigo, ulcers, cold sores, pimples, and acne. Also used in aromatherapy and as a mouthwash and shampoo. In bath form, it's used to treat vaginal infections. It can also be added to vaporizers for respiratory disorders.

DOSAGE & ADMINISTRATION
For mouth ulcers, sore gums, plaque: 3 gtt oil in water P.O. b.i.d.
For skin conditions: Concentrated tea tree oil diluted with almond or vegetable oil and applied with a cotton ball to the affected area t.i.d.
Respiratory vaporizer: A few drops of oil added to water in vaporizer.
Vaginal douche: A few drops of oil added to water for sitz bath.

ADVERSE REACTIONS
CNS: ataxia, drowsiness, weakness, confusion (if taken orally).
EENT: itching, burning (if taken orally).
Hematologic: neutrophil leukocytosis (if taken orally).
Skin: contact dermatitis, rash.

INTERACTIONS
Herb-drug. *Drugs that affect histamine release:* May alter effects. Advise patient to avoid using together.

EFFECTS ON LAB TEST RESULTS
• May increase neutrophil count.

CAUTIONS
Patients shouldn't apply tea tree products to open wounds, areas not affected by rash, or dry, cracked or broken skin. Patients shouldn't apply herb near the eyes.

NURSING CONSIDERATIONS
• Find out why patient is using the herb.
• Tea tree oil shouldn't be used internally because of systemic toxicity.
• Essential oil should be used externally only after being diluted, especially by people with sensitive skin.
• Tea tree oil may cause burns or itching in tender areas and shouldn't be used around nose, eyes, and mouth.
• Diluted essential oil, even as low as 0.25% or 0.5%, is active against microbes.
• Vaginal douches using concentrations as strong as 40% require extreme caution and supervision by a health care provider.
• Pure (100%) essential tea tree oil is rarely used and only with close supervision by a health care provider.
• Other related *Melaleuca* species are also known as tea trees, such as *M. cajeputi* and *M. dissitiflora,* but tea tree oil can be obtained only from *M. alternifolia.*

PATIENT TEACHING
• Advise patient to consult a health care provider before using an herbal preparation because a standard treatment that has been proven effective may be available.
• Tell patient that when filling a new prescription he should remind pharmacist of any herbal and dietary supplements he's taking.

• Tell patient to use very dilute tea tree oil (0.25% to 0.5%) as a topical anti-infective.

• Explain that a few drops are sufficient in mouthwash, shampoo, or sitz bath.

• Caution patient not to apply oil to wounds or to skin that is dry or cracked.

• If patient will be using the douche form of this product, stress the need for medical supervision.

• Warn patient to keep all herbal products away from children and pets.

thuja

Thuja occidentalis, American arborvitae, arborvitae, hackmatack, northern white cedar, swamp cedar, thuja oil, tree of life, white cedar

Common trade names
Fresh Thuja Leaf Oil

AVAILABLE FORMS
Available as oil, extract*, ointment, and homeopathic products.

ACTIONS & COMPONENTS
Obtained by steam distillation of leaves and twigs of *T. occidentalis.* Contains thujone, a neurotoxin. Also contains glycoproteins and polysaccharides, which have antiviral and immunostimulating properties. Thuja also has uterine-stimulant activity. Some thuja preparations are certified thujone-free.

USES
Used orally as an immune stimulant, expectorant, and diuretic.

Misused as an abortifacient. Used topically as an insect repellent and a treatment for skin diseases, infected wounds and burns, joint pain, arthritis, rheumatism, condyloma, warts, and cancers. Also used as a fragrance in personal care items and as a flavoring. Thuja is used in food items in the United States only if it's certified thujone-free.

DOSAGE & ADMINISTRATION
Extract (1:1 in 50% alcohol, 1:10 in 60% alcohol): 1 or 2 ml P.O. t.i.d.
Tincture: 100 parts thuja powder and 1,000 parts diluted spirit of wine mixed together.

ADVERSE REACTIONS
CNS: *seizures, neurotoxicity.*
CV: hypotension, tachycardia.
GI: nausea, vomiting, diarrhea.
GU: uterine stimulation and cramping, miscarriage.
Other: mucous membrane hemorrhaging.

INTERACTIONS
Herb-drug. *Anticonvulsants:* May cause seizures. Advise patient to avoid use.
Herb-herb. *Herbs that contain thuja, such as oak moss, oriental arborvitae, sage, tansy, tree moss, wormwood:* Increases risk of toxicity. Advise patient to avoid using together.
Herb-lifestyle. *Alcohol use:* May have additive CNS effects. Advise patient to avoid using together.

EFFECTS ON LAB TEST RESULTS
None reported.

Bold italic type indicates that reaction may be life-threatening.

CAUTIONS

Pregnant or breast-feeding women shouldn't use this herb. Thuja shouldn't be used by transplant patients or those with a history of seizures or immune-related diseases, such as lupus, rheumatoid arthritis, or AIDS, because it may activate the immune system and accelerate the disease.

NURSING CONSIDERATIONS

• Find out why patient is using the herb.

🗷ALERT: Thuja preparations intended for oral or topical use shouldn't contain thujone, a neurotoxin. Some thuja and thuja oil preparations are said to be thujone-free. However, if thujone toxicity is suspected, a poison control center should be notified immediately.

• For homeopathic thuja preparations, patient must not eat or drink for 15 minutes before and after taking the remedy to prevent its dilution.

• Monitor patient's response to therapy and for adverse effects.

🗷ALERT: Don't confuse this *Thuja* species with *T. orientalis,* the Oriental arborvitae.

PATIENT TEACHING

• Advise patient to consult a health care provider before using an herbal preparation because a standard treatment that has been proven effective may be available.

• Tell patient that when filling a new prescription he should remind pharmacist of any herbal and dietary supplements he's taking.

• Caution patient not to take thuja if he has a history of seizures.

• Caution patient not to take thuja if she is pregnant or breast-feeding.

• If patient intends to take thuja leaf oil by mouth, warn him to make sure it's certified thujone-free.

• If patient intends to take a homeopathic remedy, urge him not to eat or drink for 15 minutes before and after doing so.

• If patient takes a form that contains alcohol, caution him to avoid hazardous activities until full CNS effects of the herb are known.

🗷ALERT: Warn patient to immediately contact a poison control center or seek emergency treatment if he becomes ill after taking thuja orally.

• Warn patient to keep all herbal products away from children and pets.

thunder god vine

Tripterygium wilfordii, huang-t'eng ken, lei gong teng, lei-kung t'eng, threewingnut, tsao-ho-hua, yellow vine

Common trade names
None known

AVAILABLE FORMS

Available as an extract.

ACTIONS & COMPONENTS

Obtained from leaves and roots of *T. wilfordii.* Contains tripochloro-lide, tribromoline, and demethyl-zeylesteral constituents, which have immunosuppressive effects. Triptolide and tripdiolide may depress spermatogenesis and exert

---

*Liquid contains alcohol.

anti-inflammatory and immunosuppressive effects.

USES
Used for male birth control. Also
used to treat rheumatoid arthritis,
inflammation, abscesses and boils,
heavy menstrual periods, and autoimmune diseases.

DOSAGE & ADMINISTRATION
For rheumatoid arthritis: 30 mg
extract P.O. daily.
Male birth control: About ⅓ of the
dose used for anti-inflammatory
effects. Fertility usually returns 6
weeks after herb is stopped.

ADVERSE REACTIONS
CV: hypotension, *shock.*
GI: stomach upset, vomiting, diar-
rhea.
GU: amenorrhea, infertility, *renal
failure.*
Skin: rash.

INTERACTIONS
Herb-drug. *Immunosuppressants:*
Enhances immunosuppressive effects. Advise patient to avoid using
together.

EFFECTS ON LAB TEST RESULTS
• May increase BUN and creatinine levels.
• May decrease WBC and lymphocyte counts.

CAUTIONS
Patients who take immunosuppressants or have CV disease, a previous transplant, or immune disorders should avoid taking this herb.
Men trying to father a child and
women who are pregnant or breast-
feeding shouldn't use this herb.

NURSING CONSIDERATIONS
• Find out why patient is using the
herb.
⚠ **ALERT:** Herb may be fatal to
patients with a history of MI, coronary artery disease, or heart failure. The one reported death involved a patient with coexisting
cardiac damage. This patient experienced profuse vomiting, diarrhea,
decreased serum WBCs, renal failure, hypotension, and shock before
death.
• Monitor blood pressure, WBC
and lymphocyte counts, and renal
function.
• Men considering fatherhood
shouldn't use this herb because of
its infertility effect.
• When herb is taken as a male
birth control agent, fertility usually returns to normal 6 weeks after
herb is stopped.

PATIENT TEACHING
• Advise patient to consult a health
care provider before using an
herbal preparation because a standard treatment that has been
proven effective may be available.
• Tell patient that when filling a
new prescription he should remind pharmacist of any herbal
and dietary supplements he's taking.
• Tell patient not to use this herb if
he has a history of heart disease,
heart attack, or heart failure.
• Advise pregnant patients, those
trying to become pregnant, and
those not using adequate pregnancy prevention to avoid this herb.
Tell women to make sure they
aren't pregnant before use.

Bold italic type indicates that reaction may be life-threatening.

- Inform men considering fatherhood about herb's infertility effects.
- Advise against using herb if patient has a disease or condition that alters the immune system or if he takes other herbs or drugs that inhibit the immune system.
- If patient is using herb as a male contraceptive, tell him that sperm levels and activity should return to normal 6 weeks after stopping herb.
- Warn patient to keep all herbal products away from children and pets.

thyme

Thymus serpyllum, T. vulgaris, common thyme, French thyme, garden thyme, rubbed thyme, Spanish thyme, thymi herba

Common trade names
Candistroy, Dentarome Plus Toothpaste, Fenu-Thyme, Thyme Beautiful Skin Tea, Thyme Leaf & Flower, Thyme Leaf, Thyme (liquid), Ultimate Respiratory Cleanse

AVAILABLE FORMS
Available as 100% oil, dry herb, powder, liquid extract*, and dry extract.

ACTIONS & COMPONENTS
Obtained from above-ground parts of *T. serpyllum* or *T. vulgaris.* Contains thymol, flavonoids, and carvacrol, which have expectorant, antispasmodic, and antitussive effects. Thymol and carvacrol may also have antibacterial and antifungal effects. Rosmarinic acid may have antiedema and macrophage-inhibiting effects. Herb may also act as a menstrual stimulant. Common thyme (*T. vulgaris*) contains more oil than wild thyme (*T. serpyllum*) or Spanish thyme (*T. zygis*).

USES
Used for bronchitis, pertussis, laryngitis, tonsillitis, dyspepsia, diarrhea, rheumatic diseases, and pediatric enuresis. Also used as a diuretic, an antibacterial, and an antiflatulent. Used externally to treat wounds resistant to healing and as a mouthwash and gargle for mouth and throat inflammations. Also used as a spice and flavoring agent.

DOSAGE & ADMINISTRATION
Average daily dose: 1 or 2 g dried leaf or flower P.O. several times a day. Maximum, 10 g of dried leaf daily.
Bath: 0.004 g thyme oil (the minimum dose) added to 1 L water, filtered, and then added to warm bath water (95° to 100.4° F [35° to 38° C]. Or, 500 g of herb added to 4 L boiling water, filtered, and then added to bath water as directed above.
Liquid extract: 1 or 2 g P.O. up to t.i.d.
Tea: 1 or 2 g dried leaf or flower in 150 ml boiling water, steeped for 10 minutes, strained, and taken several times daily.
Topical: 5 g in 100 ml boiling water (5% infusion), steeped for 10 minutes, strained, cooled slightly, and used as gargle or applied as a compress.

*Liquid contains alcohol.

ADVERSE REACTIONS
Skin: irritation, mild sensitivity reactions.

INTERACTIONS
None known.

EFFECTS ON LAB TEST RESULTS
None reported.

CAUTIONS
Pregnant or breast-feeding women should avoid this herb, as should patients allergic to oregano. Patients with GI disorders such as ulcers and those with urinary tract inflammation should use thyme cautiously. Patients with widespread skin injuries or skin disease, high fever, infectious disease, or cardiac problems should be very cautious when using any herb as an ingredient in a whole-body bath.

NURSING CONSIDERATIONS
• Find out why patient is using the herb.
• Although no chemical interactions have been reported, consider the pharmacologic properties of the herb and its potential to interfere with therapeutic effects of conventional drugs.
• Monitor patient's response to herbal therapy.

PATIENT TEACHING
• Advise patient to consult a health care provider before using an herbal preparation because a standard treatment that has been proven effective may be available.
• Tell patient that when filling a new prescription he should remind pharmacist of any herbal and dietary supplements he's taking
• Advise patients who are pregnant or breast-feeding not to use thyme in medicinal quantities.
• Tell patient who uses thyme as an expectorant that the herb may work better if he adds honey as a sweetener, provided he has no sugar restrictions in his diet.
• Advise patient not to use herb if he is allergic to oregano.
• Warn patient not to take herb for persistent bronchitis or cough before seeking medical attention because doing so may delay diagnosis of a potentially serious medical condition.
• Instruct patient to contact a health care provider if he develops a skin reaction.
• If patient has urinary tract inflammation, urge him to be cautious when taking thyme because the herb may aggravate the inflammation.
• Instruct patient to be cautious when using herb in a whole-body bath if he has widespread skin injuries or skin disease, high fever, infectious disease, or heart problems
• Instruct patient to promptly notify health care provider about adverse effects or changes in symptoms.
• Warn patient to keep all herbal products away from children and pets.

Bold italic type indicates that reaction may be life-threatening.

tonka bean

*Dipteryx odorata, Coumarouna
odorata,* cumaru, Dutch tonka,
English tonka, tonca seed,
tongo bean, tonka, tonka seed,
tonquin bean, torquin bean

Common trade names
None known

AVAILABLE FORMS
Beans aren't used medicinally. No
longer available in the United
States.

ACTIONS & COMPONENTS
Obtained from beans of *D. odorata*
(C. odorata). Contains 1% to 3%
coumarin, but can be as high as
10%. Also contains a fatty oil.
Coumarin may increase venous
and lymphatic return, thus reducing edema and inflammation.

USES
Used as a tonic and for cachexia,
cramps, lymphedema, spasms, tuberculosis, ulcers, earache, and
sore throat. Some people claimed
the beans had aphrodisiac properties. Coumarin has been used as a
flavoring for cakes, tobacco, soaps,
and preserves.

DOSAGE & ADMINISTRATION
Usual daily dose: 60 mg
(coumarin content) P.O. daily.

ADVERSE REACTIONS
CNS: insomnia, dizziness, stupor,
headache.
CV: *cardiac arrest* with large dos-
es.
GI: nausea, vomiting, diarrhea.
GU: testicular atrophy.

Hepatic: *hepatotoxicity,* liver
damage.
Other: growth retardation.

INTERACTIONS
Herb-drug. *Anticoagulants, antiplatelets such as aspirin, clopidogrel bisulfate, warfarin:* May cause
coagulation disturbances. Monitor
PT, INR, and patient closely. Advise patient to avoid using together.
Herb-herb. *Angelica, anise, arnica, bogbean, boldo, capsicum, celery, chamomile, clove, danshen,
fenugreek, feverfew, garlic, ginger,
ginkgo, ginseng, horse chestnut,
horseradish, licorice, meadowsweet, onion, passion flower,
poplar, prickly ash, red clover,
turmeric, wild carrot, wild lettuce,
willow:* May cause coagulation
disturbances. Advise patient to
avoid using together.

EFFECTS ON LAB TEST RESULTS
• May increase liver enzyme lev-
els.
• May increase PT and INR.

CAUTIONS
Pregnant or breast-feeding women
and patients with a history of liver
disease shouldn't use this herb.

NURSING CONSIDERATIONS
• Find out why patient is using the
herb.
• High doses or long-term consumption of tonka bean should be
avoided because of the risk of liver
damage and cardiac arrest.
• Take a careful history that includes any recent foreign travel or
purchase and use of foodstuffs
abroad.

*Liquid contains alcohol.

- Take a thorough drug history to assess the patient's use of anti-platelet drugs or anticoagulants.
- Don't confuse coumarin with such anticoagulants as warfarin, dicumarol, or bishydroxycoumarin, but do recognize the potential for additive antiplatelet or anticoagulant effects.
- Vanilla extract and possibly other flavoring extracts purchased in foreign countries may contain coumarin impurities and are unsafe for consumption.
- Monitor patient for signs of bleeding, such as easy bruising and gum bleeding.
- Monitor patient for signs of liver damage, including abdominal pain, anorexia, nausea, jaundice, fatigue, and change in color of urine or stool.

PATIENT TEACHING
- Advise patient to consult a health care provider before using an herbal preparation because a standard treatment that has been proven effective may be available.
- Tell patient that when filling a new prescription he should remind pharmacist of any herbal and dietary supplements he's taking.
- Caution patient not to buy or consume flavorings, preservatives, or beverages that contain tonka beans or their chemical component (coumarin) when traveling outside the United States.
- Warn patient to avoid tonka bean if he takes blood thinners of any type, including anticoagulants or antiplatelet drugs.
- Warn pregnant and breastfeeding patients to avoid tonka bean.

- Explain the signs of bleeding, and urge patient to promptly notify a health care provider if bleeding or other adverse effects develop.
- Tell patient to avoid high doses and long-term use of tonka bean.
- Instruct patient to seek emergency medical care if he develops heart symptoms, such as chest pain, shortness of breath, or excess sweating, while taking tonka bean.

tormentil

Potentilla erecta, Tormentillae rhizoma, biscuits, bloodroot, cinquefoil, earthbank, English sarsaparilla, ewe daisy, flesh and blood, potentilla, septfoil, shepherd's knapperty, shepherd's knot, thormantle, tormentilla

Common trade names
Immune Master

AVAILABLE FORMS
Available as root, powder, tincture*, and fluidextract.

ACTIONS & COMPONENTS
Obtained from *P. erecta*. Contains tannins, flavonoids, resins, ellagic acid, and kinovic acid. Tannins are probably responsible for pharmacologic actions.

USES
Used orally to treat diarrhea, mild gastroenteritis, and fever. Used topically as a mouth rinse for mild oral inflammation and mild superficial bleeding. Fluidextract is also used to promote wound healing. Used with galangal, marshmallow

---

Bold italic type indicates that reaction may be life-threatening.

root, and powdered ginger to treat diarrhea and dysentery.

DOSAGE & ADMINISTRATION
Tea for diarrhea: 2 or 3 g of root in 150 ml boiling water, steeped for 10 to 15 minutes, strained, and taken b.i.d. to q.i.d. One teaspoon powdered root = 4 g of drug.
Tincture: 10 to 20 gtt (1:10) in a glass of water P.O., swished as a mouth rinse once daily.

ADVERSE REACTIONS
GI: nausea, vomiting, abdominal complaints.

INTERACTIONS
Herb-drug. *Disulfiram, metronidazole:* Herbal products that contain alcohol may cause a disulfiram-like reaction. Advise patient to avoid using together.
Herb-food. *Milk products:* Decreases antidiarrheal effect. Advise patient to avoid using together.

EFFECTS ON LAB TEST RESULTS
None reported.

CAUTIONS
Pregnant or breast-feeding women should avoid this herb, as should alcoholic patients and those with liver disease.

NURSING CONSIDERATIONS
• Find out why patient is using the herb.
• Milk products may bind the tannins in tormentil used as an antidiarrheal, thus decreasing both beneficial and adverse effects.
• Monitor patient's response to herbal therapy.

PATIENT TEACHING
• Advise patient to consult a health care provider before using an herbal preparation because a standard treatment that has been proven effective may be available.
• Tell patient that when filling a new prescription he should remind pharmacist of any herbal and dietary supplements he's taking.
• Tell pregnant and breast-feeding patients not to use tormentil.
• Inform patient that milk products may bind the active ingredient in tormentil when used to treat diarrhea, thus reducing its effectiveness.
• Urge patient to stop using tormentil and to contact his health care provider if diarrhea gets worse or continues for longer than 2 days.
• Tell patient to promptly notify a health care provider about adverse effects or changes in symptoms.
• Warn patient to keep all herbal products away from children and pets.

tragacanth

Astragalus gummifer, goat's thorn, green dragon, gum dragon, gum tragacanth, hog gum, Syrian tragacanth, tragacanth gum

Common trade names
Normacol, Tragacanth Mucilage

AVAILABLE FORMS
Available as powder.

ACTIONS & COMPONENTS
Obtained from *A. gummifer.* Contains tragacanthin and bassorin,

---

*Liquid contains alcohol.

which form a colloidal solution and a thick gel, respectively, when wet. Tragacanth promotes peristaltic movement, has adhesive properties, and may inhibit cancer cell growth.

USES

Used for diarrhea and constipation. Also used as a stabilizer, a thickener, a suspending agent in food and pharmaceutical products, a binder, an emulsifier, and an ingredient in denture adhesives. Mucilage is used as an adjunct for burns.

DOSAGE & ADMINISTRATION

Average daily dose: 1 teaspoon granulated herb added to 250 to 300 ml liquid, P.O.

ADVERSE REACTIONS

GI: esophageal pain or blockage, *intestinal obstruction.*
Skin: contact dermatitis.

INTERACTIONS

None known.

EFFECTS ON LAB TEST RESULTS

None reported.

CAUTIONS

Patients allergic to quillaja bark (*Quillaja saponaria*) may be sensitive to tragacanth preparations. Pregnant or breast-feeding women should avoid this herb, as should patients with esophageal strictures or intestinal obstructions.

NURSING CONSIDERATIONS

• Find out why patient is using the herb.
• Tragacanth is relatively safe, but should be taken P.O. with a full glass of water to avoid expansion of the compound in the esophagus and potential blockage or esophageal damage.
• Tragacanth may inhibit absorption of oral drugs, herbs, and foods. Doses of preparations that contain large amounts of tragacanth should be separated from other oral intake by 2 hours.
• Monitor patient for adverse effects, including difficulty swallowing and esophageal pain.

PATIENT TEACHING

• Advise patient to consult a health care provider before using an herbal preparation because a standard treatment that has been proven effective may be available.
• Tell patient that when filling a new prescription he should remind pharmacist of any herbal and dietary supplements he's taking.
• Instruct patient to drink a full glass of water with each dose of tragacanth to avoid expansion of the compound in the esophagus, which could lead to blockage or damage.
• **ALERT:** Warn patient to seek medical help immediately if he can't swallow or has significant pain, vomiting, or esophageal bleeding after taking tragacanth.
• Warn patient to keep all herbal products away from children and pets.

Bold italic type indicates that reaction may be life-threatening.

tree of heaven

Ailanthus altissima, ailanto,
ailanthus, Chinese sumach,
heaven tree, paradise tree,
vernis du Japon

Common trade names
Chun Pi

AVAILABLE FORMS
Available as trunk or root bark,
tincture*, tea, and infusion.

ACTIONS & COMPONENTS
Obtained from *A. altissima.*
Quassinoid constituents, such as
ailanthin and quassin, may have
cytotoxic effects. Tannins and
alkaloids may have astringent,
antipyretic, and antispasmodic
properties. Herb also has cardiac
depressant activity and purgative
action, and it may have antimalarial properties.

USES
Used for pathologic leukorrhea, diarrhea, chronic dysentery, dysmenorrhea, cramps, asthma, tachycardia, gonorrhea, epilepsy, and
tapeworm infestation.

DOSAGE & ADMINISTRATION
Infusion: 1 teaspoon taken b.i.d.
Prepared by adding 50 g bark to
75 g hot water, straining, and cooling.
Tincture: 5 to 60 gtt (about 7 to
20 grains)/dose P.O. b.i.d. to q.i.d.

ADVERSE REACTIONS
CNS: headache, limb tingling,
dizziness.
CV: decreased cardiac function.
GI: nausea, diarrhea.

Skin: dermatitis after contact with
leaves.

INTERACTIONS
Herb-drug. *Disulfiram:* Herbal
products that contain alcohol may
cause a disulfiram-like reaction.
Advise patient to avoid using together.

EFFECTS ON LAB TEST RESULTS
None reported.

CAUTIONS
Pregnant or breast-feeding women
should avoid this herb, as should
patients with compromised cardiac
function, such as heart failure,
coronary artery disease, or a history of MI.

NURSING CONSIDERATIONS
• Find out why patient is using the
herb.
• Bark preparations have an offen-
sive smell commonly described as
burnt peanuts.
• Although no chemical interactions have been reported, consider
the pharmacologic properties of
the herb and its potential to interfere with therapeutic effects of
conventional drugs.
• Monitor patient's response to
herb.
• Monitor patient carefully for adverse GI or CNS effects, or decreased cardiac function.
• If patient has diarrhea, monitor
intake and output as indicated.
☑ **ALERT:** Don't confuse tree of
heaven *(Ailanthus)* with tree of life
(Thuja occidentalis).

---

*Liquid contains alcohol.

PATIENT TEACHING
• Advise patient to consult a health care provider before using an herbal preparation because a standard treatment that has been proven effective may be available.
• Tell patient that when filling a new prescription he should remind pharmacist of any herbal and dietary supplements he's taking.
• Advise women to avoid using herb if pregnant or breast-feeding.
• Caution parents not to give this herb to children.
• Warn patient not to take herb for diarrhea, painful menstrual periods, or other undiagnosed symptoms before seeking medical attention because doing so may delay diagnosis of a potentially serious medical condition.
• Inform patient that bark preparations smell something like burnt peanuts.
• Tell patient to store herb in a dry, well-ventilated area away from moths.
• Warn patient to keep all herbal products away from children and pets.

true unicorn root

Aletris farinosa, ague grass, ague-root, aloe-root, bettie grass, bitter grass, black-root, blazing star, colic-root, crow corn, devil's bit, star grass, starwort, true unicorn star-grass, unicorn root, whitetube stargrass

Common trade names
Extraction Aletridis Alcoholicum, Menopause Support

AVAILABLE FORMS
Available as powdered or dried root, fluidextract*, and infusion.

ACTIONS & COMPONENTS
Obtained from *A. farinosa.* Contains some steroidal components that may have estrogenic properties. Also contains alkaloids, oil, saponin, and resins.

USES
Used for rheumatism, gynecologic disorders (particularly dysmenorrhea and amenorrhea), miscarriage, and symptoms caused by a prolapsed vagina. Also used as a sedative, a general tonic, a laxative, an antiflatulent, an antidiarrheal, a diuretic, and an antispasmodic.

DOSAGE & ADMINISTRATION
Fluidextract (1:1 in 45% alcohol): 0.3 to 0.6 g P.O. t.i.d.
Infusion: 1.5 g of herb to 100 ml water; 0.3 to 0.6 g P.O. t.i.d.

ADVERSE REACTIONS
CNS: vertigo.
GI: colic.

INTERACTIONS
Herb-drug. *Antacids, histamine H_2-antagonists, proton pump inhibitors, sucralfate:* May increase gastric acidity and reduce drug effects. Monitor patient closely.
Disulfiram, metronidazole: Herbal products that contain alcohol may cause a disulfiram-like reaction. Advise patient to avoid using together.
Estrogens, hormonal contraceptives: May have additive effect. Patient may need dosage adjustment

---

Bold italic type indicates that reaction may be life-threatening.

or a change to nonhormonal birth control. Advise patient to avoid using together.

Pitocin: May antagonize effects. If drug and herb must be used together, monitor patient closely.

EFFECTS ON LAB TEST RESULTS
None reported.

CAUTIONS
Pregnant or breast-feeding women should avoid this herb, as should patients being treated for alcoholism or liver disease. Women with hormone-sensitive conditions, such as breast, uterine, or ovarian cancer, uterine fibroids, or endometriosis, should avoid this herb.

NURSING CONSIDERATIONS
• Find out why patient is using the herb.
• Some patients may use true unicorn for repeated miscarriage despite repeated warnings against such use.
• Monitor patient's response to herb.
• Monitor patient for adverse CNS or GI effects.

PATIENT TEACHING
• Advise patient to consult a health care provider before using an herbal preparation because a standard treatment that has been proven effective may be available.
• Tell patient that when filling a new prescription he should remind pharmacist of any herbal and dietary supplements he's taking.
• Advise patient that true unicorn root may increase stomach acid and interfere with the action of antacids and other drugs used to limit or stop stomach acid production.
• Caution women of childbearing age and those attempting to conceive that using herb while pregnant or breast-feeding may have adverse effects.
• Warn patient not to take herb before seeking medical attention because doing so may delay diagnosis of a potentially serious medical condition.
• Instruct patient to promptly notify his health care provider about adverse effects or changes in symptoms.

turmeric

Amomum curcuma, Curcuma domestica, C. longa, C. rotunda, Indian saffron, turmeric root

Common trade names
Inflam-Aid, Lipolytics Plus, Phyto Quench Supreme, Pitta Balancing Elixir, Stone Free, Turmeric Catechu Supreme

AVAILABLE FORMS
Available as powdered root or tincture*.

ACTIONS & COMPONENTS
Obtained from *C. longa* and other species. Root contains volatile oils and diaryl heptanoids thought to have anti-inflammatory effects. Diaryl heptanoids may have bile-stimulating and liver-protecting effects. Antispasmodic activity has also been noted. Other components include turmerone, atlantone, zingiberone, and more than six minor components of the oil. Two com-

pounds, ukonon A and ukonon D, may possess anticancer activity via activation of phagocytosis and the reticuloendothelial system.

USES
Used orally for dyspepsia, abdominal bloating, flatulence, liver and gallbladder complaints, headaches, and chest infections. Used topically for analgesia, oral mucosa inflammation, inflammatory skin conditions, and ringworm. Also used as a flavoring and coloring agent in foods.

DOSAGE & ADMINISTRATION
Average daily dose: 0.5 to 1 g of powdered root P.O. several times a day between meals. Usual maximum dose is 1.5 to 3 g P.O. daily.
Infusion: 2 or 3 cups taken P.O. between meals. Prepared by scalding 0.5 to 1 g powdered root in boiling water, covering and steeping for 5 minutes, and then straining. Infusion isn't the preferred method of administration because turmeric contains volatile oils that aren't water soluble.
Tincture: 10 to 15 gtt P.O. t.i.d. or b.i.d.

ADVERSE REACTIONS
GI: indigestion.
GU: increased weight of sexual organs, increased sperm motility.

INTERACTIONS
Herb-drug. *Antiplatelet drugs, including aspirin, clopidogrel, dipyridamole:* May have additive effects. Monitor patient for increased bleeding tendencies. Advise patient to use together cautiously.

Herb-herb. *Angelica, anise, arnica, bogbean, boldo, capsicum, celery, chamomile, clove, danshen, fenugreek, feverfew, garlic, ginger, ginkgo, ginseng, horse chestnut, horseradish, licorice, meadowsweet, onion, passion flower, poplar, prickly ash, red clover, wild carrot, wild lettuce, willow:* May have additive antiplatelet activity. Advise patient to use together cautiously.

EFFECTS ON LAB TEST RESULTS
• May decrease WBC and RBC counts.
• May depress clotting factors.

CAUTIONS
Patients with bile duct obstruction, gallstones, gastric ulcers, or hyperacidity shouldn't use turmeric. Turmeric should be used cautiously in patients taking other herbs or drugs that have antiplatelet activity.

NURSING CONSIDERATIONS
• Find out why patient is using the herb.
• Patients who take indomethacin or reserpine may have a reduced risk of drug-induced gastric or duodenal ulcers when they also take turmeric.
• Monitor patient's response to herb.
• Monitor patient for increased bleeding tendencies or bruising.

PATIENT TEACHING
• Advise patient to consult a health care provider before using an herbal preparation because a standard treatment that has been proven effective may be available.

Bold italic type indicates that reaction may be life-threatening.

• Tell patient that when filling a new prescription he should remind pharmacist of any herbal and dietary supplements he's taking.

• Advise patient to be cautious about taking an antiplatelet drug with turmeric.

• Tell patient to contact his health care provider immediately if he develops frequent nosebleeds or other evidence of problems with blood clotting.

• Warn patient not to take herb before seeking medical attention because doing so may delay diagnosis of a potentially serious medical condition.

• Instruct patient to protect turmeric from light and to keep all herbal products away from children and pets.

*Liquid contains alcohol.

V

valerian

Valeriana officinalis, all-heal, amantilla, baldrian, Belgium valerian, capon's tail, garden heliotrope, Indian valerian, Mexican valerian, Pacific valerian, radix, setewale, setwall, vandal root

Common trade names
Herbal Sure Valerian Root, NuVeg Valerian Root, Quanterra Sleep, Valerian Root

AVAILABLE FORMS
Available as dried root, essential oil, tea, tincture*, extract, capsules, tablets, and combination products.
Capsules: 100 mg, 250 mg, 380 mg, 400 mg, 445 mg, 475 mg, 493 mg, 495 mg, 500 mg, 530 mg, 550 mg, 1,000 mg
Tablets: 160 mg, 550 mg

ACTIONS & COMPONENTS
Obtained from *V. officinalis.* Multiple constituents, including essential oils, seem to contribute to sedating properties of valerian. Valeric acid, the main component of the root, inhibits the enzyme system responsible for breaking down the neurotransmitter GABA, thus increasing its level in the brain. Valerian may also have mild pain relief properties and some hypotensive effects.

USES
Used to treat menstrual cramps, restlessness and sleep disorders from nervous conditions, and other symptoms of psychological stress, such as anxiety, nervous headaches, and gastric spasms. Used topically as a bath additive for restlessness and sleep disorders.

DOSAGE & ADMINISTRATION
Bath additive: 100 g of root mixed with 2 L of hot water and added to one full bath.
For hastening sleep and improving sleep quality: 400 to 800 mg root P.O. up to 2 hours before bedtime. Some patients need 2 to 4 weeks of use for significant improvement. Maximum dosage is 15 g daily.
For restlessness: 220 mg of extract P.O. t.i.d.
Tea: 1 cup P.O. b.i.d. to t.i.d., and h.s.
Tincture (1:5 in 45% to 50% alcohol): 15 to 20 gtt in water several times daily.

ADVERSE REACTIONS
CNS: headache, morning drowsiness, uneasiness, restlessness.
CV: cardiac disturbances.
GI: GI complaints.
Skin: contact allergies.
Other: withdrawal symptoms, including increased agitation and decreased sleep.

INTERACTIONS
Herb-drug. *Barbiturates, benzodiazepines:* May have additive CNS effects. Monitor patient closely.
Herb-herb. *Herbs with sedative effects, such as catnip, hops, kava, passion flower, skullcap:* May po-

---

Bold italic type indicates that reaction may be life-threatening.

tentiate sedative effects. Monitor patient closely.

Herb-lifestyle. *Alcohol use:* May potentiate sedative effects. Advise patient to avoid using together.

EFFECTS ON LAB TEST RESULTS
None reported.

CAUTIONS
Pregnant or breast-feeding women should avoid this herb. Patients with acute or major skin injuries, fever, infectious diseases, cardiac insufficiency, or hypertonia shouldn't bathe with valerian products.

NURSING CONSIDERATIONS
• Find out why patient is using the herb.
• Valerian seems to have a more pronounced effect on those with disturbed sleep or sleep disorders.
⚠️**ALERT:** Evidence of valerian toxicity includes difficulty walking, hypothermia, and increased muscle relaxation.
• Withdrawal symptoms, such as increased agitation and decreased sleep, can occur if valerian is abruptly stopped after prolonged use.
• Monitor CNS status and patient response to herb.
• Monitor patient for cardiac disturbances and GI complaints.

PATIENT TEACHING
• Advise patient to consult a health care provider before using an herbal preparation because a standard treatment that has been proven effective may be available.

• Tell patient that when filling a new prescription he should remind pharmacist of any herbal and dietary supplements he's taking.
• If patient takes valerian, tell him to do so 1 or 2 hours before his desired bedtime. Explain that patient may not feel herb's effect for 2 to 4 weeks.
• Inform patient that most adverse effects occur only after long-term use.
• Instruct patient to promptly notify a health care provider about adverse effects.
• Warn patient not to take herb for insomnia before seeking medical attention because doing so may delay diagnosis of a potentially serious medical condition.
• If patient takes valerian for a long time, caution that amount should be tapered to avoid withdrawal symptoms, which may include increased agitation and decreased sleep.
• Instruct patient to avoid hazardous activities until he knows how herb affects his CNS.
• Tell patient to protect herb from light and to keep tincture in a tightly closed plastic container at room temperature.
• Warn patient to keep all herbal products away from children and pets.

vervain

Verbena officinalis, common vervain, eisenkraut, enchanter's plant, herb of grace, herb of the cross, holywort, Juno's tears, pigeon's grass, pigeonweed, verbena

Common trade names
Quanterra Sinus, Sinupret, Verbena, Vervain

AVAILABLE FORMS
Available as tablets, liquid extract*, tincture*, and combination products.
Quanterra Sinus
Combination containing 29 mg verbena
Sinupret
Tablets: Combination containing 36 mg verbena

ACTIONS & COMPONENTS
Obtained from aboveground parts of *V. officinalis.* Contains iridoid glycosides, including verbascoside, verbenalin, and verbenin. Actions are many and varied. Small amounts of verbenin appear to stimulate sympathetic activity; larger amounts inhibit it. Verbenin may also stimulate milk secretion. Verbenalin may be a uterine stimulant and abortifacient. Verbascoside may have analgesic and antihypertensive action and may enhance the antitremor action of levodopa.

USES
Used to treat sore throats and other oral and pharyngeal inflammation, asthma, whooping cough, and sinusitis. Also used to stimulate secretion of breast milk. Used topically to treat wounds, abscesses, arthritis pain, contusions, itching, and minor burns. Used as a gargle for cold symptoms.

DOSAGE & ADMINISTRATION
Liquid extract (1:1 in 25% alcohol): 2 to 4 ml P.O. daily.
Tea: 1 cup P.O. t.i.d. Prepared by adding 2 to 4 g dried herb to 150 ml boiling water.
Tincture (1:1 in 40% alcohol): 5 to 10 ml P.O. t.i.d.

ADVERSE REACTIONS
CNS: paralysis, stupor, *seizures,* sedation.
CV: hypotension.
GI: vomiting.
GU: uterine stimulation.

INTERACTIONS
Herb-drug. *Antihypertensives, drugs used for hypotension:* Large amounts of herb may interfere with drug therapy for hypertension or hypotension. Advise patient to avoid use. Question patient regarding herbal use. Drug dosages may need adjustment.
Disulfiram: Herbal products that contain alcohol may cause a disulfiram-like reaction. Advise patient to avoid using together.
Hormone therapy: Excessive amounts of vervain can interfere with hormone therapy. Advise patient to avoid using together.
Levodopa: May enhance antitremor action of levodopa. Advise patient of this effect; monitor patient closely.
Herb-lifestyle. *Alcohol use:* May cause additive sedative effects. Advise patient to avoid using together.

Bold italic type indicates that reaction may be life-threatening.

EFFECTS ON LAB TEST RESULTS
None reported.

CAUTIONS
Pregnant or breast-feeding women and patients using hormone therapies should avoid this herb.

NURSING CONSIDERATIONS
• Find out why patient is using the herb.
• Monitor patient closely for adverse CNS effects, hypotension, or vomiting and response to herb.
⚠ALERT: Evidence of excessive intake of the verbenalin component includes CNS paralysis, stupor, and seizures.

PATIENT TEACHING
• Advise patient to consult a health care provider before using an herbal preparation because a standard treatment that has been proven effective may be available.
• Tell patient that when filling a new prescription he should remind pharmacist of any herbal and dietary supplements he's taking
• Warn patients using hormone therapy not to use this herb.
• Caution patient not to take this herb if pregnant or breast-feeding.
• Tell patient to refrain from using alcohol and other sedatives because they may cause increased sedative effects.
• Warn patient taking disulfiram and an herbal product that contains alcohol about possible adverse reactions.
• Advise patient that taking excessive amounts of vervain can depress the CNS.

• Warn patient to keep all herbal products away from children and pets.

---

*Liquid contains alcohol.

W

wahoo

Euonymus atropurpureus, arrow wood, bitter ash, bleeding heart, burning bush, bursting heart, fusanum, fusoria, gatten, Indian arrowroot, pigwood, spindle tree

Common trade names
Wahoo, Wahoo Root

AVAILABLE FORMS
Available as dried bark and seeds.

ACTIONS & COMPONENTS
Obtained from stems, root bark, and berries of *E. atropurpureus.* Seeds and bark contain cardioactive steroid glycosides similar to digoxin. Also contains various alkaloids, caffeine, and theobromine. Wahoo is thought to stimulate bile flow and to have laxative and diuretic effects. In larger amounts, it can affect the heart.

USES
Bark is used orally to treat indigestion and stimulate bile production. Also used as a laxative, a diuretic, and a tonic.

DOSAGE & ADMINISTRATION
No consensus exists.

ADVERSE REACTIONS
CNS: stupor, severe tonic-clonic spasms with tetanus, *coma.*
CV: *circulatory collapse.*
GI: upset stomach, severe bloody diarrhea.
Respiratory: dyspnea.

Other: fever.

INTERACTIONS
Herb-drug. *Digoxin, other cardioactive drugs:* Increases risk of cardiac or cardiac glycoside toxicity. Advise patient to avoid using together.
Macrolide antibiotics, tetracyclines: May increase the risk of cardiac glycoside toxicity. Advise patient to avoid using together.
Potassium-depleting diuretics: Increases risk of cardiac glycoside toxicity. Advise patient to avoid using together.
Stimulant laxatives: Potassium depletion can increase glycoside toxicity. In addition, stimulant laxatives may also increase potential action of the herb. Advise patient to avoid using together.
Herb-herb. *Horsetail, licorice, stimulant laxative herbs (including aloe, cascara bark, yellow dock):* May increase the risk of cardiac toxicity from potassium depletion. Advise patient to avoid using together.

EFFECTS ON LAB TEST RESULTS
• May decrease potassium level.

CAUTIONS
Patients with obstructive biliary disease should avoid use because wahoo can stimulate the flow of bile.

NURSING CONSIDERATIONS
• Find out why patient is using the herb.

Bold italic type indicates that reaction may be life-threatening.

⚠ **ALERT:** Wahoo is poisonous. Ingesting just 36 berries can be fatal. Signs of toxicity include upset stomach, bloody diarrhea, fever, shortness of breath, collapse, stupor increasing to unconsciousness, severe tonic-clonic spasms with locked jaw muscles, and coma.
• Wahoo interacts with many drugs.
• Monitor patient's response to herb and patient's cardiac status closely.

PATIENT TEACHING
• Advise patient to consult a health care provider before using an herbal preparation because a standard treatment that has been proven effective may be available.
• Tell patient that when filling a new prescription he should remind pharmacist of any herbal and dietary supplements he's taking.
• Warn patient of potential dangers of using wahoo, and discourage its use.
• Inform patient that safer, clinically proven treatments may be available for his condition.
• Warn patient not to take herb before seeking medical attention because doing so may delay diagnosis of a potentially serious medical condition.
• Warn patient to keep all herbal products away from children and pets.

watercress

Nasturtium officinale, berro, brunnenkressenkraut, crescione di fonte, Indian cress, nasilord, nasturtii herba, oranda-garashi, scurvy grass, tall nasturtium

Common trade names
Watercress

AVAILABLE FORMS
Available as fresh or dried herb, juice, and capsules.
Capsules: 500 mg

ACTIONS & COMPONENTS
Obtained from *N. officinale.* Contains mustard oil, vitamin C, beta-carotene, minerals, and vitamins B_1, B_2, E, and K. Herb has diuretic and slight antibiotic activity; both may be due to mustard oil.

USES
Used for treating catarrh (an inflammation of the air passages usually involving the nose, throat, or lungs), chronic bronchitis, and respiratory tract mucous membrane inflammation. Also used as a poultice for skin irritation, a detoxifying agent, a diuretic, a spring tonic, and an appetite stimulant. Watercress is also widely cultivated as a salad herb.

DOSAGE & ADMINISTRATION
Average daily dose: 4 to 6 g of dried herb, 20 to 30 g fresh herb, or 60 to 150 g freshly pressed juice.
Tea: 150 ml boiling water poured over 2 g of drug (about 1 or 2 teaspoons), covered for 10 to 15 min-

---

*Liquid contains alcohol.

utes, and then strained. 2 or 3 cups taken P.O. daily before meals.

ADVERSE REACTIONS
GI: GI irritation.
GU: kidney damage.
Skin: irritation.

INTERACTIONS
Herb-drug. *Chlorzoxazone, orphenadrine citrate:* May potentiate effects. Monitor patient closely.
Diuretics: May cause additive effects. Monitor patient closely.
Warfarin: May antagonize anticoagulant effects of warfarin because of high vitamin K content. Monitor PT and INR closely.

EFFECTS ON LAB TEST RESULTS
• May increase BUN and creatinine levels.
• May decrease PT and INR.

CAUTIONS
Pregnant or breast-feeding women should avoid this herb, as should children younger than age 4 and patients with gastric ulcers, intestinal ulcers, or inflammatory kidney disease.

NURSING CONSIDERATIONS
• Find out why patient is using the herb.
• Patient also taking an anticoagulant should use watercress cautiously because of high vitamin K content.
• Consuming large amounts of watercress may cause GI irritation.
• Watercress can be used topically as a poultice or compress, but skin irritation can occur.
• Monitor patient's response to herb.

• Monitor patient for GI irritation or kidney damage.

PATIENT TEACHING
• Advise patient to consult a health care provider before using an herbal preparation because a standard treatment that has been proven effective may be available.
• Tell patient that when filling a new prescription he should remind pharmacist of any herbal and dietary supplements he's taking.
• Caution patient about possible GI irritation from effects of mustard oil on mucous membranes.
• If patient takes a blood thinner, warn that herb's vitamin K content may decrease the anticlotting effect of the drug. Instruct patient to have PT and INR checked, as ordered.
• Warn patient not to take herb before seeking medical attention because doing so may delay diagnosis of a potentially serious medical condition.
• Warn patient to keep all herbal products away from children and pets.

wild cherry

Prunus serotina, black cherry, black choke, choke cherry, rum cherry bark, Virginian prune, wild black cherry

Common trade names
Black Cherry, Wild Cherry

AVAILABLE FORMS
Available as dried bark, liquid extract*, and combination products.

Bold italic type indicates that reaction may be life-threatening.

ACTIONS & COMPONENTS

Obtained from stem bark of *P. serotina* or *P. virginiana.* Contains prunasin, a cyanogenic glycoside that's hydrolyzed to toxic hydrocyanic acid (HCN) and benzaldehyde. Herb has astringent, antitussive, and sedative effects. Bark collected in the fall has higher HCN content (about 0.15%) than bark collected in the spring (about 0.05%).

USES

Widely used in cough syrups because of its sedative, expectorant, and antitussive effects. Also used for colds, bronchitis, whooping cough, other lung problems, nervous digestive disorders, and diarrhea. It's used in foods and beverages as a flavoring agent.

DOSAGE & ADMINISTRATION

Liquid extract (alcohol 12% to 14% by volume): 5 to 12 gtt in water P.O. t.i.d. or b.i.d.

ADVERSE REACTIONS

Other: *fatal poisoning* with ingestion of large amounts.

INTERACTIONS

None known.

EFFECTS ON LAB TEST RESULTS

None reported.

CAUTIONS

Pregnant or breast-feeding women shouldn't use this herb because prunasin, one of its constituents, may be teratogenic.

NURSING CONSIDERATIONS

● Find out why patient is using the herb.

☒**ALERT:** Wild cherry should be avoided because of its HCN content. Deaths have occurred in children who ate fruit or leaves.

● Wild cherry is best used only in very small amounts as a component of cough syrups because of the risk of poisoning at larger doses.

● Although no chemical interactions have been reported, consider the pharmacologic properties of the herb and its potential to interfere with therapeutic effects of conventional drugs.

● Monitor patient's response to herbal therapy.

PATIENT TEACHING

● Advise patient to consult a health care provider before using an herbal preparation because a standard treatment that has been proven effective may be available.

● Tell patient that when filling a new prescription he should remind pharmacist of any herbal and dietary supplements he's taking.

● Instruct patient to use wild cherry only in combination cough syrups, as directed by a health care provider or pharmacist.

● Caution patient about dangers of excessive use of wild cherry.

● Warn patient who is pregnant or breast-feeding to avoid herb because it may cause birth defects.

● Warn patient not to take herb for respiratory problems before seeking medical attention because doing so may delay diagnosis of a potentially serious medical condition.

---

*Liquid contains alcohol.

• Warn patient to keep all herbal products away from children and pets.

wild ginger

Asarum canadense, A. europaeum, asarabacca, cat's foot, false coltsfoot, hazelwort, Indian ginger, public house plant, snakeroot, wild nard

Common trade names
Wild Ginger Extract
Combination products:
Bronchaid, Immunaid

AVAILABLE FORMS
Available as dried root, dried rhizome, and liquid extract*.
Liquid extract: 45% alcohol

ACTIONS & COMPONENTS
Obtained from *A. canadense* or *A. europaeum.* Contains phenylpropanol, transisoasarone, and aristolochic acid. Mode of action unknown, but constituents of rhizome may have antibiotic, antiseptic, antispasmodic, anti-inflammatory, expectorant, and sedative properties. Phenylpropanol may be responsible for effects on bronchitis and bronchial asthma. Some products are standardized for this constituent. Transisoasarone may cause emetic and spasmolytic effects. Aristolochic acid may be carcinogenic and nephrotoxic.

USES
A. canadense is used for GI spasms, gas, and chronic pulmonary conditions such as bronchitis. Also used to produce sweating and promote menstruation. May be added to multiple-ingredient products and promoted for chronic cough, bronchitis, or immune system support.

Extract of *A. europaeum* is used in Europe for acute and chronic bronchitis, bronchial spasms, and bronchial asthma. Also used as a menstrual stimulant and antitussive and to treat angina pectoris, migraines, liver disease, jaundice, and pneumonia.

DOSAGE & ADMINISTRATION
Typical doses of A. canadense:
½ ounce of powdered root in 1 pint boiling water as tea; taken hot.
Typical doses of A. europaeum:
30 mg dry extract P.O. for adults and children older than age 13.

ADVERSE REACTIONS
CNS: partial paralysis.
EENT: burning of tongue.
GI: nausea, vomiting, gastroenteritis, diarrhea.
GU: *acute renal failure.*
Skin: dermatitis.

INTERACTIONS
Disulfiram, metronidazole: Herbal products that contain alcohol may cause a disulfiram-like reaction. Advise patient to avoid using together.

EFFECTS ON LAB TEST RESULTS
• May increase BUN and creatinine levels.

CAUTIONS
Pregnant or breast-feeding women should avoid this herb, as should patients with kidney disorders or infectious or inflammatory GI conditions.

Bold italic type indicates that reaction may be life-threatening.

NURSING CONSIDERATIONS
• Find out why patient is using the herb.
• Although no chemical interactions have been reported, consider the pharmacologic properties of the herb and its potential to interfere with therapeutic effects of conventional drugs.
• Monitor kidney function with long-term use.
• Monitor patient for GI distress.
• Monitor patient's response to herb.
⚠ALERT: Don't confuse wild ginger with bitter milkwort *(Polygala amara)* or senega *(P. senega),* also known as snake root.

PATIENT TEACHING
• Advise patient to consult a health care provider before using an herbal preparation because a standard treatment that has been proven effective may be available.
• Tell patient that when filling a new prescription he should remind pharmacist of any herbal and dietary supplements he's taking
• Caution patient that long-term use may cause possible kidney problems and cancer because of the aristolochic acid in the herb.
• Warn patient to keep all herbal products away from children and pets.

wild indigo

Baptisia tinctoria, American indigo, false indigo, horse-fly weed, rattlebush, rattleweed, yellow broom, yellow indigo

Common trade names
Wild Indigo Extract, Wild Indigo Root Caps
Combination products:
Echinacea & Baptisia, Echinacea Throat Relief, Esberitox, Immune Boost, Re-Zist

AVAILABLE FORMS
Available as dried root, root powder, capsules, tablets, suppositories, drops, homeopathic injection, and liquid extracts*.

ACTIONS & COMPONENTS
Obtained from *B. tinctoria.* Contains polysaccharides, glycoproteins, quinolizidine alkaloids, isoflavonoids, and hydroxycoumarins. Herb may have immunostimulant properties and a mild estrogenic effect.

USES
Used to treat such infections as typhoid and scarlet fever. Large doses used to induce bowel evacuation and vomiting. Also used for ear, nose, and throat infections and for inflamed lymph glands and fever. Used as a mouthwash to treat mouth sores and gum disease. Herb is thought to stimulate the immune system when combined with herbs such as echinacea. In homeopathic medicine, wild indigo has been used to treat confusion and blood poisoning.

*Liquid contains alcohol.

DOSAGE & ADMINISTRATION
Decoction: ½ to 1 teaspoon of root in a cup of water, boiled, and then simmered 10 to 15 minutes. Taken P.O. t.i.d.
Homeopathic dose: 5 to 10 gtt, 1 tablet, or 5 to 10 globules P.O. up to t.i.d.; for injection solution, 1 ml twice weekly S.C.
Liquid extract or tincture (1:1 in 60% alcohol): 1 or 2 ml P.O. t.i.d.
Ointment: 1:8 parts liquid extract to ointment base; applied topically to affected area.

ADVERSE REACTIONS
GI: vomiting, diarrhea, inflammation of the GI tract, spasms.
Skin: irritation.

INTERACTIONS
Disulfiram, metronidazole: Herbal products that contain alcohol may cause a disulfiram-like reaction. Advise patient to avoid using together.

EFFECTS ON LAB TEST RESULTS
None reported.

CAUTIONS
Pregnant or breast-feeding women should avoid this herb, as should patients with inflammatory GI conditions.

NURSING CONSIDERATIONS
• Find out why patient is using the herb.
• Although no chemical interactions have been reported, consider the pharmacologic properties of the herb and its potential to interfere with therapeutic effects of conventional drugs.
• Monitor patient's response to herbal therapy.
🖉 **ALERT:** Don't confuse wild indigo with the root of false blue indigo *(B. australis)* or *B. alba*.

PATIENT TEACHING
• Advise patient to consult a health care provider before using an herbal preparation because a standard treatment that has been proven effective may be available.
• Tell patient that when filling a new prescription he should remind pharmacist of any herbal and dietary supplements he's taking.
• Warn patient not to take herb before seeking medical attention because doing so may delay diagnosis of a potentially serious medical condition.
• Tell patient who uses herb as an ointment to watch for adverse effects, including local reactions, and to promptly notify health care provider about any change in symptoms.
• Warn patient to keep all herbal products away from children and pets.

wild lettuce

Lactuca canadensis, L. virosa, bitter lettuce, green endive, lactucarium, lettuce opium, poison lettuce

Common trade names
Spirit Walk, Turkhash, Vision Quest, Wild Lettuce Extract
Combination product: *Hypericum Pro (contains multiple ingredients)*

AVAILABLE FORMS

Available as dried or powdered herb, oil, dried sap, and extracts*.

ACTIONS & COMPONENTS

Obtained from *L. canadensis* and *L. virosa*. The milky latex can cause mydriasis. Lactucin, a component of the latex, may have sedative and CNS depressant properties. Trace amounts of morphine have been found in *Lactuca* species, but not enough to exert pharmacologic effects.

USES

Latex is used as a sedative and a treatment for colic and cough. Seed oil is used for arteriosclerosis and as a substitute for wheat germ oil. Leaf is used for insomnia, restlessness, dry irritated cough, and muscle or joint pain. Latex and leaf are used for excitability in children, priapism, painful menses, swollen genitals, and as an opium substitute in cough preparations. Leaf and dried sap are smoked recreationally as legal substitutes for marijuana and hashish. Crude extract has been injected I.V. for the same purpose. Also used as an analgesic and a GI aid.

DOSAGE & ADMINISTRATION

Infusion: 1 or 2 teaspoons leaves to 1 cup boiling water, steeped for 10 to 15 minutes. Taken P.O. t.i.d.
Tincture: 1 or 2 ml P.O. t.i.d.

ADVERSE REACTIONS

CNS: dizziness, somnolence, ***coma.***
CV: tachycardia.
EENT: pupil dilation, tinnitus.
Respiratory: tachypnea.

Skin: contact dermatitis.
Other: *allergic reaction.*

INTERACTIONS

Herb-drug. *Antihistamines, OTC cold medicines, sedatives:* May have additive sedative effects. Monitor patient closely. Advise patient to avoid using together.
Disulfiram, metronidazole: Herbal products that contain alcohol may cause a disulfiram-like reaction. Advise patient to avoid using together.
Herb-herb. *Herbs with anticoagulant or antiplatelet effects:* Increases risk of bleeding. Monitor patient for bleeding. Monitor PT and INR, as indicated.
Herbs with sedative effects: May enhance adverse effects. Advise patient to avoid using together.
Herb-lifestyle. *Alcohol use:* May cause additive CNS effects. Advise patient to avoid using together.

EFFECTS ON LAB TEST RESULTS

None reported.

CAUTIONS

Patients who are pregnant or breast-feeding, those sensitive to members of the Compositae family, and those with a history of glaucoma or BPH should avoid this herb.

NURSING CONSIDERATIONS

- Find out why patient is using the herb.
- Monitor patient's response to herbal therapy.
- Monitor patient for bleeding, and check PT and INR, if indicated.

*Liquid contains alcohol.

PATIENT TEACHING
• Advise patient to consult a health care provider before using an herbal preparation because a standard treatment that has been proven effective may be available.
• Tell patient that when filling a new prescription he should remind pharmacist of any herbal and dietary supplements he's taking.
• Advise patient to use caution if combining wild lettuce with other sedating drugs or with alcohol.
• Caution patient to avoid hazardous activities until CNS effects of herb are fully known.
• Warn patient not to take herb before seeking medical attention because doing so may delay diagnosis of a potentially serious medical condition.
• Tell patient to promptly notify a health care provider about adverse effects or changes in symptoms.
• Warn patient to keep all herbal products away from children and pets.

wild yam

Dioscorea composita, D. villosa, Atlantic yam, China root, colic root, devil's bones, Mexican wild yam, rheumatism root, yuma

Common trade names
Combination products: *Bone Strengthener Formula, Born Again Wild Yam Gel, Ease Wild Yam Extract, FemPro, MexiYam, Mexican Wild Yam, Progesterone Plus, Prostan, Resolve, Super Female Formula, Ultra Diet Pep, Wild Yam & Chaste Tree, Wild Yamcon, Wild Yam/Dong Quai Formula, Wild Yam EFX, Wild Yam Extract, Wild Yam-False Unicorn Virtue, Wild Yam Root, Yamcon Pro, Yamcon Vaginal, Yam Extract Plus 30*

AVAILABLE FORMS
Available as capsules, creams, gels, and liquid extracts*.
Cream and gel: 3% to 10% yam extract with or without added progesterone or other herbs. Added progesterone content runs from 0.5% to 1.5%, about 24 to 72 mg per teaspoon, depending on the product.
Liquid extracts: 1:1, 1:2; 250 mg/ml
Root powder capsules: 400 mg, 500 mg
Standardized extract capsules: 200 mg, usually standardized to 10% diosgenin

ACTIONS & COMPONENTS
Obtained from *D. composita* or *D. villosa.* Contains a glycoside, diosgenin, saponins, and tannins. Diosgenin is a steroid precursor used in the first commercial production of oral contraceptives, topical hormones, estrogens, progestogens, androgens, and other sex hormones. However, compounds in wild yam can't be used as hormones by the human body. Diosgenin may have some weak estrogenic effects, but not progesterogenic actions. Progesterogenic effects are sometimes obtained from wild yam cream by adding "natural" progesterone, which is absorbed through the skin. Diosegenin prevents estrogen-induced bile flow suppression. It may stimulate the growth of mammary tissue.

Bold italic type indicates that reaction may be life-threatening.

USES

Commercial wild yam cream and oral preparations may have hormonal properties and are used to relieve menopausal symptoms, premenstrual syndrome (PMS), and other gynecologic symptoms. However, wild yam doesn't contain hormones or compounds such as dihydroepiandrosterone (DHEA) that are converted into hormones in the human body. Orally, wild yam is used as a "natural alternative" for estrogen replacement, postmenopausal vaginal dryness, PMS, osteoporosis, increasing energy and libido in men and women, and breast enlargement. It may also be used for diverticulosis, gallbladder colic, painful menstruation, cramps, and rheumatoid arthritis.

Wild yam cream with progesterone added from other sources does exert physiologic effects from the absorbed progesterone. Progesterone cream may be useful in treating menopausal symptoms. However, progesterone has been shown to be an ineffective treatment for PMS even at much higher doses.

Wild yam is also used in multiple-ingredient commercial formulas promoted for menopause, osteoporosis prevention, PMS, threatened abortion, weight loss, women's general health, and men's prostate health. Diosgenin is promoted as a natural precursor to DHEA to increase athletic performance and slow the aging process.

DOSAGE & ADMINISTRATION

Oral dosage: No consensus exists. For adults, 1 to 6 g powder P.O. daily or 6 to 12 ml P.O. daily of liquid extract, in divided doses. *Topical dosage:* No consensus exists. Yam cream without progesterone, ¼ to ½ teaspoon daily. Cream with progesterone, ⅛ to ½ teaspoon daily (progesterone dose of 4 to 33 mg daily) depending on the product. Rubbed onto belly, breasts, inner thighs, or under the upper arms. Some manufacturers recommend using their product only 14 to 21 days per month.

ADVERSE REACTIONS

CNS: dizziness, headache, fatigue.
GI: nausea, vomiting, diarrhea, abdominal pain.
GU: abnormal menstrual flow, including amenorrhea, spotting, breakthrough bleeding.
Other: breast pain, infection.

INTERACTIONS

Herb-drug. *Disulfiram, metronidazole:* Herbal products that contain alcohol may cause a disulfiram-like reaction. Advise patient to avoid using together. *Estrogen-containing drugs, progesterone:* May increase glucose level and adverse effects of prescribed progestins. Advise patient to avoid using together and to consult a health care provider. *Indomethacin:* Decreases antiinflammatory effect. If used together, monitor patient for lack of therapeutic effect.

EFFECTS ON LAB TEST RESULTS

None reported.

CAUTIONS

The addition of progesterone and the amount added may not be obvi-

---

* Liquid contains alcohol.

ous on package labeling. Pregnant or breast-feeding women should avoid wild yam. Progesterone-containing products shouldn't be used by patients with breast cancer, liver disease, liver cancer, or undiagnosed uterine or urinary tract bleeding.

NURSING CONSIDERATIONS
• Find out why patient is using the herb.
• The term *natural progesterone* means that it's identical to human progesterone. It's produced synthetically from soybeans or other plant sources.
• Topical creams that contain progesterone may increase the adverse effects of prescribed progestins.
• Topical progesterone alone may not reduce the risk of osteoporosis.
• Breast examinations should be performed routinely, especially with prolonged progestin use.
• Monitor patient for adverse effects.

PATIENT TEACHING
• Advise patient to consult a health care provider before using an herbal preparation because a standard treatment that has been proven effective may be available.
• Tell patient that when filling a new prescription she should remind pharmacist of any herbal and dietary supplements she's taking.
• Instruct patient to have appropriate medical evaluation before beginning any new herbal or dietary supplement.
• Urge patient to talk to her health care provider before using products containing progesterone.

• Warn patient not to take herb before seeking medical attention because doing so may delay diagnosis of a potentially serious medical condition.
• Instruct patient to apply cream to alternate body areas daily to ensure optimum absorption.
• Tell patient to promptly notify a health care provider about adverse effects or changes in symptoms.
• Caution pregnant and breast-feeding women that effects of this herb are unknown.
• Warn patient to keep all herbal products away from children and pets.

willow

Salix alba, S. nigra, bay willow, black American willow, black willow, brittle willow, crack willow, Daphne willow, laurel willow, purple osier, pupurweide, violet-willow, white willow

Common trade names
Black Willow Bark Caps, White Willow Liquid Extract, Willow Bark Caps, Willowprin
Combination products: *Allerelief, Arth-Plus, Cold Control, Coldrin, Congest Ease, Menstrual-Ease, Migracin, PMSOS*

AVAILABLE FORMS
Available as crude inner bark, capsules, and dry and liquid extracts*. Extracts are often combined with root powder in commercial products.
Capsules: Powdered bark, 400 mg
Dry extract: 1:5 strength or standardized to 15% salicin

Bold italic type indicates that reaction may be life-threatening.

ACTIONS & COMPONENTS

Obtained from *S. alba* or *S. nigra*. Bark contains 2% to 11% salicin, which is converted by the body into salicylic acid—similar to aspirin in its analgesic, anti-inflammatory, and fever-reducing properties. Also contains 10% to 20% tannins, which have astringent properties, and flavonoids.

USES

Used for reducing fever, treating inflamed joints, easing GI disorders, and relieving pain. Also used in combination products for colds, flu, allergies, menstrual pain, premenstrual syndrome, migraines, arthritis, and general pain and inflammation.

DOSAGE & ADMINISTRATION

Capsules: One 400-mg capsule of willow bark with high salicin content equals $\frac{1}{10}$ of a 300-mg aspirin tablet. One capsule of a high-potency dry willow extract may equal $\frac{1}{4}$ aspirin tablet. Amount of willow in combination products would be much less.

Decoction: 1 or 2 teaspoons of bark added to 1 cup water, boiled, and then simmered 10 to 15 minutes; taken P.O. t.i.d. Manufacturers typically recommend 600 to 3,000 mg of bark equivalent up to six times daily.

ADVERSE REACTIONS

GI: stomach upset, esophageal cancer.
GU: kidney damage.
Hepatic: *liver necrosis.*
Skin: rash.
Other: bleeding episodes.

INTERACTIONS

Herb-drug. *Anticoagulants:* Increases bleeding risk. Monitor patient for bleeding and for PT and INR, as indicated. Advise patient to use together cautiously.
Disulfiram, metronidazole: Herbal products that contain alcohol may cause a disulfiram-like reaction. Advise patient to avoid using together.
NSAIDs, including aspirin, ibuprofen: May cause GI bleeding and ulceration. Monitor patient closely. Advise patient to avoid using together.

EFFECTS ON LAB TEST RESULTS

• May increase BUN, creatinine, and liver enzyme levels.
• May increase PT and INR.

CAUTIONS

Willow shouldn't be used by patients sensitive to aspirin or salicylates or by those with gastritis, peptic ulcer disease, or kidney or liver dysfunction. It shouldn't be given to feverish children or adolescents because salicylates may cause Reye's syndrome. Pregnant women shouldn't use willow because it contains salicylates similar to aspirin, which are usually contraindicated in pregnancy.

NURSING CONSIDERATIONS

• Find out why patient is using the herb.
✍ **ALERT:** Willow bark products may be marketed as "aspirin-free" but may cause some of the same adverse reactions as aspirin, such as Reye's syndrome and salicylate hypersensitivity.

*Liquid contains alcohol.

- Problems in breast-fed infants with usual analgesic doses of aspirin or willow haven't been documented. However, salicylates appear in breast milk and may cause macular rashes in breast-fed infants.
- Monitor patient for adverse reactions and signs of bleeding. Routinely check PT and INR, as indicated.
- Watch for sedative effects if patient takes a form that contains alcohol.

PATIENT TEACHING
- Advise patient to consult a health care provider before using an herbal preparation because a standard treatment that has been proven effective may be available.
- Tell patient that when filling a new prescription he should remind pharmacist of any herbal and dietary supplements he's taking.
- Ask whether patient has had adverse reactions to aspirin.
- Advise pregnant and breast-feeding women that effects of this herb are unknown and that aspirin, which is similar to some components in willow, is usually contraindicated in pregnancy.
- Caution parents not to give willow-containing products to feverish children or adolescents.
- Tell patient that taking willow with meals may reduce stomach upset.
- Instruct patient to separate doses of willow from other oral drugs to avoid interactions.
- Urge patient to have an appropriate medical evaluation before beginning an herbal supplement.

- Warn patient not to take herb before seeking medical attention because doing so may delay diagnosis of a potentially serious medical condition.
- Tell patient to promptly notify a health care provider about adverse effects or changes in symptoms.
- Warn patient to keep all herbal products away from children and pets.

wintergreen

Gaultheria procumbens, boxberry, Canada tea, checkerberry, deerberry, gaultheria oil, ground berry, hillberry, mountain tea, partridge berry, spiceberry, teaberry, wax cluster

Common trade names
Koong Yick Hung Fa Oil (KYHFO), Olbas Oil, Wintergreen Oil

AVAILABLE FORMS
Available as oil, cream, lotion, gel, and liniment*.

ACTIONS & COMPONENTS
Obtained from *G. procumbens*. Contains a volatile oil and a monotropitoside, gaultherin. The volatile oil is 96% to 98% methyl salicylate, and during steam distillation of the leaves, gaultherin is enzymatically hydrolyzed to methyl salicylate. Topical counterirritant and analgesic effects result from methyl salicylate, which is percutaneously absorbed and inhibits prostaglandin synthesis.

Bold italic type indicates that reaction may be life-threatening.

USES
Used as an anodyne, analgesic, antasthmatic, digestive stimulant, antiseptic, and aromatic. Used to treat neuralgia, gastralgia, pleurisy, pleurodynia, ovarialgia, orchitis, epididymitis, diaphragmitis, uratic arthritis, and dysmenorrhea. Used topically as an antiseptic and to treat musculoskeletal pain and rheumatoid arthritis. Also used as a flavoring agent in candies and foods.

DOSAGE & ADMINISTRATION
Gels, lotions, ointments, liniments containing 10% to 60% methyl salicylate: For adults and children older than age 2, herb is applied t.i.d. to q.i.d. topically to affected area.
Oil: 1 teaspoon wintergreen oil = about 7,000 mg salicylate or 21.5 adult aspirin (325 mg) tablets.
Tea: 1 teaspoon dried leaves added to 1 cup boiling water P.O. daily.

ADVERSE REACTIONS
CNS: confusion.
CV: *pulmonary edema and collapse.*
EENT: tinnitus.
GI: GI distress, nausea, vomiting.
GU: *renal failure.*
Hepatic: *liver failure.*
Metabolic: metabolic acidosis.
Musculoskeletal: *rhabdomyolysis.*
Respiratory: hyperventilation, respiratory alkalosis.
Skin: contact dermatitis, diaphoresis.

INTERACTIONS
Herb-drug. *Anticoagulants, antiplatelet drugs:* Increases bleeding risk. Monitor PT, INR, and patient closely.

Antidiabetics, salicylates: Large doses of topical or oral wintergreen may increase hypoglycemia. Monitor glucose level and patient closely.
Herb-lifestyle. *Alcohol use:* Use of oral wintergreen with alcohol may increase the risk of GI irritation. Advise patient to avoid using together.

EFFECTS ON LAB TEST RESULTS
• May increase BUN, creatinine, liver enzyme, and creatinine kinase levels.
• May increase PT and INR. May increase or decrease pH. May alter electrolyte balance.

CAUTIONS
Wintergreen should be avoided by patients who are or wish to become pregnant or who are breastfeeding, or who have severe asthma, nasal polyps, peptic or duodenal ulcers, or allergies to salicylates. Because methyl salicylate may play a role in Reye's syndrome, wintergreen shouldn't be used in infants, children, or adolescents during or after flulike symptoms.

NURSING CONSIDERATIONS
• Find out why patient is using the herb.
⚠ **ALERT:** Ingestion of more than small amounts of methyl salicylate is hazardous. Although the average lethal dose of methyl salicylate is estimated to be 10 ml for children and 30 ml for adults, as little as 4 ml has caused death in infants and 5 ml in children. Because of this toxicity, no drug product may contain more than 5% methyl sali-

---

*Liquid contains alcohol.

cylate or it will be regarded as misbranded. The FDA requires child-resistant containers for liquid forms that contain more than 5% methyl salicylate.

• The highest concentration of methyl salicylate used in candy flavoring is 0.04%.

• Monitor glucose level in patients who take large doses of wintergreen.

• Assess patient's response to herb.

PATIENT TEACHING

• Advise patient to consult a health care provider before using an herbal preparation because a standard treatment that has been proven effective may be available.

• Tell patient that when filling a new prescription he should remind pharmacist of any herbal and dietary supplements he's taking.

• Advise patient to inform health care provider before using wintergreen.

• Caution patient not to use a heating pad with topical wintergreen and not to apply topical wintergreen after strenuous exercise, especially on a hot, humid day. These situations increase absorption of wintergreen through the skin.

• Warn parents not to use wintergreen in infants, children, or adolescents during or after flulike symptoms.

• Instruct patient with diabetes to closely monitor glucose level and to report changes to a health care provider. Review the signs and symptoms of a low blood glucose level.

• If patient is taking wintergreen oil orally, stress the importance of proper dosing because amounts from 4 to 10 ml of the oil have been fatal.

• Explain the sign and symptoms of salicylism, including ringing in the ears (tinnitus), nausea, vomiting, sweating, and hyperventilation. Tell patient to seek medical attention immediately if symptoms occur.

• Caution patient not to consume alcohol while taking this herb.

• Warn patient to keep all herbal products away from children and pets.

witch hazel

Hamamelis virginiana, hamamelis water, hazel nut, snapping hazel, spotted alder, striped alder, tobacco wood, winter bloom

Common trade names
Grandpa Soap Witch Hazel, Superhazel Medicate, Superhazel Medicated Pads, Thayer's Herbal Astringent, Tucks Medicated Pads, Witch Hazel Aftershave, Witch Hazel & Aloe Face Pads, Witch Hazel Beauty Gel/Lotion, Witch Hazel Leaf Low Alcohol, Witch Hazel Protective Gel

AVAILABLE FORMS
Available as poultices, medicated pads and toilettes, soap, shampoo, aftershave, ointment and gel, decoction, suppositories, liquid*, liquid extract*, and gargle.
Extracts: Semisolid and liquid preparations corresponding to 5% to 10% drug
Liquid extract: 1:1 with 45% alcohol

Bold italic type indicates that reaction may be life-threatening.

Ointment, gel: 5 g witch hazel extract in 100-g ointment base
Poultices: 20% to 30% in a semisolid preparation
Suppositories: 0.1 to 1 g

ACTIONS & COMPONENTS
Obtained from dried or fresh bark, leaves, and roots of *H. virginiana.* Contains flavonoids such as kaempferol and quercetin, tannins (up to 8%), and a volatile oil (about 0.5%). Oil contains small amounts of safrole and eugenol, sesquiterpenes, resin, wax, and choline. Witch hazel's astringent and hemostatic properties result from high levels of tannins in leaf, bark, and extract. Extracts may cause vasoconstriction, decrease vascular permeability, tighten distended vessels, restore vessel tone, and stop bleeding immediately. Hamamelis water, or witch hazel water, doesn't contain tannins, so its astringent properties may result from other constituents or from alcohol content.

USES
Used orally for diarrhea, mucous colitis, hematemesis, and hemoptysis. Primarily used topically for itching, insect bites, minor burns, local inflammation of skin and mucous membranes, varicose veins, hemorrhoids, and bruises. Witch hazel may enhance solar protection factor when combined with other skin protective agents.

DOSAGE & ADMINISTRATION
Compress: 5 to 10 g leaf or bark simmered in 250 ml of water.
For anorectal disorders: Applied up to six times daily or after each bowel movement (hamamelis water in 14% to 15% alcohol).
For minor cuts, burns, and wounds: Affected area is soaked b.i.d. to q.i.d. for 15 to 30 minutes, or a compress is applied, soaked in the solution, and reapplied every few minutes for 20 to 30 minutes four to six times daily (hamamelis water in 14% to 15% alcohol).
Hamamelis liquid extract (1:1 in 45% alcohol): 2 to 4 ml P.O. t.i.d.
Ointment: 5 g witch hazel extract in 100-g ointment base. Applied topically.
Suppository: 1 suppository P.R. taken once daily to t.i.d.
Tea: 150 ml boiling water poured over 2 to 3 g drug and strained after 10 minutes. Taken P.O. t.i.d.

ADVERSE REACTIONS
GI: nausea, vomiting, constipation, fecal impaction.
Hepatic: *liver damage.*
Other: contact allergy.

INTERACTIONS
Herb-drug. *Disulfiram:* Herbal products that contain alcohol may cause a disulfiram-like reaction. Advise patient to avoid using together.

EFFECTS ON LAB TEST RESULTS
• May increase liver enzyme levels.

CAUTIONS
Pregnant or breast-feeding women shouldn't use this herb. Although extracts of witch hazel are available commercially, internal use isn't recommended because of tannin and safrole content.

---

*Liquid contains alcohol.

NURSING CONSIDERATIONS
• Find out why patient is using the herb.
• Witch hazel water (hamamelis water) isn't intended for internal use.
• In doses of 1 g, witch hazel has caused nausea, vomiting, or constipation, possibly leading to fecal impaction.
• Long-term use may cause liver damage, possibly from tannin content.
• Monitor patient for adverse effects.

PATIENT TEACHING
• Advise patient to consult a health care provider before using an herbal preparation because a standard treatment that has been proven effective may be available.
• Tell patient that when filling a new prescription he should remind pharmacist of any herbal and dietary supplements he's taking.
• Advise pregnant or breast-feeding patient to avoid oral use of this herb.
• Warn patient against taking more than 1 g of witch hazel to reduce the risk of nausea, vomiting, or constipation, possibly leading to fecal impaction.
• Inform patient that long-term oral use may lead to liver damage, possibly because of herb's tannin content.
• Warn patient not to take herb before seeking medical attention because doing so may delay diagnosis of a potentially serious medical condition.
• Tell patient to promptly notify a health care provider about adverse effects or changes in symptoms.

• Warn patient to keep all herbal products away from children and pets.

wormwood

Artemisia absinthium, absinth, absinthe, absinthii herba, absinthium, ajenjo, armoise, green ginger, herbe d'absinthe, wermut, wermutkraut, wurmkraut

Common trade names
Wormwood Capsules, Wormwood Combo, Wormwood Organo Capsules, Wormwood Tincture

AVAILABLE FORMS
Available as fresh or dried herb, powder, extract, and tincture*.

ACTIONS & COMPONENTS
Obtained from fresh or dried shoots and leaves of *A. absinthium.* Contains bitter principles absinthine, anabsinthin, artabsin, and others; a volatile oil containing up to 12% thujone; and flavones. Bitter principles may stimulate receptors in the taste buds of the tongue, triggering increased stomach acid secretion. Flavones may have spasmolytic activity. Thujone acts as an anthelmintic, causing expulsion of roundworms. It also acts on the same receptor in the brain as tetrahydrocannabinol, the active principle of marijuana. Interaction with these receptors may contribute to appetite stimulation and to the CNS toxicity seen with higher doses.

USES
Used orally for anthelmintic and diaphoretic effects and to treat ap-

---

Bold italic type indicates that reaction may be life-threatening.

petite loss, dyspepsia, bloating, and biliary dyskinesia. Used topically for wounds, skin ulcers, and insect bites. Also used as a flavoring agent for foods and aromatic alcoholic beverages such as vermouth. Extracts have been investigated for antimalarial, antimicrobial, and antifungal properties. The FDA has classified wormwood as an unsafe herb, although thujone-free derivatives have been approved for use in foods.

DOSAGE & ADMINISTRATION

Total oral daily dose shouldn't exceed 3 g of the herb as an aqueous extract.

Decoction: 1 handful of herb added to 1 L of boiling water for 5 minutes.

Infusion: 150 ml boiling water poured over ½ teaspoon of herb and strained after 10 minutes.

Liquid extract: 1 or 2 ml P.O. t.i.d.

Tea: 1 g of herb in 1 cup of water P.O. 30 minutes before each meal.

Tincture: 10 to 30 gtt in sufficient water P.O. t.i.d.

ADVERSE REACTIONS

CNS: headache, dizziness, restlessness, vertigo, trembling of the limbs, numbness of extremities, loss of intellect, paralysis, **seizures,** delirium, unconsciousness.
GI: vomiting, stomach and intestinal cramping, thirst.
GU: renal dysfunction.
Skin: topical eruptions.

INTERACTIONS

Herb-drug. *Acid-inhibitors, such as antacids, H_2 antagonists, proton pump inhibitors, sucralfate:* Increases stomach acidity; decreases drug action. If used together, monitor patient's response closely.

Anticoagulants, antiplatelet drugs: May increase bleeding risk. Monitor PT, INR, and patient closely.

Anticonvulsants: May decrease effectiveness. Advise patient to avoid using together.

Disulfiram, metronidazole: Herbal products that contain alcohol may cause a disulfiram-like reaction. Advise patient to avoid using together.

Hypoglycemics: May potentiate hypoglycemic effect. Monitor glucose level closely.

Herb-herb. *Thujone-containing herbs, such as oak moss, oriental arborvitae, sage, tansy, thuja, yarrow:* May increase risk of CNS toxicity. Advise patient to avoid using together.

Herb-lifestyle. *Alcohol use:* May cause CNS toxicity, especially with large doses or continuous use of wormwood. Advise patient to avoid using together.

EFFECTS ON LAB TEST RESULTS

• May increase BUN, creatinine, and liver enzyme levels. May decrease glucose level.
• May increase PT and INR.

CAUTIONS

Because of thujone content, consumption of large doses or continuous use of wormwood isn't recommended. Pregnant or breastfeeding women should avoid this herb, as should children, patients allergic to members of the Compositae family (such as sunflower seeds, chamomile, pistachios, hazelnuts, ragweed, chrysanthemums, marigolds, and daisies), and

---

*Liquid contains alcohol.

patients with seizure disorders, bile duct obstruction, gallbladder inflammation, gallstones, liver disease, renal dysfunction, or gastric or duodenal ulcers.

NURSING CONSIDERATIONS
- Find out why patient is using the herb.
- Many tinctures contain significant levels of alcohol, up to 20%, and may not be suitable for children, alcoholic patients, patients with liver disease, or patients who take disulfiram or metronidazole.
- **ALERT:** The FDA has classified wormwood as an unsafe herb, although thujone-free derivatives have been approved for use in foods.
- Wormwood is aromatic and has a very bitter taste.
- Monitor INR and PT closely if patient takes an anticoagulant.
- Monitor glucose level and check for signs of hypoglycemia.
- If patient has a seizure disorder, watch for lack of anticonvulsant effectiveness and lack of seizure control.
- Monitor patient for adverse effects, such as absinthism, a CNS disorder characterized by vertigo, restlessness, and delirium.

PATIENT TEACHING
- Advise patient to inform health care provider before using wormwood.
- Tell patient not to use wormwood in large doses or for continuous periods of time.
- Caution pregnant and breastfeeding women to avoid herb.
- Warn patient not to drink alcohol with this herb.

- Tell patient to promptly notify a health care provider about adverse effects or changes in symptoms.
- Instruct patient to store wormwood in a sealed container, protected from light.
- Warn patient to keep all herbal products away from children and pets.

woundwort

Anthyllis vulneraria, kidney vetch, ladies' fingers, lamb's toes, staunchwort

Common trade names
None known

AVAILABLE FORMS
Available as dried flowers and extract*.

ACTIONS & COMPONENTS
Obtained from *A. vulneraria.* Contains tannins, saponins, flavonoids, isoflavonoids, and lectins. Tannins provide astringent, hemostatic, anti-inflammatory, and antibacterial properties. Tannins may also exert vasoconstriction, decrease vascular permeability, tighten distended vessels, restore vessel tone, and stop bleeding immediately. Alcohol extract may have antiherpetic properties. Flavonoids in other herbs have been found to exert spasmolytic properties, which may account for woundwort's effect in controlling vomiting.

USES
Used internally for oropharyngeal disorders and both externally and internally for ulcers and wounds. Also used for cramps, dizziness,

---

Bold italic type indicates that reaction may be life-threatening.

fever, gout, and menstrual disorders. Combined with other herbs to purify blood and to treat coughs and vomiting.

DOSAGE & ADMINISTRATION
Extract, poultice: Applied externally.
Tea: 9 ml flowers to 250 ml of water.

ADVERSE REACTIONS
GI: digestive complaints, nausea, vomiting, constipation, impaction. **Hepatic:** *liver toxicity.*

INTERACTIONS
None known.

EFFECTS ON LAB TEST RESULTS
• May increase liver enzyme levels.

CAUTIONS
Because of tannin content, excessive ingestion of woundwort isn't recommended. Woundwort shouldn't be taken by children and patients who are pregnant, planning to become pregnant, or breast-feeding.

NURSING CONSIDERATIONS
• Find out why patient is using the herb.
• Although no chemical interactions have been reported, consider the pharmacologic properties of the herb and its potential to interfere with therapeutic effects of conventional drugs.
• Monitor patient for GI symptoms, including nausea, vomiting, and constipation.
• Monitor patient's response to herb.

⏀ **ALERT:** Don't confuse woundwort with other herbs, such as *Stachys palustris,* marsh woundwort, or *S. sylvatica,* hedge woundwort. Other plants called woundwort include *Prunella vulgaris* and *Achillea millefolium.*

PATIENT TEACHING
• Advise patient to consult a health care provider before using an herbal preparation because a standard treatment that has been proven effective may be available.
• Tell patient that when filling a new prescription he should remind pharmacist of any herbal and dietary supplements he's taking.
• Tell patient to consult with health care provider before using woundwort.
• Inform patient that if woundwort is taken orally in large amounts, the tannin content may lead to nausea, vomiting, constipation, and fecal impaction.
• Warn patient not to take herb before seeking medical attention because doing so may delay diagnosis of a potentially serious medical condition.
• Inform patient that long-term use of herbs containing tannins may lead to liver toxicity.
• Warn patient to keep all herbal products away from children and pets.

---

*Liquid contains alcohol.

Y

yarrow

Achillea millefolium, achilee, Achillea, acuilee, band man's plaything, bauchweh, birangasifa, bloodwort, carpenter's weed, civan percemi, devil's plaything, erba da cartentieri, erba da falegname, gemeine schafgarbe, green arrow, herbe aux charpentiers, katzenkrat, milefolio, milfoil, millefolii flos, millefolii herba, millefolium, millefuille, noble yarrow, nosebleed, old man's pepper, roga mari, sanguinary, soldier's woundwort, staunchweed, tausendaugbram, thousand leaf, woundwort

Common trade names
Alcohol-Free Yarrow Flowers, Tincture of Yarrow, Yarrow Capsules, Yarrow Dock Tea, Yarrow Extract, Yarrow Flower

AVAILABLE FORMS
Available as dried flower or herb, liquid extract*, tincture*, tea, or capsules.
Capsules: 340 mg, 350 mg
Liquid: 1:1, 250 mg/ml

ACTIONS & COMPONENTS
Obtained from dried flowers and dried or fresh above-ground parts of *A. millefolium.* Contains a volatile oil (0.2% to 1%) composed of sesquiterpene lactones, terpinen-4-ol, polyenes, alkamids, flavonoids, tannins, thujone, and betaines. The sesquiterpene lactones found in the volatile oil are azulenes and chamazulenes. Azulenes may have antispasmodic and anti-inflammatory effects; tannins may have astringent effects. Terpinen-4-ol may have diuretic effects. Alcohol extracts and chamazulene may be active against *Staphylococcus aureus, Bacillus subtilis, Candida albicans, Mycobacterium smegmatis, Escherichia coli, Shigella sonnei,* and *Shigella flexneri.* These properties would explain the benefit of yarrow in controlling diarrhea and dysentery. Bitter principles found in yarrow may stimulate receptors in taste buds of the tongue, triggering increased stomach acid secretion.

Thujone, found in small amounts in yarrow, may contribute to appetite stimulation. The antipyretic and hypotensive effects of yarrow may be caused by alkaloids. Yarrow's volatile oil may exert CNS depressant effects.

USES
Used orally for inducing sweating and for fever, common cold, hypertension, amenorrhea, dysentery, diarrhea, loss of appetite, mild or spasmodic GI tract discomfort, and specifically for thrombotic conditions with hypertension, including cerebral and coronary thromboses. Used topically for antibacterial and astringent properties in wound healing. Also used to treat bleeding hemorrhoids, menstrual complaints, and as a bath to remove perspiration. In the United States, yarrow is approved for use only in

---

Bold italic type indicates that reaction may be life-threatening.

alcoholic beverages, and the finished product must be thujone-free.

DOSAGE & ADMINISTRATION

Total oral daily dose shouldn't exceed 4.5 g of yarrow herb, 3 g of yarrow flower, or 3 teaspoons of pressed juice from fresh plants.

Liquid extract (1:1 in 25% alcohol): 2 to 4 ml P.O. t.i.d.

Partial bath: 100 g of herb in 20 L water.

Tea: 2 g of herb added to boiling water; covered, steeped for 10 to 15 minutes, and then strained. 1 cup freshly made tea, taken t.i.d. to q.i.d.

Tincture (1:5 in 45% alcohol): 2 to 4 ml P.O. t.i.d.

ADVERSE REACTIONS

CNS: sedation, CNS toxicities, headache, dizziness.
GI: vomiting, stomach and intestinal cramping.
GU: diuresis, renal dysfunction.
Metabolic: *hypoglycemia.*
Skin: contact dermatitis.

INTERACTIONS

Herb-drug. *Acid-inhibiting drugs, such as antacids, H₂ antagonists, proton pump inhibitors, sucralfate:* Increased stomach acid may decrease effectiveness. Advise patient to avoid using together.

Anticoagulants: May decrease effectiveness. Monitor PT, INR, and patient closely.

Antidiabetics: May potentiate hypoglycemic effect. Monitor blood glucose level closely.

Antihypertensives, hypotensives: May reduce effects. Monitor blood pressure closely.

Barbiturates, benzodiazepines: May increase sedative effects. Advise patient to avoid using together.

Disulfiram, metronidazole: Herbal products that contain alcohol may cause a disulfiram-like reaction. Advise patient to avoid using together.

Sedative-hypnotics: May increase sedative effects. Advise patient to avoid using together.

Herb-herb. *Sedative herbs:* May increase sedative effects. Advise patient to avoid using together.

Thujone-containing herbs, such as oak moss, oriental arborvitae, sage, tansy, thuja, wormwood: May increase risk of CNS toxicity. Advise patient to avoid using together.

Herb-lifestyle. *Alcohol use:* May increase CNS toxicity. Advise patient to avoid using together.

EFFECTS ON LAB TEST RESULTS

• May increase BUN and creatinine levels. May decrease glucose level. May alter electrolyte levels.
• May decrease PT and INR.

CAUTIONS

Pregnant and breast-feeding women should avoid this herb, as should patients allergic to members of the Compositae family, such as wormwood, honey, sunflower seeds, chamomile, pistachios, hazelnuts, ragweed, chrysanthemums, marigolds, and daisies.

NURSING CONSIDERATIONS

• Find out why patient is using the herb.
• Closely monitor INR and PT in patients who take anticoagulants with this herb.

---

*Liquid contains alcohol.

• Closely monitor patient's blood pressure and serum electrolyte and glucose levels.

PATIENT TEACHING
• Advise patient to consult his health care provider before using an herbal preparation because a treatment with proven efficacy may be available.
• Tell patient to remind pharmacist of any herbal and dietary supplements that he's taking, when filling a new prescription.
• Advise patient to consult his health care provider before using yarrow.
• Caution patient not to drink alcohol with this herb.
• Tell patient that taking yarrow with sedatives or other CNS depressant drugs may cause increased sedation or lethargy.
• Tell patient to avoid hazardous activities until full CNS effects of herb are known.
• Advise patient to protect yarrow from light and moisture and not to store essential oil in a synthetic container.
• Warn patient to keep all herbal products away from children and pets.

yellow root

Xanthorrhiza simplicissima, parsley-leaved yellow root, shrub yellow root, yellow wort

Common trade names
Yellowroot Liquid Extract

AVAILABLE FORMS
Available as a tincture*.

ACTIONS & COMPONENTS
Obtained from roots of *X. simplicissima.* Contains several alkaloids: berberine, jatrorrhizine, and mognoflorine. Berberine is the most abundant. Two isoquinoline alkaloids, iriodenine and palmitin, also have been identified. Most pharmacologic activity is from berberine, which may have antihypertensive, antitumor, antibacterial, antifungal, and antiprotozoal effects.

USES
Used to treat diabetes, hypertension, and infections. Recent studies documenting antineoplastic effects may lead to expanded interest in berberine-containing plants such as yellow root in treating cancer.

DOSAGE & ADMINISTRATION
Not well documented.

ADVERSE REACTIONS
CNS: tremors, sedation.
CV: reflex tachycardia.
GI: GI irritation, vomiting.
Other: *arsenic poisoning.*

INTERACTIONS
Herb-drug. *Heparin:* Reduces effectiveness. Monitor PTT and patient closely if used together. *Paclitaxel:* Reduces effectiveness. Advise patient to avoid using together.

EFFECTS ON LAB TEST RESULTS
None reported.

CAUTIONS
Pregnant or breast-feeding women shouldn't use this herb. Patients

---

Bold italic type indicates that reaction may be life-threatening.

with cardiac conditions or diabetes should use it cautiously.

NURSING CONSIDERATIONS
• Find out why patient is using the herb.
• Monitor patient's response to herbal therapy.

⚠ALERT: Don't confuse yellow root with goldenseal, which is also known as yellow root and also contains berberine.

PATIENT TEACHING
• Advise patient to consult his health care provider before using an herbal preparation because a treatment with proven efficacy may be available.
• Tell patient to remind pharmacist of any herbal and dietary supplements that he's taking when filling a new prescription.
• Explain the berberine content of this herb and its effects on blood pressure and blood clotting.
• Warn patient not to take herb before seeking medical attention because doing so may delay diagnosis of a potentially serious medical condition.
• Caution patient not to confuse yellow root with other herbs with similar common names, such as goldenseal.
• Tell patient to promptly notify a health care provider about adverse effects or changes in symptoms.
• Warn patient to keep all herbal products away from children and pets.

yerba maté

Ilex paraguariensis,
Bartholomew's tea, campeche, gaucho, ilex, jaguar, Jesuit's tea, la hoja, la mulata, mate, oro verde, Paraguay tea, payadito

Common trade names
None known

AVAILABLE FORMS
Available as dried leaves and as liquid extract*.
Extract: 1:1 in 25% alcohol

ACTIONS & COMPONENTS
Obtained from *I. paraguariensis.* Leaves contain several methylxanthines, chiefly caffeine (0.2% to 2%) theobromine (0.1% to 0.2%), and theophylline (0.05%). Leaves also contain flavonoids kaempferol and quercetin, as well as terpenoids, ursolic acid, beta-amyrin, ilexides A and B, and tannins (4% to 16%). Carotene, vitamins A and D, riboflavin, ascorbic acid, and nicotinic acid are present as well. Hepatotoxic pyrrolizidine alkaloids have also been reported. Most pharmacologic effects, including diuresis, appetite suppression, smooth-muscle relaxation, and CNS, respiratory, skeletal, and cardiac muscle stimulation, are caused by the methylxanthines, especially caffeine.

USES
Used as a CNS stimulant for drowsiness or fatigue and as a mild analgesic for headaches caused by fatigue. It's also been used as a diuretic and appetite suppressant.

---

*Liquid contains alcohol.

DOSAGE & ADMINISTRATION

Average effective daily dose of caffeine in adults is 100 to 200 mg, about 1 to 2 cups of coffee.

Infusion: 1 teaspoon or 2 to 4 g dried leaves steeped in 1 cup hot water for 5 to 10 minutes and then strained. 3 cups taken P.O. daily.

Tincture (1:1 in 25% alcohol): 2 to 4 ml P.O. t.i.d.

ADVERSE REACTIONS

CNS: sleeplessness, restlessness, irritability, anxiety, tremor, headache and sleep disturbances.
CV: palpitations.
EENT: *esophageal cancer.*
GU: *bladder cancers.*
Hepatic: *liver toxicity.*

INTERACTIONS

Herb-drug. *CNS stimulants:* Causes additive stimulatory and diuretic effects. Advise patient to avoid using together.
Herb-food. *Caffeine:* Causes additive stimulatory and diuretic effects. Advise patient to avoid using together.

EFFECTS ON LAB TEST RESULTS

• May increase liver enzyme levels.

CAUTIONS

Pregnant or breast-feeding women should avoid this herb, as should patients with CV disease (such as hypertension), ischemic heart disease, or chronic liver disease.

NURSING CONSIDERATIONS

• Find out why patient is using the herb.

• Watch for evidence of excessive stimulation, such as hypertension, restlessness, and sleeplessness.
• Headache and sleep disturbances are signs of withdrawal from yerba maté.
• Consumption of products containing caffeine may cause additive effects.
• Monitor patient's response to herb.

PATIENT TEACHING

• Advise patient to consult his health care provider before using an herbal preparation because a treatment with proven efficacy may be available.
• Tell patient to remind pharmacist of any herbal and dietary supplements that he's taking when filling a new prescription.
• Inform patient that this herb is a source of caffeine and theophylline, and combining with other caffeine-containing beverages or other stimulants could lead to excessive stimulation.
• Caution patient about possible liver toxicity and possible increased cancer risk.
• If evidence of excessive stimulation arises, suggest that patient decrease or eliminate consumption of herb.
• Urge patient to promptly notify a health care provider about adverse effects or changes in symptoms.
• Tell patient that he may have withdrawal symptoms, such as headache and sleep disturbances, when he stops taking yerba maté.
• Warn patient to keep all herbal products away from children and pets.

Bold italic type indicates that reaction may be life-threatening.

yerba santa

Eriodictyon californicum, bear's weed, consumptive's weed, gum bush, gum plant, holy weed, mountain balm, sacred herb, tarweed

Common trade names
Feminease, Respirtone

AVAILABLE FORMS
Available as fresh or dried herb, powdered herb, liquid, and ointment.

ACTIONS & COMPONENTS
Obtained from *E. californicum.* Contains at least 12 flavonoids, including eriodictyonine (6%), eriodictyol (0.5%), and eriodictine, as well as four flavones: cirsimaritin, chrysoeriol, hispidulin, and chrysin. Eriodictyol is a mild expectorant. Resins in the plant have a pleasant taste and aroma, explaining why it's used to mask the bitter taste of certain drugs or as a flavoring in foods and beverages. Several flavones and flavonoids inhibit formation of active metabolites of the carcinogen benzopyrene, thus showing chemopreventive potential. Herb is also a mild diuretic.

USES
Used orally to treat coughs, colds, asthma, and bronchitis. Used topically to treat bruises, sprains, skin wounds, poison ivy, and insect bites.

DOSAGE & ADMINISTRATION
Fresh leaves: Chewed p.r.n.

Tea: 1 teaspoon dried or fresh leaves added to 1 cup hot water, taken P.O. 30 minutes before bedtime.

ADVERSE REACTIONS
Other: sticky residue on teeth after chewing fresh leaves.

INTERACTIONS
None reported.

EFFECTS ON LAB TEST RESULTS
None reported.

CAUTIONS
Pregnant or breast-feeding women shouldn't use this herb.

NURSING CONSIDERATIONS
• Find out why patient is using the herb.
• Although no chemical interactions have been reported, consider the pharmacologic properties of the herb and its potential to interfere with therapeutic effects of conventional drugs.
• Monitor patient's response to herbal therapy.

PATIENT TEACHING
• Advise patient to consult his health care provider before using an herbal preparation because a treatment with proven efficacy may be available.
• Tell patient to remind pharmacist of any herbal and dietary supplements that he's taking when filling a new prescription.
• Advise patient that chewing the fresh leaves will leave a sticky residue on his teeth.
• Warn patient not to take herb for a chronic cough or cold before

---

*Liquid contains alcohol.

seeking medical attention because doing so may delay diagnosis of a potentially serious medical condition.

• Instruct patient to promptly notify a health care provider about adverse effects or changes in symptoms.

• Warn patient to keep all herbal products away from children and pets.

yew

Taxus baccata, T. brevifolia, T. canadensis, T. cuspidata, T. cuspididata, T. floridana, American yew, chinwood, English yew, Japanese yew, Oregon yew, Pacific yew, Western yew

Common trade names
Vital Yew, Yew Tea

AVAILABLE FORMS
Available as a tincture*, capsules, and a salve of yew bark.

ACTIONS & COMPONENTS
Obtained from bark and branch tips of *T. brevifolia.* Contains a mixture of about 19 taxane-type diterpene esters referred to as taxines. Most prominent of these are paclitaxel and taxine A and B. Other constituents include taxicatin, milossine, and ephedrine. Paclitaxel inhibits cell division by binding to the β-tubulin subunit of microtubules, which prevents the disassembly of microtubules. Cells are thus arrested in mitosis.

USES
Used for promoting menstruation, eliminating tapeworms, and treating tonsillitis. Taxol is the trade name for the drug paclitaxel, which is isolated from the bark of *T. brevifolia.* Taxotere is the trade name of docetaxel, a more potent analogue of paclitaxel. Paclitaxel is FDA-approved for treating metastatic, ovarian, and breast cancers. Pending results of clinical trials, it may be approved for other cancers, such as melanoma and lung and esophageal cancers.

DOSAGE & ADMINISTRATION
For cancers: Optimal doses and administration protocols are still being determined in ongoing clinical trials.
Infusion: Bark or needles are added to 1 cup hot water and taken P.O. once daily.
Tinctures: Doses of yew bark tinctures vary widely.

ADVERSE REACTIONS
CNS: dizziness, *unconsciousness.*
CV: *bradycardia,* tachycardia, hypotension, *heart failure.*
EENT: mydriasis, dry mouth, reddened lips.
GI: abdominal cramps, nausea, vomiting.
GU: miscarriage.
Respiratory: dyspnea, *respiratory failure.*
Skin: rash, pallor, cyanosis.

INTERACTIONS
Herb-drug. *Chemotherapeutic drugs:* Potentiates myelosuppression and interactions with other chemotherapeutic drugs. Advise patient to use together only with

---

Bold italic type indicates that reaction may be life-threatening.

extreme caution and only under direct supervision of a health care provider.

EFFECTS ON LAB TEST RESULTS
• May increase liver enzyme levels.
• May decrease hemoglobin, hematocrit, and neutrophil, WBC, and platelet counts.

CAUTIONS
Women who are pregnant or breast-feeding shouldn't use this herb. Because of the potential toxicity of multiple constituents, herbal formulations of the yew tree should be used only with extreme caution, if at all.

NURSING CONSIDERATIONS
• Find out why patient is using the herb.
⚠ **ALERT:** Most parts of the yew plant are highly poisonous. Ingestion of 50 to 100 g of yew needles or berries has been fatal and is especially dangerous in children. Treatment for poisoning includes digoxin-specific fragment antigen-binding antibodies and gastric lavage followed by administration of charcoal. Supportive measures to treat cardiac effects and other symptoms may also be indicated.
• Keep emergency equipment readily available.
• Monitor vital signs and ECG if large amounts of the herb are ingested.
• Because of the potential extreme toxicity of this herb, only prescription forms of paclitaxel should be used, and then only under the careful guidance of an oncologist.
• Some common hypersensitivity reactions to paclitaxel have been

reduced by giving the drug as a slow infusion over 6 to 24 hours.
• Monitor patient's level of consciousness, and report changes immediately to a health care provider.

PATIENT TEACHING
• If patient wants to use this herb for a cancerous condition, warn him to use it only on the recommendation of an oncologist.
• Advise patient of the need for regular follow-up care with an oncologist if taking this herb for cancer.
• Urge patient to report adverse effects promptly to a health care provider.
• Tell patient to seek emergency medical care if he develops adverse effects or a toxic response.
• Warn patient of the danger of taking this toxic herb without medical supervision.
• Warn patient to keep all herbal products away from children and pets.

yohimbe

Corynanthe yohimbi,
Pausinystalia yohimbe,
corynine, yohimbehe,
yohimbine

Common trade names
Aphrodyne, Dayto Himbin,
Potensan, Yobinol, Yocon,
Yohimbine HCl, Yohimbehe,
Yohimbe Power MAX for Women,
Yohimex

AVAILABLE FORMS
Available as tablets and tinctures*.
Tablets: Yohimbine hydrochlorothiazide 3 mg, 5.4 mg

*Liquid contains alcohol.

Tinctures: Standardized to yohimbine

ACTIONS & COMPONENTS
Obtained from bark of *P. yohimbe.* Contains tannins and 2.7% to 5.9% indole alkaloids, especially yohimbine. Other alkaloids include ajamalicin, dihydroyohimbine, corynanthein, and others. Effects of yohimbine are mediated mostly via selective blockade of alpha$_2$-receptors, primarily in CNS. At higher levels, yohimbine acts as an agonist at alpha$_1$, serotonin, and dopamine receptors. Yohimbine may also inhibit MAO and slow L-type calcium channels in heart and blood vessels.

Yohimbe increases penile cavernous blood flow in men with erectile dysfunction. It also increases autonomic nerve activity from the brain to genital tissues and increases reflex excitability in the sacral region of the spinal cord.

USES
Primarily used as an aphrodisiac and to treat organic and psychogenic erectile dysfunction in men. Also used at higher doses to treat orthostatic hypotension.

DOSAGE & ADMINISTRATION
For erectile dysfunction: 5.4 mg P.O. t.i.d. Doses of 20 to 30 mg have been shown to significantly increase blood pressure. Yohimbe bark alcoholic extracts are usually standardized to contain a certain amount of yohimbine.

ADVERSE REACTIONS
CNS: nervousness, anxiety, irritability, increased motor activity, headache, anorexia, dizziness, insomnia, manic or psychotic episodes, paralysis.
CV: tachycardia, hypotension, hypertension.
GI: abdominal discomfort, diarrhea, nausea.
GU: *acute renal failure.*

INTERACTIONS
Herb-drug. *Antihypertensives, including adrenergics and clonidine:* May precipitate clonidine withdrawal hypertensive crisis. Advise patient to avoid using together.
Anxiolytics: May block action of these drugs. Advise patient to avoid using together.
CNS-stimulating drugs: Enhances effects. Advise patient to avoid using together.
Naltrexone: Increases sensitivity to yohimbe, potentiating adverse reactions. Advise patient to avoid using together.
Selective serotonin reuptake inhibitors, tricyclic antidepressants: May cause serum serotonin levels to increase dangerously. Advise patient to avoid using together.
Herb-food. *Caffeine:* Enhances effect. Advise patient to avoid using together.
Tyramine-containing foods: Because of its reported weak MAO-inhibiting activity, yohimbe may interact with tyramine-containing foods. Advise patient to avoid using together.
Herb-lifestyle. *Alcohol use:* May have additive effects. Advise patient to avoid using together.

EFFECTS ON LAB TEST RESULTS
• May increase BUN and creatinine levels.

Bold italic type indicates that reaction may be life-threatening.

CAUTIONS

Yohimbe shouldn't be used by children, geriatric patients, pregnant women, breast-feeding women, or people with psychiatric disorders, liver disease, kidney disease, hyperthyroidism, angina pectoris, or CV disease, especially hypertension.

NURSING CONSIDERATIONS

• Find out why patient is using the herb.

• Herb is used mainly by men to help with impotence, but some women may also take it for an aphrodisiac effect.

• Be alert for possible CNS and blood pressure changes.

• Herb can significantly increase blood pressure in patients with orthostatic hypotension caused by autonomic failure or multisystem atrophy.

• Monitor patient's vital signs and ECG closely.

• Monitor patient for adverse effects or changes in condition.

PATIENT TEACHING

• Advise patient to consult his health care provider before using an herbal preparation because a treatment with proven efficacy may be available.

• Tell patient to remind pharmacist of any herbal and dietary supplements that he's taking, when filling a new prescription.

• Inform patient that herb is considered by many to have a high risk-to-benefit ratio.

• Instruct patient not to take caffeine products while taking this herb.

• Warn patient not to take herb for erectile dysfunction before seeking medical attention because doing so may delay diagnosis of a potentially serious medical condition.

• Instruct patient to report adverse effects promptly to a health care provider.

• Warn patient to keep all herbal products away from children and pets.

*Liquid contains alcohol.

acidophilus

Lactobacillus acidophilus

Common trade names
Acidophilus, Bacid, Kala, Lactinex, More-Dophilus, Pro-Bionate, Probiotics, Superdophilus

AVAILABLE FORMS
Available as capsules, granules, milk, powders, tablets, and yogurt.

ACTIONS & COMPONENTS
L. acidophilus grows naturally in the human GI tract along with *Bacteroides, Escherichia coli, Streptococcus faecalis,* and other microorganisms. Each bacterial strain prevents the others from overgrowth in the intestine. Acidophilus produces hydrogen peroxide and lactic acid to suppress pathogenic bacteria.

USES
Used for lactose intolerance, digestive disorders, and antibiotic-induced diarrhea because it helps replace intestinal flora. Also used to ease the pain of a sore mouth caused by oral candidiasis, and to treat fever blisters, canker sores, hives, and acne. Lactobacillus products have also been used to treat vaginal yeast or bacterial infections and uncomplicated lower UTIs. They're administered intra-vaginally to treat bacterial vaginosis in pregnant women in the first trimester, thus restoring normal vaginal flora and acidity.

When antibiotics are given, growth of susceptible bacteria may decline, allowing for overgrowth of other bacteria; acidophilus is taken to restore intestinal flora and, thus, homeostasis.

Some herbal practitioners claim acidophilus may also retard the growth of tumors and reduce cholesterol levels, but no data support this.

Although sometimes used to treat irritable bowel syndrome and inflammatory bowel disease, acidophilus probably isn't effective for these conditions.

DOSAGE & ADMINISTRATION
Bacid
2 capsules P.O. b.i.d. to q.i.d.
Lactinex
1 packet added to or taken P.O. with food, milk, juice, or water b.i.d. or q.i.d.
More-Dophilus
1 teaspoon P.O. daily with liquid.
Pro-Bionate
1 capsule P.O. daily to t.i.d. Or ¼ to 1 teaspoon powder P.O. daily to t.i.d.
Superdophilus
¼ to 1 teaspoon P.O. daily to t.i.d.
To decrease recurrence of vaginal candidiasis: 1 cup of yogurt containing *L. acidophilus* P.O.

ADVERSE REACTIONS
GI: flatulence.

INTERACTIONS
None reported.

EFFECTS ON LAB TEST RESULTS
None reported.

Bold italic type indicates that reaction may be life-threatening.

CAUTIONS

Patients sensitive to dairy foods and children younger than age 3 should avoid using acidophilus.

Those with high fevers should use acidophilus cautiously.

NURSING CONSIDERATIONS

• Find out why patient is using the herb.
• *L. acidophilus* is found in such dairy products as milk and yogurt. Some products may contain other strains of *Lactobacillus*, such as *L. bulgaricus.*
• Some products labeled as containing *L. acidophilus* contain little to no active ingredient, whereas others contain contaminants such as *Clostridium sporogenes, Enterococcus faecium,* and *Pseudomonas.*
• Products may be administered orally or intravaginally, depending on intended use.
• The strength of an acidophilus product is commonly quantified by the number of living organisms per capsule, typically ranging from 1 to 10 billion viable organisms in three to four divided doses every day.
• Flatulence is prevalent with initial dosing but decreases with continued use.
• Acidophilus shouldn't be used for longer than 2 days.
• Refrigeration is recommended to maintain potency.

PATIENT TEACHING

• Advise patient to consult a health care provider before using this product because a standard treatment that has been proven effective may be available.

• Tell patient that when filling a new prescription he should remind pharmacist of any herbal or dietary supplement he's taking.
• Inform patient that if he delays seeking medical diagnosis and treatment, conditions such as inflammatory bowel disease, vaginal infections, UTIs, thrush, high levels of fat in the blood, antibiotic-associated diarrhea, and developing tumors could worsen.
• Advise patient not to use acidophilus for longer than 2 days or while he has a high fever, unless his health care provider has instructed him to do so.
• Advise patient sensitive to dairy products to avoid oral use of *L. acidophilus.*
• Inform patient that flatulence may occur initially but usually decreases with continued use.
• Advise patient to store acidophilus in the refrigerator.

agar

Gelidium amansii, agar-agar, Chinese gelatin, colle du Japon, E-406, gelose, Japanese gelatin, Japanese isinglass, layor carang, vegetable gelatin

Common trade names
Gelatin, Gelosa, and various multi-ingredient preparations including Agarol, Diet Fibre Complex 1500, Emulsione, Paragar, Pseudophage

AVAILABLE FORMS

Available as a dry powder and as thin, odorless, and colorless to pale yellow, orange, or gray translucent strips, flakes, and granules.

*Liquid contains alcohol.

ACTIONS & COMPONENTS

Made up of two major polysaccharides—neutral agarose and charged agaropectin—that are extracted from various species of *Rhodophyceae algae*.

Agarose is the gelling component of agar. Agar aids peristalsis by increasing bulk in the intestines and by swelling the intestines, stimulating the intestinal muscles.

USES

Used as an oral bulk laxative to treat chronic constipation. It's also used to make dental impressions and is added to other drugs in compounding emulsions, suspensions, gels, and hydrophilic suppositories.

DOSAGE & ADMINISTRATION

Laxative: 1 or 2 teaspoons of powder P.O. with liquid, fruit, or jam before meals, daily to t.i.d.
Oral use: 4 to 16 g daily or b.i.d. with at least 8 ounces of water.

ADVERSE REACTIONS

GI: *esophageal or bowel obstruction.*
Metabolic: hypercholesterolemia.

INTERACTIONS

Herb-drug. *Oral drugs:* May impair absorption of oral drugs. Encourage patient to separate administration times.

EFFECTS ON LAB TEST RESULTS

• May increase cholesterol levels.

CAUTIONS

Patients with bowel obstruction or difficulty swallowing shouldn't use agar.

NURSING CONSIDERATIONS

• Find out why patient is using agar.
• Dry powder is soluble in boiling water and produces a clear liquid that gels when cooled.
• Agar strips, flakes, and granules are tough when damp but become brittle when dried.
• Monitor patient for chest pain, vomiting, and difficulty swallowing or breathing.

PATIENT TEACHING

• Advise patient to consult a health care provider before using this product because a standard treatment that has been proven effective may be available.
• Tell patient that when filling a new prescription he should remind pharmacist of any herbal or dietary supplement he's taking.
• Advise any patient who has difficulty swallowing not to use agar.
• Inform patient that agar may alter the effectiveness of oral drugs, and encourage him to notify his health care provider if he's taking agar.
• Advise patient to take agar with plenty of fluids (at least 8 ounces) to prevent blockage of the throat or esophagus, which could cause choking.
• Advise patient to seek immediate medical attention if he experiences chest pain, vomiting, or difficulty swallowing or breathing.

Bold italic type indicates that reaction may be life-threatening.

androstenedione

4-androstene-3,17-dione;
androst-4-ene-3, 17-dione

Common trade names
Andro, Androstene

AVAILABLE FORMS
Available as capsules.
Capsules: 50 mg, 100 mg

ACTIONS & COMPONENTS
Androstenedione is a steroid hormone produced by the adrenal glands, testes, and ovaries, and is a direct precursor of testosterone and estrone in both men and women. In young healthy men, androstenedione increases estradiol levels at low doses (100 mg/day), but has no significant effect on testosterone levels and no anabolic effect on muscle protein metabolism. Higher single doses (300 mg/day) increase both testosterone and estradiol in young men. A divided dose of 300 mg/day raises estradiol but not testosterone levels and doesn't enhance skeletal muscle adaptations to resistance training.

USES
Orally, androstenedione is used to increase endogenous testosterone production for enhanced athletic performance, to increase energy, to keep RBCs healthy, to enhance recovery and growth from exercise, and to heighten sexual arousal and function.

DOSAGE & ADMINISTRATION
Oral: 50 to 100 mg b.i.d. or 300 mg daily.

ADVERSE REACTIONS
CNS: aggression.
GU: priapism.
Hepatic: *hepatotoxicity,* liver abnormalities.

INTERACTIONS
Herb-drug. *Estrogenic drugs:* May increase the activity and incidence of adverse events associated with androgenic drugs, which can affect the activity of estrogenic drugs. Advise patient to avoid use together.

EFFECTS ON LAB TEST RESULTS
• May increase testosterone, estrone, and liver transaminase levels.

CAUTIONS
Androstenedione may stimulate prostate tumor growth. Patients with prostate problems should avoid use.

Androstenedione may cause premature closure of the bone growth plates; therefore, children shouldn't use this herb. Pregnant women shouldn't use this herb because some evidence suggests the herb may induce labor. Patients with hepatic dysfunction or any liver abnormalities should also avoid use.

NURSING CONSIDERATIONS
☑**ALERT:** Data suggest that androstenedione use can increase the risk of CV disease by increasing estrogen levels and decreasing high-density lipoprotein levels.
• Androstenedione can lead to breast enlargement and feminizing effects in men.

*Liquid contains alcohol.

- Androstenedione may increase the risk of breast cancer, pancreatic cancer, and prostate cancer.
- The long-term effects of androstenedione are unknown.
- Routinely monitor liver function test results in patients who choose to use androstenedione.
- Until further information is known, androstenedione should be considered a testosterone derivative with all the possible side effects, drug interactions, and precautions associated with this drug class.

PATIENT TEACHING
- Advise patient to consult a health care provider before using this product because a standard treatment that has been proven effective may be available.
- Tell patient that when filling a new prescription he should remind pharmacist of any herbal or dietary supplement he's taking.
- Warn patient that potency and purity of androstenedione products may differ from the product label.

benzoin

Styrax benzoin, S. paralleloneurus, Benjamin tree, gum Benjamin, gum benzoin, Siam benzoin, Sumatra benzoin

Common trade names
Benzoin Spray, Tincture of Benzoin

AVAILABLE FORMS
Available as compound tincture of benzoin* and tincture of benzoin spray*. Also available in combination products.

ACTIONS & COMPONENTS
Siam benzoin contains benzoate, alcohol, benzoic acid, *d*-siaresinolic acid, and cinnamyl benzoate. Sumatra benzoin contains benzoic acid and cinnamic esters of benzoresorcinol and coniferyl alcohol, free benzoic acid, cinnamic acids, and other ingredients. These components give benzoin its skin protectant, expectorant, and soothing properties. Benzoic acid also has antifungal and antibacterial properties.

USES
Used topically as a skin protectant. It's mixed with glycerin and water and applied to cutaneous ulcers, bedsores, cracked nipples, and fissures of the lips or anus. Also combined with zinc oxide in baby ointments.

Benzoin is administered on sugar or added to hot water and inhaled as a vapor to treat throat and bronchial inflammation, acute laryngitis, and croup.

DOSAGE & ADMINISTRATION
As an inhalant: 1% in hot water.

ADVERSE REACTIONS
Skin: irritation, urticaria at application site.

INTERACTIONS
None reported.

EFFECTS ON LAB TEST RESULTS
None reported.

CAUTIONS
Patients sensitive to benzoin should avoid use.

Bold italic type indicates that reaction may be life-threatening.

NURSING CONSIDERATIONS
• Find out why patient is using benzoin.
• Mild irritation may occur at the application site.
• Benzoin should be stored in a cool, dry place, away from excessive heat.

PATIENT TEACHING
• Advise patient to consult a health care provider before using this product because a standard treatment that has been proven effective may be available.
• Tell patient that when filling a new prescription he should remind pharmacist of any herbal or dietary supplement he's taking.
• Inform patient that mild irritation may occur at application site.
• Instruct patient to store benzoin in a cool, dry place, away from excessive heat.

chondroitin

CDS, chondroitin sulfate, chondroitin sulfate A, chondroitin sulfate C, chondroitin sulfuric acid, chonsurid, CSA, galacosaminoglucuronoglycan sulfate, structum

Common trade names
Oral (in combination with glucosamine): *ChondroFlex, Cosamin DS, OsteoBiflex*
Topical: *Humatrix*

AVAILABLE FORMS
Available as a capsule containing bovine or shark cartilage, as a gel, or as a synthetic preparation.

ACTIONS & COMPONENTS
Natural, biologic, high-viscosity polymer found in the matrix between joints. It helps maintain water content and elasticity of the cartilage between joints, allowing for easy, painless movement. Proper supplement of chondroitin may enhance repair of degenerative injuries and inflammation. Chondroitin attracts fluid and nutrients into the synovial space and thus may help protect that area.

Chondroitin is a minor component in the low-molecular-weight heparin derivative, danaparoid.

Chondroitin may help improve symptoms of osteoarthritis when it's used with glucosamine and manganese ascorbate; however, the American College of Rheumatology doesn't recommend substituting the traditional treatment with chondroitin.

USES
Used to decrease pain and inflammation after extravasation with ifosfamide, vindesine, doxorubicin, or vincristine. Chondroitin is being studied for treatment of interstitial cystitis.

DOSAGE & ADMINISTRATION
To treat osteoarthritis: 200 to 400 mg P.O. b.i.d. to t.i.d.; 1,200 mg P.O. daily; 1 tablet of Cosamin DS (contains chondroitin sulfate, glucosamine hydrochloride, manganese ascorbate) P.O. t.i.d.

ADVERSE REACTIONS
GI: epigastric pain, nausea.
Other: allergic reaction.

*Liquid contains alcohol.

INTERACTIONS
None reported.

EFFECTS ON LAB TEST RESULTS
None reported.

CAUTIONS
Patients sensitive to chondroitin or its components should avoid use.

NURSING CONSIDERATIONS
• Find out why patient is using chondroitin.
• Chondroitin may alter the effects of conventional drugs.
• Monitor patient for allergic reactions, such as shortness of breath or rash.

PATIENT TEACHING
• Advise patient to consult a health care provider before using this product because a standard treatment that has been proven effective may be available.
• Tell patient that when filling a new prescription he should remind pharmacist of any herbal or dietary supplement he's taking.
• Instruct patient not to discontinue other arthritis treatment without discussing it with his health care provider.
• Little information exists about chondroitin's long-term effects.
• Instruct patient to notify his health care provider if he experiences any allergic reactions, such as shortness of breath or rash.

coenzyme Q10

ubiquinone

Common trade names
Maxi Cardio Co-Q10, Maxi-Sorb Co-Q10, Mega Co Q10, My Fav Coenzyme Q10

AVAILABLE FORMS
Available as capsules, softgels, tablets, liquid, chewable tablets, and troches.

ACTIONS & COMPONENTS
A lipid-soluble benzoquinone that is structurally related to vitamin K. It's found in every cell in the body; it acts as a free radical scavenger and membrane stabilizer and is an important cofactor in mitochondrial transport.

USES
Used to treat ischemic heart disease, hypertension, cardiomyopathy, angina, mitral valve prolapse, and heart failure. Used to guard against doxorubicin cardiotoxicity and to protect the myocardium during invasive cardiac surgery. Used as a weight loss aid and to enhance athletic performance. Also used in chronic fatigue syndrome, fibromyalgia, diabetes, Alzheimer's disease, periodontal disease, muscular dystrophy, cancer, and immunodeficiencies.

DOSAGE & ADMINISTRATION
Oral use: 30 to 300 mg daily, divided b.i.d. to t.i.d.; however, dosages above 100 mg/day should be taken in two or three divided doses.

Bold italic type indicates that reaction may be life-threatening.

ADVERSE REACTIONS
GI: epigastric discomfort, loss of appetite, nausea, and diarrhea.

INTERACTIONS
Herb-drug. *Beta blockers:* May inhibit coenzyme Q10–dependent enzymes. Monitor patient closely.
Gemfibrozil, HMG-CoA reductase inhibitors: May decrease levels of coenzyme Q10. Advise patient taking coenzyme Q10 to supplement with oral coenzyme Q10 daily.
Insulin: May decrease insulin requirements in patients with type 1 diabetes mellitus. Monitor glucose levels closely and adjust insulin dosage, as needed.
Warfarin: May affect INR. Monitor INR and PT closely.
Herb-food. *Any food:* Food will maximize absorption. Advise patient taking coenzyme Q10 to take it with food.

EFFECTS ON LAB TEST RESULTS
• May decrease glucose level.
• May increase PT and INR.

CAUTIONS
Pregnant and breast-feeding women should avoid coenzyme Q10. Patients sensitive to coenzyme Q10 should also avoid use.

NURSING CONSIDERATIONS
• Find out why patient is using coenzyme Q10.
• Monitor vital signs and ECG, as needed.
• If patient has diabetes, monitor glucose level regularly.
• Adverse reactions to coenzyme Q10 are rare.

• Monitor PT and INR closely if patient is also taking warfarin.

PATIENT TEACHING
• Advise patient to consult a health care provider before using this product because a standard treatment that has been proven effective may be available.
• Tell patient that when filling a new prescription he should remind pharmacist of any herbal or dietary supplement he's taking.
• Advise patient to take coenzyme Q10 with food.
ALERT: Warn patient not to treat signs and symptoms of heart failure (such as increasing shortness of breath, swelling, or chest pain) with coenzyme Q10 before seeking medical evaluation because doing so may delay diagnosis of a potentially serious medical condition.
• If patient is pregnant, advise her not to use coenzyme Q10.
• If patient has diabetes, alert him to the signs and symptoms of both low and high glucose levels, and instruct him to monitor his glucose level.
• Teach patients signs and symptoms of excessive blood thinning if he is also taking warfarin.
• Instruct patient to inform his health care provider if he's taking a cholesterol or cardiac drug, a blood thinner, or insulin.

*Liquid contains alcohol.

creatine monohydrate

creatine

Common trade names
Available in numerous combination products

AVAILABLE FORMS
Available as pills, liquid, and powder.

ACTIONS & COMPONENTS
Naturally occurring substance. Can be obtained in red meat and other dietary sources. Creatine also may have an anti-inflammatory effect and may reduce blood triglyceride levels.

USES
Used as a dietary supplement to increase strength and endurance, produce energy, enhance muscle size, improve stamina, and promote faster muscle recovery.

DOSAGE & ADMINISTRATION
Adults: 20 g P.O. daily for 3 days, then 5 g P.O. daily for the next 8 weeks followed by 4 weeks with no supplementation. Cycle is then repeated.
Powder: Mixed with 4 to 8 ounces of orange or grape juice, up to q.i.d.

ADVERSE REACTIONS
GI: abdominal pain, bloating, diarrhea.
Metabolic: dehydration, electrolyte imbalances, increased body weight.
Musculoskeletal: muscle cramps.
Renal: altered renal function.

INTERACTIONS
Herb-drug. *Cimetidine, probenecid, trimethoprim:* May inhibit the tubular secretion of creatine, causing an increase in creatinine levels. Monitor creatinine levels closely.
Glucose: May increase creatine storage in muscle. Advise patient to avoid use together.
NSAIDs: May adversely affect renal function. Advise patient to use cautiously.
Herb-food. *Caffeine:* May reduce creatine's effects. Advise patient to avoid caffeine-containing products.

EFFECTS ON LAB TEST RESULTS
• May increase creatinine and potassium levels.

CAUTIONS
Pregnant and breast-feeding women and those with a history of renal disease should avoid use.

NURSING CONSIDERATIONS
• Find out why patient is using creatine monohydrate.
• If muscle cramping occurs, patient should stop taking creatine and contact health care provider. A smaller dose may be needed.
• Monitor electrolyte levels and renal function, as needed.
• Monitor youths involved in sports for overuse or abuse of creatine.

PATIENT TEACHING
• Advise patient to consult a health care provider before using this product or dietary supplement because a standard treatment that has been proven effective may be available.

Bold italic type indicates that reaction may be life-threatening.

• Tell patient that when filling a new prescription he should remind pharmacist of any herbal or dietary supplement he's taking.

• If patient is a young athlete, discuss creatine's use and adverse effects with both parents and the patient. Advise parents to monitor young athlete's use of creatine and to promptly report adverse effects to the health care provider.

• If patient is taking cimetidine, probenecid, or an NSAID, advise him to consult his health care provider before taking creatine.

• Advise patient to drink plenty of fluids while taking creatine.

• Advise patient to watch for adverse reactions, especially muscle cramps, and to promptly report such reactions to his health care provider.

• Caution patient that this product is useful only for intense exercise of short duration or when short bursts of strength are needed.

dehydroepiandrosterone

Common trade names
DHEA Fuel, DHEA Power
Combination products: *Andro-Stack 850, EAS Andro-6, Twinlab Growth Fuel, Twinlab 7-Ketofuel, Twinlab Tribulus Fuel Stack*

AVAILABLE FORMS
Available as tablets, capsules, sustained-release tablets, micronized tablets, chewing gum, liquid, S.L. drops, herbal tea, and cream.

ACTIONS & COMPONENTS
Dehydroepiandrosterone (DHEA) is a precursor of both estrogen and testosterone; it's secreted mainly by the adrenal glands. Both DHEA and its sulfate conjugate, DHEA-S, are converted in the periphery to androgens. Related compounds include androstenedione, a metabolite of DHEA, and pregnenolone, a precursor to DHEA. Circulating levels of DHEA increase during childhood into early adulthood. These levels drop with age; by age 60, levels are only 5% to 15% of what they are at age 20. Those with autoimmune and CV disease also have lower DHEA levels.

Responses to DHEA appear to be gender-specific. In women, supplementation increases both DHEA and testosterone levels; in men, it may have no effect on testosterone or estrogen levels.

DHEA may be useful as treatment for depression and as an anti-aging supplement to restore neuroendocrine function, thus improving mood and increasing feelings of well-being.

It may also be useful in treating systemic lupus erythematosus (SLE) and adrenal insufficiency. It has been reported to cause a change in response to insulin; because it decreases insulin requirements, it may be useful in treating diabetes.

USES
Used to treat osteoporosis, depression, Alzheimer's disease, Tourette syndrome, chronic fatigue syndrome, AIDS, migraines, erectile dysfunction, seizure disorders, and cancer. Also used to increase feel-

ings of well-being, slow or reverse the aging process, increase sex drive, increase lean body mass, and decrease fat mass.

DOSAGE & ADMINISTRATION
Creams (10%): 3 to 5 g applied topically to skin daily.
Oral use: 25 to 200 mg P.O. daily.

ADVERSE REACTIONS
CNS: severe mood swings.
CV: *cardiac arrhythmias.*
Skin: acne.
Other: androgenic or masculinizing effects, including hirsutism, in women; estrogenic effects, including gynecomastia, in men; male-pattern baldness.

INTERACTIONS
None known.

EFFECTS ON LAB TEST RESULTS
• May decrease glucose levels.
• May alter liver function test values.

CAUTIONS
Those with cancers that are stimulated by estrogen or testosterone (such as breast or prostate cancer) and those at risk for heart disease should avoid taking DHEA. Pregnant women also should avoid use because DHEA may have androgenic effects on female fetuses, may induce spontaneous abortion, or may inhibit fetal development. Use cautiously in patients with hepatic dysfunction.

NURSING CONSIDERATIONS
• Find out why patient is using DHEA.

• DHEA isn't a natural supplement. It's a hormone, synthetically manufactured from soybeans or wild yams. Contrary to advertising claims, wild yams don't contain DHEA. They contain diosgenin, a precursor of DHEA, which may not be converted to DHEA in the body.
• DHEA isn't intended for patients younger than age 40 unless circulating levels of DHEA are less than 130 mg/dl if patient is a woman, or less than 180 mg/dl if patient is a man.
• DHEA has orphan drug status for the treatment of corticosteroid-dependent SLE and for the treatment of severe burns in those who require skin grafting.
• The typical dosage range is 50 to 200 ml daily, depending on the intended use and the person's response.
• DHEA may increase levels of insulin-like growth factor, which may represent a risk for those with prostate cancer.
• Monitor patient for adverse hormonal effects.
• Long-term safety of DHEA supplementation is unknown.

PATIENT TEACHING
• Advise patient to consult a health care provider before using this product because a standard treatment that has been proven effective may be available.
• Tell patient that when filling a new prescription he should remind pharmacist of any herbal or dietary supplement he's taking
• Advise women to inform their health care provider if they be-

---

Bold italic type indicates that reaction may be life-threatening.

come pregnant or plan to do so in the near future.
• Instruct women to report to their health care provider any weight gain, hair loss, growth of facial hair, or other masculinizing effects.
• Instruct men to report signs of breast growth and development.

glucosamine sulfate

chitosamine

Common trade names
Glucosamine, Once-a-Day Joint Health, Osteojoint Triple Formula for Healthy Joints

AVAILABLE FORMS
Available as tablets. Often combined with chondroitin.
Tablets: 500 mg

ACTIONS & COMPONENTS
Glucosamine, an endogenous aminomonosaccharide, is a simple molecule found in mucopolysaccharides, mucoproteins, and chitin.
  Stimulates the synthesis of glycosaminoglycans and proteoglycans, both of which are considered building blocks of the cartilage. Has weak anti-inflammatory effects. May inhibit degenerative enzymes responsible for destruction of the cartilage. Appears to be effective in reducing pain and improving range of motion in patients with osteoarthritis. May also slow the process of joint damage.

USES
Used to treat osteoarthritis.

DOSAGE & ADMINISTRATION
Tablets: 500 mg P.O. t.i.d.; duration of therapy ranges from 2 weeks to 3 months. For obese patients, 20 mg/kg body weight P.O. daily.

ADVERSE REACTIONS
CNS: drowsiness, headache, insomnia.
CV: peripheral edema, tachycardia.
GI: nausea, vomiting, abdominal pain, diarrhea.
Respiratory: bronchopulmonary complications.
Skin: skin rash.

INTERACTIONS
Herb-drug. *Antidiabetics, insulin:* Increases resistance to these drugs. Adjust dosage of these drugs, as needed.
Diuretics: Decreases effectiveness of glucosamine. Dosage may need to be increased for full effect.

EFFECTS ON LAB TEST RESULTS
• May increase glucose level.

CAUTIONS
Patients with a history of an allergic reaction to glucosamine or its components should avoid use.
  Patients with diabetes mellitus should use cautiously.

NURSING CONSIDERATIONS
• Find out why patient is using glucosamine.
• Glucosamine may increase the adverse effects of diabetes mellitus.
• Monitor patient for possible adverse effects, such as peripheral edema, tachycardia, drowsiness,

---

*Liquid contains alcohol.

headache, insomnia, nausea, vomiting, abdominal pain, diarrhea, and skin rash.

PATIENT TEACHING
• Advise patient to consult a health care provider before using this product because a standard treatment that has been proven effective may be available.
• Tell patient that when filling a new prescription he should remind pharmacist of any herbal or dietary supplement he's taking.
• Advise patient to obtain glucosamine from a reliable source because its therapeutic and toxic components can vary significantly from product to product.
• Advise patient that, although limited drug interactions have been reported with use of this product, more potential interactions may exist.
• Inform patient that it may take 4 to 6 weeks before maximum benefits are achieved.
• Warn patient to keep all herbal products and nutraceuticals away from children and pets.

glycine

pangamic acid

Common trade names
None known

AVAILABLE FORMS
Available as powder and capsules.

ACTIONS & COMPONENTS
Glycine is a simple amino acid. There is no standard chemical identity for glycine and formulations can include one or more of the following: sodium gluconate, calcium gluconate, diisopropylamine dichloroacetate, dimethylglycine, calcium chloride, dicalcium phosphate, stearic acid, cellulose, or other constituents.

Diisopropylamine acts on the smooth muscle to reduce blood pressure. The high phosphate content of dicalcium phosphate has been suspected to cause upper GI lesions and death in experimental animals. Dimethylglycine can react with nitrates and form potent carcinogens called dimethylnitrosamines.

USES
Glycine is used as a nutrient and dietary supplement to detoxify the body; to treat conditions of the skin such as eczema, respiratory tract conditions such as asthma, and painful nerve and joint afflictions such as arthritis or neuritis; and to improve oxygenation of the heart, brain, and other vital organs. It's also used for alcoholism, hangovers, fatigue, protecting against urban air pollution, stimulating the immune system response, lowering blood cholesterol levels, and assisting in hormone regulation.

DOSAGE & ADMINISTRATION
No consensus exists.

ADVERSE REACTIONS
GU: kidney stones.
Other: *cancer.*

INTERACTIONS
Herb-drug. *Digoxin:* Large amounts of calcium salts (calcium chloride and dicalcium phosphate) can potentiate the effects of digox-

---

Bold italic type indicates that reaction may be life-threatening.

in and increase the risk of arrhythmia. Discourage use together.
Thiazide diuretics: May increase calcium levels, resulting in hypercalcemia. Advise patient to use cautiously.
Verapamil: May decrease effects of verapamil. Monitor effects of therapy before and after use together.
Herb-herb. *Cardiac glycoside-containing herbs (black hellebore, Canadian hemp roots, digitalis leaf, figwort, lily of the valley roots, motherwort, oleander leaf, pheasant's eye plant, pleurisy root, squill bulb leaf scales, and strophanthus seeds):* Use together of cardiac glycosides and large amounts of calcium salts (calcium chloride and dicalcium phosphate) can potentiate the effects of cardiac glycosides and increase the risk of arrhythmia. Discourage use together.

EFFECTS ON LAB TEST RESULTS
• May increase calcium level.

CAUTIONS
Glycine use may cause oxalate stones and other kidney problems. Patients with renal problems should avoid this product.

NURSING CONSIDERATIONS
• Because there is no standard chemical identity for glycine, this product may be unsafe when taken orally.
• Some formulations of glycine containing dimethylglycine and dichloroacetate may be mutagenic.
• Regularly monitor vital signs and ECG, as needed.
• Monitor electrolyte levels, especially calcium.

PATIENT TEACHING
☑**ALERT:** Tell patient that claims of effectiveness are controversial.
• Advise patient to consult a health care provider before using this product because a standard treatment that has been proven effective may be available.
• Tell patient that when filling a new prescription he should remind pharmacist of any herbal or dietary supplement he's taking.
• Inform patients taking digoxin or cardiac glycosides that there may be an increased potential for abnormal heart rhythm if administered at the same time as glycine.
• There is no standard chemical identity for glycine. Some formulations of glycine contain significant amounts of calcium.

melatonin

MEL

Common trade names
Circadian (controlled-release, not available in U.S.), Mela-T, Melatonex

AVAILABLE FORMS
Available as synthetic or animal-derived (pineal tissue) products. Also available as lozenges.
Tablets: 300 mcg, 1.5 mg, 3 mg

ACTIONS & COMPONENTS
Melatonin is a hormone produced by the pineal gland. Secretion is stimulated by darkness and inhibited by light. Secretion peaks between 2:00 a.m. and 4:00 a.m., and the extent of excretion diminishes with advancing age. Melatonin administration may regulate circadian

rhythms and may also help regulate body temperature, CV function, and reproduction. It may also protect cells against oxidation caused by free-radical formation.

USES

Used for treating insomnia, jet lag, shift-work disorder, blind entrainment, immune system enhancement, tinnitus, depression, and benzodiazepine withdrawal in geriatric patients with insomnia. Also used as a cancer adjuvant therapy, anti-aging product, contraceptive, and as prophylactic therapy for cluster headaches. Topically, it's used for skin protection against ultraviolet light.

DOSAGE & ADMINISTRATION

Adjunctive therapy for metastatic lung cancer: 10 mg P.O. h.s.
Benzodiazepine withdrawal in geriatric patients with insomnia: 2 mg (controlled-release) P.O. h.s. for 6 weeks while benzodiazepine dosage is reduced by 50% during week 2, 75% during weeks 3 and 4, and discontinued during weeks 5 and 6; may continue for up to 6 months for insomnia.
Jet lag: 5 mg P.O. h.s. for 1 week, beginning 3 days before the flight.
Sleep disturbance: 0.3 to 5 mg P.O. h.s.
Topical use: Dosage not well documented.

ADVERSE REACTIONS

CNS: headache, depression, daytime fatigue and drowsiness, dizziness, irritability, reduced alertness.
GI: abdominal cramps.

INTERACTIONS

Herb-drug. *Atenolol:* May reverse negative sleep effects caused by atenolol. Monitor patient.
CNS depressants: May cause additive sedation. Warn patient of potential hazards.
Fluoxetine: May reduce sleep disturbance in patients with major depressive disorder who take fluoxetine. Monitor patient for effect.
Immunosuppressants: May interfere with immunosuppressive therapy by improving immune function. Advise patient to avoid using together.
Nifedipine: May interfere with antihypertensive effect. Monitor patient for lack of drug effect.
Verapamil: May increase melatonin secretion. Monitor patient for increased adverse melatonin effects.
Herb-herb. *Sedating herbs or supplements, such as 5-HTP, kava, valerian:* May contribute to additive sedation. Advise patient to avoid using together.
Herb-lifestyle. *Alcohol use:* May cause additive sedation. Advise patient to avoid using together.

EFFECTS ON LAB TEST RESULTS

• May increase hormone levels.

CAUTIONS

Because melatonin may worsen depression, depressed patients taking CNS depressants shouldn't used melatonin. Patients using immunosuppressants or women who are pregnant or breast-feeding shouldn't use this product. Children shouldn't use melatonin because it may inhibit gonadal development.

Bold italic type indicates that reaction may be life-threatening.

NURSING CONSIDERATIONS
- Find out why patient is using melatonin.
- Monitor patient for excessive daytime drowsiness.
- Melatonin may increase human growth hormone levels.

PATIENT TEACHING
- Advise patient to consult a health care provider before using this product or dietary supplement because a standard treatment that has been proven effective may be available.
- Tell patient that when filling a new prescription he should remind pharmacist of any herbal and dietary supplements he's taking.
- Warn patient to avoid hazardous activities until he knows the full extent of CNS depressant effects.
- Tell patient that melatonin may have a contraceptive effect, but the product shouldn't be used as a form of birth control.
- Although no chemical interactions have been reported, tell patient that melatonin may interfere with therapeutic effects of conventional drugs.
- Warn patient about possible additive effects if melatonin is taken with alcohol.
- Advise patient to use only the synthetic form (not the animal-derived product) because of concerns about contamination and viral transmission.
- Advise patient not to use melatonin for prolonged periods because safety data aren't available.

methylsulfonylmethane

MSM, dimethyl sulfone, crystalline DMSO, $DMSO_2$, methyl sulfonyl methane, sulfonyl sulfur

Common trade names
None known

AVAILABLE FORMS
Available as capsules, tablets, powder, and liquid. Also available as cream, lotion, nasal spray, EENT drops, shampoo, and conditioner formulations.
Capsules: 500 mg, 750 mg, 1,000 mg
Liquid: 390 mg/5 ml
Powder: 2,600 mg/half teaspoon
Tablets: 500 mg, 750 mg, 1,000 mg

ACTIONS & COMPONENTS
Methylsulfonylmethane is found naturally in foods, but heat or dehydration destroys it. It's found in green plants such as field horsetail *(Equisetum arvense),* some algae species, fruits, vegetables, grains, and some animal products, such as adrenal cortex of cattle, milk, and urine. It's a possible source of sulfur for formation of the amino acids cysteine and methionine.

USES
Used to treat GI upset, inflammatory disorders, musculoskeletal pain, arthritis, allergies, autoimmune diseases, cancer, and interstitial cystitis. Also used as an antimicrobial and an immune system stimulant.

*Liquid contains alcohol.

DOSAGE & ADMINISTRATION
Dosages vary from 250 to 3,000 mg P.O. daily with meals. Dosages for topical use aren't well documented.

ADVERSE REACTIONS
CNS: headache, fatigue.
GI: nausea, diarrhea.

INTERACTIONS
None reported.

EFFECTS ON LAB TEST RESULTS
None reported.

CAUTIONS
Women who are pregnant or breast-feeding should avoid this supplement, as should patients sensitive to it.

NURSING CONSIDERATIONS
• No important toxicities or contraindications have been reported.

PATIENT TEACHING
• Advise patient to consult a health care provider before using this product or dietary supplement because a standard treatment that has been proven effective may be available.
• Tell patient that when filling a new prescription he should remind pharmacist of any herbal and dietary supplements he's taking
• Tell patient to avoid use during pregnancy and breast-feeding.
• Urge patient to report adverse effects to a health care provider.
• Because heat destroys methylsulfonylmethane, advise patient to store it in a cool, dry place.

octacosanol

1-octacosanol,
14c-octacosanol,
n-octacosanol, octacosyl
alcohol, policosanol

Common trade names
*Enduraplex, Less tanol,
Octacosanol Capsules,
Octacosanol Concentrate, Octa
Power, Super Octacosanol*
**Combination products (with
other dietary supplements):**
Boost, Prometol, Stamiplex

AVAILABLE FORMS
Available as capsules, soft gels, and tablets.
Capsules: 60 mcg, 2,000 mcg, 3,000 mcg, 5,000 mcg, 8,000 mcg
Softgel capsules: 3,000 mcg
Tablets: 1,000 mcg, 6,000 mcg

ACTIONS & COMPONENTS
Octacosanol is a type of long-chain alcohol that can be extracted from wheat germ oil, sugar cane wax, and other vegetable oils. Octacosanol may have ergogenic effects and is thought to increase oxygen use by tissues during workouts; it also may improve glycogen storage in muscles.

USES
Used by athletes to improve cardiac function, stamina, strength, and reaction time. Also used to treat Parkinson's disease and amyotrophic lateral sclerosis (Lou Gehrig's disease), although little evidence exists to support its use for these disorders. Octacosanol is also being studied as an antiviral for herpes and as a treatment for

---

Bold italic type indicates that reaction may be life-threatening.

inflammatory skin disorders and hyperlipidemia.

DOSAGE & ADMINISTRATION
For Parkinson's disease: 5 mg P.O. t.i.d. with meals.
To enhance athletic performance: 40 to 80 mg P.O. daily.

ADVERSE REACTIONS
CNS: dizziness; jerky, involuntary movements; nervousness.
CV: orthostasis.

INTERACTIONS
Herb-drug. *Levodopa-carbidopa:* May have additive effects; may worsen dyskinesias. Advise patient to avoid use together.

EFFECTS ON LAB TEST RESULTS
• May alter cholesterol and lipid levels.

CAUTIONS
Patients allergic to wheat germ oil or sugar cane shouldn't take octacosanol.

NURSING CONSIDERATIONS
• Find out why patient is using the supplement.
• Patients with Parkinson's disease should use octacosanol cautiously.
✍ **ALERT:** The combination of octacosanol and levodopa-carbidopa may worsen dyskinesias.
• Patients allergic to wheat germ oil or sugar cane shouldn't take octacosanol.
• No chemical interactions have been reported, but consideration must be given to the pharmacologic properties of the supplement and their potential to interfere with the intended effect of conventional drugs.

PATIENT TEACHING
• Advise patient to consult a health care provider before using this product because a standard treatment that has been proven effective may be available.
• Tell patient that when filling a new prescription he should remind pharmacist of any herbal and dietary supplements he's taking.
• Recommend that patient consult a health care provider before taking octacosanol as part of a new exercise routine.
• Advise patient with Parkinson's disease or any undiagnosed tremor to consult a health care provider before taking octacosanol.

s-adenosylmethionine

s-adenosyl-L-methionine, SAMe, Sammy

Common trade names
SAM-e

AVAILABLE FORMS
Available as tablets.
Tablets (enteric-coated): 200 mg

ACTIONS & COMPONENTS
A naturally occurring amino acid found in all living cells that plays an integral role in methylation processes, including DNA methylation, protein methylation (critical for cell growth and repair), and phospholipid methylation, which maintains flexibility of cell membranes. Also helps produce cysteine, an amino acid needed for glutathione, the main antioxidant

in the liver, and helps limit homocysteine levels. Increased homocysteine levels may increase the risk of CV disease.

USES
Used to treat postpartum, menopausal and clinical depression, as well as osteoarthritis, fibromyalgia, fatigue, and liver disorders. Also used to prevent heart disease.

DOSAGE & ADMINISTRATION
For arthritis: 200 to 1,600 mg P.O. daily in divided doses.
For depression: 400 mg daily or 200 mg b.i.d. P.O. before breakfast and lunch. Patients sensitive to drugs or supplements may start with 200 mg daily. Increased to 800 mg daily or 400 mg b.i.d. if no improvement occurs after 2 weeks. Doses up to 800 mg b.i.d. may be required.
For fibromyalgia: 800 mg P.O. daily or 200 mg I.M. daily.
For liver disease: 1,200 mg P.O. daily.

ADVERSE REACTIONS
CNS: headache, agitation, mania.
GI: diarrhea, nausea, GI disturbances.

INTERACTIONS
Herb-drug. *Antidepressants, especially MAO inhibitors:* May cause serotonin syndrome (tremor, agitation, diarrhea, diaphoresis, hemodynamic instability). Advise patient of this potential effect.

EFFECTS ON LAB TEST RESULTS
None reported.

CAUTIONS
Patients with bipolar depression should avoid this product because of the risk of inducing mania.

NURSING CONSIDERATIONS
• Find out why patient is using the product.
• Some patients try to diagnose or treat severe or life-threatening depression on their own. Determine the extent of the patient's depression and make appropriate referrals for psychiatric help, as needed.
• Product can be stopped without adverse effects, although depression may recur.
• Product shouldn't be used within 2 weeks of discontinuing an MAO inhibitor.
• Doses up to 3,600 mg have caused no adverse effects. No deaths have been reported from overdose.

PATIENT TEACHING
• Advise patient to consult a health care provider before using this product because a standard treatment that has been proven effective may be available.
• Tell patient that when filling a new prescription he should remind pharmacist of any herbal and dietary supplements he's taking.
• Advise patient not to combine herb with other antidepressants unless approved by health care provider.
• Warn patient about the danger of treating depression on his own.
• Instruct patient to have a medical evaluation before taking this product for depression or other symptoms.

Bold italic type indicates that reaction may be life-threatening.

• Tell patient that the effects of the product may not be noticeable for 2 weeks when taken for depression or 30 days when taken for osteoarthritis.

• Recommend that patient promptly notify health care provider about new symptoms or adverse effects.

• Warn patient to keep all herbal products and nutraceuticals away from children and pets.

shark cartilage

Sphyrna lewini, Squalus acanthias and other shark species, squalamine

Common trade names
BeneFin, Cartilade

AVAILABLE FORMS
Available as powder and capsules.
Capsules: 200 g, 500 g

ACTIONS & COMPONENTS
Obtained from shredded and dried cartilage of the hammerhead shark *(S. lewini)* and the spiny dogfish shark *(S. acanthias)*. Shark cartilage is purported to have anticancer properties by inhibiting angiogenesis (new blood vessel formation) in tumors. Another hypothesis for the anticancer effect involves a class of proteins normally present in cartilage and bone called tissue inhibitors of metalloproteinases (TIMPs). TIMPs block enzymes that tumors use to invade surrounding tissue. An inhibitor, or series of inhibitors, of neovascularization present in shark cartilage has been identified as guanidine extractable protein. A family of complex carbohydrates and mucopolysaccharides may be the primary anti-inflammatory components.

USES
Used to treat or prevent cancer and to treat osteoarthritis, rheumatoid arthritis, psoriasis, lupus, eczema, and enteritis. Also used to assist in bone and wound healing and to maintain proper bone and joint function. Powder is also used as a retention enema. Data from ongoing studies may help define the role of shark cartilage in the treatment of lung cancer, AIDS-associated Kaposi's sarcoma, and prostate cancer.

DOSAGE & ADMINISTRATION
No consensus exists on the dosage for anticancer effects or other uses.
For benefit of additional cartilage protein and calcium: 6 g powder in 1 glass of water or juice P.O.
To maintain proper bone and joint function: 4 g powder in 1 glass of water or juice P.O.

ADVERSE REACTIONS
GI: nausea.

INTERACTIONS
None reported.

EFFECTS ON LAB TEST RESULTS
None reported.

CAUTIONS
Shark cartilage shouldn't be used by children or by pregnant or breast-feeding women. Patients recovering from MI or CVA shouldn't use this product because inhibition of angiogenesis may in-

*Liquid contains alcohol.

terfere with revascularization of an infarcted area.

NURSING CONSIDERATIONS
• Find out why patient is using shark cartilage.
• No data exist regarding toxicity of shark cartilage.

PATIENT TEACHING
• Advise patient to consult a health care provider before using this product because a standard treatment that has been proven effective may be available.
• Tell patient that when filling a new prescription he should remind pharmacist of any herbal and dietary supplements he's taking.
• Warn patient not to take shark cartilage before seeking medical attention because doing so may delay diagnosis of a potentially serious medical condition.
• Tell women not to use shark cartilage if pregnant or breast-feeding unless advised by a knowledgeable health care provider because effects of shark cartilage on pregnant or breast-feeding women are unknown.
• Warn patient not to take shark cartilage after a recent heart attack or stroke. Explain that shark cartilage may interfere with the body's ability to form new blood vessels, which may obstruct healing in the injured heart or brain area.

Supplemental vitamins and minerals

Name and recommended daily allowances	Actions	Special considerations
vitamin A (retinol) *Women:* 800 mcg retinol equivalents (RE), or 4,000 IU *Pregnant women:* Supplement with beta-carotene to form necessary retinol. *Men:* 1,000 mcg RE, or 5,000 IU	• Promotes growth, differentiates and maintains epithelial tissue. • Fights infection. • Aids in bone and teeth formation. • Promotes wound healing. • Maintains good vision (rod and cone function; adaptation to light changes). • Improves body's ability to utilize insulin and normalize glucose levels with higher doses.	• Best food sources include liver, fish liver oil, tuna, mackerel, eggs, egg yolks, butter, cheese, fortified milk, and fruits and vegetables containing beta-carotene that can be converted to retinol in the body. • Best if taken with B complex; vitamins C, D, and E; and calcium, phosphorus, and zinc. • Mineral oil may decrease GI absorption of vitamin A. • Supplementation of over 6,000 IU daily of retinol without beta-carotene is associated with birth defects. • Should be taken during or shortly after a meal. • Vitamin A and accutane enhance the toxicity of each. • Patients taking colestipol may need more vitamin A. • Overdose can cause serious liver toxicity and damage.
beta-carotene Forms vitamin A when retinol isn't in the diet. The amount of beta-carotene needed to meet the vitamin A requirement is roughly double that of retinol: 6 mcg beta-carotene = 1 mcg RE = 3.33 IU. Safe supplementation range is 5-25,000 IU.	• Same as retinol. • Taken with other antioxidants, may help prevent cancer. • Enhances immune system. • Useful in the treatment of cataracts and muscular degeneration.	• Best food sources include dark green and yellow fruits and vegetables, such as carrots, cantaloupe, sweet potato, papaya, apricots, red grapefruit, watermelon, peaches, and squash. • Best if taken with a meal, because fat facilitates absorption. • Should be taken with a network of other antioxidants: vitamins E and C, selenium, zinc. • Hypercarotenemia causes yellowing of the palms, nasolabial folds, and soles of the feet, but not of the sclerae, which distinguishes it from jaundice.

(continued)

Name and recommended daily allowances	Actions	Special considerations
beta-carotene *(continued)*		• For overall support of the immune system, look for supplements that contain at least six leading carotenoids.
vitamin B₁ (thiamine) *Women:* 1-1.1 mg *Pregnant women:* 1.5 mg *Men:* 1-1.5 mg	• Aids digestion, especially carbohydrates. • Improves mental attitude and maintains a healthy nervous system. • Stimulates good muscle tone and appetite.	• Best food sources include lean pork, brewer's yeast, whole brown rice, soybeans, tofu, whole wheat, oatmeal, wheat germ, milk, and most vegetables. • Best if taken with B complex, vitamin C, and manganese. • Increased physical activity combined with carbohydrate loading may promote depletion. • Allicin, a factor in onions and garlic, promotes the absorption of vitamin B_1. • No known toxic ranges with oral supplementation because B vitamins are water soluble. • Chronic alcoholism inhibits absorption of vitamin B_1 from the intestinal lumen. • Long-term use of loop diuretics depletes vitamin B_1. • Coffee and tea (both caffeinated and decaffeinated) reduce thiamine absorption.
vitamin B₂ (riboflavin) *Women:* 1.2-1.3 mg *Pregnant women:* 1.6 mg *Men:* 1.2-1.5 mg	• Needed for carbohydrate, protein, and fat metabolism. • Aids in RBC formation. • Promotes healthy vision, nails, skin. • Stimulates immune system and nerve function. • Necessary for body to use niacin and thiamine, all instrumental in energy metabolism.	• Best food sources include milk, brewer's yeast, liver, dark meat of poultry, cheese, fish, eggs, leafy green vegetables, enriched cereals and grains, broccoli, beef, and pork. • Riboflavin needs gastric acids to be released from foods. • Best if taken with B complex, folic acid, and vitamin C. • Urine will become discolored with high doses of riboflavin, which can affect urinalysis results.

Name and recommended daily allowances	Actions	Special considerations
vitamin B₂ (riboflavin) *(continued)*		• Hormonal contraceptives interfere with the metabolism of riboflavin; a woman using this method of birth control should ask her health care provider about supplementation.
vitamin B₃ (niacin, nicotinic acid) *Women:* 15 mg *Pregnant women:* 17 mg *Men:* 19-20 mg Requirements vary according to amount of protein in the diet.	• Improves circulation and reduces cholesterol level. • Needed for carbohydrate, fat, and protein metabolism. • Needed for healthy skin, nervous system, and digestive tract. • Functions as a coenzyme with B_1 and B_2 to produce energy within the cells.	• Best food sources include eggs, organ meats, fortified grains, peanuts, peanut butter, brewer's yeast, cottage cheese, broccoli, peas, lean meat, poultry, fish, whole grains, milk, nuts, seeds, and mushrooms. • Best if taken with B complex, vitamin C, magnesium, and potassium. • Hepatotoxicity is more likely with high-dose, sustained-release niacin therapy. Such therapy shouldn't be used without medical supervision and liver enzyme tests every 3 months.
vitamin B₅ (pantothenic acid) *Women, pregnant women, men:* 4-7 mg	• Aids in stress resistance. • Assists in release of energy from carbohydrates, fat, and protein metabolism. • Needed for healthy skin, nervous system, and digestive tract. • Needed to form porphyrin, a precursor of heme, to form hemoglobin. • Plays a role in glucose metabolism and immune function.	• Best food sources include meats, whole grain cereals, chicken, milk, corn, mushrooms, avocado, nuts, and eggs. • Best if taken with B complex and vitamin C.
vitamin B₆ (pyridoxamine) *Women:* 1.4-1.5 mg	• Needed for carbohydrate, fat, and protein metabolism.	• Best food sources include brewer's yeast, liver, beef, pork, *(continued)*

Name and recommended daily allowances	Actions	Special considerations
vitamin B$_6$ (pyridoxamine) *(continued)* *Pregnant women:* 1.2 mg *Men:* 1.7-2 mg	• Aids in antibody and RBC formation. • Helps maintain balance of sodium and phosphorus. • Acts as a natural diuretic. • Essential for neurotransmitter synthesis. • Maintains immune function. • Helps control homocysteine and prevent atherosclerosis.	lamb, fish, seafood, whole grains, eggs, milk, yogurt, cheese, bananas, soybeans, cabbage, brown rice, avocado, peanuts, and walnuts. • Best if taken with B complex, vitamin C, magnesium, and potassium. • Oral contraceptives, theophylline, isoniazid, cycloserine, penicillamine, and hydralazine interfere with vitamin B$_6$ metabolism or action. • High doses of vitamin B$_6$ interfere with levodopa metabolism. • Caution must be used when prescribing large daily doses for premenstrual syndrome, and nausea and vomiting of pregnancy because of potential risk of neurotoxicity.
vitamin B$_9$ (folic acid) *Women, men:* 400 mcg *Pregnant women:* 600 mcg *Breast-feeding women:* 500 mcg	• Helps prevent birth defects and improve lactation. • Important in RBC formation. • Needed for growth and division of body cells. • May relieve depression and certain headaches. • Protects against osteoporosis. • Indicated with vitamin B$_{12}$ for macrocytic anemia. • Works closely with B$_{12}$ in the metabolism of amino acids, the synthesis of proteins, and the production of	• Best food sources include green leafy vegetables, beans, liver, egg yolk, brewer's yeast, whole wheat, peanuts, beef liver, and soybean flour. • Best if taken with B complex, vitamin B$_{12}$, vitamin C, and biotin. • Vitamin C helps reduce the amount of folic acid lost to excretion. • Prolonged use of high folic acid supplementation may lead to lower plasma zinc levels. • Estrogens, alcohol, some chemotherapy drugs, sulfasalazine, aspirin, barbiturates, and anticonvulsants interfere with folate absorption. • High-dose folic acid supplementation should be used with

Name and recommended daily allowances	Actions	Special considerations
vitamin B$_9$ (folic acid) *(continued)*	genetic material (RNA and DNA). • Functions as coenzyme for neurotransmitters.	extreme caution in those with epilepsy. It may increase seizure activity. • Because folic acid supplementation can mask vitamin B$_{12}$ deficiency, which can lead to irreversible neurologic damage, folic acid supplementation should always include vitamin B$_{12}$.
vitamin B$_{12}$ (cyanocobalamin) *Women, men:* 2 mcg *Pregnant women:* 2.2 mcg	• Needed for all blood cell formation and a healthy nervous system. • Needed for maturation of RBCs. • Helps to improve the appetite and increase energy. • Needed for carbohydrate, fat, and protein metabolism. • Together with folic acid and vitamin B$_6$, vitamin B$_{12}$ has been shown to reduce high plasma levels of homocysteine, which is an independent risk factor for CV disease.	• Best food sources include liver, kidney, milk, eggs, fish, cheese, and yogurt. • Best if taken with B complex, folic acid, vitamin C, potassium, and calcium. • Vegetarians are at a higher risk for low B$_{12}$ levels than nonvegetarians. • People need adequate gastric intrinsic factor to convert oral vitamin B$_{12}$ to its active form. • Parenteral cyanocobalamin given for B$_{12}$ deficiency caused by malabsorption should be given I.M. or by deep S.C. route but never I.V.
B complex *Women, men:* 100-200 mg	• Helps nervous system function and maintains a healthy digestive tract. • Supports the immune system. • Needed for carbohydrate, fat, and protein metabolism. • Maintains the health of eyes, skin, hair, and liver.	• Best food sources include brewer's yeast, liver, wheat germ, whole grains, rice, oats, rye, poultry, fish, green leafy vegetables, nuts, and beans. • Best if taken with vitamin C, vitamin E, calcium, and phosphorus. • A balanced B complex helps to ensure proper absorption of all the B vitamins.

(continued)

Name and recommended daily allowances	Actions	Special considerations
vitamin C *Women:* 75 mg *Pregnant women:* 85 mg *Breast-feeding women:* 120 mg *Men:* 90 mg	• Helps heal wounds and burns and helps prevent hemorrhaging. • Reduces serum cholesterol level. • Aids in preventing many bacterial and viral infections. • Fights toxins caused by smoke pollution. • Useful in treating allergies. • Aids in iron absorption. • Protects against cancer and boosts immune system. • Works with other antioxidants and neutralizes free radicals. • Plays key role in the metabolism of fats, cholesterol, and certain proteins. • Needed for folic acid metabolism. • Essential for the formation of collagen; necessary to build and maintain vessels, skin, muscles, joints, bones, and teeth.	• The daily requirement for vitamin C in persons who smoke is increased by 35 mg daily. • Best food sources include citrus fruits, berries, tomatoes, broccoli, green and red pepper, dark leafy greens, kiwi, papaya, strawberries, brussels sprouts, and potatoes. • More effective with all other vitamins, minerals, calcium, and magnesium. • Interferes with blood tests for vitamin B_{12}. • High doses of more than 2,000 mg daily can cause diarrhea, gas, or stomach upset. • Persons with a history of kidney stones should use extra caution when taking high doses of vitamin C. • Buffered vitamin C is available if regular vitamin C upsets the stomach. • Cooking vegetables decreases their vitamin C content.
vitamin D *Women:* 200 IU *Pregnant women, adults ages 51-70:* 400 IU *Men:* 200 IU	• Needed for absorption and utilization of calcium and phosphorus, to form strong bones and teeth. • Helps maintain normal heart action and stable nervous system. • Helps to control blood glucose level. • Reduces cartilage damage in people with	• Best food sources include fortified milk, egg yolks, fish liver oil, sardines, halibut, tuna, salmon, and mackerel. • Sunlight is the most common natural source: a fair-skinned person needs 20 to 30 minutes daily; a dark-skinned person needs about 3 hours daily. • More than 1,000 IU of vitamin D daily can cause illness. Symptoms include excessive

Name and recommended daily allowances	Actions	Special considerations
vitamin D *(continued)*	osteoarthritis and may decrease the severity of rheumatoid arthritis. • Plays a role in fostering immunity and provides protection against some cancers.	thirst, fatigue, irregular pulse, vomiting, diarrhea, muscle problems, and itching skin. • Drug interactions that may cause mineral imbalances include: digoxin, verapamil, and thiazide diuretics.
vitamin E *Women:* 8-12 IU *Pregnant women:* 15 IU *Men:* 10-15 IU The recommended dose for disease prevention and treatment for adults is 400-800 IU/day.	• Potent antioxidant that, along with vitamin A and C, helps prevent the breakdown of cells by free radicals. • Protects lungs against air pollution. • Alleviates fatigue and protects RBCs. • Prevents blood clots. • Helps wounds heal faster and promotes circulation. • High intake of vitamin E correlates with a reduced risk of heart attacks and cataracts.	• Best food sources include salmon, tuna, shrimp, lobster, egg yolks, avocados, wheat germ, soybeans, nuts, leafy greens, sunflower, walnut, and safflower oils, sweet potato, whole wheat, and liver. • Best if taken with B complex, vitamin C, magnesium, and selenium. • Natural vitamin E (d-alpha-tocopherol) is the preferred form because it's absorbed best and most actively. • Chronic alcoholism depletes vitamin E stores in the liver. • May prolong bleeding time and enhance antiplatelet drugs. Stop vitamin E intake before surgery to reduce the risk of bleeding. • High doses may interfere with vitamin K activity. • Cholestyramine and colestipol may decrease absorption of vitamin E. • Selenium enhances antioxidant activity of vitamin E. • Improves vitamin A effectiveness. • Considered generally nontoxic. In doses of more than 1,200 IU daily, it can cause nausea, gas, diarrhea, and heart palpitations.

(continued)

Name and recommended daily allowances	Actions	Special considerations
vitamin H (biotin) *Women, pregnant women, men:* 30-100 mcg Because biotin is synthesized in the intestinal microflora, deficiency is rare.	• Needed for carbohydrate, fat, and protein metabolism • Helps fatty acid and amino acid synthesis • Improves blood glucose control in diabetic patients by enhancing insulin sensitivity • Needed for healthy hair, skin, and nails	• Best food sources include kidney, liver, almonds, peanuts, pecans, walnuts, cooked eggs, mushrooms, salmon, sardines, cauliflower, brewer's yeast, oat bran, and unpolished rice. • Works best when taken with B complex and vitamin C. • Isn't absorbed if taken with raw egg whites. • Requirements may rise if a person takes sulfa drugs or estrogen, or drinks alcohol. • Deficiency may result from prolonged use of anticonvulsant drugs or antibiotics. • Biotin is nontoxic; no adverse effects have been noted, even at high doses. • Food processing can destroy biotin.
vitamin K (phytomenadione) *Women:* 55-65 mcg *Pregnant women:* 65 mcg *Men:* 65-80 mcg	• Needed for prothrombin formation and blood coagulation; for normal liver functioning; and for the bones to use calcium • May prevent kidney stones	• Best food sources include dark green leafy vegetables, especially kale, spinach, turnip greens, broccoli, and cabbage; beef liver; egg yolk; green tea; cheese; butter; and safflower oil. • Natural vitamin K taken orally is generally nontoxic. • Large doses of the synthetic form of vitamin K, which are usually given to prevent bleeding in certain conditions, may cause anemia and liver damage. • Vitamin K can interfere with the action of anticoagulants such as warfarin. • High doses of vitamin E can interfere with vitamin K metabolism and increase the risk of bleeding. • X-rays and radiation can raise vitamin K requirements.

Name and recommended daily allowances	Actions	Special considerations
vitamin K (phytomenadione) *(continued)*		• Extended use of antibiotics may result in vitamin K deficiency. • Aspirin, cholestyramine, and mineral oil laxatives may decrease vitamin K levels. • Freezing foods may destroy vitamin K, but heating doesn't affect it.
calcium *Women:* 1,000-1,300 mg *Pregnant women:* 1,200 mg *Men:* 1,000-1,200 mg	• Needed for developing and maintaining bones and teeth, maintaining heartbeat and proper blood pressure, and transmitting nerve impulses. • Reduces pregnancy risks, such as high blood pressure and preeclampsia. • Helps maintain proper cholesterol levels. • Directly involved in the formation of blood clotting and the start of wound healiilng.	• Best food sources include milk, yogurt, cottage cheese, cheese, broccoli, dark leafy greens, canned salmon, mackerel, sardines, fortified orange juice, soymilk, dates, canteloupe, tofu, soybean nuts, hard or mineral water, almonds, and brazil nuts. • Supplements should be taken in small doses throughout the day. • High-protein diets cause calcium excretion. • Increased urinary calcium loss is also caused by sodium, phosphorus, sugar, saturated fats, caffeine, alcohol, and aluminum-containing antacids. • Excess calcium can interfere with the absorption of iron, zinc, magnesium, iodine, manganese, and copper. • Doses of 5,000 mg daily are toxic. • Doses above 2,000 mg daily may increase the risk of kidney stones and soft-tissue calcification. • Several types of calcium supplements exist; check dosage for the type of calcium ingested.

(continued)

Name and recommended daily allowances	Actions	Special considerations
copper Estimated safe and adequate daily dietary intake: *Adults:* 1.5-3 mg	• Needed for hemoglobin formation. • Involved in many reactions to produce and release energy. • Needed to develop and maintain skeletal structures. • Plays a role in proper functioning of the immune system. • Needed for taste sensitivity. • Needed for the maturing of collagen, a component of connective tissue, and the formation of elastin, a protein that forms tissue. • Forms copper complexes that facilitate or promote tissue repair. • Needed to build and maintain myelin, the protective sheath surrounding nerve fibers	• Best food sources include raw oysters, avocados, green olives, seafood, organ meats, nuts, legumes, chocolate, fruits and vegetables, black pepper, blackstrap molasses, and water that flows through copper piping. • Copper supplements should be kept away from children. A dose as little as 3.5 g may be lethal. • Excess copper can interfere with absorption of zinc. • Copper absorption may be affected by calcium, iron, manganese, zinc, vitamin B_6, high levels of vitamin C, and antacids in high amounts. • Copper deficiency may be aggravated by alcohol, eggs, and fructose. • Copper deficiency is rare. • Low copper levels may reduce thyroid function. • Low copper levels may cause significantly elevated low-density cholesterol levels.
iron *Women:* 10-15 mg *Pregnant women:* 30 mg *Men:* 10 mg	• Improves the symptoms of iron-deficient anemia. • Helps deliver oxygen from the lungs to all parts of the body. • Serves as a component of many enzymes involved in energy metabolism.	• Best food sources include liver, lean red meat, poultry, fish, dried beans, egg yolks, soybeans, vegetables, and dried apricots, raisins, and other dried fruits. • Iron supplements should be kept in childproof bottles and away from children. • Children between the ages of 12 and 24 months are at highest risk of iron poisoning from accidental ingestion. • Vitamin C enhances absorption of iron. • Antacids can reduce the absorption of iron.

Name and recommended daily allowances	Actions	Special considerations
iron *(continued)*		• Iron reduces absorption of the antibiotics ciprofloxacin, norfloxacin, ofloxacin, and tetracycline. • Tannins in tea, oxalic acid in spinach and other foods, and phytates from bran and other whole-grain products reduce iron absorption. • Supplemental oral iron may cause GI disturbances, such as nausea, diarrhea, constipation, heartburn, and upper gastric discomfort.
magnesium *Women:* 280-300 mg *Pregnant women:* 320 mg *Men:* 350-400 mg	• Needed in protein synthesis and amino acid activation • May correct heart arrhythmias • Needed for nerve transmission and muscle contraction and relaxation • Needed to develop teeth and bones • Needed for many metabolic reactions; acting as an enzyme cofactor, it produces energy, synthesizes lipids and proteins, regulates calcium flow, forms urea, and relaxes muscles.	• Best food sources include tofu, legumes, whole grains, green leafy vegetables, brazil nuts, almonds, cashews, pumpkin and squash seeds, pine nuts, oatmeal, bananas, and baked potatoes with skin. • Vitamin B_6 assists in the body's accumulation of magnesium and works with magnesium in many enzyme systems. • Magnesium and calcium don't inhibit each other's absorption, but increased magnesium intake may result in excess calcium excretion. • Magnesium should be taken with a full glass of water with each dose to avoid diarrhea. • Some foods, drinks, and drugs can cause magnesium loss. These include sodium, sugar, caffeine, alcohol, fiber, riboflavin in high doses, insulin, diuretics, and digoxin. • Dietary factors can reduce magnesium absorption; for example, high intake of calcium and phosphates, fats, bran, whole grains, *(continued)*

Name and recommended daily allowances	Actions	Special considerations
magnesium *(continued)*		spinach, rhubarb, and other foods high in axalic acid. ● Magnesium supplements shouldn't be taken by those with severe heart or kidney disease without talking to a health care provider.
manganese Estimated safe and adequate daily dietary intake: *Adults:* 2-5 mg	● Aids in forming connective tissue, fats, and cholesterol, bones, blood clotting factors, and proteins. ● Needed for normal brain function. ● Is a component of manganese superoxide dismutase, an antioxidant that protects the body from toxic substances. ● Promotes insulin utilization and glucose metabollism.	● Best food sources include pecans, almonds, wheat germ, whole grains, leafy vegetables, liver, kidney, legumes, peanuts, avocados, brown rice, rice bran, potatoes, pineapple, molasses, sunflower seeds, and dried fruits. ● There's no RDA for manganese. ● Manganese deficiency hasn't been documented. ● Manganese is the least toxic of the trace elements. Toxicity is more common in those exposed to manganese dust found in steel mills and mines and certain chemical industries. ● Excess manganese may produce iron-deficiency anemia and symptoms similar to those of schizophrenia, Parkinson's disease, and Wilson's disease.
potassium *Women, pregnant women, men:* 2,000 mg/day	● Treats symptoms of hypokalemia, which include weakness, lack of energy, stomach disturbances, irregular heartbeat, and abnormal ECG. ● Controls or prevents hypertension. ● Reduces the mortality associated with acute MI (used in	● Best food sources include fresh, unprocessed food, such as meats, fish, and vegetables, especially potatoes; soybeans and other legumes; black-strap molasses, tomatoes, and nuts; fruits, especially oranges and avocados; citrus juices; milk; and wheat and rice bran. ● Potassium supplements, other than those in a multivitamin, shouldn't be taken unless rec-

Name and recommended daily allowances	Uses	Special considerations
potassium *(continued)*	combination with glucose and insulin). • Essential for proper muscle function. • Protects against stroke. • Maintains the body's fluid and acid/base balances.	ommended by a health care provider. • Patients with renal insufficiency should use with caution. Those with severe renal impairment should avoid use of potassium. • Care should be taken when prescribing potassium supplements to geriatric patients because of decreased renal functions. • Potassium-depleting drugs include thiazides, furosemide, bumetanide, and ethacrynic acid. • Other drugs interacting with potassium include potassium-sparing diuretics, NSAIDs, ACE inhibitors, beta blockers, heparin, digoxin, and trimethoprim.
selenium *Women:* 50-55 mcg *Pregnant women:* 65 mcg *Men:* 50-70 mcg	• Acts as antioxidant to boost the immune system and prevent age-related diseases, such as cancer and cataracts. • Helps with reproductive health and needed for proper fetal development. • Prevents MI and stroke by lowering low-density lipoprotein cholesterol level. • Required for antioxidant protection of the eye lens; helps prevent cataract formation. • Promotes proper liver and metabolic function.	• Best food sources include brewer's yeast, wheat germ, soy flour, kidney beans, liver, butter, fish, shellfish, sunflower seeds, and brazil nuts. • The amount of selenium in foodstuffs corresponds directly to selenium levels in the soil. • Food-source selenium is destroyed during processing. • Selenium should be taken with vitamin E, because the two act synergistically. • Vitamin C may increase risk of selenium toxicity. • Although rare, extended high intake, exceeding 1,000 mcg daily, may lead to toxicity. • Chemotherapy drugs may increase selenium requirements.

(continued)

Name and recommended daily allowances	Uses	Special considerations
selenium *(continued)*	• Protects cellular DNA against free radicals. • Binds with toxic metals to reduce toxicity.	
zinc *Women:* 12 mg *Pregnant women, men:* 15 mg	• Needed for more than 200 enzymatic reactions in the body. • Needed for proper growth and development, especially in early life. • Needed to maintain proper vision, taste, and smell. • Improves wound healing. • Improves immune system function.	• Best food sources include poultry, wheat bran, wheat germ, oysters, shrimp, crab, and other shellfish; red meat; lima beans, pinto beans, soybeans; whole grains, miso, tofu, brewer's yeast, cooked greens, and pumpkin seeds. • Zinc sulfate can cause GI irritation. • Zinc toxicity is rare, usually occurring only after a dose of 2,000 mg or more has been ingested. • High doses of zinc interfere with the assimilation of other trace minerals, such as copper and iron. • Long-term high doses of zinc (100 mg/day) can actually impair rather than enhance immune function. • High doses of calcium may interfere with zinc absorption. • Because of the many interactions between zinc and other nutrients, people should take a balanced multiple vitamin with mineral, containing zinc, copper, iron, and folate to help prevent deficiencies of these nutrients.

Herb-drug interactions

Herb	Drug	Possible effects
aloe (dried juice from leaf [latex])	antiarrhythmics, cardiac glycosides	Ingestion of aloe juice may lead to hypokalemia, which may potentiate cardiac glycosides and antiarrhythmics.
	licorice, thiazide diuretics, other potassium-wasting drugs such as corticosteroids	May cause additive effect of potassium wasting with thiazide diuretics and other potassium-wasting drugs.
	orally administered drugs	May decrease absorption of drugs because of more rapid GI transit time.
	stimulant laxatives	May increase risk of potassium loss.
bilberry	anticoagulants, antiplatelets	Decreases platelet aggregation.
	hypoglycemics, insulin	May increase serum insulin levels, causing hypoglycemia; additive effect with diabetes drugs.
capsicum	ACE inhibitors	May cause cough.
	anticoagulants, antiplatelets	Decreases platelet aggregation and increases fibrinolytic activity, prolonging bleeding time.
	antihypertensives	May interfere with antihypertensives by increasing catecholamine secretion.
	aspirin NSAIDs	Stimulates GI secretions to help protect against NSAID-induced GI irritation.
	CNS depressants such as barbiturates, benzodiazepines, opioids	Increases sedative effect.
	cocaine	Concomitant use (including exposure to capsicum in pepper spray) may increase effects of cocaine and risk of adverse reactions, including death.

(continued)

Herb	Drug	Possible effects
capsicun (continued)	H$_2$ blockers, proton-pump inhibitors	Decreases effects resulting from the increased catecholamine secretion by capsicum.
	hepatically metabolized drugs	May increase hepatic metabolism of drugs by increasing G6PD and adipose lipase activity.
	MAO inhibitors	May decrease effectiveness because of increased acid secretion by capsicum.
	theophylline	Increases absorption of theophylline, possibly leading to higher serum levels or toxicity.
chamomile	anticoagulants	Warfarin constituents may enhance anticoagulant therapy and prolong bleeding time.
	drugs requiring GI absorption	May delay drug absorption.
	drugs with sedative properties, such as benzodiazepines	May cause additive effects and adverse reactions.
	iron	Tannic acid content may reduce iron absorption.
echinacea	hepatotoxics	Hepatotoxicity may increase with drugs known to elevate liver enzyme levels.
	immunosuppressants	Echinacea may counteract immunosuppressant drugs.
	warfarin	Increases bleeding time without increased INR.
evening primrose	anticonvulsants	Lowers seizure threshold.
	antiplatelets, anticoagulants	Increases risk of bleeding and bruising.
feverfew	anticoagulants, antiplatelets	May decrease platelet aggregation and increase fibrinolytic activity.
	methysergide	May potentiate methysergide.

Herb	Drug	Possible effects
garlic	anticoagulants, anti-platelets	Enhances platelet inhibition, leading to increased anticoagulation.
	antihyperlipidemics	May have additive lipid-lowering properties.
	antihypertensives	May cause additive hypotension.
	cyclosporine	May decrease effectiveness of cyclosporine. May induce metabolism and decrease CSA to subtherapeutic levels; may cause rejection.
	hormonal contraceptives	May decrease efficacy of contraceptives.
	insulin, other drugs causing hypoglycemia	May increase serum insulin levels, causing hypoglycemia, an additive effect with antidiabetics.
	nonnucleotide reverse transcriptase inhibitors	May affect metabolism of these drugs.
	saquinavir	Decreases saquinavir levels, causing therapeutic failure and increased viral resistance.
ginger	anticoagulants, anti-platelets	Inhibits platelet aggregation by antagonizing thromboxane synthetase and enhancing prostacyclin, leading to prolonged bleeding time.
	antidiabetics	May interfere with diabetes therapy because of hypoglycemic effects.
	antihypertensives	May antagonize antihypertensive effect.
	barbiturates	May enhance barbiturate effects.
	calcium channel blockers	May increase calcium uptake by myocardium, leading to altered drug effects.
	chemotherapy	May reduce nausea associated with chemotherapy.
	H_2 blockers, proton-pump inhibitors	May decrease effectiveness because of increased acid secretion by ginger.

(continued)

Herb	Drug	Possible effects
ginkgo	anticoagulants, anti-platelets	May enhance platelet inhibition, leading to increased anticoagulation.
	anticonvulsants	May decrease effectiveness of anticonvulsants.
	drugs known to lower seizure threshold	May further reduce seizure threshold.
	insulin	Ginkgo leaf extract can alter insulin secretion and metabolism, affecting blood glucose levels
	thiazide diuretics	Ginkgo leaf may increase blood pressure.
ginseng	alcohol	Increases alcohol clearance, possibly by increasing activity of alcohol dehydrogenase.
	anabolic steroids, hormones	May potentiate effects of hormone and anabolic steroid therapies. Estrogenic effects of ginseng may cause vaginal bleeding and breast nodules.
	antibiotics	Siberian ginseng may enhance effects of some antibiotics.
	anticoagulants, anti-platelets	Decreases platelet adhesiveness.
	antidiabetics	May enhance blood glucose–lowering effects.
	antipsychotics	Because of CNS stimulant activity, avoid use with antipsychotics.
	digoxin	May falsely elevate digoxin levels.
	furosemide	May decrease diuretic effect with furosemide.
	immunosuppressants	May interfere with immunosuppressive therapy.
	MAO inhibitors	Potentiates action of MAO inhibitors. May cause insomnia, headache, tremors, and hypomania.
	stimulants	May potentiate stimulant effects.

Herb	Drug	Possible effects
ginseng *(continued)*	warfarin	Causes antagonism of warfarin, resulting in a decreased INR.
goldenseal	antihypertensives	Large amounts of goldenseal may interfere with blood pressure control.
	CNS depressants, such as barbiturates, benzodiazepines, opioids	Increases sedative effect.
	diuretics	Causes additive diuretic effect.
	general anesthetics	May potentiate hypotensive action of general anesthetics.
	heparin	May counteract anticoagulant effect of heparin.
	H_2 blockers, proton-pump inhibitors	May decrease effectiveness because of increased acid secretion by goldenseal.
grapeseed	warfarin	Increases effects and INR because of tocopherol content of grapeseed.
green tea	acetaminophen, aspirin	May increase effectiveness of these drugs by as much as 40%.
	adenosine	May inhibit hemodynamic effects of adenosine.
	beta-adrenergic agonists (albuterol, isoproterenol, metaproterenol, terbutaline)	May increase the cardiac inotropic effect of these drugs.
	clozapine	May cause acute exacerbation of psychotic symptoms.
	disulfiram	Increases risk of adverse effects of caffeine; decreases clearance and increases half-life of caffeine.
	ephedrine	Increases risk of agitation, tremors, and insomnia.
	hormonal contraceptives	Decreases clearance by 40% to 65%. Increases effects and adverse effects.

(continued)

Herb	Drug	Possible effects
green tea (continued)	lithium	Abrupt caffeine withdrawal increases lithium levels; may cause lithium tremor.
	MAO inhibitors	Large amounts of green tea may precipitate hypertensive crisis.
	mexiletine	Decreases caffeine elimination by 50%. Increases effects and adverse effects.
	verapamil	Increases plasma caffeine levels by 25%; increases effects and adverse effects.
	warfarin	Causes antagonism resulting from vitamin content of green tea.
hawthorn berry	cardiovascular drugs	May potentiate or interfere with conventional therapies used for congestive heart failure, hypertension, angina, and arrhythmias.
	CNS depressants	Causes additive effects.
	coronary vasodilators	Causes additive vasodilator effects when used with such agents as theophylline, caffeine, papaverine, sodium nitrate, adenosine, and epinephrine.
	digoxin	Causes additive positive inotropic effect, with potential for digitalis toxicity.
kava	alcohol	Potentiates depressant effect of alcohol and other CNS depressants.
	benzodiazepines	Use with benzodiazepines has resulted in comalike states.
	CNS stimulants or depressants	May hinder therapy with CNS stimulants.
	hepatotoxic drugs	May increase risk of liver damage.
	levodopa	Decreases effectiveness because of dopamine antagonism by kava.

Herb	Drug	Possible effects
licorice	antihypertensives	Decreases effect of antihypertensive therapy. Large amounts of licorice cause sodium and water retention and hypertension.
	aspirin	May provide protection against aspirin-induced damage to GI mucosa.
	corticosteroids	Causes additive and enhanced effects of the corticosteroids.
	digoxin	Licorice causes hypokalemia, which predisposes to digitalis toxicity.
	hormonal contraceptives	Increases fluid retention and potential for increased blood pressure resulting from fluid overload.
	hormones	Interferes with estrogen or anti-estrogen therapy.
	insulin	Causes hypokalemia and sodium retention when used together.
	spironolactone	Decreases effects of spironolactone.
ma huang (ephedra)	amitriptyline	May decrease hypertensive effects of ephedrine.
	caffeine	Increases risk of stimulatory adverse effects of ephedra and caffeine and risk of hypertension, myocardial infarction, stroke, and death.
	CNS stimulants, caffeine, theophylline	Causes additive CNS stimulation.
	dexamethasone	Increases clearance and decreases effectiveness of dexamethasone.
	digoxin	Increases risk of arrhythmias.
	hypoglycemics	Decreases hypoglycemic effect because of hyperglycemia caused by ma huang.
	MAO inhibitors	Potentiates MAO inhibitors.

(continued)

Herb	Drug	Possible effects
ma huang (ephedra) *(continued)*	oxytocin	May cause hypertension.
	theophylline	May increase risk of stimulatory adverse effects.
melatonin	CNS depressants, such as barbiturates, benzodiazepines, opioids	Increases sedative effect.
	fluoxetine	Improves sleep in some patients with major depressive disorder.
	fluvoxamine	May significantly increase melatonin levels; may decrease melatonin metabolism.
	immunosuppressants	May stimulate immune function and interfere with immunosuppressive therapy.
	isoniazid	May enhance effects of isoniazid against some Mycobacterium species.
	nifedipine	May decrease effectiveness of nifedipine; increases heart rate.
	verapamil	Increases melatonin excretion.
milk thistle	drugs causing diarrhea	Increases bile secretion and often causes loose stools. May increase effect of other drugs commonly causing diarrhea. May have liver membrane-stabilization and antioxidant effects, leading to protection from liver damage from various hepatotoxic drugs, such as acetaminophen, phenytoin, ethanol, phenothiazines, butyrophenones.
nettle	anticonvulsants	May increase sedative adverse effects; may increase risk of seizure.
	anxiolytics, hypnotics, narcotics,	May increase sedative adverse effects.
	warfarin	Antagonism resulting from vitamin K content of aerial parts of nettle.
	iron	Tannic acid content may reduce iron absorption.

Herb	Drug	Possible effects
passion flower	CNS depressants, such as barbiturates, benzodiazepines, opioids	Increases sedative effect.
St. John's wort	5-HT$_1$ agonists (triptans)	Increases risk of serotonin syndrome.
	alcohol, narcotics	Enhances the sedative effect of narcotics and alcohol.
	anesthetics	May prolong effect of anesthesia drugs.
	barbiturates	Decreases barbiturate-induced sleep time.
	cyclosporine	Decreases cyclosporine levels below therapeutic levels, threatening transplanted organ rejection.
	digoxin	May reduce serum digoxin concentrations, decreasing therapeutic effects.
	HIV protease inhibitors (PIs); indinavir; non-nucleoside reverse transcriptase inhibitors (NNRTIs)	Induces cytochrome P-450 metabolic pathway, which may decrease therapeutic effects of drugs using this pathway for metabolism. Use of St. John's wort and PIs or NNRTIs should be avoided because of the potential for subtherapeutic antiretroviral levels and insufficient virologic response that could lead to resistance or class cross-resistance.
	hormonal contraceptives	Increases breakthrough bleeding when taken with hormonal contraceptives; decreases serum levels and effectiveness of contraceptives.
	irinotecan	Decreases serum irinotecan levels by 50%.
	iron	Tannic acid content may reduce iron absorption.

(continued)

Herb	Drug	Possible effects
St. John's wort *(continued)*	MAO inhibitors, nefazodone, SSRIs, trazodone	Causes additive effects with SSRIs, MAO inhibitors, and other antidepressants, potentially leading to serotonin syndrome, especially when combined with SSRIs.
	photosensitizing drugs	Increases photosensitivity.
	reserpine	Antagonizes effects of reserpine.
	sympathomimetic amines such as pseudoephedrine	Causes additive effects.
	theophylline	May decrease serum theophylline levels, making the drug less effective.
	warfarin	May alter INR. Reduces effectiveness of anticoagulant, requiring increased dosage of drug.
valerian	alcohol	Claims no risk for increased sedation with alcohol, although debated.
	CNS depressants, sedative hypnotics,	Enhances effects of sedative hypnotic drugs.
	iron	Tannic acid content may reduce iron absorption.

Common uses of herbs and nutraceuticals

Abdominal disorders
- artichoke

Abdominal pain
- bitter orange
- Chinese cucumber
- Chinese rhubarb
- ground ivy
- khella

Abortifacients
- black hellebore
- cumin
- feverfew
- pennyroyal
- pomegranate
- rosemary
- rue
- saffron
- senega
- slippery elm
- tansy
- thuja

Abscesses
- burdock
- castor bean
- Chinese cucumber
- echinacea
- kava
- thunder god vine
- vervain

Acne
- acidophilus
- arnica
- asparagus
- burdock
- cat's claw
- chaste tree
- jojoba
- marigold
- pansy
- soapwort
- tea tree

Aging
- melatonin
- morinda
- royal jelly
- wild yam

Agitation
- passion flower

AIDS
- cat's claw
- dehydroepiandrosterone

Air pollution protection
- glycine

Alcoholism
- glycine
- kudzu

Allergy symptoms
- bearberry
- bee pollen
- chaparral
- devil's claw
- fenugreek
- ginkgo
- grape seed
- methylsulfonylmethane
- nettle
- willow

Altitude sickness
- ginkgo

Alzheimer's disease
- dehydroepiandrosterone
- galanthamine
- sage

***Amanita* mushroom poisoning**
- milk thistle

Amenorrhea
- astragalus
- black hellebore
- blessed thistle
- chaste tree
- Chinese rhubarb
- false unicorn root
- mayapple
- motherwort
- parsley
- rue
- safflower
- saffron
- squaw vine
- true unicorn root
- yarrow

Amoebiasis
- pill-bearing spurge

Amyloidosis
- autumn crocus

Amyotrophic lateral sclerosis
- octacosanol

Analgesia
- aconite
- allspice
- arnica
- bethroot
- borage
- butterbur
- capsicum
- celandine
- devil's claw
- horse chestnut
- indigo
- lemongrass
- meadowsweet

Analgesia *(continued)*
- nettle
- parsley
- passion flower
- peach
- poplar
- red poppy
- safflower
- scented geranium
- turmeric
- wild lettuce
- willow
- wintergreen
- yerba maté

Anemia
- bee pollen
- dong quai
- onion
- ragwort

Angina pectoris
- celandine
- Chinese cucumber
- comfrey
- hawthorn
- khella
- kudzu
- night-blooming cereus
- onion
- sweet flag
- wild ginger

Ankylosing spondylitis
- morinda

Anogenital inflammation
- oak bark

Anorectal disorders
- aloe
- benzoin
- bitter orange
- buckthorn

- Irish moss
- senna

Antiaging
- shiitake

Antibiotic-induced diarrhea
- acidophilus

Anticoagulant effects
- blessed thistle
- clove oil
- horse chestnut

Antihistaminic effects
- agrimony

Antimicrobial effects
- acidophilus
- aloe
- anise
- barberry
- basil
- blessed thistle
- blue cohosh
- chamomile
- chaulmoogra oil
- dill
- eyebright
- galangal
- garlic
- green tea
- hops
- methylsulfonyl-methane
- olive
- scented geranium
- self-heal
- sorrel
- thyme
- wormwood
- yarrow

Antimutagenic effects
- cat's claw
- self-heal

Antioxidant effects
- astragalus
- grape seed
- self-heal

Antiseptic effects
- agrimony
- allspice
- anise
- basil
- bay
- bearberry
- boswellia
- buchu
- celandine
- clove oil
- feverfew
- lavender
- parsley
- pennyroyal
- poplar
- sassafras
- saw palmetto
- sorrel
- tea tree
- wintergreen

Antispasmodic effects
- American hellebore
- anise
- black haw
- bloodroot
- blue cohosh
- boldo
- butterbur
- cardamom
- celery
- clary
- cowslip
- dill
- fennel
- galangal
- ginger
- goldenrod
- hops
- jambolan
- lady's slipper
- lemongrass

- lovage
- madder
- parsley
- passion flower
- peppermint
- skunk cabbage
- true unicorn root

Antitumorigenic effects
- acidophilus
- agrimony
- ginger
- gotu kola

Anxiety
- betony
- black cohosh
- black hellebore
- blue cohosh
- chamomile
- clary
- hops
- Jamaican dogwood
- jambolan
- kava
- kelpware
- lemon balm
- mugwort
- rauwolfia
- St. John's wort
- valerian

Aphrodisiac effects
- burdock
- damiana
- guarana
- hops
- jambolan
- kava
- tonka bean
- yohimbe

Apocrine chromhidrosis
- capsicum

Appendicitis
- Chinese cucumber

Appetite stimulation
- bitter orange
- blessed thistle
- bogbean
- boldo
- caraway
- centaury
- cinnamon
- condurango
- coriander
- daisy
- dandelion
- devil's claw
- elecampane
- false unicorn root
- fenugreek
- galangal
- gentian
- hops
- hyssop
- Iceland moss
- juniper
- milk thistle
- nutmeg
- onion
- oregano
- Oregon grape
- peppermint
- rosemary
- sage
- sarsaparilla
- watercress
- wormwood
- yarrow

Appetite suppression
- cola
- ephedra
- guarana
- khat
- yerba maté

Aromatherapy
- clary
- coriander
- marjoram
- tea tree

Arrhythmias
- broom
- chicory
- khella
- kudzu
- motherwort
- shepherd's purse
- squill
- tree of heaven

Arthritis
- autumn crocus
- bearberry
- black pepper
- bogbean
- burdock
- capsicum
- celery
- chaparral
- chaulmoogra oil
- couch grass
- evening primrose oil
- feverfew
- fumitory
- ginger
- glycine
- guggul
- kelpware
- male fern
- mayapple
- meadowsweet
- methylsulfonyl-methane
- morinda
- nettle
- nutmeg
- oregano
- pau d'arco
- rose hip
- safflower
- sassafras

Arthritis *(continued)*
- shark cartilage
- squill
- thuja
- thunder god vine
- vervain
- willow
- wintergreen

Ascites
- pipsissewa

Asthma
- alfalfa
- anise
- betony
- black haw
- black pepper
- bloodroot
- blue cohosh
- catnip
- celandine
- chickweed
- coltsfoot
- cowslip
- cranberry
- elderberry
- elecampane
- ephedra
- evening primrose oil
- feverfew
- ginkgo
- glycine
- hyssop
- jambolan
- jimsonweed
- khella
- lobelia
- mullein
- nettle
- onion
- pill-bearing spurge
- royal jelly
- saw palmetto
- schisandra
- skunk cabbage
- St. John's wort
- sundew

- sweet cicely
- sweet violet
- tree of heaven
- vervain
- wild ginger
- wintergreen
- yerba santa

Astringent effects
- agrimony
- bayberry
- bethroot
- birch
- black catechu
- borage
- boswellia
- clary
- daffodil
- eyebright
- green tea
- ground ivy
- horse chestnut
- lady's mantle
- lungwort
- meadowsweet
- night-blooming cereus
- pipsissewa
- rose hip
- saw palmetto
- scented geranium
- sorrel
- yarrow

Atherosclerosis
- Asian ginseng
- butcher's broom
- devil's claw
- fumitory
- garlic
- green tea
- guggul
- hawthorn
- kelpware
- mistletoe
- onion
- saffron
- wild lettuce

Athlete's foot
- tea tree

Autoimmune diseases
- methylsulfonyl-methane
- thunder god vine

Autonomic dysfunction
- jimsonweed

Autonomic neuroses
- mugwort

Backache
- butterbur
- rue

Bacterial vaginosis
- acidophilus

Bacteriostatic effects
- dill

Bedsores
- balsam of Peru
- benzoin
- karaya gum

Bedwetting
- damiana
- pumpkin
- St. John's wort
- thyme

Bee sting
- ragwort

Behcet's disease
- autumn crocus

Belching
- blue flag

Bell's palsy
- rue

Benzodiazepine withdrawal
- melatonin

Bile secretion stimulation
- butterbur
- cat's foot
- dandelion
- elecampane
- goldenseal
- horehound
- mugwort
- oregano
- wahoo

Biliary disorders
- autumn crocus
- wormwood

Bilious fever
- black root

Bladder disorders
- alfalfa
- American cranesbill
- asparagus
- betony
- blackthorn
- borage
- buchu
- capsicum
- celery
- coriander
- cumin
- devil's claw
- flax
- fumitory
- horsetail
- kava
- parsley piert
- pau d'arco
- pipsissewa
- pumpkin
- Queen Anne's lace
- sea holly
- shepherd's purse
- stone root

Bleeding
- Asian ginseng
- bee pollen
- bethroot
- blessed thistle
- broom
- bugleweed
- goldenseal
- lady's mantle
- mistletoe
- night-blooming cereus
- peach
- self-heal
- shepherd's purse
- tormentil

Blepharitis
- eyebright

Blind entrainment
- melatonin

Blisters
- peach

Bloating
- anise
- bitter orange
- caraway
- cinnamon
- daisy
- oregano
- turmeric
- wormwood

Blood disorders
- chickweed
- safflower

Blood glucose regulation
- fenugreek
- fumitory
- goat's rue
- olive
- pipsissewa
- raspberry

Blood poisoning
- wild indigo

Blood pressure regulation
- aconite
- American hellebore
- astragalus
- balsam of Peru
- betony
- blue cohosh
- broom
- capsicum
- celery
- coenzyme Q10
- cucumber
- dong quai
- elecampane
- gotu kola
- hawthorn
- lemon balm
- mistletoe
- morinda
- olive
- onion
- peach
- prickly ash
- rauwolfia
- rosemary
- rue
- sassafras
- self-heal
- shepherd's purse
- Siberian ginseng
- yarrow
- yellow root
- yohimbe

Blood purification
- blackthorn
- blue flag
- burdock
- fumitory
- indigo
- kelpware
- mistletoe
- nettle
- sarsaparilla

Blood purification
(continued)
- sassafras
- sweet cicely
- woundwort

Body composition
- dehydroepiandros-
  terone

Boils
- black catechu
- blessed thistle
- castor bean
- peach
- thunder god vine

Bowel preparation
- aloe
- senna

Bradycardia
- hawthorn

Brain damage
- bee pollen

Breast cancer
- astragalus
- yew

Breast disorders
- bugleweed
- celandine
- chaste tree
- Chinese cucumber

Breast enlargement
- wild yam

Breathing difficulty
- sweet cicely

Bronchitis
- anise
- balsam of Peru
- benzoin
- betony

- black pepper
- bloodroot
- boswellia
- broom
- catnip
- celery
- chickweed
- clove oil
- coltsfoot
- couch grass
- elderberry
- elecampane
- fennel
- galangal
- horehound
- jambolan
- jimsonweed
- juniper
- kelpware
- lungwort
- mallow
- meadowsweet
- mullein
- onion
- peach
- pill-bearing spurge
- saffron
- sassafras
- saw palmetto
- sea holly
- senega
- skunk cabbage
- St. John's wort
- sundew
- sweet violet
- thyme
- watercress
- wild cherry
- wild ginger
- yerba santa

Bronchospasm
- butterbur
- ephedra
- wild ginger

Bruises
- arnica
- balsam of Peru
- blue flag
- chaulmoogra oil
- comfrey
- daisy
- grape seed
- hyssop
- mullein
- onion
- passion flower
- peach
- ragwort
- rue
- St. John's wort
- vervain
- witch hazel
- yerba santa

Burns
- aloe
- balsam of Peru
- bloodroot
- chamomile
- daffodil
- echinacea
- figwort
- ginger
- gotu kola
- horsetail
- hyssop
- kelpware
- lavender
- marigold
- marshmallow
- mullein
- olive
- onion
- peach
- ragwort
- slippery elm
- St. John's wort
- tea tree
- thuja
- tragacanth
- vervain
- witch hazel

Bursitis
- nettle

Cachexia
- tonka bean

Calculosis
- American cranesbill
- celery

Cancer
- Asian ginseng
- asparagus
- astragalus
- autumn crocus
- black hellebore
- bloodroot
- buckthorn
- burdock
- carline thistle
- celandine
- chaparral
- comfrey
- condurango
- dehydroepiandros-terone
- echinacea
- garlic
- ginger
- ginkgo
- grape seed
- green tea
- indigo
- marigold
- mayapple
- melatonin
- methylsulfonyl-methane
- mistletoe
- morinda
- pau d'arco
- peach
- Queen Anne's lace
- red clover
- safflower
- sassafras
- self-heal
- shark cartilage
- Siberian ginseng
- soy
- spirulina
- squill
- thuja
- yellow root
- yew

Canker sores
- acidophilus
- raspberry
- rhatany
- sage

Capillary insufficiency
- bilberry
- bloodroot

Carbuncles
- castor bean
- ground ivy

Cardiac depressant effects
- aconite
- American hellebore

Cardiac surgery
- coenzyme Q10

Cardiotonic effects
- agrimony
- balsam of Peru
- borage
- ephedra
- figwort
- hawthorn

Cardiovascular disorders
- arnica
- broom
- coenzyme Q10
- cowslip
- garlic
- grape seed
- hawthorn
- khella
- lily-of-the-valley
- motherwort
- night-blooming cereus
- oleander
- pipsissewa
- raspberry
- S-adenosylmeth-ionine
- shepherd's purse
- soy
- squill

Catarrh
- acacia gum
- agrimony
- betony
- boneset
- burdock
- lemon balm
- pill-bearing spurge
- pipsissewa
- plantain
- sassafras
- senega
- shepherd's purse
- watercress

Cathartic effects
- aloe
- bloodroot
- blue flag
- broom
- mayapple
- Oregon grape

Celiac disease
- carob

Cerebral hemorrhage
- bee pollen

Cerebral insufficiency
- ginkgo

Cerebral thrombosis
- yarrow

Cervical cancer
- astragalus
- bee pollen

Cervical ripening
- evening primrose oil

Chemotherapy adverse effects
- chondroitin
- coenzyme Q10

Chest complaints
- coriander
- safflower
- skunk cabbage
- sweet cicely
- turmeric

Chilblains
- rhatany

Chills
- ephedra

Chinese rhubarb
- clove oil
- coriander
- elderberry
- male fern
- mallow
- marigold
- meadowsweet
- prickly ash
- rosemary
- tansy

Cholecystitis
- celandine

Cholera
- barberry
- birch
- black pepper

Chronic fatigue syndrome
- dehydroepiandros-terone
- evening primrose oil
- morinda
- schisandra

Circulation
- arnica
- barberry
- bayberry
- broom
- butcher's broom
- capsicum
- condurango
- coriander
- ginkgo
- hyssop
- monascus
- mugwort
- prickly ash
- rose hip
- rosemary
- self-heal
- soy

Cirrhosis
- autumn crocus
- cat's claw
- milk thistle

Cluster headaches
- melatonin

Coagulant effects
- agrimony

Cochlear deafness
- ginkgo

Coffee substitutes
- asparagus
- blue cohosh
- dandelion

Colic
- black pepper
- blessed thistle
- blue cohosh
- boswellia
- butterbur
- calumba
- catnip
- coriander
- cumin
- ginger
- hyssop
- juniper
- marjoram
- mugwort
- nutmeg
- parsley
- Queen Anne's lace
- rauwolfia
- rue
- sea holly
- sweet cicely
- sweet flag
- wild lettuce

Colitis
- Asian ginseng
- bee pollen
- carob
- cat's claw
- ginkgo
- peppermint
- squaw vine
- witch hazel

Colostomy care
- karaya gum

Common cold
- anise
- balsam of Peru
- bay
- bayberry
- blackthorn
- boneset
- boswellia
- burdock
- catnip

- chickweed
- cinnamon
- clove oil
- coltsfoot
- couch grass
- echinacea
- ephedra
- galangal
- garlic
- hyssop
- Iceland moss
- kava
- kudzu
- linden
- marjoram
- meadowsweet
- onion
- pau d'arco
- pennyroyal
- peppermint
- rose hip
- saw palmetto
- sweet violet
- vervain
- wild cherry
- willow
- yarrow
- yerba santa

Concentration problems
- Asian ginseng
- Siberian ginseng

Condylomata acuminata
- mayapple
- thuja

Confusion
- wild indigo

Conjunctivitis
- cornflower
- eyebright
- marjoram

Constipation
- agar
- aloe
- asparagus
- barberry
- bee pollen
- black hellebore
- black pepper
- black root
- blessed thistle
- bloodroot
- blue cohosh
- boldo
- buchu
- buckthorn
- burdock
- butcher's broom
- cascara sagrada
- celandine
- chickweed
- chicory
- Chinese cucumber
- Chinese rhubarb
- cornflower
- couch grass
- damiana
- dandelion
- elderberry
- figwort
- flax
- glucomannan
- jambolan
- karaya gum
- kelp
- kelpware
- mallow
- marshmallow
- mayapple
- mugwort
- olive
- pansy
- pareira
- peach
- pineapple
- plantain
- rose hip
- senna
- stone root

- tragacanth
- true unicorn root
- wahoo

Contact dermatitis
- bearberry

Contraception
- asparagus
- cat's claw
- gossypol
- gotu kola
- melatonin
- thunder god vine

Cor pulmonale
- lily of the valley

Corns
- agrimony

Coronary thrombosis
- yarrow

Cosmetic products
- cacao tree
- coriander
- cucumber
- hyssop
- Irish moss
- jojoba
- juniper
- karaya gum
- lemon
- marigold
- nutmeg
- pennyroyal
- rosemary
- soapwort

Cough
- acacia gum
- aconite
- anise
- balsam of Peru
- bayberry
- betel palm
- betony

Cough *(continued)*
- borage
- boswellia
- burdock
- butterbur
- catnip
- chickweed
- Chinese cucumber
- clove oil
- coltsfoot
- coriander
- cornflower
- couch grass
- elderberry
- elecampane
- ephedra
- eyebright
- fennel
- galangal
- garlic
- horehound
- horse chestnut
- horseradish
- Iceland moss
- Irish moss
- jimsonweed
- linden
- lungwort
- mallow
- marshmallow
- meadowsweet
- mullein
- onion
- oregano
- peach
- pokeweed
- Queen Anne's lace
- ragwort
- red clover
- red poppy
- rosemary
- rue
- saw palmetto
- schisandra
- sea holly
- soapwort
- sundew
- sweet violet

- wild cherry
- wild ginger
- wild lettuce
- woundwort
- yerba santa

Cramps
- blue cohosh

Crohn's disease
- American cranesbill
- cat's claw
- peppermint

Croup
- benzoin
- bloodroot
- mullein

Cutaneous ulcers
- balsam of Peru
- benzoin
- bethroot
- black catechu
- blessed thistle
- echinacea
- fenugreek
- figwort
- gotu kola
- horse chestnut
- jambolan
- karaya gum
- papaya
- prickly ash
- Queen Anne's lace
- rhatany
- southernwood
- tea tree
- tonka bean
- wormwood

Cystitis
- American cranesbill
- betony
- buchu
- chamomile
- fumitory
- kava

- methylsulfonyl-
methane
- night-blooming
cereus
- parsley
- shepherd's purse

**Cytomegalovirus
infection**
- St. John's wort

Dandruff
- birch
- burdock
- southernwood
- squill

Deafness
- ginkgo

Decongestant effects
- betony
- bloodroot
- ephedra
- ground ivy
- horseradish
- kudzu
- linden
- parsley
- saw palmetto

Dehydration
- onion

Delirium
- black pepper
- Chinese rhubarb

Dementia
- dehydroepiandros-
terone
- galanthamine
- ginkgo
- sage

Dental health
- acacia gum
- allspice

- bay
- chaparral
- green tea

Dental impressions
- agar

Dental pain
- allspice
- arnica
- asparagus
- bloodroot

Depression
- Asian ginseng
- clary
- damiana
- dehydroepiandros-
terone
- ginger
- ginkgo
- jambolan
- khat
- marjoram
- melatonin
- mugwort
- S-adenosylmeth-
ionine
- scented geranium
- schisandra
- St. John's wort

Dermatitis herpetiformis
- autumn crocus

Detoxification
- soy
- watercress

Diabetes
- agrimony
- alfalfa
- artichoke
- Asian ginseng
- astragalus
- bitter melon
- cat's claw

- dandelion
- elecampane
- glucomannan
- jambolan
- kudzu
- morinda
- olive
- onion
- rose hip
- Siberian ginseng
- spirulina
- yellow root

Diabetic neuropathy
- capsicum
- evening primrose oil

Diabetic retinopathy
- ginkgo

Diaphoretic effects
- angelica
- birch
- blackthorn
- blessed thistle
- blue cohosh
- borage
- burdock
- carline thistle
- catnip
- jaborandi
- kudzu
- linden
- skunk cabbage
- soapwort
- sweet flag
- wild ginger
- wormwood
- yarrow

Diaphragmitis
- wintergreen

Diarrhea
- acacia gum
- acidophilus
- agrimony
- American cranesbill

- avens
- barberry
- bayberry
- bethroot
- betony
- bilberry
- birch
- bistort
- black catechu
- black haw
- black pepper
- blessed thistle
- calumba
- carob
- catnip
- chamomile
- Chinese rhubarb
- cinnamon
- comfrey
- coriander
- cumin
- flax
- green tea
- ground ivy
- horse chestnut
- Irish moss
- kudzu
- jaborandi
- jambolan
- lady's mantle
- lungwort
- marshmallow
- meadowsweet
- monascus
- mugwort
- nutmeg
- oak bark
- pau d'arco
- plantain
- quince
- raspberry
- rhatany
- rose hip
- rue
- schisandra
- self-heal
- shepherd's purse
- squaw vine

Diarrhea (continued)
- thyme
- tormentil
- tragacanth
- tree of heaven
- true unicorn root
- wild cherry
- witch hazel
- yarrow

Dietary supplement
- glycine

Dietary stimulation
- evening primrose oil

Digestive stimulation
- bloodroot

Diphtheria
- betel palm

Diuresis
- agrimony
- alfalfa
- American hellebore
- angelica
- artichoke
- asparagus
- astragalus
- basil
- bearberry
- black haw
- blackthorn
- blue flag
- boldo
- broom
- buchu
- butcher's broom
- carline thistle
- catnip
- cat's foot
- chicory
- coffee
- condurango
- cornflower
- couch grass
- cowslip

- dandelion
- elderberry
- elecampane
- false unicorn root
- figwort
- goat's rue
- goldenrod
- green tea
- hops
- horsetail
- jambolan
- lemon
- lovage
- madder
- marigold
- meadowsweet
- mullein
- nettle
- onion
- oregano
- papaya
- pareira
- parsley
- parsley piert
- pipsissewa
- pumpkin
- rose hip
- saw palmetto
- scented geranium
- soapwort
- sorrel
- thuja
- thyme
- true unicorn root
- wahoo
- watercress
- yerba maté

Diverticulitis
- flax
- slippery elm

Diverticulosis
- cat's claw
- wild yam

Dizziness
- cowslip
- marjoram
- woundwort

Doxorubicin adverse effects
- chondroitin
- coenzyme Q10

Dropsy
- pipsissewa

Drug additives
- acacia gum
- agar
- Irish moss
- licorice
- sarsaparilla
- tragacanth

Drug extravasation
- chondroitin

Drunkenness
- kudzu

Dyes
- agrimony
- indigo
- tansy

Dysentery
- American cranesbill
- birch
- bitter orange
- calumba
- cat's foot
- coriander
- ground ivy
- guarana
- jambolan
- kudzu
- peach
- Queen Anne's lace
- quince
- self-heal
- tormentil

- tree of heaven
- yarrow

Dysmenorrhea
- black cohosh
- black haw
- black pepper
- butterbur
- caraway
- catnip
- chaparral
- daisy
- dong quai
- false unicorn root
- feverfew
- guarana
- Jamaican dogwood
- lady's mantle
- marigold
- night-blooming cereus
- parsley
- passion flower
- peach
- peppermint
- ragwort
- shepherd's purse
- squaw vine
- squill
- tree of heaven
- true unicorn root
- valerian
- wild lettuce
- wild yam
- willow
- wintergreen

Dyspepsia
- acidophilus
- allspice
- artichoke
- avens
- bee pollen
- bitter orange
- black pepper
- blackthorn
- blessed thistle
- bogbean

- boldo
- capsicum
- cardamom
- carline thistle
- carob
- catnip
- centaury
- chaparral
- chicory
- condurango
- coriander
- damiana
- dandelion
- dill
- elecampane
- feverfew
- galangal
- ginger
- goldenseal
- guarana
- horehound
- hyssop
- Iceland moss
- juniper
- kelpware
- milk thistle
- monascus
- mugwort
- nutmeg
- onion
- oregano
- parsley
- peach
- peppermint
- pineapple
- rosemary
- rue
- stone root
- sweet violet
- thyme
- turmeric
- wahoo
- wormwood

Dysuria
- parsley piert
- rauwolfia
- squaw vine

Ear cancer
- bloodroot

Ear infection
- betel palm
- castor bean
- kava
- rue
- wild indigo

Ear wax softening
- olive

Earache
- male fern
- mullein
- peach

Eclampsia
- black hellebore
- rauwolfia

Eczema
- balsam of Peru
- borage
- burdock
- celandine
- chaulmoogra oil
- chickweed
- cornflower
- echinacea
- evening primrose oil
- figwort
- fumitory
- glycine
- marigold
- nettle
- pansy
- peach
- red clover
- rosemary
- shark cartilage
- soapwort

Edema
- broom
- Chinese rhubarb
- ephedra

Edema *(continued)*
- grape seed
- horse chestnut
- horseradish
- horsetail
- lovage
- night-blooming cereus
- papaya
- parsley piert
- peach
- pineapple
- Queen Anne's lace
- rose hip
- sea holly
- stone root

Emetic effects
- black root
- bloodroot
- blue flag
- bogbean
- broom
- false unicorn root
- indigo
- lobelia
- pokeweed
- skunk cabbage
- wild indigo

Emphysema
- coltsfoot
- kelpware

Encephalitis
- black hellebore

Endometriosis
- evening primrose oil

Energy enhancement
- androstenedione
- bee pollen
- creatine monohydrate
- damiana
- spirulina
- wild yam

Enuresis
- damiana
- pumpkin
- St. John's wort
- thyme

Epididymitis
- wintergreen

Epilepsy
- black hellebore
- blue cohosh
- dehydroepiandrosterone
- elderberry
- mistletoe
- mugwort
- rue
- tree of heaven

Erectile dysfunction
- dehydroepiandrosterone
- yohimbe

Erysipelas
- mullein

Esophageal cancer
- yew

Euphoric effects
- broom
- corkwood
- damiana
- jimsonweed
- khat

Exanthema
- pansy

Excitability
- wild lettuce

Exercise recovery
- androstenedione

Expectoration
- bethroot
- betony
- blackthorn
- blessed thistle
- bloodroot
- blue cohosh
- cornflower
- cowslip
- eucalyptus
- fennel
- goldenseal
- horehound
- horse chestnut
- hyssop
- licorice
- lungwort
- nettle
- oregano
- parsley
- scented geranium
- senega
- skunk cabbage
- soapwort
- squill
- sweet cicely
- sweet violet
- thuja
- wild cherry

Extrasystoles
- khella

Eye disorders
- bilberry
- corkwood
- cornflower
- cumin
- eyebright
- flax
- ginkgo
- jaborandi
- marigold
- quince
- ragwort
- rue
- sassafras
- schisandra

Facial dressing
- betel palm

Familial Mediterranean fever
- autumn crocus

Fatigue
- bee pollen
- cola
- dehydroepiandrosterone
- evening primrose oil
- ginseng
- glycine
- jambolan
- khat
- morinda
- onion
- S-adenosylmethionine
- sage
- schisandra
- Siberian ginseng
- yerba maté

Fever
- aconite
- American hellebore
- avens
- balsam of Peru
- barberry
- bayberry
- blessed thistle
- bloodroot
- boneset
- burdock
- catnip
- Chinese cucumber
- cinnamon
- coriander
- cornflower
- couch grass
- cranberry
- daisy
- elderberry
- ephedra
- eucalyptus

- galangal
- garlic
- goat's rue
- horse chestnut
- hyssop
- Iceland moss
- indigo
- kudzu
- linden
- marigold
- onion
- pau d'arco
- prickly ash
- saffron
- southernwood
- sweet flag
- tormentil
- wild indigo
- willow
- woundwort
- yarrow

Fever blisters or cold sores
- acidophilus
- tea tree

Fibrocystic breast disease
- chaste tree

Fibromyalgia
- S-adenosylmethionine

Fish-spine wounds
- onion

Fistulas
- gotu kola

Flatulence
- allspice
- anise
- black pepper
- blessed thistle
- boswellia
- calumba

- capsicum
- caraway
- cardamom
- celery
- chamomile
- cinnamon
- coriander
- cumin
- dandelion
- fennel
- galangal
- ginger
- hyssop
- jambolan
- juniper
- lemon
- lemon balm
- lovage
- marjoram
- motherwort
- nutmeg
- onion
- parsley
- peppermint
- Queen Anne's lace
- rauwolfia
- rosemary
- sweet cicely
- sweet violet
- thyme
- true unicorn root
- turmeric
- wild ginger

Flavoring agents
- agrimony
- allspice
- anise
- bitter orange
- black pepper
- blessed thistle
- caraway
- carob
- coriander
- dill
- galangal
- guarana
- horseradish

Flavoring agents
(continued)
- hyssop
- Iceland moss
- juniper
- lemon
- mullein
- onion
- pennyroyal
- pipsissewa
- sarsaparilla
- sassafras
- scented geranium
- sweet flag
- thyme
- tonka bean
- turmeric
- wild cherry
- wintergreen
- wormwood

Fluid retention
- burdock

Food and beverage products
- acacia gum
- asparagus
- bitter orange
- cacao tree
- caraway
- carob
- chicory
- coffee
- coriander
- dandelion
- guarana
- hops
- hyssop
- juniper
- karaya gum
- lemon
- lemongrass
- licorice
- madder
- papaya
- pokeweed

- red poppy
- rosemary
- safflower
- slippery elm
- thuja
- tragacanth
- watercress
- yarrow

Fractures
- butcher's broom
- royal jelly
- shark cartilage

Fragrances
- clary
- coriander
- cucumber
- hyssop
- juniper
- lemon
- lemongrass
- marigold
- marjoram
- pennyroyal
- scented geranium
- tansy
- thuja

Frostbite
- balsam of Peru
- horsetail
- hyssop
- mullein
- poplar

Fungal infection
- acidophilus
- bitter orange
- bloodroot
- cornflower
- elderberry
- garlic
- olive
- pau d'arco
- sage
- tea tree

Furuncles
- marigold
- onion

Gallbladder disorders
- agrimony
- American cranesbill
- artichoke
- black root
- blessed thistle
- boldo
- broom
- carline thistle
- celandine
- cornflower
- dandelion
- fumitory
- galangal
- hyssop
- milk thistle
- onion
- pennyroyal
- peppermint
- pipsissewa
- rose hip
- rosemary
- St. John's wort
- turmeric
- wild yam

Gastric secretion stimulation
- bogbean
- gentian
- mugwort

Gastrointestinal disorders
- acacia gum
- acidophilus
- agrimony
- alfalfa
- allspice
- American cranesbill
- angelica
- anise
- artichoke
- avens

- barberry
- bee pollen
- betel palm
- bistort
- bitter melon
- bitter orange
- black catechu
- black pepper
- blackthorn
- blessed thistle
- blue flag
- buchu
- burdock
- calumba
- capsicum
- caraway
- cardamom
- carline thistle
- catnip
- cat's claw
- centaury
- chaparral
- chicory
- cinnamon
- comfrey
- condurango
- coriander
- cumin
- daisy
- dandelion
- devil's claw
- dill
- elecampane
- fennel
- fenugreek
- feverfew
- flax
- fumitory
- galangal
- ginger
- green tea
- ground ivy
- hops
- hyssop
- Irish moss
- jambolan
- juniper
- kava

- kudzu
- lavender
- lemon balm
- lemongrass
- marjoram
- marshmallow
- meadowsweet
- methylsulfonyl-
methane
- monascus
- morinda
- mugwort
- nutmeg
- oregano
- Oregon grape
- papaya
- parsley
- pennyroyal
- peppermint
- pulsatilla
- Queen Anne's lace
- quince
- raspberry
- rose hip
- rosemary
- rue
- saffron
- shark cartilage
- slippery elm
- soapwort
- stone root
- sweet cicely
- sweet flag
- sweet violet
- tansy
- tormentil
- wild cherry
- wild ginger
- wild lettuce
- willow
- wintergreen
- yarrow

Genitourinary disorders
- boldo
- kava
- kelpware

- pulsatilla
- wild lettuce

Gingivitis
- avens
- rhatany
- sage
- sweet flag
- wild indigo

Glaucoma
- jaborandi

Goiter
- kelp
- kelpware

Gonorrhea
- autumn crocus
- black pepper
- cat's claw
- pipsissewa
- quince
- tree of heaven

Gout
- autumn crocus
- betony
- bogbean
- boldo
- broom
- buchu
- burdock
- celandine
- celery
- chickweed
- Chinese rhubarb
- cowslip
- daisy
- elderberry
- fenugreek
- horsetail
- mistletoe
- pennyroyal
- Queen Anne's lace
- ragwort
- rose hip
- rosemary

Gout *(continued)*
- rue
- soapwort
- squill
- St. John's wort
- sweet cicely
- woundwort

Guillain-Barré syndrome
- capsicum

Gynecologic wounds
- gotu kola

Hair dryness
- olive

Hair growth
- asparagus
- burdock
- jojoba
- parsley
- rosemary
- royal jelly
- sage
- southernwood

Halitosis
- avens
- basil
- chaparral
- coriander
- parsley
- peach
- sage

Hallucinogenic effects
- corkwood
- damiana
- jimsonweed
- nutmeg
- peyote
- wild lettuce

Hand soak
- mugwort

Hangovers
- glycine
- kudzu

Hay fever
- nettle

Headache
- black pepper
- blue flag
- butterbur
- castor bean
- catnip
- Chinese rhubarb
- clary
- cola
- cowslip
- cumin
- daisy
- damiana
- dehydroepiandros-
terone
- dong quai
- elderberry
- ephedra
- feverfew
- ginkgo
- green tea
- guarana
- Jamaican dogwood
- kava
- lady's slipper
- lemon balm
- marjoram
- meadowsweet
- melatonin
- morinda
- passion flower
- peach
- peppermint
- pulsatilla
- ragwort
- rosemary
- rue
- saffron
- shepherd's purse
- stone root
- tansy

- turmeric
- valerian
- wild ginger
- willow
- yerba maté

Heart failure
- astragalus
- coenzyme Q10
- motherwort
- squaw vine
- squill

Heartburn
- betony
- blessed thistle
- blue flag
- devil's claw
- juniper
- meadowsweet
- Oregon grape
- sweet violet

Helminthic infection
- false unicorn root
- morinda
- onion
- wormwood

Hematemesis
- shepherd's purse
- witch hazel

Hematoma
- bethroot

Hematuria
- shepherd's purse

Hemoglobin A_{1C} reduction
- fenugreek

Hemophilia
- broom

Hemoptysis
- night-blooming cereus
- witch hazel

Hemorrhoids
- aloe
- balsam of Peru
- bethroot
- bilberry
- buckthorn
- butcher's broom
- cat's claw
- celandine
- coriander
- figwort
- ground ivy
- horse chestnut
- lungwort
- mullein
- pomegranate
- poplar
- rhatany
- senna
- St. John's wort
- stone root
- witch hazel
- yarrow

Hepatitis
- dong quai
- rue
- self-heal
- St. John's wort

Herpesvirus infection
- capsicum
- goldenseal
- motherwort
- octacosanol
- peach
- pokeweed
- sage
- senna
- slippery elm
- St. John's wort

Hiccups
- blue cohosh
- Queen Anne's lace

HIV infection
- cat's claw
- dehydroepiandrosterone

Hives
- acidophilus
- catnip
- kudzu
- nettle

Hoarseness
- eyebright
- mallow

Hormone regulation
- glycine

Hot flushes
- black cohosh

Hyperactivity
- evening primrose oil

Hypercholesterolemia
- acacia gum
- acidophilus
- alfalfa
- artichoke
- celandine
- evening primrose oil
- fenugreek
- garlic
- ginger
- glucomannan
- glycine
- guggul
- monascus
- oats
- olive
- onion
- plantain
- royal jelly

- safflower
- shiitake

Hyperglycemia
- goat's rue
- pipsissewa

Hyperlipidemia
- artichoke
- glucomannan
- green tea
- royal jelly

Hypersensitivity reactions
- bearberry

Hypertension
- aconite
- American hellebore
- basil
- betony
- blue cohosh
- broom
- capsicum
- celery
- coenzyme Q10
- cucumber
- dong quai
- elecampane
- gotu kola
- kudzu
- lemon balm
- mistletoe
- morinda
- olive
- onion
- peach
- rauwolfia
- rue
- sassafras
- self-heal
- yarrow
- yellow root

Hyperthyroidism
- bugleweed
- motherwort

Hypertonia
- khella

Hypertriglyceridemia
- garlic
- guggul
- monascus

Hyperuricuria
- stone root

Hypnotic effects
- cowslip
- lady's slipper
- passion flower

Hypochondriasis
- mugwort

Hypoglycemia
- fumitory

Hypotension
- astragalus
- balsam of Peru
- broom
- cucumber
- mistletoe
- prickly ash
- shepherd's purse
- Siberian ginseng
- yohimbe

Hysteria
- blue cohosh
- celery
- mistletoe
- passion flower
- rue

Ifosfamide extravasation
- chondroitin

Ileitis
- peppermint

Ileostomy care
- karaya gum

Immune suppression
- astragalus

Immune system enhancement
- black hellebore
- cat's claw
- echinacea
- figwort
- glycine
- marigold
- melatonin
- methylsulfonyl-methane
- morinda
- rose hip
- royal jelly
- shiitake
- skullcap
- thuja
- wild ginger
- wild indigo

Impetigo
- pansy

Impotence
- ginger
- ginkgo

Incontinence
- caraway
- sweet violet

Infection
- acidophilus
- asparagus
- astragalus
- balsam of Peru
- birch
- bloodroot
- blue cohosh
- burdock
- chaparral

- cinnamon
- clove oil
- couch grass
- cranberry
- echinacea
- eucalyptus
- fumitory
- galangal
- garlic
- Iceland moss
- indigo
- kava
- linden
- male fern
- marigold
- olive
- onion
- pau d'arco
- pulsatilla
- senna
- slippery elm
- southernwood
- St. John's wort
- wild indigo
- yellow root

Infertility
- chaste tree
- Siberian ginseng

Inflammation
- agrimony
- American cranesbill
- arnica
- astragalus
- balsam of Peru
- betel palm
- bilberry
- blackthorn
- blue cohosh
- blue flag
- boldo
- boneset
- borage
- boswellia
- buchu
- butcher's broom

- castor bean
- chamomile
- chaulmoogra oil
- Chinese rhubarb
- clary
- coffee
- comfrey
- couch grass
- daisy
- devil's claw
- fenugreek
- flax
- gentian
- ginger
- goldenrod
- ground ivy
- indigo
- jambolan
- lemon
- marigold
- marshmallow
- meadowsweet
- methylsulfonyl-methane
- nettle
- oak bark
- octacosanol
- onion
- pansy
- papaya
- pau d'arco
- peach
- pineapple
- plantain
- prickly ash
- pulsatilla
- rue
- sassafras
- skullcap
- sorrel
- St. John's wort
- thunder god vine
- turmeric
- willow
- witch hazel

Inflammatory bowel disease
- acidophilus
- cat's claw
- evening primrose oil

Influenza
- boneset
- boswellia
- chickweed
- ephedra
- jimsonweed
- kudzu
- lungwort
- pau d'arco
- peppermint
- pokeweed
- rose hip
- St. John's wort
- sweet violet
- willow

Injuries
- arnica
- cat's claw
- papaya
- quince

Insect bites and stings
- kelpware
- ragwort
- sage
- sassafras
- southernwood
- witch hazel
- wormwood
- yerba santa

Insect repellents
- basil
- elderberry
- lemongrass
- pennyroyal
- rosemary
- rue
- scented geranium
- southernwood

- tansy
- thuja

Insecticides
- false unicorn root
- feverfew

Insulin regulation
- fenugreek

Intermittent claudication
- ginkgo

Intervertebral disc herniation
- papaya

Iodine sources
- kelp
- kelpware

Irrigation
- asparagus
- carline thistle
- nettle

Irritability
- mugwort

Irritable bowel syndrome
- acidophilus
- flax
- marshmallow
- meadowsweet
- peppermint
- plantain

Ischemic heart disease
- coenzyme Q10

Jaundice
- broom
- celandine
- Chinese rhubarb
- ground ivy

Jaundice (continued)
- pineapple
- self-heal
- wild ginger

Jet lag
- melatonin

Joint symptoms
- comfrey
- daffodil
- daisy
- glycine
- juniper
- Queen Anne's lace
- quince
- ragwort
- rosemary
- thuja
- wild lettuce
- willow

Kaposi's sarcoma
- shark cartilage

Keloids
- papaya

Keratoses
- mayapple

Kidney disorders
- alfalfa
- American cranesbill
- angelica
- astragalus
- blackthorn
- borage
- buchu
- celery
- devil's claw
- dill
- elecampane
- horsetail
- lungwort
- pareira
- parsley
- peach

- pipsissewa
- royal jelly
- sarsaparilla
- sassafras
- schisandra
- soapwort
- squill

Kidney stones
- asparagus
- betony
- birch
- broom
- burdock
- butterbur
- Chinese rhubarb
- couch grass
- cranberry
- cumin
- goldenrod
- horseradish
- juniper
- lovage
- madder
- nettle
- parsley piert
- pipsissewa
- Queen Anne's lace
- rose hip
- sarsaparilla
- sea holly
- stone root

Labor
- blue cohosh

Lactation
- blessed thistle
- caraway
- chaste tree
- goat's rue
- parsley
- raspberry
- squaw vine
- vervain

Lactose intolerance
- acidophilus

Larvicidal effects
- nutmeg

Laryngeal papilloma
- mayapple

Laryngeal spasm
- pill-bearing spurge

Laryngitis
- benzoin
- bloodroot
- boswellia
- coltsfoot
- mallow
- nettle
- pokeweed
- poplar
- sage
- thyme

Leg pain and edema
- horse chestnut

Leg ulcers
- balsam of Peru
- bethroot
- rhatany

Leprosy
- chaulmoogra oil
- cumin
- gotu kola
- kava

Leukorrhea
- buchu
- tree of heaven

Lice
- anise

Liniments
- aconite

Lip conditions
- benzoin
- marigold

Liver disorders
- American cranesbill
- astragalus
- autumn crocus
- black root
- blessed thistle
- boldo
- celandine
- cornflower
- daisy
- dandelion
- devil's claw
- dong quai
- elderberry
- fumitory
- galangal
- ginger
- gotu kola
- hyssop
- milk thistle
- morinda
- parsley
- peach
- pennyroyal
- peppermint
- pineapple
- rauwolfia
- rosemary
- royal jelly
- rue
- S-adenosylmethionine
- schisandra
- soapwort
- squaw vine
- St. John's wort
- turmeric
- wild ginger

Liver protectant effects
- artichoke
- bilberry
- indigo
- milk thistle
- self-heal

Locked jaw
- peach

Lung cancer
- astragalus
- mayapple
- shark cartilage
- yew

Lung disorders
- Chinese cucumber
- peach
- pennyroyal
- schisandra
- senega
- wild cherry
- wild ginger

Lupus
- shark cartilage

Lymphadenopathy
- pokeweed
- wild indigo

Lymphedema
- figwort
- horse chestnut
- tonka bean

Macular degeneration
- bilberry
- ginkgo

Malaria
- guarana

Mania
- galanthamine

Mastectomy pain
- capsicum

Mastitis
- Chinese cucumber
- evening primrose oil

Measles
- coriander
- kudzu

Melanoma
- yew

Memory enhancement
- blessed thistle
- blue cohosh

Meningitis
- black hellebore

Menopausal symptoms
- black cohosh
- borage
- chaste tree
- clary
- devil's claw
- dong quai
- red clover
- soy
- wild yam

Menorrhagia
- broom
- bugleweed
- chaste tree
- horsetail
- lungwort
- night-blooming cereus
- raspberry
- shepherd's purse
- thunder god vine

Menstrual disorders
- bethroot
- blessed thistle
- blue cohosh
- broom
- bugleweed
- caraway
- catnip
- cat's claw

Menstrual disorders
(continued)
- celery
- chaste tree
- Chinese rhubarb
- cornflower
- cumin
- devil's claw
- dong quai
- elecampane
- false unicorn root
- feverfew
- ground ivy
- guarana
- horsetail
- kava
- lady's mantle
- lovage
- lungwort
- mugwort
- night-blooming cereus
- onion
- oregano
- pareira
- parsley
- peach
- raspberry
- rosemary
- safflower
- saffron
- shepherd's purse
- southernwood
- squaw vine
- tansy
- thunder god vine
- true unicorn root
- wild ginger
- woundwort
- yarrow
- yew

Mental alertness
- schisandra

Mental disorders
- black hellebore
- clary

- damiana
- dehydroepiandrosterone
- galanthamine
- ginger
- ginkgo
- ginseng
- hops
- jambolan
- mugwort
- St. John's wort

Mental fatigue
- clary
- cola

Metabolic enhancement
- capsicum
- pansy
- soapwort

Metrorrhagia
- shepherd's purse

Migraine
- butterbur
- castor bean
- catnip
- clary
- cola
- daisy
- dehydroepiandrosterone
- dong quai
- feverfew
- Jamaican dogwood
- kudzu
- lemon balm
- passion flower
- peppermint
- pulsatilla
- tansy
- wild ginger
- willow

Miscarriage
- true unicorn root
- wild yam

Moles
- Chinese cucumber

Mood disturbances
- hops

Morning sickness
- cola
- false unicorn root
- ginger

Motility-enhancing effects
- cardamom

Motion sickness
- chamomile
- galangal
- ginger
- marjoram

Mucolytic agents
- lovage
- onion

Multiple sclerosis
- autumn crocus
- rue

Mumps
- cat's foot

Muscle pain
- allspice
- eucalyptus
- fenugreek
- horseradish
- juniper
- male fern
- marjoram
- methylsulfonylmethane
- peppermint
- prickly ash

- rosemary
- St. John's wort
- wild lettuce
- wintergreen

Muscle spasms
- bay
- blue cohosh
- rue
- tonka bean

Muscle strains
- daffodil

Mushroom poisoning
- milk thistle

Myalgia
- kudzu

Myocardial infarction
- garlic

Myocardial protectant effects
- coenzyme Q10

Myocarditis
- astragalus

Myxedema
- kelpware

Nail disorders
- horsetail
- tea tree

Nasal cancer
- bloodroot

Nasal infection
- wild indigo

Nasal inflammation
- boneset
- sorrel

Nasal polyps
- bloodroot

Nausea and vomiting
- artichoke
- black hellebore
- black pepper
- blue flag
- caraway
- carob
- cola
- false unicorn root
- galangal
- ginger
- lemon balm
- mugwort
- rauwolfia
- saffron
- woundwort

Neck stiffness
- kudzu
- lemon balm

Nephritis
- aconite
- astragalus

Nerve disorders
- glycine

Nervousness
- betony
- bugleweed
- celery
- cowslip
- hops
- lady's slipper
- lemon balm
- lemongrass
- linden
- passion flower
- peach
- rauwolfia

Neuralgia
- aconite
- angelica

- betony
- black pepper
- capsicum
- cowslip
- daisy
- devil's claw
- dong quai
- elderberry
- hops
- Jamaican dogwood
- lemon balm
- male fern
- passion flower
- peppermint
- pulsatilla
- rosemary
- wintergreen

Neurasthenia
- mugwort

Neuritis
- glycine

Neurodermatitis
- borage
- evening primrose oil

Neurogenic bladder
- capsicum

Neuromuscular blockade reversal
- galanthamine

Neuromuscular disorders
- galanthamine

Nicotine addiction
- oats

Nicotine poisoning
- devil's claw

Night sweats
- schisandra

Nipple disorders
- balsam of Peru
- benzoin
- marigold
- quince
- squaw vine

Nocturnal seminal emissions
- schisandra

Nosebleed
- bugleweed
- shepherd's purse

Nutritional supplements
- carob
- glycine
- soy
- spirulina

Obesity
- carob
- evening primrose oil
- glucomannan
- kelp
- kelpware
- khat
- mugwort
- spirulina

Obstetric patients
- barberry
- bee pollen
- black hellebore
- blue cohosh
- broom
- carob
- cola
- evening primrose oil
- false unicorn root
- ginger
- mistletoe
- olive
- parsley
- raspberry
- rauwolfia

- slippery elm
- squaw vine

Oophoralgia
- wintergreen

Opium addiction
- oats

Oral cancer
- spirulina

Oral inflammation
- agrimony
- American cranesbill
- arnica
- balsam of Peru
- bilberry
- blackthorn
- boneset
- clove oil
- coltsfoot
- jambolan
- oak bark
- peppermint
- plantain
- rhatany
- thyme
- tormentil
- turmeric
- vervain

Oral pain
- acidophilus

Oral rinses and gargles
- American cranesbill
- arnica
- bayberry
- bistort
- bitter orange
- black catechu
- blackthorn
- caraway
- carline thistle
- chaparral
- feverfew

- pomegranate
- poplar
- ragwort
- raspberry
- self-heal
- soapwort
- St. John's wort
- tea tree
- thyme
- tormentil
- vervain
- wild indigo

Orchitis
- wintergreen

Osteoarthritis
- bogbean
- capsicum
- glucosamine sulfate
- nettle
- S-adenosylmethionine
- shark cartilage

Osteogenesis imperfecta
- rose hip

Osteoporosis
- dehydroepiandrosterone
- soy
- wild yam

Otitis
- betel palm
- castor bean
- kava

Ovarian cancer
- indigo
- mayapple
- yew

Ovulation inhibition
- blue cohosh

Oxygenation
- glycine

Palmoplantar pustulosis
- autumn crocus

Palpitations
- hawthorn
- lemon balm

Pancreatic cancer
- ginkgo

Pancreatic disorders
- jambolan
- papaya
- royal jelly

Paralytic disorders
- black pepper

Parasitic infection
- betel palm
- black hellebore
- blue cohosh
- chaparral
- false unicorn root
- feverfew
- male fern
- morinda
- mugwort
- onion
- papaya
- pau d'arco
- peach
- pomegranate
- pumpkin
- rue
- santonica
- southernwood
- tansy
- tree of heaven
- wormwood
- yew

Parkinson's disease
- octacosanol

Peptic ulcers
- capsicum
- cat's claw
- comfrey
- ginger
- Irish moss
- khat
- licorice
- lungwort
- marigold
- meadowsweet
- Oregon grape
- papaya
- pau d'arco
- royal jelly
- slippery elm

Performance enhancement
- bee pollen
- borage
- creatine monohydrate
- damiana
- guarana
- octacosanol
- wild yam

Periodontal health
- acacia gum
- allspice
- avens
- broom
- chaparral
- sage
- sweet flag
- wild indigo

Peripheral arterial disease
- ginkgo

Personal defense products
- capsicum

Pertussis
- black pepper
- cowslip

horehound
- horehound
- khella
- red clover
- sundew
- thyme
- vervain
- wild cherry

Phantom limb pain
- capsicum

Pharyngeal inflammation
- agrimony
- arnica
- balsam of Peru
- bilberry
- blackthorn
- bloodroot
- boneset
- clove oil
- coltsfoot
- jambolan
- oak bark
- peppermint
- plantain
- rhatany
- thyme
- vervain

Phlebitis
- borage
- horse chestnut

Plague
- goat's rue

Pleurisy
- wintergreen

Pleuritis with effusion
- self-heal

Pleurodynia
- wintergreen

Pneumonia
- peach
- pennyroyal
- senega
- wild ginger

Poison ivy
- soapwort
- yerba santa

Poisoning
- devil's claw
- milk thistle
- senega

Polio
- pokeweed
- St. John's wort

Polydipsia
- jambolan

Postherpetic neuralgia
- capsicum

Postpartum complications
- coriander
- bethroot
- broom
- goldenseal

Pregnancy symptoms
- blue cohosh
- carob
- cola
- false unicorn root
- ginger
- olive

Premenstrual symptoms
- black cohosh
- bugleweed
- chaste tree
- clary
- couch grass

- dong quai
- evening primrose oil
- ginkgo
- morinda
- nettle
- shepherd's purse
- wild yam
- willow

Prenatal health
- bee pollen

Pressure ulcers
- balsam of Peru
- benzoin
- karaya gum

Priapism
- wild lettuce

Prostaglandin synthesis inhibition
- galangal

Prostate cancer
- shark cartilage

Prostate disorders
- alfalfa
- autumn crocus
- bee pollen
- buchu
- cat's claw
- evening primrose oil
- horse chestnut
- motherwort
- nettle
- poplar
- pumpkin
- saw palmetto
- sea holly
- wild yam

Pruritus
- balsam of Peru
- capsicum
- kudzu
- motherwort

- pansy
- peppermint
- pokeweed
- sage
- vervain
- witch hazel

Pseudogout
- autumn crocus

Psoriasis
- anise
- autumn crocus
- burdock
- capsicum
- chaulmoogra oil
- chickweed
- feverfew
- figwort
- fumitory
- gotu kola
- jojoba
- khella
- kudzu
- lavender
- olive
- Oregon grape
- red clover
- sage
- sarsaparilla
- shark cartilage
- soapwort

Pulmonary embolism
- arnica

Purgative effects
- allspice
- blackthorn
- mayapple

Quinsy
- cat's foot

Radiation sickness
- bee pollen

Raynaud's disease
- evening primrose oil

Rectal prolapse
- bitter orange

Red blood cells
- androstenedione

Reflex sympathetic dystrophy
- capsicum

Relaxation
- boswellia
- broom
- chamomile
- lavender
- sweet violet

Renal colic
- sea holly

Reptile bites
- broom
- cat's foot
- goat's rue
- pareira
- rauwolfia

Respiratory tract disorders
- angelica
- blackthorn
- blue flag
- boswellia
- chickweed
- coltsfoot
- elecampane
- ephedra
- fenugreek
- glycine
- ground ivy
- hyssop
- mallow
- mullein
- oregano
- pansy

- raspberry
- red poppy
- sea holly
- soapwort
- tea tree
- watercress

Respiratory tract infection
- astragalus
- echinacea
- eyebright
- fennel
- Irish moss
- kava
- peach
- pennyroyal
- poplar
- rose hip
- senega
- wild ginger

Restlessness
- chamomile
- hops
- kava
- mugwort
- pulsatilla
- valerian
- wild lettuce

Retention enema
- shark cartilage

Rheumatic diseases
- aconite
- angelica
- arnica
- asparagus
- autumn crocus
- birch
- blessed thistle
- bloodroot
- blue cohosh
- bogbean
- boldo
- boneset
- borage

- broom
- capsicum
- cat's claw
- celery
- chaparral
- chaulmoogra oil
- chickweed
- cumin
- daisy
- elderberry
- eucalyptus
- evening primrose oil
- feverfew
- fumitory
- galangal
- horsetail
- juniper
- kava
- kelpware
- lemon balm
- mayapple
- meadowsweet
- mullein
- nettle
- night-blooming cereus
- nutmeg
- parsley
- pau d'arco
- pokeweed
- poplar
- prickly ash
- ragwort
- rue
- sarsaparilla
- shark cartilage
- St. John's wort
- sweet flag
- thuja
- thunder god vine
- thyme
- true unicorn root
- wild yam
- wintergreen

Rhinitis
- dong quai
- grape seed

Rhinitis *(continued)*
- marjoram
- nettle

Ringworm
- turmeric

Rodenticide
- squill

Rubefacients
- pipsissewa

Scabies
- anise
- balsam of Peru
- birch
- black pepper
- celandine
- ground ivy
- safflower
- tansy

Scarlatina
- black pepper

Scarlet fever
- wild indigo

Schizophrenia
- ginkgo

Sciatica
- aconite
- broom
- male fern
- nettle
- ragwort
- rose hip
- rosemary
- St. John's wort

Scleroderma
- autumn crocus

Scrofulosus
- celandine
- oregano

Scurvy
- peach
- rose hip

Seborrhea
- pansy
- squill

Secretion reduction
- balsam of Peru
- cowslip

Sedation
- agrimony
- American hellebore
- betony
- borage
- celery
- chamomile
- chicory
- cowslip
- feverfew
- hawthorn
- kava
- lady's slipper
- lavender
- lemon balm
- lovage
- morinda
- mugwort
- mullein
- oregano
- papaya
- passion flower
- red poppy
- saffron
- scented geranium
- skullcap
- skunk cabbage
- sweet violet
- true unicorn root
- wild cherry
- wild lettuce

Seizure disorders
- black hellebore
- blue cohosh

- dehydroepiandrosterone
- elderberry
- kava
- mistletoe
- mugwort
- passion flower
- skullcap
- squaw vine
- tree of heaven

Sexual function
- androstenedione
- celery
- damiana
- dehydroepiandrosterone
- ginger
- ginkgo
- royal jelly
- wild yam
- yohimbe

Shift-work disorder
- melatonin

Shingles
- capsicum
- motherwort
- peach
- sage

Shortness of breath
- night-blooming cereus

Sinusitis
- betony
- kudzu
- vervain

Sjögren's syndrome
- evening primrose oil

Skin conditions
- agrimony
- aloe
- anise

- arnica
- autumn crocus
- balsam of Peru
- bearberry
- benzoin
- birch
- black catechu
- blackthorn
- blessed thistle
- bloodroot
- bogbean
- borage
- burdock
- capsicum
- carline thistle
- castor bean
- celandine
- chamomile
- chaulmoogra oil
- chickweed
- Chinese rhubarb
- echinacea
- fenugreek
- feverfew
- figwort
- flax
- fumitory
- glycine
- green tea
- hyssop
- jambolan
- jojoba
- kava
- kelpware
- lavender
- mallow
- marigold
- mullein
- nettle
- oak bark
- oats
- octacosanol
- oleander
- olive
- onion
- Oregon grape
- pansy
- passion flower

- peach
- pennyroyal
- peppermint
- plantain
- poplar
- pulsatilla
- ragwort
- red clover
- royal jelly
- rue
- sage
- sassafras
- sea holly
- slippery elm
- soapwort
- St. John's wort
- sweet cicely
- tea tree
- thuja
- turmeric
- vervain
- watercress
- witch hazel
- wormwood
- yerba santa

Skin masks
- acacia gum

Sleep disturbances
- black cohosh
- black pepper
- bugleweed
- catnip
- dill
- hops
- Jamaican dogwood
- lemon balm
- marjoram
- melatonin
- mugwort
- nutmeg
- passion flower
- rauwolfia
- red poppy
- royal jelly
- squaw vine

- valerian
- wild lettuce

Smoking cessation
- black pepper
- lobelia

Snakebite
- broom
- goat's rue
- pareira
- rauwolfia

Sore throat
- acacia gum
- agrimony
- avens
- bayberry
- benzoin
- bistort
- bitter orange
- black catechu
- bloodroot
- blue cohosh
- borage
- burdock
- galangal
- garlic
- horehound
- hyssop
- linden
- mallow
- marigold
- marshmallow
- mullein
- onion
- peach
- pomegranate
- rue
- saffron
- sage
- sweet cicely
- sweet flag
- tea tree
- vervain
- wild indigo

Spermicidal effects
- gossypol

Spleen disorders
- broom
- dandelion
- milk thistle
- monascus
- parsley

Sprains
- arnica
- chaulmoogra oil
- comfrey
- daisy
- meadowsweet
- ragwort
- rue
- tansy
- yerba santa

Sprue
- carob

Stenocardia
- night-blooming cereus

Stimulant effects
- acacia gum
- arnica
- bay
- betel palm
- birch
- buchu
- coffee
- cola
- corkwood
- galangal
- green tea
- guarana
- yerba maté

Stingray wounds
- onion

Stomach cancer
- celandine
- condurango
- indigo
- safflower

Stomatitis
- chamomile
- rhatany

Stress
- kava
- valerian

Stretch marks in pregnancy
- olive

Stroke
- garlic

Styes
- eyebright

Styptics
- lady's mantle
- shepherd's purse

Sunburn
- cucumber
- jojoba
- poplar
- tansy
- tea tree

Sunscreens
- buckthorn
- cascara sagrada
- jojoba
- melatonin
- witch hazel

Surgical patients
- aloe
- buckthorn
- coenzyme Q10
- gotu kola

Sweating
- black cohosh
- sage
- schisandra

Swelling
- catnip
- comfrey
- horse chestnut
- pineapple
- ragwort

Syphilis
- condurango
- sarsaparilla
- sassafras
- slippery elm

Tachycardia
- khella
- motherwort
- tree of heaven

Teething pain
- mallow

Tendinitis
- meadowsweet
- nettle

Tension
- clary
- hops
- lady's slipper
- rauwolfia

Testicular cancer
- mayapple

Testosterone production
- androstenedione

Thirst
- kudzu

Thirst suppression
- cola
- guarana

Thrombocytopenic purpura
- alfalfa

Thrombophlebitis
- arnica

Thrombosis
- yarrow

Thrush
- quince

Thyroid function
- alfalfa
- blue flag
- bugleweed
- kelp
- kelpware
- motherwort

Tinea lesions
- mayapple
- tea tree
- turmeric

Tinnitus
- ginkgo
- melatonin

Tongue cancer
- carline thistle

Tongue inflammation
- boneset

Tonics
- bloodroot
- boneset
- buchu
- buckthorn
- calumba
- horse chestnut
- Irish moss

- motherwort
- mugwort
- nettle
- pareira
- royal jelly
- sarsaparilla
- sassafras
- tonka bean
- true unicorn root
- wahoo
- watercress

Tonsillitis
- burdock
- figwort
- mallow
- pokeweed
- sage
- soapwort
- St. John's wort
- thyme
- yew

Toothache
- allspice
- asparagus
- Chinese rhubarb
- coriander
- elderberry
- male fern
- marigold
- meadowsweet
- prickly ash
- rosemary
- tansy

Tourette syndrome
- dehydroepiandrosterone

Trauma
- kudzu

Tremors
- cowslip

Tuberculosis
- agrimony
- black pepper
- chaparral
- chaulmoogra oil
- chickweed
- kava
- lungwort
- mullein
- pipsissewa
- self-heal
- tonka bean

Typhoid
- wild indigo

Ulcerative colitis
- avens

Urethritis
- buchu

Uric acid metabolism disorders
- rose hip

Urinary retention
- sea holly

Urinary tract disorders
- angelica
- buchu
- burdock
- butterbur
- dill
- elecampane
- goldenrod
- hyssop
- lovage
- lungwort
- night-blooming cereus
- oregano
- parsley piert
- ragwort
- rose hip
- sarsaparilla

Urinary tract disorders *(continued)*
- sea holly
- sweet cicely

Urinary tract infection
- acidophilus
- asparagus
- birch
- blue cohosh
- couch grass
- cranberry
- echinacea
- horseradish
- juniper
- parsley piert
- sea holly

Urinary tract irrigation
- nettle

Uterine contractions
- barberry
- blue cohosh
- broom
- mistletoe
- parsley
- rauwolfia

Uterine fibroids
- chaste tree

Uterine inflammation
- blue cohosh
- kava

Uterine prolapse
- bitter orange

Uterine tonic during pregnancy
- false unicorn root

Vaginal disorders
- acidophilus
- buchu

- cornflower
- kava
- mallow

Vaginal infection
- pau d'arco
- sage
- tea tree

Vaginal prolapse
- true unicorn root

Varicose veins
- bethroot
- horse chestnut
- marigold
- rue
- witch hazel

Vascular disorders
- bilberry
- bloodroot
- borage
- broom
- butcher's broom
- gotu kola
- grapeseed
- horse chestnut
- witch hazel

Vasodilation
- astragalus
- barberry

Venereal disease
- autumn crocus
- black pepper
- buchu
- cat's claw
- chaparral
- condurango
- ephedra
- kava
- pipsissewa
- quince
- sarsaparilla
- sassafras

- slippery elm
- tree of heaven

Venous insufficiency
- bilberry
- butcher's broom
- gotu kola
- grapeseed
- horse chestnut

Vertigo
- black pepper
- ginkgo

Vincristine extravasation
- chondroitin

Vindesine extravasation
- chondroitin

Vitiligo
- capsicum
- St. John's wort

Vulvar pruritus
- pansy

Vulvar vestibulitis
- capsicum

Warts
- agrimony
- bloodroot
- mayapple
- onion
- pansy
- peach
- squill
- sundew
- thuja

Water retention
- stone root

Weakness
- bee pollen

Weight loss
- bee pollen
- capsicum
- glucomannan
- guarana
- guggul
- Irish moss
- wild yam

Well-being
- dehydroepiandros-
terone

Whooping cough
- black pepper
- cowslip
- horehound
- khella
- red clover
- sundew
- thyme
- vervain
- wild cherry

Worm infestation
- betel palm
- black hellebore
- blue cohosh
- male fern
- mugwort
- peach
- pomegranate
- pumpkin
- rue
- southernwood
- tansy
- tree of heaven
- yew

Wound debridement
- bloodroot
- feverfew
- pineapple

Wound healing
- acacia gum
- aloe
- balsam of Peru

- bistort
- blessed thistle
- burdock
- chamomile
- chaparral
- Chinese rhubarb
- comfrey
- daisy
- echinacea
- fenugreek
- figwort
- goldenseal
- gotu kola
- green tea
- ground ivy
- horsetail
- juniper
- kava
- lungwort
- marigold
- peach
- poplar
- prickly ash
- quince
- raspberry
- rauwolfia
- rosemary
- rue
- safflower
- self-heal
- senega
- shark cartilage
- slippery elm
- southernwood
- sweet cicely
- thuja
- thyme
- tormentil
- vervain
- wormwood
- woundwort
- yarrow

Wound irrigation
- carline thistle

Monitoring patients using herbs

Altered laboratory values and changes in a patient's condition can signal unwanted effects of an herb. This table helps you focus your assessments so that you can better meet the needs of a patient who is using an alternative medicine.

Herb	What to monitor	Explanation
aloe	• Serum electrolyte levels • Weight patterns • BUN and creatinine levels • Heart rate • Blood pressure • Urinalysis	Aloe possesses cathartic properties that inhibit water and electrolyte reabsorption, which may lead to potassium depletion, weight loss, and diarrhea. Long-term use may lead to nephritis, albuminuria, hematuria, and cardiac disturbances.
bilberry	• Weight patterns • CBC • Blood glucose level • Triglyceride level • Liver function tests • INR, PT, PTT	Bilberry contains flavonoids and chromium, which are thought to have blood glucose- and triglyceride-lowering effects. Continued intoxication may lead to wasting, anemia, and jaundice.
capsicum	• Liver function tests • BUN and creatinine levels • PT, PTT	Oral administration of capsicum can lead to gastroenteritis and hepatic or renal damage.
cat's claw	• Blood pressure • Lipid panel • Serum electrolyte levels	Cat's claw can potentially cause hypotension through inhibition of the sympathetic nervous system and its diuretic properties. May also lower cholesterol level.
chamomile (German, Roman)	• Menstrual changes • Pregnancy	Chamomile has been reported to cause changes in menstrual cycle and is a known teratogen in animals.
echinacea	• Temperature	When echinacea is used parenterally, dose-dependent, short-term fever, nausea, and vomiting can occur.

Herb	What to monitor	Explanation
ephedra	• Blood pressure • Heart rate • BUN and creatinine levels • Weight patterns	Ephedra's active ingredient, ephedrine, stimulates the CNS in a similar manner to that of amphetamine. Adverse effects include hypertension, tachycardia, and kidney damage.
evening primrose	• Pregnancy • CBC • Lipid profile	Evening primrose elevates plasma lipid levels and reduces platelet aggregation. It may increase the risk of pregnancy complications, including rupture of membranes, oxytocin augmentation, arrest of descent, and vacuum extraction.
fennel	• Liver function tests • Blood pressure • Serum calcium level • Blood glucose level	Fennel contains trans-anethole and estrogole. Trans-anethole has estrogenic activity, whereas estrogole is a procarcinogen with the potential to cause liver damage. Adverse effects include photodermatitis and allergic reactions, particularly in those sensitive to carrots, celery, and mugwort.
feverfew	• CBC • Pregnancy • Sleep patterns • INR, PT, PTT	Feverfew may inhibit blood platelet aggregation and decrease neutrophil and platelet secretory activity. It can cause uterine contractions in full-term, pregnant women. Adverse effects include mouth ulceration, tongue irritation and inflammation, abdominal pain, indigestion, diarrhea, flatulence, nausea, and vomiting. Post-feverfew syndrome includes nervousness, headache, insomnia, joint pain, stiffness, and fatigue.
flaxseed	• Lipid panel • Blood pressure • Serum calcium level • Blood glucose level	Flaxseed possesses weak estrogenic and antiestrogenic activity. May cause a reduction in *(continued)*

Herb	What to monitor	Explanation
flaxseed *(continued)*	• Liver function tests	platelet aggregation and serum cholesterol level. Oral administration with inadequate fluid intake can cause intestinal blockage.
garlic	• Blood pressure • Lipid panel • Blood glucose level • CBC • PT and PTT	Garlic is associated with hypotension, leukocytosis, inhibition of platelet aggregation, and decreased blood glucose and cholesterol levels. Postoperative bleeding and prolonged bleeding time can occur.
ginger	• Blood glucose level • Blood pressure • Heart rate • Respiratory rate • Lipid panel • ECG • INR, PT, PTT	Ginger contains gingerols, which have positive inotropic properties. Adverse effects include platelet inhibition, hypoglycemia, hypotension, hypertension, and stimulation of respiratory centers. Overdoses cause CNS depression and arrhythmias.
ginkgo	• Respiratory rate • Heart rate • PT and PTT	Consumption of ginkgo seed may cause difficulty breathing, weak pulse, seizures, loss of consciousness, and shock. Ginkgo leaf is associated with infertility, as well as GI upset, headache, dizziness, palpitations, restlessness, lack of muscle tone, weakness, bleeding, subdural hematoma, subarachnoid hemorrhage, and a bleeding iris.
ginseng (American, Panax, Siberian)	• BUN and creatinine levels • Blood pressure • Serum electrolyte levels • Liver function tests • Serum calcium level • Blood glucose level • Heart rate • Sleep patterns	Ginseng contains ginsenosides and eleutherosides that can affect blood pressure, CNS activity, platelet aggregation, and coagulation. A reduction in glucose and hemoglobin A_{1C} levels has also been reported. Adverse effects include drowsiness, mastalgia, vaginal bleeding, tachycardia, mania, cere-

Herb	What to monitor	Explanation
ginseng *(continued)*	• Menstrual changes • Weight patterns • PT, PTT, and INR • Blood pressure	bral arteritis, Stevens-Johnson syndrome, cholestatic hepatitis, amenorrhea, decreased appetite, diarrhea, edema, hyperpyrexia, pruritus, hypotension, palpitations, headache, vertigo, euphoria, and neonatal death.
goldenseal	• Respiratory rate • Heart rate • Blood pressure • Liver function tests • Mood patterns	Goldenseal contains berberine and hydrastine. Berberine improves bile secretion and bilirubin level, increases coronary blood flow, and stimulates or inhibits cardiac activity. Hydrastine causes hypotension, hypertension, increased cardiac output, exaggerated reflexes, seizures, paralysis, and death from respiratory failure. Other adverse effects include digestive disorders, constipation, excitatory states, hallucinations, delirium, GI upset, nervousness, depression, dyspnea, and bradycardia.
kava	• Weight patterns • Lipid panel • CBC • Blood pressure • Liver function tests • Urinalysis • Mood changes • Sleep patterns	Kava contains arylethylene pyrone constituents that have CNS activity. It also has antianxiety effects. Long-term use may lead to weight loss, increased HDL cholesterol levels, hematuria, increased RBCs, decreased platelet count, decreased lymphocyte levels, reduced protein levels, and pulmonary hypertension.
milk thistle	• Liver function tests	Milk thistle contains flavonolignans, which have liver-protective and antioxidant effects.
nettle	• Blood glucose level • Blood pressure • Weight patterns	Nettle contains significant amounts of vitamin C, vitamin K, potassium, and calcium. *(continued)*

Herb	What to monitor	Explanation
nettle *(continued)*	• BUN and creatinine levels • Serum electrolyte levels • Heart rate • PT and INR	Nettle may cause hyperglycemia, decreased blood pressure, decreased heart rate, weight loss, and diuretic effects.
passion flower	• Liver function tests • Amylase level • Lipase level	Passion flower may contain cyanogenic glycosides, which can cause liver and pancreas toxicity.
St. John's wort	• Vision • Menstrual changes • INR, PT, PTT • Sleep patterns	Changes in menstrual bleeding and a reduction in fertility may be caused by St. John's wort. Other adverse effects include GI upset, fatigue, dry mouth, dizziness, headache, delayed hypersensitivity, phototoxicity, and neuropathy. St. John's wort may also increase the risk of cataracts.
SAM-e	• Blood pressure • Heart rate • BUN and creatinine levels	SAM-e contains homocysteine, which requires folate, cyanocobalamin, and pyridoxine for metabolism. Increased levels of homocysteine are associated with CV and renal disease.
saw palmetto	• Liver function tests	Saw palmetto inhibits conversion of testosterone to dihydrotestosterone and may cause inhibition of growth factors. Adverse effects include cholestatic hepatitis, erectile or ejaculatory dysfunction, and altered libido.
valerian	• Blood pressure • Heart rate • Sleep patterns • Liver function tests	Valerian contains valerenic acid, which increases gamma-butyric acid and decreases CNS activity. Adverse effects include cardiac disturbances, insomnia, chest tightness, and hepatotoxicity.

Food and Drug Administration's list of toxic herbs

The following herbs have been declared unsafe by the FDA because the plants contain poisonous components.

Common name	Botanical name
arnica	*Arnica montana*
belladonna	*Atropa belladonna*
bittersweet	*Solanum dulcamara*
bloodroot	*Sanguinaris canadensis*
broom-tops	*Cytisus scoparius*
buckeye	*Aesculus hippocastanum*
heliotrope	*Heliotropium eropaeum*
hemlock	*Conium maculatum*
henbane	*Hyoscyamus niger*
jimsonweed	*Datura stramonium*
lily of the valley	*Convallaria majalis*
lobelia	*Lobelia inflata*
mandrake	*Mandragora officinarum*
mayapple	*Podophyllum peltatum*
mistletoe	*Phoradendron flavescens*
periwinkle	*Vinca major, Vinca minor*
snakeroot	*Eupatorium rugosum*
tonka bean	*Dipteryx odorata, Coumarouna odorata*
wahoo bark	*Euonymus atropurpureus*
wormwood	*Artemisia absinthium*
yohimbe	*Corynanthe yohimbe*

Selected references

Blumenthal, M., et al., eds. *The Complete German Commission E Monographs: Therapeutic Guide to Herbal Medicines.* Translated by Klein, S. Boston: Integrated Medicine Communications, 1998.

Boullata, J.I., and Nace, A.M. "Safety Issues with Herbal Medicine," *Pharmacotherapy* 20:257-69, 2000.

Brinker, F. Herb *Contraindications and Drug Interactions,* 3rd ed. Sandy, Ore: Eclectic Medical Publications, 2001.

Castleman, M. *The Healing Herbs. The Ultimate Guide to the Curative Power of Nature's Medicines.* Emmaus, Pa: Rodale Press, 1991.

Chevallier, A. *The Encyclopedia of Medicinal Plants.* New York: DK Publishing, 1996.

Culpeper, N. *Culpeper's Complete Herbal: A Book of Natural Remedies for Ancient Ills.* London: Foulsham & Co. Ltd., 1995.

DerMarderosian, A., et al, eds. *Facts and Comparisons: The Review of Natural Products.* St. Louis: Wolters Kluwer, 1999.

Duke, J.A. *Handbook of Medicinal Herbs.* Boca Raton, Fla: CRC Press, 1985.

Duke, J.A. *The Green Pharmacy.* Emmaus, Pa: Rodale Press, 1997.

Dukes, M.N.G., ed. *Meyler's Side Effects of Drugs: An Encyclopedia of Adverse Reactions and Interactions,* 13th ed. Amsterdam: Elsevier, 1996.

Fleming, T., et al, eds. *PDR for Herbal Medicines,* 2nd ed. Montvale, NJ: Medical Economics Co., 2000.

Foster, S., and Tyler, V.E. *Tyler's Honest Herbal. A Sensible Guide to the Use of Herbs and Related Remedies,* 4th ed. Binghamton, NY: Haworth Herbal Press, 1999.

Fugh-Berman, A. "Herb-Drug Interactions," *Lancet* 355:134-38, 2000.

A Guide to Popular Natural Products. St. Louis, Mo: Facts & Comparisons, A Wolters Kluwer Company, 1999.

Grieve, M., and Leyel, C.F. *A Modern Herbal.* New York: Dover Publications, 1978.

Harbone, J.B., and Baxter, H. *Dictionary of Plant Toxins.* Chichester, NJ: John Wiley & Sons, 1996.

Hoffman, D. T*he Complete Illustrated Holistic Herbal. A Safe and Practical Guide to Making and Using Herbal Remedies.* Rockport, Mass: Element Books, 1996.

Hoffmann, D. *The New Holistic Herbal.* New York: Barnes & Noble Books, 1995.

Hoffmann, D., ed. *The Herbal Handbook: A User's Guide to Medical Herbalism* (revised edition). Rochester, Vt: Healing Arts Press, 1998.

Jellin, J.M., ed. *Natural Medicines Comprehensive Database,* 2nd ed. Compiled by the Editors of Pharmacist's Letter and Physician's Letter. Stockton, Calif: Therapeutic Research Faculty, 2000.

Klepser, T.B., and Klepser, M.E. "Unsafe and Potentially Safe Herbal Therapies," *Am J Health-Syst Pharm* 56:125-37, 1999.

Leung, A.Y., and Foster, S. *Encyclopedia of Common Natural Ingredients Used in Food, Drugs, and Cosmetics,* 2nd ed. New York: John Wiley & Sons, 1996.

Liberman, S., and Bruning, N. *The Real Vitamin and Mineral Book.* New York: Avery, 1997.

Mabey, R. *The New Age Herbalist: How to Use Herbs for Healing, Nutrition, Body Care, and Relaxation.* New York: Simon & Schuster, 1988.

Macdonald, H.G. *A Dictionary of Natural Products.* Medford, NJ: Plexus Publishing, 1997.

McGuffin, M., et al., eds. *American Herbal Products Association's Botanical Safety Handbook.* Boca Raton, Fla: CRC Press, 1997.

Miller, L.G. "Herbal Medicinals: Selected Clinical Considerations Focusing on Known or Potential Drug-Herb Interactions," *Arch Intern Med* 158:2200-11, 1998.

Miller, L.G., and Murray, W.J., eds. *Herbal Medicinals: A Clinician's Guide.* Binghamton, NY: Pharmaceutical Products Press, 1998.

Mowrey, D.B. *Herbal Tonic Therapies.* New Canaan, Conn: Keats Publishing, 1993.

Murray, M. *The Healing Power of Herbs,* 2nd ed. Rocklin, Calif: Prima Publishing, 1995.

Murray, M., and Pizzorno, J. *Encyclopedia of Natural Medicine,* 2nd ed. Rocklin, Calif: Prima Publishing, 1998.

Newall, C.A., et al. *Herbal Medicines: A Guide for Health Care Professionals.* London: Pharmaceutical Press, 1996.

Nutriceutica. Database on CD-ROM. San Clemente, Calif: JAG Group, 1999.

Parfitt, K., ed. *Martindale's Complete Drug Reference,* 32nd ed. Micromedex Healthcare Series, vol. 103, Pharmaceutical Press, 2000.

Peirce, A. *The American Pharmaceutical Association. Practical Guide to Natural Medicines.* New York: Stonesong Press, 1999.

Peirce, A., and Gans, J.A. *The American Pharmaceutical Association Practical Guide to Natural Medicines.* New York: William Morrow and Co, 1999.

Reynolds, J., ed. *Martindale: The Extra Pharmacopoeia,* 32nd ed. London: Royal Pharmaceutical Society of Great Britain, 1996.

Ritchason, J. *The Little Herb Encyclopedia,* 3rd ed. Pleasant Grove, Utah: Woodland Health Books, 1995.

Robbers, J.E., and Tyler, V.E. *Tyler's Herbs of Choice: The Therapeutic Use of Phytomedicinals.* Binghamton, NY: Haworth Herbal Press, 1999.

Robbers, J.E., et al. *Pharmacognosy and Pharmacobiotechnology.* Baltimore, Philadelphia: Williams & Wilkins, 1996.

Roberts, A., et al. *Nutraceuticals: The Complete Encyclopedia of Supplements, Herbs, Vitamins, and Healing Foods.* New York: The Berkley Publishing Group, 2001.

Schulz, V., et al. *Rational Phytotherapy: A Physician's Guide to Herbal Medicine,* 3rd ed. Translated by Telger, T.C. Berlin: Springer, 1998.

Squier, T.B.B. *Herbal Folk Medicine.* New York: Henry Holt and Company, 1997.

Tyler, V.E. *Herbs of Choice: The Therapeutic Use of Phytomedicinals,* 2nd ed. Binghamton, NY: Pharmaceutical Press, 1999.

Tyler, V.E. *Rational Phytotherapy.* Berlin: Springer, 1998.

Wichtl, M.W. *Herbal Drugs and Phytopharmaceuticals: A Handbook for Practice on a Scientific Basis,* 2nd ed. Edited by Bisset, N.G. Stuttgart: Medpharm Scientific Publishers, 1994.

Wren, R.C., et al. *Potter's New Cyclopaedia of Botanical Drugs and Preparations.* Saffron Waldron, Essex, England: C.W. Daniel Company Ltd, 1988.

Herbal resource list

Alternative Medicine
www.alternativemedicine.com
Burton Goldberg
1650 Tiburon Blvd., Suite 2
Tiburon, CA 94920
Phone (800) 515-4325

Alternative Medicine Foundation, Inc.
www.amfoundation.org
P.O. Box 60016
Potomac, MD 20859-0016

American Botanical Council
www.herbalgram.org
P.O. Box 144345
Austin, TX 78714-4345
Phone (512) 926-4900

American Herbal Pharmacopoeia
www.herbal-ahp.org
Box 5159
Santa Cruz, CA 95063
Phone (831) 461-6318

American Holistic Health Association
www.ahha.org
P.O. Box 17400
Anaheim, CA 92817-7400
Phone (714) 779-6152

Association of Natural Medicine Pharmacists
www.anmp.org
P.O. Box 150727
San Rafael, CA 94915-0727
Phone (415) 868-1909

Botanical Society of America
www.botany.org
BSA Business Manager
P.O. Box 299
St. Louis, MO 63166-0299
Phone (314) 577-9566

Centers for Disease Control and Prevention
www.cdc.gov
1600 Clifton Road
Atlanta, GA 30333
Phone (404) 639-3311

Longwood Herbal Task Force
www.mcp.edu/herbal
Massachusetts College of Pharmacy and Health Sciences
179 Longwood Avenue
Boston, MA 02115

Healthy Alternatives
www.health-alt.com
4532 W. Kennedy Blvd. #312
Tampa, FL 33609-3042

Herb Research Foundation
www.herbs.org
1007 Pearl Street, Suite 200
Boulder, CO 80302
Phone (800) 748-2617 or (303) 449-2265

Office of Dietary Supplements
http://ods.od.nih.gov
National Institutes of Health
6100 Executive Blvd.
Room 3B01, MSC 7517
Bethesda, MD 20892-7517

MedHerb.com
www.medherb.com
Editor: Paul Bergner
P.O. Box 20512
Boulder, CO 80308

National Center for Homeopathy
www.homeopathic.org
801 N. Fairfax Street, Suite 306
Alexandria, VA 22314
Phone (877) 624-0613 or (703) 548-7790

Rosenthal Center for Complementary and Alternative Medicine
http://cpmcnet.columbia.edu/dept/rosenthal
Columbia University, College of Physicians and Surgeons
630 W. 168th Street
P.O. Box 75
New York, NY 10032
Phone (212) 342-0101

United States Department of Agriculture
www.usda.gov/welcome.html
14th and Independence Avenue, SW
Washington, DC 20250
Phone (202) 720-2791

Glossary

abortifacient A substance capable of inducing a miscarriage.

adaptogen A substance used to strengthen the body and increase resistance to disease.

alkaloid A substance found in plants that acts like a drug in the body. Examples include caffeine, morphine, nicotine, quinine, and strychnine. The term also applies to synthetic substances whose structures resemble that of plant alkaloids.

anthelmintic An agent that destroys worms.

antioxidant A substance such as vitamin E that works alone or in a group to destroy disease-causing substances called free radicals.

antisialagogue An agent that prevents or opposes the formation of saliva.

astringent A substance that causes tissues to contract. It's usually used locally, as on the skin.

Ayurvedic medicine The ancient traditional Indian system of medicine based on Hindu philosophy. This system shares some fundamental concepts with traditional Chinese medicine: the interconnectedness of body, mind, and spirit; the belief that the cosmos is composed of five basic elements (earth, air, fire, water, and space); and the belief in a human energy field that must be kept in balance to maintain health. Ayurvedic medicine also emphasizes the importance of a person's metabolic body type *(dosha)* in determining

his health, personality, and susceptibility to disease.

binder A substance added to a drug or herbal product to hold together the product's ingredients.

bioflavonoid One of a group of naturally occurring plant compounds needed to strengthen tiny blood vessels called capillaries. Some researchers believe bioflavonoids may help protect against cancer and infection.

biomedicine A system of medicine based on the principles of the natural sciences.

bitter A preparation often used to promote appetite or digestion.

carminative A preparation used to relieve intestinal gas.

catarrh Inflammation of the air passages of the nose, throat, and lungs.

Chinese medicine, traditional A sophisticated, complex health care system based on the belief that good health depends largely on a person's lifestyle, thoughts, and emotions. It has expanded over the centuries to embrace many theories, methods, and approaches. The cornerstone of traditional Chinese medicine, which evolved from Taoism, Confucianism, and Buddhism, is the concept of *qi,* defined as a vital life force, or energy, that flows through the body along channels called meridians.

cholagogue A preparation that stimulates the flow of bile from the gallbladder.

choleretic A preparation that stimulates the production of bile.

Commission E A government committee in Germany that evaluates and reviews the safety and effectiveness of herbal products.

decoction A drug or other substance prepared by boiling.

diaphoretic An agent that induces sweating or perspiration.

Doctrine of Signatures In herbal medicine, the archaic method of determining which plants should be used for which ailments, based on the plant's resemblance to the ailment—for example, heart-shaped leaves for heart conditions and plants with red flowers for bleeding disorders.

dram A unit of weight equivalent to ⅛ ounce or 60 grains.

elixir A mixture of a drug or herb, alcohol, water, and sugar.

emmenagogue A preparation that stimulates menstrual flow.

essential oil A naturally occurring pure oil obtained from distillation of a plant.

extract A concentrate prepared by extracting—that is, removing all or nearly all of the solvent and adjusting the residual amount to a prescribed standard. Most extracts are solutions of essential constituents of a plant or other complex material placed in alcohol.

febrifuge An antipyretic.

free radical A molecule containing an odd number of electrons. Some researchers believe free radicals may play a role in cancer development by interacting with DNA (the cell's genetic material) and impairing normal cell function.

glycerite A solution or mixture of a medicinal substance in glycerin. Usually sweet to the taste and warm on the tongue, glycerites are an alternative to alcohol extracts and better suited to some people.

glycoside An active component in plants that yields sugars when it decomposes.

herbal medicine The use of plants for healing purposes, dating back to the ancient cultures of Egypt, China, and India, and possibly even prehistoric times. Today, more than a quarter of conventional drugs are derived from herbs and about 80% of the world's population uses herbal remedies.

homeopathy A method of healing in which minute amounts of a substance that causes symptoms in a healthy person are given to a sick person to cure the same symptoms. Homeopathic remedies are thought to stimulate the body's ability to heal itself.

infusion A method of making an herbal tea in which a dried herb is steeped in hot water for 3 to 5 minutes before drinking.

inhalation treatment A type of herbal treatment used mainly to open congested sinuses and lung passages, help discharge mucus, and ease breathing. In one inhalation method, 2 to 5 drops of an herbal oil are placed in a sink filled with very hot water; the steam is then inhaled for 5 minutes. In another method, dried or fresh herbs (or an aromatic oil) are added to a large pot of hot water, which is then brought to a boil, allowed to simmer for 5 minutes, and removed from the heat to cool. Then the person drapes a towel over his head to form a tent, leans over the pot, and inhales the steam for 5 minutes.

maceration The softening of a solid agent by soaking in liquid.

muscarinic Producing effects similar to postganglionic parasympathetic stimulation, including smooth-muscle contraction, abdominal colic, and excessive perspiration, salivation, and bronchial secretions.

naturopathy An alternative system of medical practice that combines a mainstream understanding of human physiology and disease with alternative remedies, such as herbal and nutritional therapies, acupuncture, hydrotherapy, and counseling. Naturopathic practitioners favor natural treatments aimed at stimulating the body's own healing ability over drugs and surgery.

nutraceutical A natural, bioactive chemical compound that possesses medicinal properties, including disease prevention and health promotion.

pharmacognosy The study of the natural sources of drugs, such as plants, animals, and minerals and their products.

phytomedicine Herbal medicine.

phytotherapy Treatment by use of plants.

poultice A moist paste made from crushed herbs that's applied directly to the affected area or wrapped in cloth and then applied.

purgative A substance that causes bowel evacuation.

rhizome A plant's underground stem, commonly thickened by deposits of reserve food material, that produces shoots above and roots below. Unlike a true root, a rhizome typically has buds, nodes, and (usually) scalelike leaves.

spirit A volatile liquid, especially one that has been distilled; a volatile substance dissolved in alcohol.

stomachic A preparation that improves appetite and digestion.

tincture A liquid preparation that contains a drug or herb and alcohol (alcoholic solution) or a drug or herb, alcohol, and water (hydroalcoholic solution).

tonic A drug or herb that restores, invigorates, refreshes, or stimulates.

tuberous root A thick, fleshy storage root that lacks buds or scale leaves.

volatile oil An oil that evaporates quickly. (In contrast, a fixed oil, such as castor oil or olive oil, doesn't easily evaporate.) Volatile oils occur in aromatic plants, giving them odor and other characteristics. Examples include peppermint, spearmint, and juniper. Also called distilled oil or essential oil.

Index

t refers to a table.